THE DIABETES CARBOHYDRATE & FAT GRAM GUIDE

—— 5TH EDITION ——

Quick, Easy Meal Planning Using Carbohydrate and Fat Gram Counts

LEA ANN HOLZMEISTER, RD, CDE

A.American Diabetes Association.

Director, Book Publishing, Abe Ogden; *Managing Editor,* Rebekah Renshaw; *Acquisitions Editor,* Victor Van Beuren; *Project Manager,* Lauren Wilson; *Production Manager and Composition,* Melissa Sprott; *Cover Design,* Vis-á-Vis Creative; *Printer,* Data Reproductions.

Printed in the United States of America
1 3 5 7 9 10 8 6 4 2

The suggestions and information contained in this publication are generally consistent with the *Standards of Medical Care in Diabetes* and other policies of the American Diabetes Association, but they do not represent the policy or position of the Association or any of its boards or committees. Reasonable steps have been taken to ensure the accuracy of the information presented. However, the American Diabetes Association cannot ensure the safety or efficacy of any product or service described in this publication. Individuals are advised to consult a physician or other appropriate health care professional before undertaking any diet or exercise program or taking any medication referred to in this publication. Professionals must use and apply their own professional judgment, experience, and training and should not rely solely on the information contained in this publication before prescribing any diet, exercise, or medication. The American Diabetes Association—its officers, directors, employees, volunteers, and members—assumes no responsibility or liability for personal or other injury, loss, or damage that may result from the suggestions or information in this publication.

⊚ The paper in this publication meets the requirements of the ANSI Standard Z39.48-1992 (permanence of paper).

ADA titles may be purchased for business or promotional use or for special sales. To purchase more than 50 copies of this book at a discount, or for custom editions of this book with your logo, contact the American Diabetes Association at the address below or at booksales@diabetes.org.

American Diabetes Association
2451 Crystal Drive, Suite 900
Arlington, VA 22202

DOI: 10.2337/9781580405553

Library of Congress Cataloging-in-Publication Data

Names: Holzmeister, Lea Ann.
Title: The diabetes carbohydrate & fat gram guide : quick, easy meal planning using carbohydrate and fat counts / Lea Ann Holzmeister.
Other titles: Diabetes carbohydrate and fat gram guide | Quick, easy meal planning using carbohydrate and fat gram counts
Description: 5th edition. | Alexandria : American Diabetes Association, [2017]
Identifiers: LCCN 2016043602 | ISBN 9781580405553 (paperback)
Subjects: LCSH: Diabetes--Diet therapy. | Food exchange lists. | Food--Carbohydrate content--Tables. | Food--Fat content--Tables.
Classification: LCC RC662 .H66 2017 | DDC 641.5/6314--dc23
LC record available at https://lccn.loc.gov/2016043602

Dedication

To all people with diabetes, who I count on for inspiration.

Table of Contents

Preface to the Fifth Edition

Since the fourth edition of *The Diabetes Carbohydrate & Fat Gram Guide* was published, many new food products have been introduced, many new fast-food restaurants have opened, and other fast-food restaurants have revised their menus. This fifth edition includes over 7,300 listings, as well as one additional nutrient category. The 2015 Dietary Guidelines for Americans recommend that intake from added sugars be less than 10% of total calories. To help consumers know the sugar content of foods, the grams of sugar for each food have been added.

To prepare the updates for this new edition we obtained current product information from product labels and food company websites and scanned grocery store shelves for the newest products. The result is a more complete resource for anyone who is concerned about their nutrition intake.

Introduction

Since its discovery hundreds of years ago, diabetes has been linked with what people eat. What people with diabetes are advised to eat and how they plan their meals has changed over the years. The latest American Diabetes Association Nutrition Therapy Recommendations for the Management of Adults with Diabetes (published each January in Supplement 1 of the journal *Diabetes Care*) emphasizes promoting and supporting healthful eating patterns to improve overall health and, more specifically, advises people with diabetes to:

- Attain individualized blood glucose, blood pressure, and lipid goals
- Achieve and maintain body weight goals
- Delay or prevent the complications of diabetes
- Address individual nutrition needs while maintaining the pleasure of eating

Many people with diabetes use some type of meal-planning system to help them meet their individual nutrition goals. Just as there is no one diet that is right for everyone with diabetes, there is also no one meal planning approach that meets everyone's needs. It is important to know your own nutrition goals. A registered dietitian (RD) can help you determine your individual nutrition goals and develop a meal plan based on your food preferences, lifestyle, blood glucose and blood lipid (fat) levels, overall health, and abilities. If you're not currently seeing a dietitian, your doctor may be able to recommend one. Or you can visit the Academy of Nutrition and Dietetics website at www.eatright.org.

Types of Meal-Planning Approaches

Three types of meal-planning approaches are described in this book:

- Carbohydrate counting
- *Choose Your Foods: Food Lists for Diabetes,* published by the American Diabetes Association and the Academy of Nutrition and Dietetics
- Calorie counting

The advantages and disadvantages of each approach are discussed, and information about where to learn more is provided.

It is important to select a meal-planning approach that you are comfortable using and that will work toward achieving your goals. You do not have to use the same approach your entire life. As your individual nutrition goals change, so may your meal-planning approach. Before switching to a different approach, though, it is a good idea to consult with your dietitian or healthcare provider.

Carbohydrate Counting

Carbohydrate counting has been a popular meal-planning tool in Europe and in the U.S. for many years. The three main nutrients in the foods we eat are carbohydrate, protein, and fat. The carbohydrate in foods affects your blood glucose level more than protein or fat. In carbohydrate counting, you count only carbohydrate. Carbohydrate-containing foods and beverages and your body's own insulin production are the greatest determinant of your postmeal blood glucose. The two main types of carbohydrate are sugars and starches. According to the American Diabetes Association's nutrition recommendations, both the amount (grams) of carbohydrate as well as the type of carbohydrate in a food affect blood glucose levels. However, monitoring total grams of carbohydrate and eating the same amount of carbohydrate at meals and snacks each day, remains a key strategy in achieving good blood glucose control.

To use the carbohydrate counting approach, you must know your total carbohydrate allotment for the day. A dietitian can help you determine this. Together, you and your dietitian will make a carbohydrate counting meal plan based on your usual food intake, lifestyle, diabetes medications, and physical activity. Once you have your carbohydrate counting meal plan, you'll need to become familiar with the carbohydrate content in foods. Carbohydrate is found in many foods, such as grains, vegetables, fruits, milk, and table sugar. It is important to count all carbohydrate regardless of its source. When choosing carbohydrate-containing foods, choose nutrient-dense, high-fiber foods whenever possible instead of processed foods with added sodium, fat, and sugars.

Carbohydrate counting can provide some advantages over other meal-planning approaches. Some people feel that focusing on only one nutrient makes this system easier. With the focus on carbohydrate, food and insulin can be matched more precisely. Matching food and insulin increases flexibility in meal and snack times. This can be particularly helpful when your appetite varies or your schedule changes. Also, insulin can be matched to carbohydrate eaten at specific times during the day. For example, some people need more insulin at breakfast for each gram of carbohydrate eaten. Thus, carbohydrate counting may be most appropriate for people who take insulin.

One disadvantage of carbohydrate counting is that when you focus only on carbohydrate, it is easy to lose sight of the overall nutritional quality of foods. For example, counting the carbohydrate in foods like bacon or sausage but ignoring their fat content may lead you to eat these fatty foods more often. Too much fat in the diet increases your risk of heart disease, cancer, and weight gain. If you don't pay attention to the overall nutritional quality of foods, including the type of carbohydrate, you may end up eating a diet that is too high in fat or sugar. To learn more about carbohydrate counting, contact your dietitian.

Choose Your Foods: Food Lists for Diabetes

For many years, the food exchange system was used as a meal-planning approach for people with diabetes. This system has been revised and is now called *Choose Your Foods: Food Lists for Diabetes*. This system groups foods with similar nutritional value into lists, with the goal of helping people with diabetes eat consistent amounts of nutrients. Each food on a list has approximately the same number of calories and amount of carbohydrate, protein, and fat as the other foods on the same list. Any food on a list can be traded or "exchanged" for any other food on the same list.

To use *Choose Your Foods* you need an individualized meal plan that tells you how many choices from each list to select for your meals and snacks. Your dietitian can help you design your individualized meal plan and teach you how to use this system.

The American Diabetes Association and the Academy of Nutrition and Dietetics' booklet *Choose Your Foods: Food Lists for Diabetes* groups food into four broad lists: the carbohydrate list, the protein list, the fat list, and the alcohol list. The carbohydrate list includes five sublists: the starch list, the fruit list, the milk list, the sweets, desserts, and other carbohydrates list, and the non-starchy vegetables list. The protein list includes four sublists: the lean list, the medium-fat list, the high-fat list, and plant-based protein list. The fat list includes a monounsaturated (unsaturated) fat list, a polyunsaturated fat list, and a saturated fat list. In addition to these lists, there is a free foods list, a combination foods list, a fast foods list, and an alcohol list.

One advantage of the *Choose Your Foods* system is its emphasis on more than one nutrient and the importance of the overall nutritional content of foods. This system also encourages consistency in the timing and amount of your meals and snacks. People wanting to lose weight might find this approach useful for learning the caloric and fat values of foods. *Choose Your Foods* can also be used as a reference for those using carbohydrate counting. Each serving of a food in the carbohydrate group counts as 15 grams of carbohydrate.

One disadvantage of this system is the level of understanding needed to grasp the concept of grouping or "exchanging" foods. It also requires learning where a food that is not listed fits. To learn more about using *Choose Your Foods: Food Lists for Diabetes* for meal planning, contact your dietitian.

Calorie Counting

Calorie counting has been used for many years as a way to achieve weight loss, weight gain, or weight maintenance. This approach is most appropriate for people with diabetes who are overweight and do not take insulin. For people who are overweight, even modest weight loss can improve blood glucose levels.

To use calorie counting, you and your dietitian need to establish a calorie goal that will help you achieve your weight goal. Your weight goal will be based on your current weight, height, and activity level. If you desire to lose weight, your calorie goal will be set lower than your usual intake of calories. If you wish to maintain your current weight, your calorie goal will be set at a calorie level similar to your current intake of calories. You should keep records of the foods you eat and their calorie content. A periodic comparison of your food records and weekly weight can give you feedback on how you are progressing toward your weight goal. These records can also help you identify problem areas. For example, you might realize after reviewing your records that you tend to overeat when away from home. Knowing this information will help you and your dietitian develop strategies for changing this behavior.

The main advantage of calorie counting is the expanded choice of foods, which gives you more flexibility in what you eat. You decide if and how a food might fit into your meal plan. For example, say your daily calorie goal is 1,500 calories, and a food you want to eat contains 600 calories. You can eat that food as long as you plan what other foods you'll eat that day to add up to the remaining 900 calories. Your serving size, too, is based on how you want to "spend" your calories. You might decide you can work in only half a serving of pasta salad, or you might choose to have a double serving of pasta salad depending on your calorie goals.

One disadvantage of calorie counting might be the amount of time involved in keeping records and calculating the calorie content of foods. Also, because this approach does not guide you toward making nutritionally balanced choices, you may end up with a high-fat diet or one low in essential vitamins and minerals. Your dietitian can provide you with basic nutrition guidelines by which to select your foods to ensure that you meet your nutrition goals as well.

Estimating Serving Sizes

The success of any meal-planning approach depends on how accurately you estimate your serving sizes. Therefore, it is essential to train your eyes to do this. Equip your kitchen with measuring spoons, measuring cups, and a food scale. Use these tools to measure and weigh your food consistently for 2 weeks or until you have trained your eyes to recognize the correct serving sizes for your favorite foods. You should know, for example, what a cup of pasta looks like on your plate or how much 1 cup of milk fills your favorite glass.

Without some practice, it is surprisingly easy to mistakenly pour yourself 1 cup instead of a 1/2 cup of juice. A cup of juice has twice the carbohydrate and calories of 1/2 cup of juice. This might tip you over your calorie or carbohydrate goal. If you did this with just two to three foods each day, it could spoil your efforts at weight loss and blood glucose control.

Of course, it is not practical to measure servings when you eat out in a restaurant, but training your eyes will help. Fortunately, the serving sizes of fast foods are fairly standardized among restaurants, e.g., a taco at any Taco Bell restaurant is likely to be the same size.

How Food Counts Can Work for You

The meal-planning approach you select will determine what you will "count" in your diet. But using a meal-planning approach to guide your food choices is only a starting point. To reach your individual goals (such as blood glucose, blood lipid, blood pressure, weight, or general health goals), you need to respond every day to changes in your blood glucose levels and periodically to other indicators of your progress (such as blood lipid levels, blood pressure changes, weight gain, or weight loss).

Food Counts and Blood Glucose

Making the connection between what you eat and how it affects your blood glucose level can be a very powerful step toward achieving your blood glucose goals. Once you have recorded your food intake and blood glucose values, you can learn to analyze the data to see how individual foods and meals affect your blood glucose. You can then try adjusting food intake, physical activity, and diabetes medications (with the help of your physician) as needed to optimize your blood glucose control.

Food Counts and Blood Lipids

Counting saturated fat and trans fat in your diet while keeping tabs on your blood lipid levels (total cholesterol, HDL cholesterol, LDL cholesterol, and triglycerides) allows you to determine whether your meal plan is helping you to achieve your blood lipid goals. Suppose you have been advised to follow a diet with minimal trans fat and less than 25 grams of saturated fat per day in an attempt to reduce your total cholesterol from 250 to 200 mg/dL. By comparing your food records of saturated fat and trans fat intake to your blood lipid levels over time, you can determine how close you are coming to your blood lipid goals.

Using This Book of Food Counts

This book is intended to be a comprehensive listing of both generic and brand name foods and fast foods that are available nationally. The nutrition information in this fifth edition comes from several sources, including:

- U.S. Department of Agriculture, Agricultural Research Service, National Nutrient Database for Standard Reference Release 28
- Food manufactures and fast-food restaurants' websites
- Nutrition Facts from food labels

Foods are listed alphabetically by food category and manufacturer. Nutrient information for foods from mixes (for example, puddings and cakes) reflect values after the food has been prepared according to package directions.

This book lists the calories, fat, calories from fat, saturated fat, trans fat, cholesterol, sodium, carbohydrate, sugar, fiber, and protein of many foods. These particular nutrients were selected because they are the most commonly monitored by people with diabetes (see Table 1, page xviii).

The nutrient values you use will depend on your meal-planning approach. You may need one, two, or even more of the values to figure out how a food fits into your plan. The serving sizes listed in this book are those most commonly used. Similar foods will have the same serving sizes. The serving size may be very different from the amount you serve yourself or eat. If your serving size is different, ask your dietitian to help you recalculate the numbers.

The exchange values of foods have been calculated using the "rounding off method" (Wheeler ML, Franz M, Barrier PH, Holler H, Cronmiller N, Delahanty LM. Macronutrient and energy database for the 1995 Exchange Lists for Meal Planning: a rationale for clinical practice decisions. *J Am Diet Assoc* 1996;96:1167–1171). Table 2 (page xx) shows the amount of nutrients in one serving from each list.

Some of the foods in this book have a nutrient claim, such as "reduced-fat" or "low-calorie," as part of their name. These claims have standard meanings set by the Food and Drug Administration (FDA). Some of these terms and their meanings are listed in Table 3 (page xxi).

TABLE 1. American Diabetes Association Nutrient Recommendations

Energy balance: For overweight or obese adults with type 2 diabetes, reducing calorie intake while maintaining a healthful eating pattern is recommended to promote weight loss.

Carbohydrate: Carbohydrate raises your blood glucose level, therefore monitoring carbohydrate intake is recommended. For good health, carbohydrate intake from fruits, vegetables, whole grains, legumes, and dairy products is recommended over intake from carbohydrate sources containing added fats, sugars, or sodium. The 2015 Dietary Guidelines for Americans, from the U.S. Department of Health and Human Services and the U.S. Department of Agriculture, recommends that intake from added sugars be less than 10% of total calories. Your dietitian can help you determine how much carbohydrate you need in a day.

Fat: Fat is a concentrated source of calories. There is no ideal amount of fat intake for all people with diabetes; it varies by individual. Generally, the type of fat you eat is more important than how much fat you eat. Your dietitian can help you determine your ideal amount of fat intake.

Monounsaturated Fat/Omega-3 Fats: In people with diabetes, a diet high in monounsaturated fats (Mediterranean-style eating pattern) may benefit blood glucose control and lower cardiovascular risk. In addition, people with diabetes may benefit from consuming foods containing long-chain omega-3 fatty acids (EPA and DHA) from fatty fish and omega-3 linolenic acid (ALA). The recommendation for the general public to eat fish, particularly fatty fish, at least two times (two servings) per week is also appropriate for people with diabetes.

Saturated Fat/Dietary Cholesterol/Trans Fat: The amount of dietary saturated fat, cholesterol, and trans fat recommended for people with diabetes is the same as that recommended for the general population. The 2015 Dietary Guidelines for Americans recommends consuming less than 10% of calories from saturated fat, aiming for less than 200 mg of dietary cholesterol per day, and limiting trans fat as much as possible to reduce cardiovascular disease risk.

Sodium: Sodium has been linked to higher blood pressure and cardiovascular health risks. The recommendation for the general population to reduce sodium intake to less than 2,300 mg per day is also appropriate for people with diabetes. For individuals with both diabetes and hypertension, consult with your dietitian for individual recommendations.

Fiber: For most adults, including people with diabetes, daily consumption of 25 grams of dietary fiber for adult women and 38 grams of dietary fiber for adult men, consisting of both soluble and insoluble fibers from a wide variety of food sources, is recommended. Dietary fiber may be helpful in the treatment and prevention of constipation and several gastrointestinal disorders. Soluble fiber has a beneficial effect on serum lipids and provides satiety value to your diet.

Protein: Most adults, including people with diabetes, require approximately 15–20% of their calories from protein. Some individuals with diabetes and those with kidney disease may require a reduction of protein intake.

Alcohol: If adults choose to use alcohol, daily intake should be limited to a moderate amount—one drink per day or fewer for adult women and two drinks per day or fewer for adult men. For individuals with diabetes who take diabetes medication, alcohol should be consumed with food.

TABLE 2. Nutrient Content of Food Lists

Food List	Carbohy-drate (g)	Protein (g)	Fat (g)	Calories
Carbohydrates				
Starch	15	3	1	80
Fruits	15	0	0	60
Milk and Milk Substitutes				
Fat-Free, Low-Fat, 1%	12	8	0–3	100
Reduced-Fat, 2%	12	8	5	120
Whole	12	8	8	160
Sweets, Desserts, and Other Carbohydrate	15	Varies	Varies	Varies
Nonstarchy Vegetables	5	2	0	25
Proteins				
Lean	0	7	2	45
Medium-Fat	0	7	5	75
High-Fat	0	7	8	100
Plant-Based	Varies	7	Varies	Varies
Fats	0	0	5	45
Free Foods	5 or less	Varies	Varies	Less than 20
Alcohol	Varies	0	0	~100

Source: Adapted from the American Diabetes Association and the Academy of Nutrition and Dietetics. *Choose Your Foods: Food Lists for Diabetes.* Alexandria, VA, 2014, p. 4.

TABLE 3. Nutrient Claims on Food Labels

Term	Meaning
Calorie-Free	Less than 5 calories per serving
Cholesterol-Free	Less than 2 mg of cholesterol per serving and 2 g or less of saturated fat per serving
Extra-Lean	Less than 5 g of fat, 2 g of saturated fat, and 95 mg of cholesterol per serving
Fat-Free	Less than 0.5 g of fat per serving
High-Fiber	5 g of fiber or more per serving
Good Source of Fiber	2.5 g to 4.9 g of fiber per serving
Lean	Less than 10 g of fat, 4.54 g of saturated fat, and 95 mg of cholesterol per serving
Light	33.3% fewer calories or 50% less fat per serving than comparison food
Low-Calorie	40 calories or less per serving
Low-Cholesterol	20 mg or less of cholesterol per serving and 2 g or less of saturated fat per serving
Low-Fat	3 g or less of fat per serving
Low–Saturated Fat	1 g or less of saturated fat per serving and 15% or less of calories from saturated fat
Low-Sodium	140 mg or less of sodium per serving
Reduced (Calories/ Sugar/Sodium/ Fat/Saturated Fat/Cholesterol)	25% less per serving than comparison food
Salt-Free	Less than 5 mg sodium per serving
Saturated Fat– Free	Less than 0.5 g of saturated fat and 0.5 g of trans fatty acids per serving
Sodium-Free	Less than 5 mg of sodium per serving
Sugar-Free	Less than 0.5 g of sugar per serving
Very Low Sodium	35 mg of sodium or less per serving

ALCOHOLIC BEVERAGES & MIXERS

	Serving	Calories	Fat (g)	Cal. from Fat	Sat. Fat (g)	Trans Fat (g)	Chol. (mg)	Sod. (mg)	Carb. (g)	Sugar (g)	Fiber (g)	Prot. (g)	Servings/Exchanges
BEER													
Beer, Light	12 oz	104	0	0	0	0	0	14	6	0	0	1	1/2 carb, 1 alcohol
Beer, Regular	12 oz	155	0	0	0	0	0	14	13	0	0	2	1 carb, 1 alcohol
Beer, Non-alcoholic	12 oz	70	0	0	0	0	0	8	13	0	0	1	1 alcohol
Bud Light	12 oz	110	0	0	0	0	0	11	7	0	0	1	1/2 carb, 1 alcohol
Budweiser	12 oz	145	0	0	0	0	0	11	11	0	0	1	1/2 carb, 1 alcohol
Michelob Light	12 oz	123	0	0	0	0	0	NA	9	0	0	1	1/2 carb, 1 alcohol
Michelob Ultra	12 oz	95	0	0	0	0	0	9	3	0	0	<1	1 alcohol
Miller Genuine Draft Light	12 oz	110	0	0	0	0	0	NA	7	0	0	0	1/2 carb, 1 alcohol
Miller Light	12 oz	95	0	0	0	0	0	NA	3	0	0	<1	1 alcohol
Blue Moon, Belgian White, ABV 5.4	12 oz	168	0	0	0	0	0	16.3	14.1	0	0	1.9	1 carb, 1 alcohol
Deschutes Inversion IPA, ABV 6.9	12 oz	226	0	0	0	0	0	6.6	20	0	<1	<1	1 carb, 1 alcohol
Deschutes, Mirror Pond Pale Ale, ABV 5.2	12 oz	172	0	0	0	0	0	6.6	16	0	<0.5	<1	1 carb, 1 alcohol
Deschutes Obsidian Stout, ABV 6.4	12 oz	212	0	0	0	0	0	7.7	19	0	<1	<1	1 carb, 1 alcohol

ALCOHOLIC BEVERAGES & MIXERS

	Serving	Calories	Fat (g)	Cal. from Fat	Sat. Fat (g)	Trans Fat (g)	Chol. (mg)	Sod. (mg)	Carb. (g)	Sugar (g)	Fiber (g)	Prot. (g)	Servings/Exchanges
Deschutes, Black Butte Porter, ABV 5.3	12 oz	195	0	0	0	0	0	7	20	0	1	2.84	1 carb, 1 alcohol
COCKTAILS													
Daiquiri, Mix, from frozen	4 oz	153	0	0	0	0	0	7	38	NA	0	0	2 1/2 carb
Piña Colada	4 oz	228	2	18	2	0	0	6	32	NA	0	0	2 carb
Tequila Sunrise	4 oz	140	0	0	0	0	0	6	11	NA	0	0	1 carb
Whiskey Sour	4 oz	164	0	0	0	0	0	13	7	NA	0	0	1/2 carb
LIQUEURS													
Coffee Liqueur (Kahlúa Original)	1.5 oz	80	0	0	0	0	0	NA	11	NA	0	0	1 carb
Liqueur with Cream (Bailey's)	1.5 oz	153	5	45	3	0	0	29	6	NA	0	1	1/2 carb
Triple Sec Liqueur	1.5 oz	120	0	0	0	0	0	0	3	0	0	0	1 alcohol
SPIRITS (GIN, RUM, VODKA, WHISKEY)													
100 Proof	1.5 oz	124	0	0	0	0	0	0	0	0	0	0	1 alcohol
86 Proof	1.5 oz	105	0	0	0	0	0	0	0	0	0	0	1 alcohol
80 Proof	1.5 oz	97	0	0	0	0	0	0	0	0	0	0	1 alcohol
WINE													
Cooking Wine	5 oz	73	0	0	0	0	0	7	9	NA	0	1	1/2 carb, 1 alcohol

Light Wine	5 oz	72	0	0	0	0	10	2	NA	0	0	1 alcohol
Non-Alcoholic Wine	5 oz	9	0	0	0	0	10	2	NA	0	1	1 alcohol
Red Table Wine	5 oz	125	0	0	0	0	6	4	NA	1	0	1 alcohol
Sake	1 oz	39	0	0	0	0	1	1	NA	0	0	1/2 alcohol
Sweet Dessert Wine	5 oz	236	0	0	0	0	13	20	NA	0	0	1 carb, 1 alcohol
White Table Wine	5 oz	121	0	0	0	0	7	4	NA	0	0	1 alcohol
Wine Cooler	11.2 oz	116	0	0	0	0	15	14	NA	0	0	1 carb, 1 alcohol
MIXERS (NON-ALCOHOLIC)												
Finest Call												
Grenadine	1 oz	90	0	0	0	0	0	22	NA	0	0	1 1/2 carb
Margarita Mix	4 oz	180	0	0	0	0	15	45	NA	0	0	3 carb
Sweet & Sour Mix	4 oz	110	0	0	0	0	25	28	NA	0	0	2 carb
Rose's												
Sweetened Lime Juice	1 tsp	10	0	0	0	0	0	2	NA	0	0	free
Jose Cuervo												
Lite Margarita Mix	4 oz	0	0	0	0	0	65	0	NA	0	0	free
Margarita Mix	4 oz	110	0	0	0	0	55	28	NA	0	0	2 carb
Master of Mixes												
Classic Bloody Mary Mix	4 oz	25	0	0	0	0	0	720	NA	6	1	1/2 carb
Margarita Mixer	4 oz	140	0	0	0	0	50	35	NA	32	0	2 carb

ALCOHOLIC BEVERAGES & MIXERS

	Serving	Calories	Fat (g)	Cal. from Fat	Sat. Fat (g)	Trans Fat (g)	Chol. (mg)	Sod. (mg)	Carb. (g)	Sugar (g)	Fiber (g)	Prot. (g)	Servings/Exchanges
Piña Colada Mixer	4 oz	230	1.5	1.5	0	0	0	55	53	NA	50	0	3 1/2 carb
Strawberry Daiquiri Margarita Mixer	4 oz	190	0	0	0	0	0	20	47	NA	44	0	3 carb
Sweet 'N Sour Mixer On the House	3 oz	80	0	0	0	0	0	35	21	NA	19	0	1 1/2 carb
Margarita Mix	4 oz	100	0	0	0	0	0	20	25	NA	23	0	1 1/2 carb
Piña Colada Mix	4 oz	160	0	0	0	0	0	15	39	NA	35	0	2 1/2 carb
Stirrings													
5 Calorie Cosmopolitan	3 oz	5	0	0	0	0	0	0	2	NA	0	0	free
5 Calorie Margarita Mix	3 oz	5	0	0	0	0	0	0	2	NA	0	0	free
Simple Apple Martini Mix	3 oz	90	0	0	0	0	0	0	22	NA	0	0	1 1/2 carb
Simple Bloody Mary Mix	3 oz	30	0	0	0	0	0	570	8	NA	<1	1	1/2 carb
Simple Blood Orange Martini Mixer	3 oz	70	0	0	0	0	0	0	17	NA	0	0	1 carb
Simple Margarita Mix	3 oz	60	0	0	0	0	0	0	17	NA	0	0	1 carb
Simple Mojito Mix	2 oz	50	0	0	0	0	0	0	13	NA	0	0	1 carb

BEANS, PEAS, LENTILS

	Serving	Calories	Fat (g)	Cal. from Fat	Sat. Fat (g)	Trans Fat (g)	Chol. (mg)	Sod. (mg)	Carb. (g)	Sugar (g)	Fiber (g)	Prot. (g)	Servings/Exchanges
Baked Beans (Boston)	1/2 cup	195	6	54	2	0	6	576	28	9	5	8	2 carb, 1 fat
Baked Beans, Vegetarian, Canned	1/2 cup	119	0	0	0	0	0	436	27	10	5	6	2 carb
Black Beans, Canned	1/2 cup	99	0	0	0	0	0	184	18	0	4	6	1 carb, 1/2 lean protein
Black Beans, Cooked (no salt or fat added)	1/2 cup	99	0	0	0	0	0	9	18	1	4	6	1 carb, 1/2 lean protein
Fava/Broadbeans, Canned	1/2 cup	93	0	0	0	0	0	201	17	2	5	6	1 carb, 1/2 lean protein
Fava/Broadbeans, Cooked (no salt or fat added)	1/2 cup	93	0	0	0	0	0	4	17	2	5	6	1 carb, 1/2 lean protein
Garbanzo Beans/Chickpeas, Canned	1/2 cup	148	2	18	0	0	0	199	25	4	7	8	1 1/2 carb, 1/2 lean protein
Garbanzo Beans/Chickpeas, Cooked (no salt or fat added)	1/2 cup	148	2	18	0	0	0	6	25	4	7	8	1 1/2 carb, 1/2 lean protein

BEANS, PEAS, LENTILS

	Serving	Calories	Fat (g)	Cal. from Fat	Sat. Fat (g)	Trans Fat (g)	Chol. (mg)	Sod. (mg)	Carb. (g)	Sugar (g)	Fiber (g)	Prot. (g)	Servings/Exchanges
Great Northern Beans, Canned	1/2 cup	121	0	0	0	0	0	207	22	0	6	8	1 1/2 carb, 1/2 lean protein
Hummus	1/2 cup	218	11	100	1	0	0	298	25	0	5	6	1 1/2 carb, 2 fat
Kidney Beans, Canned	1/2 cup	108	0	0	0	0	0	200	19	0	6	7	1 carb, 1 lean protein
Kidney Beans, Cooked (no salt or fat added)	1/2 cup	108	0	0	0	0	0	2	19	0	6	7	1 carb, 1 lean protein
Lentils, Cooked (no salt or fat added)	1/2 cup	110	0	0	0	0	0	2	19	2	8	9	1 carb, 1 lean protein
Lima Beans, Canned	1/2 cup	105	0	0	0	0	0	214	19	3	6	7	1 carb, 1 lean protein
Lima Beans, Cooked from dry (no salt or fat added)	1/2 cup	105	0	0	0	0	0	2	19	3	6	7	1 carb, 1 lean protein
Pink Beans, Canned	1/2 cup	125	0	0	0	0	0	165	23	0	4	8	1 1/2 carb, 1/2 lean protein
Pink Beans, Cooked (no salt or fat added)	1/2 cup	125	0	0	0	0	0	2	23	0	4	8	1 1/2 carb, 1/2 lean protein
Pinto Beans, Canned	1/2 cup	99	0	0	0	0	0	187	18	0	4	6	1 carb, 1/2 lean protein

Food	Serving	Cal.	Fat (g)	% Cal. Fat	Sat. Fat (g)	Trans Fat (g)	Chol. (mg)	Sodium (mg)	Carb. (g)	Sugars (g)	Fiber (g)	Prot. (g)	Exchanges/Choices
Pinto Beans, Cooked (no salt or fat added)	1/2 cup	99	0	0	0	0	0	10	18	1	4	6	1 carb, 1/2 lean protein
Peas, Black-Eyed, Canned	1/2 cup	86	0	0	0	0	0	256	18	3	5	3	1 carb
Peas, Black-Eyed, Cooked (no salt or fat added)	1/2 cup	97	0	0	0	0	0	3	17	3	5	6	1 carb, 1/2 lean protein
Pork & Beans, generic	1/2 cup	119	1	0	0	0	9	553	24	11	5	7	1 1/2 carb
Refried Beans (no fat added)	1/2 cup	91	1	0	0	0	0	506	16	1	5	6	1 carb, 1/2 lean protein
Refried Beans (with animal fat)	1/2 cup	177	6	2	0	0	5	485	24	1	8	8	1 1/2 carb, 1/2 lean protein, 1 fat
Split Peas, Cooked (no salt or fat added)	1/2 cup	115	0	0	0	0	0	2	21	3	8	8	1 1/2 carb, 1/2 lean protein
White Beans, Canned	1/2 cup	121	0	0	0	0	0	207	22	0	6	8	1 1/2 carb, 1/2 lean protein
White Beans, Cooked (no salt or fat added)	1/2 cup	121	0	0	0	0	0	5	22	0	6	8	1 1/2 carb, 1/2 lean protein
CANNED BEANS (BRANDS)													
B & M													
Baked Beans, Bacon & Onion	1/2 cup	190	2	20	1	0	<5	450	36	13	8	8	2 1/2 carb

BEANS, PEAS, LENTILS

	Serving	Calories	Fat (g)	Cal. from Fat	Sat. Fat (g)	Trans Fat (g)	Chol. (mg)	Sod. (mg)	Carb. (g)	Sugar (g)	Fiber (g)	Prot. (g)	Servings/Exchanges
Baked Beans, Boston's Best	1/2 cup	170	2	15	1	0	<5	440	32	12	8	7	2 carb
Baked Beans, Country Style	1/2 cup	170	2	15	1	0	<5	570	35	13	6	6	2 carb
Baked Beans, Homestyle	1/2 cup	190	1	10	0	0	0	620	39	16	8	8	2 1/2 carb
Baked Beans, Maple Flavor	1/2 cup	150	1	10	0	0	0	340	28	12	6	6	2 carb
Baked Beans, Original	1/2 cup	170	2	20	1	0	<5	400	31	10	5	7	2 carb
Baked Beans, Vegetarian	1/2 cup	160	1	10	0	0	0	383	28	12	8	7	2 carb
Bush's													
Baked Beans, Bold & Spicy	1/2 cup	140	1	10	0	0	0	560	24	9	5	6	1 1/2 carb
Baked Beans, Boston Style	1/2 cup	150	1	10	0	0	0	440	31	11	5	6	2 carb
Baked Beans, Country Style	1/2 cup	170	1	10	0	0	0	600	33	14	6	7	2 carb

Food	Serving	Cal.	Fat (g)	Fat Cal.	Sat. Fat (g)	Chol. (mg)	Sod. (mg)	Carb. (g)	Fiber (g)	Sugar (g)	Prot. (g)	Choices/Exchanges
Baked Beans, Homestyle	1/2 cup	140	1	10	0	0	550	29	12	5	6	2 carb
Baked Beans, Honey	1/2 cup	170	2	15	0	0	520	32	15	5	7	2 carb
Baked Beans, Maple Cured Bacon	1/2 cup	150	2	15	0	0	570	27	10	6	7	2 carb
Baked Beans, Onion	1/2 cup	140	1	10	0	0	550	29	12	5	6	2 carb
Baked Beans, Original	1/2 cup	140	1	10	0	0	550	29	12	5	6	2 carb
Baked Beans, Vegetarian	1/2 cup	130	0	0	0	0	550	29	12	5	6	2 carb
Baked Beans, Vegetarian Reduced Sodium	1/2 cup	140	0	0	0	0	410	29	12	6	6	2 carb
Black Beans	1/2 cup	100	0	0	0	0	490	18	1	4	6	1 carb, 1/2 lean protein
Black-Eyed Peas	1/2 cup	80	0	0	0	0	480	15	0	3	5	1 carb
Black-Eyed Peas with Bacon	1/2 cup	110	2	15	0	0	370	17	0	3	6	1 carb, 1/2 lean protein
Butter Beans, Baby	1/2 cup	110	0	0	0	0	470	21	1	5	6	1 1/2 carb
Cannellini Beans	1/2 cup	100	0	0	0	0	270	19	0	6	7	1 carb, 1 lean protein
Crowder Peas	1/2 cup	90	0	0	0	0	460	18	0	5	5	1 carb
Field Peas with Snaps	1/2 cup	80	0	0	0	0	430	16	0	2	5	1 carb

BEANS, PEAS, LENTILS

	Serving	Calories	Fat (g)	Cal. from Fat	Sat. Fat (g)	Trans Fat (g)	Chol. (mg)	Sod. (mg)	Carb. (g)	Sugar (g)	Fiber (g)	Prot. (g)	Servings/Exchanges
Garbanzo Beans	1/2 cup	120	2	20	0	0	0	470	20	0	5	6	1 carb, 1/2 lean protein
Great Northern Beans	1/2 cup	90	0	0	0	0	0	460	17	0	6	6	1 carb, 1/2 lean protein
Grillin' Beans, Bourbon & Brown Sugar	1/2 cup	170	1	5	0	0	0	480	35	15	6	7	2 carb
Grillin' Beans, Smoke-house Tradition	1/2 cup	160	1	10	0	0	0	550	33	14	4	5	2 carb
Grillin' Beans, Southern Pit BBQ	1/2 cup	170	1	5	0	0	0	550	35	16	6	6	2 carb
Grillin' Beans, Steak-house Recipe	1/2 cup	180	1	5	0	0	0	510	39	21	5	6	2 1/2 carb
Kidney Beans, Dark Red	1/2 cup	120	0	0	0	0	0	260	22	3	8	7	1 1/2 carb
Mixed Beans	1/2 cup	90	0	0	0	0	0	470	18	0	7	5	1 carb
Navy Beans	1/2 cup	90	0	0	0	0	0	470	17	0	7	6	1 carb, 1/2 lean protein
Pinto Beans	1/2 cup	100	0	0	0	0	0	310	18	0	7	6	1 carb, 1/2 lean protein
Pinto Beans with Pork	1/2 cup	110	1	10	0	0	0	450	17	0	7	6	1 carb, 1/2 lean protein

Food	Serving	Cal					Sodium	Carb				Exchanges
Purple Hull Peas	1/2 cup	90	0	0	0	0	460	19	0	5	6	1 carb, 1/2 lean protein
Red Beans	1/2 cup	100	0	0	0	0	480	20	2	7	6	1 carb, 1/2 lean protein
Refried Beans, Fat Free	1/2 cup	130	0	0	0	0	480	24	0	7	9	1 1/2 carb, 1 lean protein
Refried Beans, Traditional	1/2 cup	150	3	25	1	0	480	24	0	7	9	1 1/2 carb, 1 lean protein
White Beans	1/2 cup	90	0	0	0	0	470	17	0	7	6	1 carb, 1/2 lean protein
Eden Organic												
Aduki Beans	1/2 cup	110	0	0	0	0	10	19	0	5	7	1 carb, 1 lean protein
Black Beans	1/2 cup	110	1	10	0	0	15	18	0	6	7	1 carb, 1 lean protein
Black-Eyed Peas	1/2 cup	90	1	10	0	0	25	16	<1	4	6	1 carb, 1/2 lean prctein
Black Soy Beans	1/2 cup	120	6	50	1	0	30	8	1	7	11	1/2 carb, 1 med-fat protein
Butter Beans (Baby Lima)	1/2 cup	100	1	10	0	0	35	17	0	4	6	1 carb, 1/2 lean protein
Cannellini (White Kidney)	1/2 cup	100	1	10	0	0	40	17	<1	5	6	1 carb, 1/2 lean protein
Garbanzo Beans	1/2 cup	130	1	10	0	0	30	21	<1	5	7	1 1/2 carb
Great Northern Beans	1/2 cup	130	1	10	0	0	45	20	1	8	5	1 carb

BEANS, PEAS, LENTILS

	Serving	Calories	Fat (g)	Cal. from Fat	Sat. Fat (g)	Trans Fat (g)	Chol. (mg)	Sod. (mg)	Carb. (g)	Sugar (g)	Fiber (g)	Prot. (g)	Servings/Exchanges
Kidney Beans	1/2 cup	100	0	0	0	0	0	15	18	<1	10	8	1 carb, 1 lean protein
Pinto Beans	1/2 cup	100	1	0	0	0	0	15	18	<1	6	6	1 carb, 1/2 lean protein
Refried Beans, Pinto	1/2 cup	90	1	10	0	0	0	180	19	1	7	6	1 carb, 1/2 lean protein
Gebhardt													
Fat Free Refried Beans	1/2 cup	80	0	0	0	0	0	500	17	<1	5	6	1 carb, 1/2 lean protein
Refried Beans	1/2 cup	100	2	20	1	0	0	490	16	0	4	6	1 carb, 1/2 lean protein
Old El Paso													
Refried Beans, Fat-Free	1/2 cup	90	0	0	0	0	0	440	16	0	6	6	1 carb, 1/2 lean protein
Refried Beans with Green Chili	1/2 cup	90	1	5	0	0	0	440	16	<1	5	5	1 carb
Refried Beans, Traditional	1/2 cup	110	3	25	1	0	0	440	16	0	5	5	1 carb
Refried Beans, Vegetarian	1/2 cup	90	1	5	0	0	0	440	15	0	5	5	1 carb
Progresso													
Black Beans	1/2 cup	100	1	5	0	0	0	400	17	0	5	6	1 carb, 1/2 lean protein

Chick Peas	1/2 cup	100	2	15	0	0	0	280	17	2	4	5	1 carb
Dark Red Kidney Beans	1/2 cup	110	0	0	0	0	0	340	20	2	6	8	1 carb, 1 lean protein
Fava Beans	1/2 cup	100	1	5	0	0	0	250	17	0	5	6	1 carb, 1/2 lean protein
Ranch Style													
Beans with Jalapeño Peppers	1/2 cup	140	3	30	0	0	0	500	22	2	7	6	1 1/2 carb
Beans, Original	1/2 cup	140	3	30	1	0	0	460	22	2	7	6	1 1/2 carb
Black Beans	1/2 cup	110	1	5	0	0	0	390	19	<1	7	6	1 carb, 1/2 lean protein
Pinto Beans	1/2 cup	120	0	0	0	0	0	240	22	1	7	6	1 1/2 carb
Rosarita													
Low Fat Refried Black Beans	1/2 cup	110	1	5	0	0	0	560	19	<1	6	6	1 carb, 1/2 lean protein
No Fat Refried Beans	1/2 cup	100	0	0	0	0	0	540	18	<1	5	6	1 carb, 1/2 lean protein
No Fat Refried Beans with Green Chili & Lime	1/2 cup	100	0	0	0	0	0	580	19	<1	6	6	1 carb, 1/2 lean protein
Refried Beans, Traditional	1/2 cup	120	3	27	1	0	0	540	18	<1	6	6	1 carb, 1/2 lean protein
Refried Beans, Vegetarian	1/2 cup	120	2	20	0	0	0	540	19	<1	6	6	1 carb, 1/2 lean protein

BEANS, PEAS, LENTILS

	Serving	Calories	Fat (g)	Cal. from Fat	Sat. Fat (g)	Trans Fat (g)	Chol. (mg)	Sod. (mg)	Carb. (g)	Sugar (g)	Fiber (g)	Prot. (g)	Servings/Exchanges
Simple Truth Organic													
Black Beans	1/2 cup	110	0	0	0	0	0	130	20	1	5	7	1 carb, 1 lean protein
Cannellini Beans	1/2 cup	110	0	0	0	0	0	90	19	1	5	8	1 carb, 1 lean protein
Garbanzo Beans	1/2 cup	120	2	20	0	0	0	130	20	3	6	6	1 carb, 1/2 lean protein
Great Northern Beans	1/2 cup	110	0	0	0	0	0	125	20	1	6	7	1 carb, 1 lean protein
Kidney Beans, Dark Red	1/2 cup	110	0	0	0	0	0	130	20	1	8	8	1 carb, 1 lean protein
Pinto Beans	1/2 cup	110	0	0	0	0	0	125	21	1	5	7	1 1/2 carb
Refried Black Beans	1/2 cup	120	0	0	0	0	0	410	19	1	5	7	1 carb, 1 lean protein
Tri-Bean Blend	1/2 cup	100	0	0	0	0	0	130	19	1	5	7	1 carb, 1 lean protein
S & W													
Black Beans	1/2 cup	120	0	0	0	0	0	370	22	1	9	7	1 1/2 carb
Black Beans, 50% Less Sodium	1/2 cup	110	1	5	0	0	0	180	22	1	9	7	1 1/2 carb
Chili Beans, Pinto	1/2 cup	130	2	10	0	0	0	620	23	3	7	7	1 1/2 carb

Food	Serving												Exchanges
Chili Beans, Pinto, 50% Less Sodium	1/2 cup	130	2	10	0	0	0	190	23	3	7	7	1 1/2 carb
Garbanzo Beans	1/2 cup	120	2	15	0	0	0	430	20	0	6	7	1 carb, 1 lean protein
Garbanzo Beans, 50% Less Sodium	1/2 cup	110	2	15	0	0	0	180	20	3	6	7	1 carb, 1 lean protein
Kidney Beans	1/2 cup	110	0	0	0	0	0	380	21	3	8	7	1 1/2 carb
Kidney Beans, 50% Less Sodium	1/2 cup	110	0	0	0	0	0	180	21	3	8	7	1 1/2 carb
Pinquitos	1/2 cup	110	1	5	0	0	0	490	20	2	6	6	1 carb, 1/2 lean protein
Pinto Beans	1/2 cup	100	0	0	0	0	0	540	20	1	7	6	1 carb, 1/2 lean protein
White Beans	1/2 cup	100	0	0	0	0	0	480	19	1	6	7	1 carb, 1 lean protein
Trader Joe's													
Black Beans	1/2 cup	110	0	0	0	0	0	430	20	2	8	7	1 carb, 1 lean protein
Cannellini White Kidney Beans	1/2 cup	120	0	0	0	0	0	260	21	<1	10	8	1 1/2 carb, 1/2 lean protein
Cuban Style Black Beans	1/2 cup	100	1	5	0	0	0	370	19	1	6	6	1 carb, 1/2 lean protein
Fat Free Refried Pinto Beans	1/2 cup	120	0	0	0	0	0	520	22	<1	7	7	1 1/2 carb

BEANS, PEAS, LENTILS

	Serving	Calories	Fat (g)	Cal. from Fat	Sat. Fat (g)	Trans Fat (g)	Chol. (mg)	Sod. (mg)	Carb. (g)	Sugar (g)	Fiber (g)	Prot. (g)	Servings/Exchanges
Garbanzo Beans	1/2 cup	120	1	10	0	0	0	380	22	<1	6	6	1 1/2 carb
Organic Baked Beans	1/2 cup	140	0	0	0	0	0	450	29	10	7	7	2 carb
Organic Black Beans	1/2 cup	100	0	0	0	0	0	140	19	0	4	7	1 carb, 1 lean protein
Organic Pinto Beans	1/2 cup	110	0	0	0	0	0	140	21	0	8	6	1 1/2 carb
Refried Black Beans with Jalapeño Peppers	1/2 cup	120	1	5	0	0	0	440	22	1	7	8	1 1/2 carb, 1/2 lean protein
Van Camps													
Baked Beans, Country Maple	1/2 cup	170	1	5	0	0	0	530	35	13	8	6	2 carb
Baked Beans, Hickory & Bacon	1/2 cup	170	1	10	0	0	0	470	32	12	5	7	2 carb
Baked Beans, Original	1/2 cup	160	1	10	0	0	0	510	30	14	5	7	2 carb
New Orleans Red Kidney Beans	1/2 cup	90	0	0	0	0	0	450	19	1	6	6	1 carb, 1/2 lean protein
Pork & Beans	1/2 cup	120	1	10	0	0	0	390	23	7	6	6	1 1/2 carb

BEVERAGES, SODAS, SPORTS/ENERGY DRINKS, MEAL REPLACEMENT DRINKS, COCOA, COFFEE/CREAMER, TEA

	Serving	Calories	Fat (g)	Cal. from Fat	Sat. Fat (g)	Trans Fat (g)	Chol. (mg)	Sod. (mg)	Carb. (g)	Sugar (g)	Fiber (g)	Prot. (g)	Servings/Exchanges
SODA DRINKS													
Average (All Brands)													
Club Soda	12 oz	0	0	0	0	0	0	75	0	0	0	0	free
Diet Cola/Coke with Aspartame	12 oz	7	0	0	0	0	0	28	1	0	0	0	free
Soft Drink, Cola	12 oz	136	0	0	0	0	0	15	35	33	0	0	2 carb
Soft Drink, Cream Soda	12 oz	189	0	0	0	0	0	45	49	49	0	0	3 carb
Soft Drink, Ginger Ale	12 oz	124	0	0	0	0	0	26	32	32	0	0	2 carb
Soft Drink, Lemon-Lime	12 oz	148	0	0	0	0	0	33	38	33	0	0	2 1/2 carb
Soft Drink, Root Beer	12 oz	152	0	0	0	0	0	48	39	39	0	0	2 1/2 carb
Tonic Water	12 oz	124	0	0	0	0	0	15	32	31	0	0	2 carb
SODA BRANDS													
7-Up	20 oz	240	0	0	0	0	0	70	64	63	0	0	4 carb

BEVERAGES, SODAS, SPORTS/ENERGY DRINKS, MEAL REPLACEMENT DRINKS, COCOA, COFFEE/CREAMER, TEA

	Serving	Calories	Fat (g)	Cal. from Fat	Sat. Fat (g)	Trans Fat (g)	Chol. (mg)	Sod. (mg)	Carb. (g)	Sugar (g)	Fiber (g)	Prot. (g)	Servings/Exchanges
7-Up, Cherry	20 oz	240	0	0	0	0	0	65	64	62	0	0	4 carb
7-Up, Diet	20 oz	0	0	0	0	0	0	75	0	0	0	0	free
A&W Cream Soda	8 oz	120	0	0	0	0	0	30	31	31	0	0	2 carb
A&W Root Beer	8 oz	120	0	0	0	0	0	30	31	31	0	0	2 carb
Barq's Root Beer	12 oz	160	0	0	0	0	0	70	45	45	0	0	3 carb
Canada Dry Ginger Ale	20 oz	230	0	0	0	0	0	80	60	59	0	0	4 carb
Coca-Cola													
Cherry Coke	12 oz	150	0	0	0	0	0	35	42	42	0	0	3 carb
Coca-Cola Classic	12 oz	140	0	0	0	0	0	45	39	39	0	0	2 1/2 carb
Coca-Cola Life	12 oz	90	0	0	0	0	0	35	24	24	0	0	1 1/2 carb
Coca-Cola Zero	12 oz	0	0	0	0	0	0	40	0	0	0	0	free
Diet Coke	12 oz	0	0	0	0	0	0	40	0	0	0	0	free
Diet Coke with Lime	12 oz	0	0	0	0	0	0	40	0	0	0	0	free
Fanta Orange	12 oz	160	0	0	0	0	0	60	45	44	0	0	3 carb
Fresca	12 oz	0	0	0	0	0	0	35	1	0	0	0	free

Pibb Xtra	12 oz	160	0	0	0	0	40	39	39	0	0	2 1/2 carb
Seagram's Ginger Ale	12 oz	100	0	0	0	0	35	26	26	0	0	2 carb
Vanilla Coke	12 oz	150	0	0	0	0	35	42	42	0	0	3 carb

Hansen's Natural Cane Soda

Cherry Vanilla Créme	12 oz	160	0	0	0	0	0	43	43	0	0	3 carb
Creamy Root Beer	12 oz	160	0	0	0	0	0	43	43	0	0	3 carb
Diet Black Cherry	12 oz	0	0	0	0	0	0	0	0	0	0	free
Mandarin Lime	8 oz	150	0	0	0	0	0	39	39	0	0	2 1/2 carb
Orange	12 oz	170	0	0	0	0	0	44	44	0	0	3 carb

Pepsi

Diet Pepsi	12 oz	0	0	0	0	0	60	0	0	0	0	free
Mountain Dew	12 oz	170	0	0	0	0	65	46	46	0	0	3 carb
Mountain Dew Code Red	12 oz	170	0	0	0	0	105	46	46	0	0	3 carb
Mountain Dew Diet	12 oz	0	0	0	0	0	50	0	0	0	0	free
MUG Root Beer	12 oz	160	0	0	0	0	65	43	43	0	0	3 carb
Pepsi	12 oz	150	0	0	0	0	30	41	41	0	0	3 carb
Pepsi Max	12 oz	0	0	0	0	0	65	0	0	0	0	free

BEVERAGES, SODAS, SPORTS/ENERGY DRINKS, MEAL REPLACEMENT DRINKS, COCOA, COFFEE/CREAMER, TEA

	Serving	Calories	Fat (g)	Cal. from Fat	Sat. Fat (g)	Trans Fat (g)	Chol. (mg)	Sod. (mg)	Carb. (g)	Sugar (g)	Fiber (g)	Prot. (g)	Servings/Exchanges
Sierra Mist	12 oz	120	0	0	0	0	0	35	30	29	0	0	2 carb
Wild Cherry Pepsi	12 oz	160	0	0	0	0	0	30	42	42	0	0	3 carb
Sprite													
Sprite	12 oz	140	0	0	0	0	0	65	38	38	0	0	2 1/2 carb
Sprite Zero	12 oz	0	0	0	0	0	0	35	0	0	0	0	free
Squirt	12 oz	140	0	0	0	0	0	50	39	39	0	0	2 1/2 carb
Sunkist Grape	12 oz	170	0	0	0	0	0	60	46	45	0	0	3 carb
Sunkist Orange	12 oz	170	0	0	0	0	0	70	44	43	0	0	3 carb
TAB	12 oz	0	0	0	0	0	0	40	0	0	0	0	free
SPORTS/NUTRITION/ENERGY DRINKS													
Accelerade, Lemon Lime	1 scoop (makes 12 oz)	120	1	5	0	0	5	210	21	20	0	5	1 1/2 carb
All Sport Body Quencher	20 oz	150	0	0	0	0	0	140	40	40	0	0	2 1/2 carb
All Sport Naturally Zero	20 oz	0	0	0	0	0	0	140	2	0	0	0	free

Food	Amount												Exchanges
AMP Energy Drink	16 oz	220	0	0	0	0	0	140	58	51	0	0	4 carb
AMP Energy Drink, Sugar Free	16 oz	10	0	0	0	0	0	150	<1	0	0	0	free
Boost	8 oz	240	4	35	1	0	10	150	41	20	3	10	3 carb
Boost Calorie Smart	8 oz	190	7	60	1	0	10	220	16	4	3	16	1 carb, 2 lean protein, 1 fat
Boost Glucose Control	8 oz	190	7	60	1	0	10	220	16	4	3	16	1 carb, 2 lean protein, 1 fat
Boost High Protein	8 oz	240	6	50	1	0	10	200	33	27	0	15	2 carb, 1 med-fat protein
Boost Plus	8 oz	360	14	130	2	0	10	200	45	24	3	14	3 carb, 1 med-fat protein, 2 fat
Carnation Instant Breakfast Essentials Powder Mix (All Varieties)	1 pkt	130	0–1	0–10	0–0.5	0	<5	90–160	26–27	18–20	<1	5	2 carb
Carnation Instant Breakfast Essentials, High Protein Ready-to-Drink	8 oz bottle	220	6	50	1	0	10	200	28	12	3	15	2 carb, 1 med-fat protein
Carnation Instant Breakfast Essentials, Ready-to-Drink	8 oz bottle	240	4	35	1	0	10	150	41	15	0	10	3 carb

BEVERAGES, SODAS, SPORTS/ENERGY DRINKS, MEAL REPLACEMENT DRINKS, COCOA, COFFEE/CREAMER, TEA

	Serving	Calories	Fat (g)	Cal. from Fat	Sat. Fat (g)	Trans Fat (g)	Chol. (mg)	Sod. (mg)	Carb. (g)	Sugar (g)	Fiber (g)	Prot. (g)	Servings/Exchanges
Carnation Instant Breakfast Essentials, Sugar-Free (All Varieties)	1 pkt	60	0–0.5	0–5	0	0	<5	60–70	12	7–8	3–4	5	1 carb
Core Power, Chocolate	11.5 oz	240	3.5	30	2	0	15	140	28	26	2	26	2 carb, 3 lean protein
CytoSport Muscle Milk Powder	1 scoop	150	6	50	2	0	10	80	9	2	2	16	1/2 carb, 2 lean protein
CytoSport Muscle Milk Ready-to-Drink	11 oz	180	7	60	1.5	0	10	300	9	3	1	20	1/2 carb, 2 lean protein
CytoSport Muscle Milk 100 Calories Ready-to-Drink	11 oz	100	1.5	15	0	0	10	230	3	0	2	20	3 lean protein
Gatorade (All Varieties)	12 oz	80	0	0	0	0	0	160	21	21	0	0	1 1/2 carb
Gatorade G2	12 oz	30	0	0	0	0	0	160	7	7	0	0	1/2 carb
Monster Energy Drink	8 oz	110	0	0	0	0	0	180	27	27	0	0	2 carb
Powerade (All Varieties)	20 oz	130	0	0	0	0	0	250	36	35	0	0	2 1/2 carb
Powerade Zero	20 oz	0	0	0	0	0	0	250	0	0	0	0	free

Propel Body Fitness Water, Peach Mango	12 oz	0	0	0	0	0	0	0	0	0	free

Abbot Products

Ensure	8 oz	220	6	50	1	<5	190	33	15	1	9	2 carb, 1 fat
Ensure Complete	8 oz	350	11	100	1	5	240	52	20	3	13	3 1/2 carb, 2 1/2 fat
Ensure High Protein	8 oz	160	2	20	<5	20	190	19	4	1	16	1 carb, 2 lean protein
Ensure Plus	8 oz	350	11	100	1	10	220	50	20	<1	13	3 carb, 1 med-fat protein, 1 fat
Glucerna Shake, Vanilla	8 oz	190	7	60	1	5	210	23	6	3	10	1 1/2 carb, 1 lean protein, 1 fat

Arizona

Natural Energy Fruit Punch	8 oz	70	0	0	0	0	10	18	16	0	0	1 carb
Natural Energy Watermelon	8 oz	70	0	0	0	0	10	18	17	0	0	1 carb

RW Knudsen

Just Concord Grape	8 oz	160	0	0	0	0	15	37	31	0	2	2 1/2 carb
Just Cranberry	8 oz	70	0	0	0	0	25	18	9	0	0	1 carb

BEVERAGES, SODAS, SPORTS/ENERGY DRINKS, MEAL REPLACEMENT DRINKS, COCOA, COFFEE/CREAMER, TEA

	Serving	Calories	Fat (g)	Cal. from Fat	Sat. Fat (g)	Trans Fat (g)	Chol. (mg)	Sod. (mg)	Carb. (g)	Sugar (g)	Fiber (g)	Prot. (g)	Servings/Exchanges
Recharge Sports Beverage (All Varieties)	8 oz	70	0	0	0	0	0	25	18	18	0	0	1 carb
Simply Nutritious Mega C	8 oz	120	0	0	0	0	0	15	30	26	0	0	2 carb
Simply Nutritious Mega Green	8 oz	120	0	0	0	0	0	25	29	25	0	1	2 carb
Sparkling Blueberry	8 oz	110	0	0	0	0	0	15	28	23	0	0	2 carb
Slim Fast													
Advance Creamy Chocolate Shake	11 oz	180	8	80	1.5	0	10	220	6	1	5	20	1/2 carb, 3 lean protein
High Protein Creamy Milk Chocolate	11 oz	180	9	80	1.5	0	15	260	4	2	2	20	3 lean protein, 1 fat
Original Rich Chocolate Royale	11 oz	190	6	50	2	0	10	210	24	18	4	14	1 1/2 carb, 1 med-fat protein
SoBe													
Citrus Energy	20 oz	250	0	0	0	0	0	55	64	63	0	0	4 carb
Energize Green Tea	20 oz	200	0	0	0	0	0	55	52	51	0	0	3 1/2 carb

Energize Mango Melon	20 oz	250	0	0	0	0	55	65	64	0	0	4 carb
Lifewater, Pacific Coconut	20 oz	80	0	0	0	0	70	21	20	0	0	1 1/2 carb
Lifewater, Strawberry Kiwi	20 oz	100	0	0	0	0	55	26	26	0	0	2 carb
Lifewater, Zero Calorie	20 oz	0	0	0	0	0	60	7–10	0	0	0	1/2 carb
Starbucks												
Refreshers, Blueberry Açaí	12 oz can	90	0	0	0	0	5	26	20	0	0	2 carb
Refreshers, Raspberry Pomegranate	12 oz can	90	0	0	0	0	5	27	20	0	0	2 carb
Vitaminwater												
Vitaminwater (All Flavors)	20 oz bottle	120	0	0	0	0	0	32–34	31–32	0	0	2 carb
Vitaminwater Zero (All Flavors)	20 oz bottle	0	0	0	0	0	0	4–5	0	0	0	free
Taste Nirvana												
Real Coco Aloe	16.2 oz can	100	0	0	0	0	100	25	19	3	0	1 1/2 carb

BEVERAGES, SODAS, SPORTS/ENERGY DRINKS, MEAL REPLACEMENT DRINKS, COCOA, COFFEE/CREAMER, TEA

	Serving	Calories	Fat (g)	Cal. from Fat	Sat. Fat (g)	Trans Fat (g)	Chol. (mg)	Sod. (mg)	Carb. (g)	Sugar (g)	Fiber (g)	Prot. (g)	Servings/Exchanges
Real Coconut Water	16.2 oz can	100	0	0	0	0	0	100	26	19	0	0	1 1/2 carb
Real Coconut Water with Pulp	16.2 oz can	120	1.5	15	0	0	0	100	26	12	2	0	1 1/2 carb
Vita Coco													
Pure Coconut Water with Pineapple	8 oz	60	0	0	0	0	0	40	15	15	0	0	1 carb
Pure Coconut Water	8 oz	45	0	0	0	0	0	70	11	11	0	0	1 carb
Zico													
Coconut Water	8.45 oz box	50	0	0	0	0	0	70	11	9	0	0	1 carb
FRUIT PUNCH & LEMONADE													
Capri Sun													
Original (All Flavors)	6 oz	50	0	0	0	0	0	15	13–14	13	0	0	1 carb

Food	Serving											Carb Choices
Roarin Waters (All Flavors)	6 oz	30	0	0	0	0	15	8	8	0	0	1/2 carb
Country Time												
Lemonade, Prepared from Powder (Lemonade, Pink Lemonade, and Half & Half Varieties)	8 oz	60	0	0	0	0	25	16	16	0	0	1 carb
Crystal Light												
Crystal Light Fruit Flavored Drinks or Lemonades, and Teas	8 oz	5	0	0	0	0	0–35	0	0	0	0	free
Crystal Light Liquid Drops	2 ml per 8 oz	0	0	0	0	0	0	0	0	0	0	free
Kool-Aid												
Drink Mix from Powder (All Varieties)	8 oz	60	0	0	0	0	0	16	16	0	0	1 carb
Kool-Aid Bursts (All Flavors)	6.75 oz bottle	20	0	0	0	0	25–35	5	5	0	0	free

BEVERAGES, SODAS, SPORTS/ENERGY DRINKS, MEAL REPLACEMENT DRINKS, COCOA, COFFEE/CREAMER, TEA

	Serving	Calories	Fat (g)	Cal. from Fat	Sat. Fat (g)	Trans Fat (g)	Chol. (mg)	Sod. (mg)	Carb. (g)	Sugar (g)	Fiber (g)	Prot. (g)	Servings/Exchanges
Kool-Aid Jammers (All Flavors)	5.9 oz pouch	30	0	0	0	0	0	15	8	8	0	0	free
Kool-Aid Soft Drink (All Flavors)	12 oz	150	0	0	0	0	0	25–30	13	13	0	0	1 carb
Tang													
Orange Drink Mix, Prepared from Powder	8 oz	90	0	0	0	0	0	40	22	22	0	0	1 1/2 carb
Orange Liquid	2 ml per 8 oz	0	0	0	0	0	0	30	0	0	0	0	free
True Time													
Lemonade Powder Packets (All Varieties)	1 packet	10	0	0	0	0	0	0	3	1	0	0	free
COCOA/HOT CHOCOLATE/CHOCOLATE MILK													
Hot Chocolate (Cocoa)	1 envelope	113	1	10	1	0	0	150	24	19	1	2	1 1/2 carb

	Serving											
Hot Chocolate (Cocoa), Sugar Free	1 envelope	57	0	0	0	0		0	142	11	6	1	2	1 carb
Hershey's												
Chocolate Syrup	1 Tbsp	45	0	0	0	0		5	12	10	1	0	1 carb
Chocolate Syrup, Sugar Free	1 Tbsp	5	0	0	0	0		30	3	0	0	0	free
Nestlé												
Carnation Malted Milk	3 Tbsp	90	2	20	1	0	5	100	15	10	0	2	1 carb
Hot Chocolate, Dark Chocolate	1 envelope	80	1	10	1	0	0	80	18	15	0	<1	1 carb
Hot Chocolate, No Sugar Added, Fat-Free Rich Chocolate	1 envelope	20	0	0	0	0	0	120	5	4	<1	1	free
Hot Chocolate, Rich Chocolate	1 envelope	80	2.5	20	2	0	0	180	16	12	<1	<1	1 carb
Hot Cocoa with Mini Marshmallows	1 envelope	80	2	20	2	0	0	170	16	16	<1	<1	1 carb
Nesquik Chocolate	2 Tbsp	50	0.5	5	0	0	0	35	12	11	<1	<1	1 carb

BEVERAGES, SODAS, SPORTS/ENERGY DRINKS, MEAL REPLACEMENT DRINKS, COCOA, COFFEE/CREAMER, TEA

	Serving	Calories	Fat (g)	Cal. from Fat	Sat. Fat (g)	Trans Fat (g)	Chol. (mg)	Sod. (mg)	Carb. (g)	Sugar (g)	Fiber (g)	Prot. (g)	Servings/Exchanges
Nesquik No Sugar Added Chocolate	2 Tbsp	35	0.5	5	0	0	0	5	12	3	1	1	1 carb
Ovaltine													
Malted Milk Drink, Chocolate Malt	2 Tbsp	40	0	0	0	0	0	70	9	8	<1	0	1/2 carb
Malted Milk Drink, Rich Chocolate	2 Tbsp	40	0	0	0	0	0	70	10	9	0	0	1/2 carb
Swiss Miss													
Hot Chocolate Marshmallow Lovers	1 envelope	90	2	20	1.5	0	0	150	16	8	0.5	1	1 carb
Hot Chocolate, No Sugar Added	1 envelope	25	0	0	0	0	0	160	4	2	1	2	free
Milk Chocolate Hot Cocoa	1 envelope	90	2	20	1.5	0	0	150	16	8	0.5	1	1 carb
Simply Dark Chocolate Hot Cocoa	1 envelope	110	1	5	0	0	0	125	23	12	2	2	1 1/2 carb

COFFEE

Coffee, Brewed	8 oz	2	0	0	0	0	0	5	0	0	0	0	free
Coffee, Instant	8 oz	5	0	0	0	0	0	10	<1	0	0	0	free
Nestlé												
Taster's Choice Vanilla/Hazelnut	1 packet	5	0	0	0	0	0	0	1	0	0	0	free
Maxwell House												
International Café French Vanilla	1 1/3 Tbsp	60	2.5	25	2.5	0	0	55	10	8	0	0	1/2 carb
International Café Sugar Free	1 1/3 Tbsp	30	2.5	20	2	0	0	55	1	0	0	0	free
International Café Suisse Mocha	1 1/3 Tbsp	60	2	15	2	0	0	40	10	8	0	0	1/2 carb
Starbucks												
Coffee Frappuccino Drink	13.7 oz bottle	290	4.5	45	3	0	20	160	53	46	0	9	3 1/2 carb
Doubleshot Coffee Drink	15 oz	210	2.5	20	1.5	0	15	170	36	26	0	12	2 1/2 carb, 1 lean protein

BEVERAGES, SODAS, SPORTS/ENERGY DRINKS, MEAL REPLACEMENT DRINKS, COCOA, COFFEE/CREAMER, TEA

	Serving	Calories	Fat (g)	Cal. from Fat	Sat. Fat (g)	Trans Fat (g)	Chol. (mg)	Sod. (mg)	Carb. (g)	Sugar (g)	Fiber (g)	Prot. (g)	Servings/Exchanges
Doubleshot Coffee & Protein, Coffee	11 oz can	200	2.5	25	1.5	0	10	120	32	20	2	20	2 carb, 2 lean protein
Doubleshot Coffee & Protein, Dark Chocolate	11 oz can	210	2.5	25	1.5	0	10	115	33	20	2	20	2 carb, 2 lean protein
Doubleshot Coffee & Protein, Vanilla Bean	11 oz can	200	2.5	25	1.5	0	10	120	34	21	2	20	2 carb, 2 lean protein
Doubleshot Espresso	6.4 oz can	140	6	50	3.5	0	20	70	18	17	0	4	1 carb, 1 fat
Mocha Frappuccino Coffee Drink	13.7 oz bottle	260	4.5	40	3	0	20	140	47	45	1	9	3 carb
Vanilla Frappuccino Coffee Drink	13.7 oz bottle	290	4.5	40	3	0	20	150	53	46	0	9	3 1/2 carb
White Chocolate Mocha Coffee Drink	13.7 oz bottle	300	5	45	3	0	20	150	55	47	1	9	3 1/2 carb

COFFEE CREAMER

Cremora

Lite & Creamy	1 tsp	10	0	0	0	0	5	1	0	0	0	free
Original	1 tsp	10	0.5	5	0.5	0	10	1	0	0	0	free

International Delight Coffee House

French Vanilla	1 Tbsp	35	1.5	15	1	0	0	5	5	0	0	free
Fat-Free French Vanilla	1 Tbsp	30	0	0	0	0	5	7	5	0	0	1/2 carb
Sugar-Free French Vanilla	1 Tbsp	20	2	15	1	0	0	1	0	0	0	free

Nestle Coffee-Mate

Hazelnut, Liquid	1 Tbsp	35	1.5	15	0	0	5	5	5	0	0	free
Hazelnut, Sugar Free Liquid	1 Tbsp	15	1	10	0	0	10	2	0	0	0	free
Hazelnut, Powder	4 tsp	60	2.5	25	2.5	0	15	9	7	0	0	1/2 carb
Hazelnut, Sugar Free Powder	4 tsp	30	2.5	25	2.5	0	20	1	0	0	0	free
Original, Liquid	1 Tbsp	20	1	10	0	0	5	2	<1	0	0	free

BEVERAGES, SODAS, SPORTS/ENERGY DRINKS, MEAL REPLACEMENT DRINKS, COCOA, COFFEE/CREAMER, TEA

	Serving	Calories	Fat (g)	Cal. from Fat	Sat. Fat (g)	Trans Fat (g)	Chol. (mg)	Sod. (mg)	Carb. (g)	Sugar (g)	Fiber (g)	Prot. (g)	Servings/Exchanges
Original, Fat Free Liquid	1 Tbsp	10	0	0	0	0	0	10	2	0	0	0	free
Original, Powder	1 tsp	10	0.5	5	0.5	0	0	0	1	0	0	0	free
Original, Fat Free Powder	1 tsp	10	0	0	0	0	0	5	2	0	0	0	free
TEA													
Tea, Black, Brewed	8 oz	2	0	0	0	0	0	7	1	0	0	0	free
Tea, Herbal, Brewed	8 oz	2	0	0	0	0	0	2	0	0	0	0	free
Tea, Instant, Unsweetened	8 oz	5	0	0	0	0	0	9	1	0	0	0	free
Arizona Brand													
Arnold Palmer Half & Half	8 oz	80	0	0	0	0	0	10	22	21	0	0	1 1/2 carb
Green Tea with Ginseng & Honey	8 oz	60	0	0	0	0	0	10	17	16	0	0	1 carb
Iced Tea with Lemon Flavor	8 oz	70	0	0	0	0	0	10	22	21	0	0	1 1/2 carb

Food	Serving	Cal	Fat (g)	Sat Fat (g)	Chol (mg)	Sodium (mg)	Carb (g)	Fiber (g)	Sugar (g)	Prot (g)	Carb Choices
Mucho Mango Cowboy Cocktail	8 oz	80	0	0	0	10	20	0	19	0	1 carb
Southern Style Sweet Tea	8 oz	80	0	0	0	21	21	0	21	0	1 1/2 carb
Crystal Light											
Crystal Light Iced Tea Mixes (All Varieties)	8 oz	5	0	0	0	0	0	0	0	0	free
Gold Peak											
Lemonade Tea	12 oz	140	0	0	0	35	36	0	36	0	2 1/2 carb
Lemon Iced Tea	12 oz	120	0	0	0	25	30	0	29	0	2 carb
Sweet Tea	12 oz	120	0	0	0	35	32	0	32	0	2 carb
Honest Tea											
Half Tea & Half Lemonade	16.9 oz bottle	100	0	0	0	35	25	0	25	0	1 1/2 carb
Honest Tea, Lemon	16.9 oz bottle	80	0	0	0	0	21	0	21	0	1 1/2 carb
Honey Green Tea	16.9 oz bottle	70	0	0	0	15	19	0	19	0	1 carb

BEVERAGES, SODAS, SPORTS/ENERGY DRINKS, MEAL REPLACEMENT DRINKS, COCOA, COFFEE/CREAMER, TEA

	Serving	Calories	Fat (g)	Cal. from Fat	Sat. Fat (g)	Trans Fat (g)	Chol. (mg)	Sod. (mg)	Carb. (g)	Sugar (g)	Fiber (g)	Prot. (g)	Servings/Exchanges
Orange Mango Flavored Herbal Tea	16.9 oz bottle	100	0	0	0	0	0	35	25	22	0	0	1 1/2 carb
Peach Tea	16.9 oz bottle	100	0	0	0	0	0	35	25	25	0	0	1 1/2 carb
Pomegranate Blue Flavored Herbal Tea	16.9 oz bottle	100	0	0	0	0	0	35	24	23	0	0	1 1/2 carb
Nestea													
Diet Iced Tea with Lemon	8 oz	0	0	0	0	0	0	45	0	0	0	0	free
Liquid Water Enhancer (All Flavors)	2 ml	0	0	0	0	0	0	0	0	0	0	0	free
Sweetened Iced Tea with Lemon	8 oz	50	0	0	0	0	0	45	12	11	0	0	1 carb
Lipton													
Citrus Green Tea	20 oz bottle	120	0	0	0	0	0	180	33	32	0	0	2 carb

	Serving											Exchange
Diet Peach Tea Mix, Powder	1 Tbsp	5	0	0	0	0	0	0	1	0	0	free
Half & Half	20 oz bottle	120	0	0	0	0	210	31	30	0		2 carb
Instant Unsweetened Tea	1 1/2 Tbsp	0	0	0	0	0	0	0	0	0		free
Lemon Iced Tea	20 oz bottle	120	0	0	0	0	220	31	30	0		2 carb
Lemon Iced Tea Mix, Powder	1 1/3 Tbsp	70	0	0	0	0	0	18	18	0		1 carb
Liquid Iced Tea Go Packets (All Flavors)	1/2 packet	5	0	0	0	0	0	1	0	0		free
Sparkling Citrus Green Tea	12 oz can	70	0	0	0	0	125	18	18	0		1 carb
White Tea with Raspberry	16.9 oz bottle	110	0	0	0	0	170	29	28	0		2 carb
PepsiCo												
Brisk Raspberry Iced Tea	12 oz can	70	0	0	0	0	80	19	19	0		1 carb

BEVERAGES, SODAS, SPORTS/ENERGY DRINKS, MEAL REPLACEMENT DRINKS, COCOA, COFFEE/CREAMER, TEA

	Serving	Calories	Fat (g)	Cal. from Fat	Sat. Fat (g)	Trans Fat (g)	Chol. (mg)	Sod. (mg)	Carb. (g)	Sugar (g)	Fiber (g)	Prot. (g)	Servings/Exchanges
Brisk Sweet Tea	12 oz can	70	0	0	0	0	0	100	19	19	0	0	1 carb
Pure Leaf Iced Tea Lemon	18.5 oz bottle	160	0	0	0	0	0	0	41	41	0	0	2 1/2 carb
Pure Leaf Sweet Tea	18.5 oz bottle	160	0	0	0	0	0	0	42	42	0	0	3 carb
Pure Leaf Extra Sweet Tea	18.5 oz bottle	250	0	0	0	0	0	0	65	65	0	0	4 carb
Pure Leaf Not Too Sweet Peach Tea	18.5 oz bottle	100	0	0	0	0	0	0	26	26	0	0	2 carb
Pure Leaf Tea & Lemonade	18.5 oz bottle	160	0	0	0	0	0	15	42	42	0	0	3 carb
Snapple													
All Natural Half 'n Half	16 oz	210	0	0	0	0	0	10	51	50	0	0	3 1/2 carb
All Natural Lemon Tea	16 oz	150	0	0	0	0	0	10	37	36	0	0	2 1/2 carb
Sweet Straight Up Tea	18.5 oz bottle	180	0	0	0	0	0	10	45	44	0	0	3 carb

BREAD, BAGELS, ROLLS, BISCUITS, TORTILLAS, PANCAKES, WAFFLES, STUFFING, CROUTONS

	Serving	Calories	Fat (g)	Cal. from Fat	Sat. Fat (g)	Trans Fat (g)	Chol. (mg)	Sod. (mg)	Carb. (g)	Sugar (g)	Fiber (g)	Prot. (g)	Servings/Exchanges
Bagel, 100% Whole Wheat	4 oz regular	263	2	20	0	0	0	461	51	6	4	11	3 1/2 carb
Bagel, Plain, Wheat	4 oz regular	270	2	20	0	0	0	501	53	5	2	11	3 1/2 carb
Biscuit	3-inch across	204	7	65	2	0	3	577	29	7	1	5	2 carb, 1 fat
Bread, Butter Croissant	1 medium	231	12	110	7	0	38	424	26	6	1	5	2 carb, 2 fat
Bread, Corn	2, 3/4-inch across	174	5	45	1	0	15	297	29	10	2	3	2 carb, 1 fat
Bread, Cracked Wheat	1 slice	70	1	10	0	0	0	135	13	2	1	3	1 carb
Bread, French, Vienna, or Sourdough	1 small slice	92	1	10	0	0	0	208	18	1	1	4	1 carb

BREAD, BAGELS, ROLLS, BISCUITS, TORTILLAS, PANCAKES, WAFFLES, STUFFING, CROUTONS

	Serving	Calories	Fat (g)	Cal. from Fat	Sat. Fat (g)	Trans Fat (g)	Chol. (mg)	Sod. (mg)	Carb. (g)	Sugar (g)	Fiber (g)	Prot. (g)	Servings/Exchanges
Bread, Italian	1 large slice	81	1	10	0	0	0	175	15	0	1	3	1 carb
Bread, Multigrain	1 slice	69	1	10	0	0	0	109	11	2	2	3	1 carb
Bread, Oat Bran	1 slice	68	1	10	0	0	0	118	11	2	1	3	1 carb
Bread, Oatmeal	1 slice	102	2	20	0	0	0	228	18	3	2	3	1 carb
Bread, Pita	6.5-inch large	234	1	10	0	0	0	456	47	1	2	8	3 carb
Bread, Pita, Whole-Wheat	6.5-inch large	226	2	20	0	0	0	452	47	1	6	8	3 carb
Bread, Pumpernickel	1 slice	65	1	10	0	0	0	174	12	0	2	2	1 carb
Bread, Raisin	1 slice	71	1	10	0	0	0	101	14	1	1	2	1 carb
Bread, Rye	1 slice	67	1	10	0	0	0	172	13	1	2	2	1 carb
Bread, Wheat Bran	1 slice	89	1	10	0	0	0	175	17	3	1	3	1 carb
Bread, White	1 slice	69	1	10	0	0	0	177	13	1	1	2	1 carb
Bread, Whole-Wheat	1 slice	69	1	10	0	0	0	132	12	1	2	4	1 carb

Food	Serving											Choices/Exchanges
Bread Sticks, Plain	1 large	139	4	35	0	0	143	20	1	1	4	1 carb, 1 fat
Bread Sticks with Garlic & Parmesan Cheese	1 large	225	12	120	2	0	395	23	1	1	7	1 1/2 carb, 2 fat
Bun, Hamburger	1	120	2	20	0	0	206	21	2	1	4	1 1/2 carb
Bun, Hot Dog	1	120	2	20	0	0	206	21	2	1	4	1 1/2 carb
Croutons	1 cup	186	7	65	2	0	495	25	2	2	4	1 1/2 carb, 1 fat
Egg Bread/Challah	1 slice	65	1	10	0	0	113	11	0	1	2	1 carb
English Muffin	1	132	1	10	0	0	247	26	2	2	5	2 carb
French Toast, Plain	1 regular slice	156	6	55	2	89	320	20	5	1	6	1 carb, 1 fat
French Toast Sticks, Plain	1 stick	71	4	40	1	0	90	9	2	0	1	1/2 carb, 1 fat
Naan	1/4 large	137	3	30	1	0	224	22	2	2	5	1 1/2 carb, 1 fat
Pancakes, Plain	1, 5-inch diameter	93	3	30	0	7	184	15	3	0	2	1 carb, 1 fat
Roll, White, Soft	1	100	2	20	0	0	172	18	2	1	3	1 carb

BREAD, BAGELS, ROLLS, BISCUITS, TORTILLAS, PANCAKES, WAFFLES, STUFFING, CROUTONS

	Serving	Calories	Fat (g)	Cal. from Fat	Sat. Fat (g)	Trans Fat (g)	Chol. (mg)	Sod. (mg)	Carb. (g)	Sugar (g)	Fiber (g)	Prot. (g)	Servings/Exchanges
Roll, Whole-Wheat	1	96	2	20	0	0	0	172	18	3	3	3	1 carb
Taco Shells, Corn	2, 5-inch shells	119	5	45	2	0	0	99	16	0	1	2	1 carb, 1 fat
Tortilla, Corn	1, 6-inch	52	1	10	0	0	0	11	11	0	2	1	1 carb
Tortilla, Flour	1, 6-inch	94	2	20	1	0	0	191	15	1	1	2	1 carb
Tortilla, Whole-Wheat	1, 6-inch	84	3	30	1	0	0	138	12	1	3	3	1 carb, 1 fat
Waffles, Toaster Style	1, 4-inch	121	4	40	1	0	5	281	19	2	1	3	1 carb, 1 fat
BRANDS													
Aunt Hattie's													
Big BBQ Hamburger Buns	1	190	2.5	25	0.5	0	0	360	39	6	1	6	2 1/2 carb

Big Onion Hamburger Buns	1	190	2.5	25	0.5	0	390	36	5	1	6	2 1/2 carb
Big Potato Hamburger Buns	1	180	2.5	25	0	0	350	35	6	1	6	2 carb
Potato Hamburger Buns	1	140	2	20	0	0	260	26	5	<1	4	1 1/2 carb
Potato Hot Dog Buns	1	140	2	20	0	0	260	26	5	<1	4	1 1/2 carb
Texas Toast	1 slice	90	1	10	0	0	180	17	2	<1	3	1 carb
Bimbo												
100% Whole Wheat	2 slices	110	1.5	15	0	0	230	20	3	3	5	1 carb
Aunt Jemima												
Pancake/Waffle Mix, Buttermilk	1/3 cup	110	0.5	5	0	0	420	24	4	1	3	1 1/2 carb
Pancake/Waffle Mix, Original	1/3 cup	150	0.5	5	0	0	740	33	7	1	4	2 carb
Pancake/Waffle Mix, Whole Wheat	1/4 cup	120	0.5	5	0	0	620	26	4	3	4	2 carb
Ballpark												
Hamburger Buns	1	160	2	20	0.5	0	270	28	5	1	5	2 carb

BREAD, BAGELS, ROLLS, BISCUITS, TORTILLAS, PANCAKES, WAFFLES, STUFFING, CROUTONS

	Serving	Calories	Fat (g)	Cal. from Fat	Sat. Fat (g)	Trans Fat (g)	Chol. (mg)	Sod. (mg)	Carb. (g)	Sugar (g)	Fiber (g)	Prot. (g)	Servings/Exchanges
Hot Dog Buns	1	140	2	15	0	0	0	240	25	4	<1	4	1 1/2 carb
Betty Crocker													
Bisquick, Original	1/3 cup	150	3	25	0.5	0	0	380	28	2	<1	3	2 carb, 1 fat
Heart Smart	1/3 cup	140	2.5	25	0	0	0	340	27	3	<1	3	2 carb
Food for Life													
Ezekial 4:9 100% Whole Wheat Sprouted	1 slice	80	0.5	5	0	0	0	80	14	0	3	4	1 carb
Ezekiel 4:9 Low Sodium	1 slice	80	0.5	5	0	0	0	0	15	0	3	4	1 carb
Home Pride													
Butter Top White	1 slice	70	1	10	0	0	0	140	14	2	0	2	1 carb
Jiffy													
Buttermilk Biscuit Mix	1/3 cup	160	5	45	2	0	<5	420	27	2	<1	3	2 carb, 1 fat
Corn Muffin Mix	1/4 cup	160	4.5	40	2	0	<5	340	27	7	<1	2	1 carb, 1 fat
Kellogg's Eggo													
French Toast Sticks	2 sticks	230	6	60	1.5	0	20	490	38	15	<1	4	2 1/2 carb, 1 fat

Pancakes, Blueberry	3	260	8	70	1.5	0	15	500	42	11	1	6	3 carb, 2 fat
Pancakes, Buttermilk	3	280	9	80	1.5	0	15	590	45	12	1	6	3 carb, 2 fat
Waffles, Blueberry	2	180	6	50	1.5	0	10	370	29	6	<1	4	2 carb, 1 fat
Waffles, Buttermilk	2	190	8	70	2	0	15	370	27	2	<1	5	2 carb, 2 fat
Waffles, Chocolate Chip	2	200	7	60	2.5	0	15	370	31	9	1	4	2 carb, 1 fat
Waffles, Cinnamon Toast	3	300	11	100	3	0	10	480	46	17	<1	5	3 carb, 2 fat
Waffles, Gluten Free	2	170	5	50	1.5	0	25	260	27	4	2	3	2 carb, 1 fat
Waffles, Homestyle	2	190	7	70	2	0	15	360	27	2	<1	4	2 carb, 1 fat
Waffles, Minis	3	260	10	90	2.5	0	25	600	38	3	1	6	2 1/2 carb, 2 fat
Waffles, Nutri-Grain Low Fat	2	140	2.5	25	0.5	0	<5	380	27	3	3	4	2 carb
Waffles, Thick & Fluffy Blueberry Cobbler	1	160	7	60	1.5	0	15	260	23	7	<1	3	1 1/2 carb, 1 fat
Krusteaz													
Buttermilk Pancakes	2 (4-inch) pancakes	180	1.5	15	0.5	0	0	530	37	6	1	4	2 1/2 carb

BREAD, BAGELS, ROLLS, BISCUITS, TORTILLAS, PANCAKES, WAFFLES, STUFFING, CROUTONS

	Serving	Calories	Fat (g)	Cal. from Fat	Sat. Fat (g)	Trans Fat (g)	Chol. (mg)	Sod. (mg)	Carb. (g)	Sugar (g)	Fiber (g)	Prot. (g)	Servings/Exchanges
Gluten Free Pancakes	3 (4-inch) pancakes	180	3	25	1	0	5	560	36	1	1	3	2 1/2 carb, 1 fat
Marshall's													
Biscuits, Buttermilk	3	240	12	110	3	3.5	0	600	29	1	1	4	2 carb, 2 fat
Biscuits, Homestyle	1	120	6	50	2	1.5	0	330	15	1	0	2	1 carb, 1 fat
Mission													
95% Fat Free Flour Tortilla, Large Burrito Size	1	180	2.5	20	1	0	0	430	36	2	3	5	2 1/2 carb
95% Fat Free Flour Tortilla, Medium Soft Taco Size	1	130	1.5	15	0.5	0	0	320	26	2	2	4	1 1/2 carb
95% Fat Free Whole Wheat Flour Tortilla, Medium Soft Taco Size	1	130	2	15	0.5	0	0	300	24	3	4	5	1 1/2 carb

Carb Balance Flour Tortilla, Fajita Size	1	80	2	20	1	0	0	190	13	0	9	3	1 carb
Carb Balance Flour Tortilla, Medium Soft Taco Size	1	120	3	25	1.5	0	0	280	19	0	13	5	1 carb, 1 fat
Carb Balance Whole Wheat Flour Tortilla, Small Fajita Size	1	80	2	20	1	0	0	200	13	0	10	3	1 carb
Life Balance Whole Wheat Tortilla, Medium Soft Taco Size	1	130	3.5	30	1.5	0	0	270	19	1	3	4	1 carb, 1 fat
Multi-Grain Flour Tortilla, Medium Soft Taco Size	1	150	4	35	1.5	0	0	310	23	2	5	4	1 1/2 carb, 1 fat
Tortilla, Large Burrito Size	1	200	4.5	40	2	0	0	600	34	1	1	5	2 carb, 1 fat
Tortilla, Medium Soft Taco Size	1	140	3.5	30	1.5	0	0	420	24	1	1	4	1 1/2 carb, 1 fat
Tortilla, Small Fajita	1	110	2.5	20	1	0	0	310	18	0	1	3	1 carb
Tortilla Wraps, Jalapeno Cheddar	1	210	5	45	2	0	0	560	37	3	2	6	2 1/2 carb, 1 fat

BREAD, BAGELS, ROLLS, BISCUITS, TORTILLAS, PANCAKES, WAFFLES, STUFFING, CROUTONS

	Serving	Calories	Fat (g)	Cal. from Fat	Sat. Fat (g)	Trans Fat (g)	Chol. (mg)	Sod. (mg)	Carb. (g)	Sugar (g)	Fiber (g)	Prot. (g)	Servings/Exchanges
Tortilla Wraps, Multi-Grain	1	210	6	50	2.5	0	0	440	33	3	7	6	2 carb, 1 fat
Tortilla Wraps, Sun Dried Tomato Basil	1	210	4.5	40	2	0	0	480	36	3	2	5	2 1/2 carb, 1 fat
White Corn Tortilla	2	100	1.5	15	0	0	0	10	20	2	3	2	1 carb
Yellow Corn Tortilla	2	100	1.5	15	0	0	0	10	20	2	3	2	1 carb
Mrs. Cubbison's													
Caesar Salad Croutons	2 Tbsp	30	1	10	0	0	0	65	5	0	0	1	1/2 carb
Fat Free Herb Seasoned Croutons	2 Tbsp	30	0	0	0	0	0	100	5	0	0	1	1/2 carb
Nature's Own													
100% Whole Grain	1 slice	70	1.5	10	0	0	0	115	12	2	2	4	1 carb
100% Whole Wheat	1 slice	60	0.5	5	0	0	0	110	11	<1	2	4	1 carb
Butterbread	1 slice	60	0.5	5	0	0	0	95	12	1	<1	3	1 carb
Honey Oat	1 slice	70	1	10	0	0	0	110	13	2	<1	3	1 carb

Food	Serving	Cal	Fat (g)	Cal from Fat	Sat Fat (g)	Chol (mg)	Sod (mg)	Carb (g)	Fiber (g)	Sugar (g)	Pro (g)	Choices/Exch
Honey Wheat	1 slice	70	1	5	0	0	125	13	2	<1	3	1 carb
Nature's Harvest												
100% Whole Wheat	2 slices	120	1.5	15	0	0	180	27	4	3	6	2 carb
Butter Wheat	2 slices	130	1	10	0	0	240	24	3	2	5	1 1/2 carb
Honey 7 Grain	2 slices	160	2.5	25	0	0	260	28	5	2	6	2 carb
Honey Wheat	2 slices	130	1.5	15	0	0	230	25	3	2	5	1 1/2 carb
Old El Paso												
Stand n' Stuff Taco Shells, Corn	2	130	6	50	2.5	0	115	16	0	1	2	1 carb, 1 fat
Taco & Tostada Shells, Corn	3	150	7	60	3	0	135	19	0	1	2	1 carb, 1 fat
Oroweat												
12 Grain	1 slice	100	2	15	0	0	140	17	2	3	4	1 carb
100% Whole Wheat	1 slice	90	1	10	0	0	135	16	3	2	4	1 carb
Country 100% Whole Wheat	1 slice	90	1	10	0	0	135	16	2	2	4	1 carb
Country Buttermilk	1 slice	100	1	10	0	0	135	20	3	<1	3	1 carb

BREAD, BAGELS, ROLLS, BISCUITS, TORTILLAS, PANCAKES, WAFFLES, STUFFING, CROUTONS

	Serving	Calories	Fat (g)	Cal. from Fat	Sat. Fat (g)	Trans Fat (g)	Chol. (mg)	Sod. (mg)	Carb. (g)	Sugar (g)	Fiber (g)	Prot. (g)	Servings/Exchanges
Country Potato	1 slice	100	1	10	0	0	0	135	19	2	<1	3	1 carb
Country White	1 slice	100	1.5	15	0	0	0	140	19	2	<1	3	1 carb
Dark Rye	1 slice	80	1	10	0	0	0	210	15	<1	1	3	1 carb
Healthful Flax & Sun-flower	1 slice	80	2	15	0	0	0	135	14	2	3	3	1 carb
Italian	1 slice	80	0.5	5	0	0	0	240	16	<1	<1	2	1 carb
Jewish Rye	1 slice	90	1.5	15	0	0	0	180	16	1	1	3	1 carb
Oatnut	1 slice	110	2	20	0	0	0	130	19	3	2	4	1 carb
Russian Rye	1 slice	80	1	10	0	0	0	210	15	<1	<1	3	1 carb
Sandwich Thins Original	1	100	2	20	0	0	0	190	21	1	5	4	1 1/2 carb
Ortega													
Taco & Tosatda Shells, Corn	2	120	6	50	1	0	0	150–170	16	0	2	2	1 carb, 1 fat

Pepperidge Farm

100% Whole Grain Breads

All Varieties (Honey Wheat, 15 Grain, Whole Wheat, Oatmeal, Ancient Grains, German Dark Wheat)	1 slice	100–110	1.5–2	15–20	0.5	0	0	110–130	17–21	2–4	3	3–5	1–1 1/2 carb

Farm House Hearty Sliced Bread

All Varieties (Hearty White, Whole Wheat White, 100% Whole Wheat, Honey Wheat, Potato, 12 Grain, Oatmeal, Sourdough)	1 slice	100–120	1–2	10–20	0–0.5	0	0	150–240	20–22	2–5	<1–3	3–4	1–1 1/2 carb

Hearth-Baked Style Breads

Twin French	1 (4-inch) slice	150	1.5	15	0	0	0	260	29	2	1	5	1 carb

BREAD, BAGELS, ROLLS, BISCUITS, TORTILLAS, PANCAKES, WAFFLES, STUFFING, CROUTONS

	Serving	Calories	Fat (g)	Cal. from Fat	Sat. Fat (g)	Trans Fat (g)	Chol. (mg)	Sod. (mg)	Carb. (g)	Sugar (g)	Fiber (g)	Prot. (g)	Servings/Exchanges
Light Style Breads													
All Varieties (7 Grain, Oatmeal, Soft Wheat, 100% Whole Wheat)	3 slices	130–140	1	5–10	0–0.5	0	0	210–260	25–27	2–3	2–5	7–8	1 1/2–2 carb
Party Breads													
Dark Pumpernickel	5 slices	130	1.5	15	0	0	0	320	23	1	3	5	1 1/2 carb
Jewish Rye	5 slices	130	2	15	0	0	0	460	25	1	2	4	1 1/2 carb
Rye & Pumpernickel													
All Varieties (Rye & Pump, Pumpernickel, Seeded Rye, Seedless Rye, Whole Grain Seeded Rye, Soft Rye)	1 slice	80	1–1.5	0–10	0–0.5	0	0	170–230	14–16	<1–1	0–2	3	1 carb
Variety Breads													
All Varieties (100% Stoneground Whole Wheat, Oatmeal)	2 slices	130	2	20	0.5	0	0	130–170	23–24	3	2–4	5	1 1/2 carb

Very Thin Breads

100% Whole Wheat	3 slices	110	2	15	0.5	0	0	160	20	3	3	4	1 carb
White	3 slices	120	1	10	0	0	0	230	24	2	1	4	1 1/2 carb

White Breads

Family Size	2 slices	150	3	25	0.5	0	0	270	26	3	<1	4	2 carb, 1 fat
Sandwich	2 slices	130	2.5	20	0.5	0	0	230	23	3	<1	4	1 1/2 carb
Thin Sliced, Enriched	1 slice	70	1	10	0	0	0	75	13	2	1	2	1 carb

Bagels and Rolls

Bagel, Cinnamon Raisin	1	270	1	10	0	0	0	290	57	14	3	9	4 carb
Bagel, Everything	1	260	1.5	15	0.5	0	0	340	53	9	2	9	3 1/2 carb
Bagel, Mini Plain	1	110	0.5	5	0	0	0	130	22	4	1	4	1 1/2 carb
Bagel, Plain	1	260	1	10	0	0	0	330	54	10	3	9	3 1/2 carb
Buns, Classic 100% Whole Wheat Hamburger	1	130	1.5	15	0	0	0	210	22	3	3	7	1 1/2 carb
Buns, Sandwich with Sesame Seeds	1	150	2	20	0.5	0	0	220	26	4	2	6	1 1/2 carb

BREAD, BAGELS, ROLLS, BISCUITS, TORTILLAS, PANCAKES, WAFFLES, STUFFING, CROUTONS

	Serving	Calories	Fat (g)	Cal. from Fat	Sat. Fat (g)	Trans Fat (g)	Chol. (mg)	Sod. (mg)	Carb. (g)	Sugar (g)	Fiber (g)	Prot. (g)	Servings/Exchanges
English Muffin, 100% Whole Wheat	1	140	1.5	10	0.5	0	0	180	25	4	3	6	1 1/2 carb
English Muffin, Original	1	130	1.5	15	0.5	0	0	170	25	1	1	5	1 1/2 carb
Mini Bagel, Brown Sugar Cinnamon	1	120	0.5	5	0.5	0	0	140	24	6	1	3	1 1/2 carb
Rolls, French	1	120	0	0	0	0	0	300	25	<1	1	4	1 1/2 carb
Rolls, Soft Hoagie with Sesame Seeds	1	210	6	55	1.5	0	0	250	35	3	2	7	2 carb, 1 fat
Rolls, Sourdough	1	90	1.5	15	0	0	0	120	17	3	1	3	1 carb
Croutons													
Seasoned, Caesar Salad & Zesty Italian	6	30	1	10	0	0	0	55–75	5	<1	0	<1	free
Pillsbury													
Bread, Rustic French Loaf	1/8 batch	110	1.5	15	0	0	0	210	21	2	1	4	1 1/2 carb

Crescent Rolls, 90 Calorie	1	90	3	30	1	0	0	220	13	3	0	2	1 carb
Crescent Rolls, Original	1	100	5	50	2	0	0	210	12	3	0	2	1 carb, 1 fat
Crescent Rounds	1	100	5	50	2	0	0	220	12	3	0	1	1 carb, 1 fat
Pizza Crust, Classic	1/6 crust	160	2	20	0.5	0	0	380	31	4	1	5	2 carb
Pizza Crust, Thin	1/5 package	160	2	20	0.5	0	0	280	30	3	1	5	2 carb
Pillsbury Grands!													
Biscuits, Buttermilk	1	170	6	60	2.5	0	0	470	26	4	1	3	2 carb, 1 fat
Biscuits, Buttermilk Reduced Fat	1	150	4	40	1.5	0	0	470	26	4	1	3	1 1/2 carb, 1 fat
Biscuits, Flaky Layers	1	170	6	60	2.5	0	0	460	25	4	1	3	1 1/2 carb, 1 fat
Biscuits, Flaky Layers Reduced Fat	1	160	4.5	45	1.5	0	0	480	26	5	1	4	2 carb, 1 fat
Progresso													
Bread Crumbs, Italian-Style	1/4 cup	100	1	10	0	0	0	420	19	2	1	4	1 carb

BREAD, BAGELS, ROLLS, BISCUITS, TORTILLAS, PANCAKES, WAFFLES, STUFFING, CROUTONS

	Serving	Calories	Fat (g)	Cal. from Fat	Sat. Fat (g)	Trans Fat (g)	Chol. (mg)	Sod. (mg)	Carb. (g)	Sugar (g)	Fiber (g)	Prot. (g)	Servings/Exchanges
Bread Crumbs, Parmesan	1/4 cup	100	1.5	10	0	0	0	820	18	2	1	4	1 carb
Bread Crumbs, Plain	1/4 cup	110	1	10	0	0	0	160	20	2	1	4	1 carb
PSST													
Hamburger Buns	1	120	1	10	0	0	0	200	22	3	<1	4	1 1/2 carb
Hotdog Buns	1	110	1	10	0	0	0	170	21	3	<1	3	1 1/2 carb
Wheat Bread	2 slices	120	1.5	10	0	0	0	210	22	3	1	4	1 1/2 carb
White Bread	2 slices	120	1.5	15	0	0	0	220	23	3	<1	3	1 1/2 carb
Sara Lee													
100% Whole Wheat	1 slice	60	1	10	0	0	0	120	12	1	2	3	1 carb
Artesano Style	1 slice	100	1	10	0	0	0	190	20	2	<1	3	1 carb
Bagel, Plain	1	260	1	10	0	0	0	390	52	4	2	8	3 1/2 carb
Butterbread	1 slice	70	0.5	5	0	0	0	105	13	2	<1	2	1 carb
Delightful Multigrain	2 slices	90	1	10	0	0	0	170	18	1	5	6	1 carb

	Serving											
Honey Wheat	1 slice	70	0.5	5	0	0	110	13	2	<1	2	1 carb
Iron Kids	2 slices	140	1.5	15	0	0	220	28	4	4	5	2 carb
Sweet Hawaiian	1 slice	100	1.5	15	1	0	170	18	3	<1	4	1 carb
Whole Grain White	2 slices	130	1.5	15	0	0	250	26	3	3	5	1 1/2 carb
Sara Lee Hearty & Delicious												
100% Whole Wheat	1 slice	90	1	10	0	0	115	17	3	2	5	1 carb
100% Whole Wheat with Honey	1 slice	100	1	10	0	0	120	20	4	3	5	1 carb
Healthy Multi-Grain	1 slice	90	1	10	0	0	110	18	3	4	4	1 carb
Shake 'N Bake												
Coating Mix, Italian Herb	1/8 pkt	30	0	0	0	0	230	2	0	0	1	free
Coating Mix, Original Chicken	1/8 pkt	30	0.5	5	0	0	170	2	0	0	1	free
Coating Mix, Parmesan Crusted	1/8 pkt	30	0	0	0	0	230	2	0	0	1	free
Stove Top												
Stuffing Mix, Chicken Flavor	1/2 cup	110	2.5	20	0	0	450	19	2	1	3	1 carb

BREAD, BAGELS, ROLLS, BISCUITS, TORTILLAS, PANCAKES, WAFFLES, STUFFING, CROUTONS

	Serving	Calories	Fat (g)	Cal. from Fat	Sat. Fat (g)	Trans Fat (g)	Chol. (mg)	Sod. (mg)	Carb. (g)	Sugar (g)	Fiber (g)	Prot. (g)	Servings/Exchanges
Stuffing Mix, Corn Bread	1/2 cup	100	1	10	0	0	0	400	21	2	1	3	1 carb
Stuffing Mix, Lower Sodium Chicken Flavor	1/2 cup	110	1	10	0	0	0	250	21	2	1	4	1 1/2 carb
Thomas'													
Bagel, Plain	1	260	1	10	0	0	0	460	53	6	2	9	3 1/2 carb
Cinnamon Raisin English Muffin	1	140	1	10	0	0	0	170	29	8	1	4	2 carb
Double Protein Oatmeal Cinnamon English Muffin	1	150	1	10	0	0	0	210	26	2	1	7	1 1/2 carb
Light 100 Multigrain English Muffin	1	100	1	10	0	0	0	160	26	1	8	5	1 1/2 carb
Original English Muffin	1	120	1	10	0	0	0	200	25	1	1	4	1 1/2 carb
Original Sandwich Size English Muffin	1	190	1.5	10	15	0	0	310	37	2	1	6	2 1/2 carb

Whole Grain English Muffin	1	130	1	10	0	0	220	27	1	2	5	2 carb
Trader Joe's												
California Style Sprouted Wheat	1 slice	80	0	0	0	0	150	15	1	2	5	1 carb
Fat Free Organic Whole Wheat	1 slice	100	0	0	0	0	200	21	2	3	4	1 1/2 carb
Gourmet White	1 slice	120	3.5	35	0	0	260	19	2	1	3	1 carb, 1 fat
Harvest White Bread	1 slice	100	0	0	0	0	190	23	3	1	2	1 1/2 carb
Harvest Whole Wheat	1 slice	100	0.5	5	0	0	180	20	3	3	3	1 1/2 carb
Multi-Grain, Organic	1 slice	80	1	10	0	0	115	17	<1	2	4	1 carb
Organic Flourless Sprouted 7 Grain	1 slice	80	1	5	0	0	90	15	1	3	4	1 carb
Soft 10 Grain	1 slice	90	1.5	15	0	0	140	16	2	2	3	1 carb
Sprouted Flourless Whole Wheat Berry	1 slice	80	0	0	0	0	160	15	2	2	5	1 carb
Sprouted Multigrain	1 slice	90	0.5	5	0	0	170	15	2	2	5	1 carb
Whole Grain	1 slice	90	0.5	5	0	0	200	19	2	3	3	1 carb

BREAD, BAGELS, ROLLS, BISCUITS, TORTILLAS, PANCAKES, WAFFLES, STUFFING, CROUTONS

	Serving	Calories	Fat (g)	Cal. from Fat	Sat. Fat (g)	Trans Fat (g)	Chol. (mg)	Sod. (mg)	Carb. (g)	Sugar (g)	Fiber (g)	Prot. (g)	Servings/Exchanges
Whole Wheat Fiber Bread	1 slice	90	1	10	0	0	0	160	20	3	5	4	1 carb
Wonder													
100% Whole Wheat	1 slice	60	0.5	5	0	0	0	105	11	0	2	4	1 carb
Classic White	2 slices	140	1.5	15	0	0	0	180	29	5	2	4	2 carb
Made with Whole Grain White	2 slices	120	2	15	0	0	0	150	24	3	3	6	1 1/2 carb
White	2 slices	120	1.5	5	0	0	0	250	24	3	<1	4	1 1/2 carb

BREAKFAST CEREAL, READY-TO-EAT CEREAL, HOT CEREAL

	Serving	Calories	Fat (g)	Cal. from Fat	Sat. Fat (g)	Trans Fat (g)	Chol. (mg)	Sod. (mg)	Carb. (g)	Sugar (g)	Fiber (g)	Prot. (g)	Servings/Exchanges
Bran, Oat, Cooked	1/2 cup	40	1	10	0	0	0	1	11	0	3	3	1 carb
Bulgur, Cooked	1/2 cup	56	0	0	0	0	0	3	12	0	3	2	1 carb
Corn Grits, White or Yellow, Cooked	1/2 cup	54	0	0	0	0	0	2	12	0	1	1	1 carb
Cream of Rice, Cooked	1/2 cup	63	0	0	0	0	0	1	14	0	0	1	1 carb
Cream of Wheat, Cooked	1/2 cup	55	0	0	0	0	0	8	11	0	1	2	1 carb
Granola, Homemade	1/2 cup	298	15	135	2	0	0	15	32	6	5	9	2 carb, 3 fat
Kasha or Buckwheat Groats, Cooked	1/2 cup	77	1	10	0	0	0	3	17	1	2	3	1 carb
Millet, Cooked	1/4 cup	51	0	0	0	0	0	1	10	0	1	2	1/2 carb
Muesli	1/4 cup	72	1	10	0	0	0	49	17	7	2	2	1 carb
Oatmeal Cereal, Cooked	1/2 cup	71	1	10	0	0	0	5	13	0	2	2	1 carb
Puffed Rice	1 1/2 cups	80	0	0	0	0	0	1	18	0	0	1	1 carb

BREAKFAST CEREAL, READY-TO-EAT CEREAL, HOT CEREAL

	Serving	Calories	Fat (g)	Cal. from Fat	Sat. Fat (g)	Trans Fat (g)	Chol. (mg)	Sod. (mg)	Carb. (g)	Sugar (g)	Fiber (g)	Prot. (g)	Servings/Exchanges
Puffed Wheat	1 1/2 cups	66	0	0	0	0	0	1	14	0	2	3	1 carb
Shredded Wheat, Plain	1/2 cup	86	1	10	0	0	0	1	20	0	3	3	1 carb
Wheatena, Cooked	1/2 cup	57	0	0	0	0	0	0	13	0	2	2	1 carb
BRANDS													
Cascadian Farm Organic													
Ancient Grains Granola	3/4 cup	240	6	60	1	0	0	70	41	9	4	6	2 1/2 carb, 1 fat
Chocolate O's	3/4 cup	100	0.5	5	0	0	0	95	24	8	3	2	1 1/2 carb
Cinnamon Raisin Granola	2/3 cup	240	6	50	1	0	0	65	43	13	4	6	3 carb, 1 fat
Dark Chocolate Almond Granola	2/3 cup	260	8	70	1.5	0	0	70	44	12	5	7	3 carb, 2 fat
Fruitful O's	3/4 cup	100	1	10	0	0	0	130	23	8	3	2	1 1/2 carb
Gluten Free Berry Vanilla Puffs	3/4 cup	100	1	10	0	0	0	105	22	7	1	2	1 1/2 carb
Graham Crunch	3/4 cup	110	2	20	0	0	0	140	23	8	3	2	1 1/2 carb

Honey Oat Crunch	1 cup	190	1.5	15	0	0	300	41	9	2	4	2 1/2 carb
Eating Right												
Cranberry Almond	1 cup	220	3	30	0	0	280	44	13	3	4	3 carb, 1 fat
Raisin/Date/Pecan Multigrain	3/4 cup	210	2.5	0	0	0	280	42	11	5	4	3 carb
General Mills												
Basic 4	1 cup	200	2	20	1	0	280	44	13	5	4	3 carb
Cheerios	1 cup	100	2	15	0.5	0	140	20	1	3	3	1 carb
Cheerios, Ancient Grains	3/4 cup	110	2	15	0.5	0	105	22	5	2	3	1 1/2 carb
Cheerios, Frosted	3/4 cup	100	1.5	15	0	0	150	22	9	2	2	1 1/2 carb
Cheerios, Honey Nut	3/4 cup	110	1.5	15	0	0	160	22	9	2	2	1 1/2 carb
Cheerios, Multi-Grain	1 cup	110	1.5	10	0	0	115	24	6	3	2	1 1/2 carb
Cheerios, Protein Oats & Honey	1 1/4 cups	210	2.5	25	0.5	0	280	41	17	4	7	2 1/2 carb
Chex, Chocolate	3/4 cup	130	2.5	25	0.5	0	200	26	8	1	2	2 carb
Chex, Cinnamon	3/4 cup	120	2	20	0	0	180	25	8	1	1	1 1/2 carb
Chex, Clusters, Fruit & Oats	1 cup	200	1.5	10	0	0	250	45	17	2	3	3 carb

BREAKFAST CEREAL, READY-TO-EAT CEREAL, HOT CEREAL

	Serving	Calories	Fat (g)	Cal. from Fat	Sat. Fat (g)	Trans Fat (g)	Chol. (mg)	Sod. (mg)	Carb. (g)	Sugar (g)	Fiber (g)	Prot. (g)	Servings/Exchanges
Chex, Corn	1 cup	120	0.5	5	0	0	0	220	26	3	2	2	2 carb
Chex, Honey Nut	3/4 cup	120	0.5	5	0	0	0	200	28	9	1	2	2 carb
Chex, Rice	1 cup	100	0.5	5	0	0	0	220	23	2	1	2	1 1/2 carb
Chex, Vanilla	3/4 cup	120	2	15	0	0	0	190	25	8	<1	1	1 1/2 carb
Chex, Wheat	3/4 cup	160	1	10	0	0	0	270	39	5	6	5	2 1/2 carb
Cinnamon Toast Crunch	3/4 cup	130	3	30	0.5	0	0	180	25	9	2	1	1 1/2 carb, 1 fat
Cocoa Puffs	3/4 cup	100	1.5	10	0	0	0	150	23	10	2	1	1 1/2 carb
Cookie Crisp	3/4 cup	100	1	10	0	0	0	120	22	12	1	1	1 1/2 carb
Count Chocula	3/4 cup	100	1.5	15	0	0	0	130	23	9	1	1	1 1/2 carb
Dora The Explorer	3/4 cup	100	1.5	15	0	0	0	150	23	6	3	1	1 1/2 carb
Fiber One	1/2 cup	60	1	10	0	0	0	110	25	0	14	2	1 1/2 carb
Fiber One, Honey Clusters	1 cup	170	1.5	15	0	0	0	210	44	9	10	4	3 carb

Fiber One, Maple Brown Sugar	2/3 cup	220	6	50	0.5	0	0	150	40	15	5	6	2 1/2 carb, 1 fat
Fiber One, Protein Cranberry Almond	3/4 cup	210	5	45	1	0	0	150	40	15	6	6	2 1/2 carb, 1 fat
Fiber One, Raisin Bran Clusters	1 cup	170	1	10	0	0	0	200	46	14	10	3	3 carb
Frankenberry	1 cup	130	1.5	15	0	0	0	150	28	9	1	2	2 carb
Golden Grahams	3/4 cup	120	1	10	0	0	0	240	26	9	2	2	2 carb
Kix	1 1/4 cups	110	1	10	0	0	0	180	25	3	3	2	1 1/2 carb
Kix, Berry Berry	1 1/4 cups	120	1.5	15	0	0	0	160	28	7	2	2	2 carb
Kix, Honey	1 1/4 cups	120	1	10	0	0	0	190	28	6	3	2	2 carb
Lucky Charms	3/4 cup	110	1	10	0	0	0	170	22	10	2	2	1 1/2 carb
Lucky Charms, Chocolate	3/4 cup	110	1.5	15	0	0	0	150	24	10	2	1	1 1/2 carb
Oatmeal Crisp, Almond	1 cup	240	4	35	0.5	0	0	125	47	14	6	6	3 carb, 1 fat

BREAKFAST CEREAL, READY-TO-EAT CEREAL, HOT CEREAL

	Serving	Calories	Fat (g)	Cal. from Fat	Sat. Fat (g)	Trans Fat (g)	Chol. (mg)	Sod. (mg)	Carb. (g)	Sugar (g)	Fiber (g)	Prot. (g)	Servings/Exchanges
Oatmeal Crisp, HeartyRaisin	1 cup	230	2.5	20	0.5	0	0	120	50	17	5	5	3 carb
Raisin Nut Bran	3/4 cup	180	3	30	1	0	0	210	40	14	6	4	2 1/2 carb, 1 fat
Reese's Puffs	3/4 cup	120	3	30	0.5	0	0	160	22	9	1	2	1 1/2 carb, 1 fat
SpongeBob SquarePants Fruity Splash	3/4 cup	100	1	10	0	0	0	115	22	8	1	1	1 1/2 carb
Tiny Toast Blueberry	3/4 cup	120	3	30	1	0	0	120	22	9	1	2	1 1/2 carb, 1 fat
Total Raisin Bran	1 cup	160	1	5	0	0	0	180	40	17	5	3	2 1/2 carb
Total Whole-Grain	3/4 cup	100	0.5	5	0	0	0	140	23	5	3	2	1 1/2 carb
Trix	1 cup	130	1.5	15	0	0	0	160	27	10	1	1	2 carb
Wheaties	3/4 cup	100	0.5	5	0	0	0	180	23	4	3	2	1 1/2 carb
Health Valley Organic													
Organic Amaranth Flakes	1 1/4 cups	210	2	20	0	0	0	190	43	11	5	6	3 carb
Organic Oat Bran Flakes	1 cup	190	1.5	15	0.5	0	0	190	39	11	4	5	2 1/2 carb

	Serving	Cal.	Fat (g)	Cal. from Fat	Sat. Fat (g)	Trans Fat (g)	Chol. (mg)	Sod. (mg)	Carb. (g)	Fiber (g)	Sugar (g)	Prot. (g)	Exchanges
Rice Crunch-Ems	1 1/4 cups	110	0	0	0	0	0	150	26	2	2	2	2 carb
Kashi													
7 Grain Honey Puffs	1 cup	110	1	5	0	0	0	0	26	7	3	3	2 carb
7 Whole Grain Flakes	1 cup	170	0.5	5	0	0	0	150	41	6	6	6	2 1/2 carb
7 Whole Grain Nuggets	1/2 cup	210	1.5	15	0	0	0	220	46	3	6	8	3 carb
Berry Fruitful Whole Wheat Biscuits	32 biscuits	190	1.0	9	0	0	0	0	42	9	6	7	3 carb
GoLean Clusters Vanilla Pepita	1 cup	230	6	60	1	0	0	85	37	3	6	9	2 1/2 carb, 1 fat
GoLean Crunch	3/4 cup	190	3	30	0	0	0	100	38	13	8	9	2 1/2 carb, 1 fat
GoLean Crunch Honey Almond Flax	2/3 cup	200	5	45	0.5	0	0	140	35	12	8	9	2 1/2 carb, 1 fat
GoLean Original	1 1/4 cups	180	2	15	0	0	0	115	40	8	6	12	2 1/2 carb
Heart to Heart Honey Toasted	3/4 cup	120	1.5	15	0	0	0	85	26	5	4	3	1 1/2 carb
Heart to Heart Oat Flakes & Wild Blueberry Clusters	1 cup	200	2.5	20	0	0	0	125	42	11	3	5	3 carb

BREAKFAST CEREAL, READY-TO-EAT CEREAL, HOT CEREAL

	Serving	Calories	Fat (g)	Cal. from Fat	Sat. Fat (g)	Trans Fat (g)	Chol. (mg)	Sod. (mg)	Carb. (g)	Sugar (g)	Fiber (g)	Prot. (g)	Servings/Exchanges
Heart to Heart Warm Cinnamon	3/4 cup	120	1.5	15	0	0	0	75	26	5	4	3	1 1/2 carb
Indigo Morning Organic Corn	3/4 cup	100	1	10	0	0	0	125	22	6	2	2	1 1/2 carb
Island Vanilla Whole Wheat Biscuits	27 biscuits	190	1	10	0	0	0	5	44	9	6	6	3 carb
Organic Promise Sprouted Grains	1 1/4 cups	190	1	10	0	0	0	110	45	9	6	6	3 carb
Organic Promise Sweet Potato Sunshine	1 cup	180	1	10	0	0	0	160	43	7	4	5	3 carb
Simply Maize Organic Corn	3/4 cup	100	1	10	0	0	0	110	23	6	2	2	1 1/2 carb
Strawberry Fields Original	1 cup	200	0	0	0	0	0	190	46	11	3	5	3 carb
Kellogg's													
All-Bran	1/2 cup	80	1	10	0	0	0	80	23	6	10	4	1 1/2 carb

All-Bran Buds	1/3 cup	80	1	10	0	0	210	24	8	13	3	1 1/2 carb
All-Bran Complete Wheat Flakes	3/4 cup	90	0.5	5	0	0	210	24	5	5	3	1 1/2 carb
Apple Jacks	1 cup	100	1	10	0	0	150	25	10	3	1	1 1/2 carb
Cocoa Krispies	3/4 cup	120	1	5	0.5	0	130	27	12	<1	1	2 carb
Corn Flakes	1 cup	100	0	0	0	0	200	24	3	1	2	1 1/2 carb
Corn Pops	1 cup	120	0	0	0	0	105	27	9	3	1	2 carb
Cracklin' Oat Bran	3/4 cup	200	7	60	3	0	135	34	14	6	4	2 carb, 1 fat
Crispix	1 cup	110	0	0	0	0	190	25	4	0	2	1 1/2 carb
Froot Loops	1 cup	110	1	10	0.5	0	150	25	10	3	1	1 1/2 carb
Frosted Flakes	3/4 cup	110	0	0	0	0	150	26	10	<1	1	1 1/2 carb
Honey Smacks	3/4 cup	100	0.5	5	0	0	40	24	15	1	2	1 1/2 carb
Krave, Chocolate & S'Mores Flavors	3/4 cup	120	3.5	30	1	0	100–105	24	10–11	3	2	1 1/2 carb, 1 fat
Mini-Wheats, Frosted	21 biscuits	190	1	10	0	0	0	46	11	<1	5	3 carb
Mini-Wheats, Frosted Blueberry	25 biscuits	190	1	10	0	0	0	47	12	6	5	3 carb

BREAKFAST CEREAL, READY-TO-EAT CEREAL, HOT CEREAL

	Serving	Calories	Fat (g)	Cal. from Fat	Sat. Fat (g)	Trans Fat (g)	Chol. (mg)	Sod. (mg)	Carb. (g)	Sugar (g)	Fiber (g)	Prot. (g)	Servings/Exchanges
Mini-Wheats, Frosted Little Bites	1 cup	200	1	10	0	0	0	0	47	11	6	5	3 carb
Origins, Ancient Grains Blend	3/4 cup	110	0.5	5	0	0	0	150	26	9	3	3	1 1/2 carb
Origins, Fruit & Nut Blend	3/4 cup	190	4	35	0	0	0	140	38	13	3	3	2 1/2 carb, 1 fat
Raisin Bran	1 cup	190	1	10	0	0	0	210	46	18	7	5	3 carb
Raisin Bran Crunch	1 cup	190	1	10	0	0	0	200	45	19	4	4	3 carb
Raisin Bran with Cranberries	1 cup	200	1	10	0	0	0	210	50	18	5	4	3 carb
Rice Krispies	1 1/4 cups	130	0	0	0	0	0	190	29	4	0	2	2 carb
Shredded Wheat	2 biscuits	160	1	10	0	0	0	0	37	0	6	5	2 1/2 carb
Smart Start Original Antioxidants	1 cup	190	1	10	0	0	0	200	43	14	3	4	3 carb

Special K	1 cup	120	0.5	5	0	0	0	210	23	4	0	6	1 1/2 carb
Special K, Chocolate Almond	2/3 cup	110	1.5	15	0	0	0	150	23	8	3	2	1 1/2 carb
Special K, Fruit & Yogurt	3/4 cup	120	1	10	0	0	0	140	27	10	3	2	2 carb
Special K, Gluten Free Touch of Brown Sugar	1 cup	180	1	10	0	0	0	180	42	9	5	3	3 carb
Special K, Protein	3/4 cup	120	1	10	0	0	0	190	19	7	3	10	1 carb, 1 lean meat
Special K, Protein, Cinnamon Brown Sugar	3/4 cup	110	1	5	0	0	0	190	22	9	3	7	1 1/2 carb, 1/2 lean meat
Special K, Red Berries	1 cup	110	0	0	0	0	0	190	27	9	3	2	2 carb
Special K, Vanilla Almond	3/4 cup	110	1	10	0	0	0	170	25	9	3	2	1 1/2 carb
Malt-O-Meal													
Apple Zings	1 cup	130	1	10	0	0	0	150	30	16	1	1	2 carb
Berry Berry Crunch	3/4 cup	120	1	10	0	0	0	140	26	14	1	1	1 1/2 carb
Berry Colossal Crunch	3/4 cup	120	1.5	15	0	0	0	190	26	13	1	1	1 1/2 carb
Cinnamon Toasters	3/4 cup	130	3.5	30	0.5	1	0	140	24	10	1	1	1 1/2 carb, 1 fat
Cocoa Roos	3/4 cup	120	1.5	15	1	0	0	110	26	14	1	1	1 1/2 carb

BREAKFAST CEREAL, READY-TO-EAT CEREAL, HOT CEREAL

	Serving	Calories	Fat (g)	Cal. from Fat	Sat. Fat (g)	Trans Fat (g)	Chol. (mg)	Sod. (mg)	Carb. (g)	Sugar (g)	Fiber (g)	Prot. (g)	Servings/Exchanges
Creamy Hot Wheat	3 Tbsp dry	130	0	0	0	0	0	0	27	0	1	4	2 carb
Crispy Rice	1 1/4 cups	130	0	0	0	0	0	300	29	3	0	2	2 carb
Dyno Bites (Cocoa or Fruity)	3/4 cup	110	0.5	5	0	0	0	170	24	11	0	1	1 1/2 carb
Frosted Flakes	3/4 cup	120	0	0	0	0	0	140	28	12	0	1	2 carb
Frosted Mini Spooners	1 cup	190	1	10	0	0	0	10	45	11	6	5	3 carb
Golden Puffs	3/4 cup	100	0	0	0	0	0	55	24	14	0	2	1 1/2 carb
Honey Buzzers	1 1/3 cups	110	0.5	5	0	0	0	220	26	11	1	1	1 1/2 carb
Honey Graham Toasters	3/4 cup	120	3	30	0	0	0	260	23	10	1	2	1 1/2 carb, 1 fat
Honey Nut Scooters	1 cup	120	1.5	10	0	0	0	210	24	9	2	3	1 1/2 carb
Honey & Oat Blenders	3/4 cup	120	1.5	15	0	0	0	150	25	6	2	2	1 1/2 carb
Hot Wheat Cereal, Chocolate	3 Tbsp dry	130	0	0	0	0	0	0	27	7	1	4	2 carb

Hot Wheat Cereal, Maple & Brown Sugar	1/4 cup dry	170	0	0	0	0	0	37	13	1	4	2 1/2 carb
Hot Wheat Cereal, Original	3 Tbsp dry	130	0.5	5	0	0	0	27	0	1	5	2 carb
Marshmallow Mateys	1 cup	120	1	10	0	0	200	25	13	1	2	1 1/2 carb
Raisin Bran	1 cup	220	1.5	10	0	0	340	45	20	6	5	3 carb
Tootie Fruities	1 cup	130	1	10	0	0	150	28	15	1	2	2 carb
Nature's Path Organic												
Organic Flax Plus Flakes	3/4 cup	110	1.5	15	0	0	135	23	4	5	4	1 1/2 carb
Organic Flax Plus Raisin Bran	3/4 cup	190	2.5	20	0	0	190	41	12	8	6	2 1/2 carb
Organic Heritage Flakes	3/4 cup	120	1	10	0	0	130	24	4	5	4	1 1/2 carb
Organic Optimum Blueberry Cinnamon Hot Oatmeal	1 packet	160	2.5	25	0	0	120	30	8	3	5	2 carb
Organic Original Hot Oatmeal	1 packet	190	3	25	0.5	0	0	34	1	6	8	2 carb, 1 fat
Organic Pumpkin Flax Plus Granola	3/4 cup	260	10	90	1.5	0	45	37	10	5	6	2 1/2 carb, 2 fat

BREAKFAST CEREAL, READY-TO-EAT CEREAL, HOT CEREAL

	Serving	Calories	Fat (g)	Cal. from Fat	Sat. Fat (g)	Trans Fat (g)	Chol. (mg)	Sod. (mg)	Carb. (g)	Sugar (g)	Fiber (g)	Prot. (g)	Servings/Exchanges
Post													
Alpha-Bits	1 cup	120	1.5	10	0	0	0	180	24	6	2	3	1 1/2 carb
Bran Flakes	3/4 cup	100	0.5	5	0	0	0	180	24	5	5	3	1 1/2 carb
Cocoa Pebbles	3/4 cup	120	1	10	1	0	0	170	25	10	0	1	1 1/2 carb
Fruity Pebbles	3/4 cup	110	1	10	1	0	0	140	23	9	0	1	1 1/2 carb
Golden Crisp	3/4 cup	100	0	0	0	0	0	25	24	14	1	1	1 1/2 carb
Grape Nuts	1/2 cup	210	1	10	0	0	0	270	47	5	7	6	3 carb
Grape Nuts Flakes	3/4 cup	110	1	10	0	0	0	135	24	4	3	3	1 1/2 carb
Great Grains, Crunchy Pecan	3/4 cup	210	6	50	0.5	0	0	150	38	8	5	5	2 1/2 carb, 1 fat
Great Grains, Raisin/Date/Pecan	3/4 cup	210	4	35	0	0	0	135	41	13	5	4	2 1/2 carb, 1 fat
Honey Bunches of Oats, Honey Roasted	3/4 cup	120	1.5	15	0	0	0	135	25	6	2	2	1 1/2 carb

Honeycombs	1 1/2 cups	130	1	10	0	0	180	28	10	1	2	2 carb
Raisin Bran	1 cup	190	1	10	0	0	230	47	19	8	5	3 carb
Shredded Wheat	2 biscuits	160	1	10	0	0	0	37	0	6	5	2 1/2 carb
Shredded Wheat, Honey Nut	1 cup	220	2	15	0	0	60	49	12	6	5	3 carb
Shredded Wheat 'n Bran	1 1/4 cups	210	1.5	10	0	0	0	47	0	8	7	3 carb
Quaker												
Corn Bran Crunch	3/4 cup	90	1	10	0.5	0	210	23	6	4	2	1 1/2 carb
Granola, Apple, Cranberry & Almond	1/2 cup	200	5	45	0.5	0	25	37	13	5	5	2 1/2 carb, 1 fat
Granola, Honey & Almonds	1/2 cup	200	6	50	0.5	0	25	35	10	5	5	2 carb, 1 fat
Instant Grits, Butter	1 pkt	100	1.5	15	0	0	340	21	NA	1	2	1 1/2 carb
Instant Grits, Original	1 pkt	100	0	0	0	0	310	22	NA	1	2	1 1/2 carb

BREAKFAST CEREAL, READY-TO-EAT CEREAL, HOT CEREAL

	Serving	Calories	Fat (g)	Cal. from Fat	Sat. Fat (g)	Trans Fat (g)	Chol. (mg)	Sod. (mg)	Carb. (g)	Sugar (g)	Fiber (g)	Prot. (g)	Servings/Exchanges
Instant Hot Oatmeal, Classics Apples & Cranberry	1 pkt	160	2	20	0.5	0	0	170	33	12	3	4	2 carb
Instant Hot Oatmeal, Classics Maple & Brown Sugar	1 pkt	160	2	20	0.5	0	0	260	32	12	3	4	2 carb
Instant Hot Oatmeal, Classics Peaches & Cream	1 pkt	130	2	20	0.5	0	0	180	27	12	2	3	2 carb
Instant Hot Oatmeal, Classics Raisin/Date/Walnut	1 pkt	140	2.5	25	0	0	0	190	27	11	3	3	2 carb
Instant Hot Oatmeal, High Fiber Maple & Brown Sugar	1 pkt	160	2	20	0	0	0	260	34	7	10	4	2 carb
Instant Hot Oatmeal, Organic Maple & Brown Sugar	1 pkt	150	2	20	0	0	0	95	31	12	3	4	2 carb

	Serving Size	Calories	Fat (g)	% Cal. from Fat	Sat. Fat (g)	Trans Fat (g)	Chol. (mg)	Sodium (mg)	Carb. (g)	Sugar (g)	Fiber (g)	Protein (g)	Exchanges/Choices
Instant Hot Oatmeal, Organic Original	1 pkt	100	2	20	0	0	0	0	19	0	3	4	1 carb
Instant Hot Oatmeal, Protein Banana Nut	1 pkt	240	5	45	1	0	0	190	40	12	4	10	2 1/2 carb, 1 fat
Instant Hot Oatmeal, Super Grains Apple & Cinnamon	1 pkt	210	3	25	0.5	0	0	200	41	12	5	7	2 1/2 carb, 1 fat
Instant Hot Oatmeal, Super Grains Cranberry Almond	1 pkt	210	4.5	40	0.5	0	0	180	38	12	5	7	2 1/2 carb, 1 fat
Instant Hot Oatmeal, Weight Control Banana Bread	1 pkt	160	3	25	0.5	0	0	280	29	1	6	7	2 carb, 1 fat
Instant Hot Oatmeal, Weight Control Maple & Brown Sugar	1 pkt	160	3	25	0.5	0	0	290	29	1	6	7	2 carb, 1 fat
Life	3/4 cup	120	1.5	15	0	0	0	160	25	6	2	3	1 1/2 carb
Life, Cinnamon or Maple & Brown Sugar	3/4 cup	120	1.5	15	0	0	0	150	25	8	2	3	1 1/2 carb
Old-Fashioned Hot Oats	1/2 cup	150	3	25	0.5	0	0	0	27	1	4	5	2 carb, 1 fat

BREAKFAST CEREAL, READY-TO-EAT CEREAL, HOT CEREAL

	Serving	Calories	Fat (g)	Cal. from Fat	Sat. Fat (g)	Trans Fat (g)	Chol. (mg)	Sod. (mg)	Carb. (g)	Sugar (g)	Fiber (g)	Prot. (g)	Servings/Exchanges
Old Fashioned Hot Oats, 1 Minute	1/2 cup	150	3	25	0.5	0	0	0	27	1	4	5	2 carb, 1 fat
Puffed Rice	1 cup	50	0	0	0	0	0	0	12	0	NA	1	1 carb
Puffed Wheat	1 cup	50	0	0	0	0	0	0	22	NA	1	2	1 1/2 carb
Real Medleys Granola, Dark Chocolate Cranberry Almond	1/3 cup	130	3.5	30	0.5	0	0	25	22	8	2	3	1 1/2 carb, 1 fat
Real Medleys Granola, Summer Berry	1/3 cup	110	2.5	25	0	0	0	25	20	7	2	2	1 carb
Real Medleys Hot Oatmeal, Apple Walnut	1 pkg	290	8	70	1	0	0	270	53	22	5	6	3 1/2 carb, 2 fat
Real Medleys Hot Oatmeal, Steel Cut Cranberry Vanilla Almond	1 pkg	240	7	60	1	0	0	200	41	15	4	5	2 1/2 carb, 1 fat
Real Medleys Hot Oatmeal, Summer Berry	1 pkg	250	3	25	0.5	0	0	250	51	14	7	8	3 1/2 carb, 1 fat

Real Medleys Hot Oatmeal, SuperGrains Banana Walnut	1 pkg	280	8	70	1	0	0	200	49	19	5	7	3 carb, 2 fat
Real Medleys Multigrain Cereal Cherry Almond Pecan	3/4 cup	240	7	60	1	0	0	40	41	15	3	5	2 1/2 carb, 1 fat
Real Medleys Su-perGrains Granola Blueberry Pecan	1/4 cup	110	4	35	0	0	0	10	18	6	2	2	1 carb, 1 fat
Steel Cut Oats, Hot	1/4 cup	150	2.5	25	0.5	0	0	0	27	1	4	5	2 carb
Toasted Oatmeal Squares, All Varieties	1 cup	210	2.5	25	0–0.5	0	0	190	44	9	5	6	3 carb
Trader Joe's													
Banana Nut Clusters	1 cup	240	8	70	0.5	0	0	140	40	12	2	4	2 1/2 carb, 2 fat
Chocolate Almond Granola Clusters	2/3 cup	250	9	80	1.5	0	0	60	38	13	4	6	2 1/2 carb, 2 fat
Crisp Rice	1 cup	120	0	0	0	0	0	250	26	3	0	2	1 1/2 carb
Frosted Flakes	3/4 cup	120	0	0	0	0	0	140	26	10	0	2	1 1/2 carb
Fruity O's	1 cup	110	0.5	5	0	0	0	95	23	8	1	2	1 1/2 carb

BREAKFAST CEREAL, READY-TO-EAT CEREAL, HOT CEREAL

	Serving	Calories	Fat (g)	Cal. from Fat	Sat. Fat (g)	Trans Fat (g)	Chol. (mg)	Sod. (mg)	Carb. (g)	Sugar (g)	Fiber (g)	Prot. (g)	Servings/Exchanges
Gluten Free Granola Ancient Grain & Super Seed Oatmeal	1/3 cup	160	6	50	1	0	0	35	24	1	4	6	1 1/2 carb, 1 fat
High Fiber Cereal	2/3 cup	80	0.5	5	0	0	0	70	23	5	9	3	1 1/2 carb
High Fiber Fruit & Nut Medley	2/3 cup	90	1.5	15	0	0	0	55	25	8	7	2	1 1/2 carb
Honey Nut O's	3/4 cup	110	1	10	0	0	0	160	23	9	2	2	1 1/2 carb
Joe's O's	1 cup	100	2	15	0	0	0	170	20	1	3	3	1 carb
Just The Cluster's Maple Pecan Granola	2/3 cup	250	10	90	1	0	0	70	38	15	3	5	2 1/2 carb, 2 fat
Lowfat Granola with Almonds	3/4 cup	210	3	25	0	0	0	75	44	15	5	4	3 carb, 1 fat
Lowfat Granola Mixed Berry	3/4 cup	210	2.5	20	0	0	0	75	45	17	5	4	3 carb
Mango Instant Oatmeal	1 pouch	160	3	25	0	0	0	35	29	9	4	5	2 carb, 1 fat
Multigrain O's	1 cup	110	1	10	0	0	0	135	24	6	3	2	1 1/2 carb

Organic Cinnamon Spice Instant Oatmeal	1 pkt	150	1.5	15	0	0	90	30	13	2.5	4	2 carb
Organic Corn Flakes	1 cup	110	0	0	0	0	280	26	2	<1	2	2 carb
Organic Granny's Apple Granola	2/3 cup	240	7	7	1	0	55	39	11	4	5	2 1/2 carb, 1 fat
Organic High Fiber 0's	1 1/4 cups	180	1	10	0	0	110	44	9	9	6	3 carb
Organic Honey Crunch n' Oats	3/4 cup	120	1	10	0	0	135	25	6	2	2	1 1/2 carb
Organic Multigrain Hot Cereal	1/2 cup	140	1	10	0	0	0	29	0	5	5	2 carb
Organic Quick Cook Steel Cut Oats	1/4 cup dry	150	3	25	0	0	0	27	1	4	5	2 carb, 1 fat
Organic Raisin Bran Clusters	1 cup	190	3	25	0.5	0	170	41	18	9	5	2 1/2 carb, 1 fat
Pomegranate Blueberry Flakes & Clusters	1 cup	210	2	20	0	0	110	46	10	4	4	3 carb
Raisin Bran	1 cup	170	1	10	0	0	120	44	16	8	4	3 carb

BREAKFAST CEREAL, READY-TO-EAT CEREAL, HOT CEREAL

	Serving	Calories	Fat (g)	Cal. from Fat	Sat. Fat (g)	Trans Fat (g)	Chol. (mg)	Sod. (mg)	Carb. (g)	Sugar (g)	Fiber (g)	Prot. (g)	Servings/Exchanges
Shredded Bite Size Wheats	1 cup	180	1	10	0	0	0	0	38	0	5	5	2 1/2 carb
Shredded Bite Size Wheats, Frosted	1 cup	200	1	10	0	0	0	0	42	11	5	5	3 carb
Strawberry Yogurt 0's	3/4 cup	120	2.5	25	1.5	0	0	95	23	8	1	2	1 1/2 carb
Toasted Oatmeal Flakes	3/4 cup	110	1	10	0	0	0	190	23	7	3	3	1 1/2 carb
Trek Mix, Almonds, Cashews & Cranberries	2/3 cup	240	8	70	1	0	0	100	37	12	3	6	2 1/2 carb, 2 fat
Triple Berry 0's	3/4 cup	110	1	10	0	0	0	180	25	7	3	2	1 1/2 carb
Unsweetened Instant Oatmeal	1 pouch	160	3.5	30	0.5	0	0	20	27	0	5	5	2 carb, 1 fat
Vanilla Almond Clusters	1 cup	220	8	70	0.5	0	0	60	34	12	3	5	2 carb, 2 fat

BUTTER, MARGARINE, SOUR CREAM

	Serving	Calories	Fat (g)	Cal. from Fat	Sat. Fat (g)	Trans Fat (g)	Chol. (mg)	Sod. (mg)	Carb. (g)	Sugar (g)	Fiber (g)	Prot. (g)	Servings/Exchanges
Butter, Light	1 tsp	25	3	25	3	0	5	23	0	0	0	0	1 fat
Butter, Stick	1 tsp	36	4	36	3	0	11	32	0	0	0	0	1 fat
Butter, Whipped	1 Tbsp	67	8	67	5	0	21	62	0	0	0	0	2 fat
Margarine, Fat-Free/Nonfat	1 Tbsp	6	0	0	0	0	0	85	1	0	0	0	free
Margarine-Like Spread, Light or Lower Fat	1 Tbsp	49	5	49	1	NA	0	85	0	0	0	0	1 fat
Margarine, Stick	1 Tbsp	102	11	100	2	NA	0	107	0	0	0	0	2 fat
Margarine, Tub	1 tsp	34	4	34	1	NA	0	31	0	0	0	0	1 fat
Sour Cream, Fat-Free	1 Tbsp	12	0	0	0	0	1	23	2	0	0	1	free
Sour Cream, Reduced-Fat or Light	2 Tbsp	44	3	25	2	0	11	27	2	0	0	1	1 fat
Sour Cream, Regular	2 Tbsp	56	6	50	3	0	15	14	1	0	0	1	1 fat

BUTTER, MARGARINE, SOUR CREAM

	Serving	Calories	Fat (g)	Cal. from Fat	Sat. Fat (g)	Trans Fat (g)	Chol. (mg)	Sod. (mg)	Carb. (g)	Sugar (g)	Fiber (g)	Prot. (g)	Servings/Exchanges
BUTTER/MARGARINE													
Benecol Spread													
Light	1 Tbsp	50	5	50	0.7	0	0	110	0	0	0	0	1 fat
Regular	1 Tbsp	70	8	70	1	0	0	110	0	0	0	0	2 fat
Blue Bonnet Margarine													
Light Stick	1 Tbsp	50	5	50	1	1	0	80	<1	0	0	0	1 fat
Regular Stick	1 Tbsp	70	9	70	1.5	1.5	0	125	0	0	0	0	2 fat
Regular Tub	1 Tbsp	60	6	60	1.5	0	0	125	0	0	0	0	1 fat
Brummel & Brown Margarine Spread with Yogurt													
Tub	1 Tbsp	45	5	45	1.5	0	0	90	0	0	0	0	1 fat
Butter Buds													
Butter Replacement, Dry	1 tsp	5	0	0	0	0	0	75	6	0	0	0	free
Canoleo													
100% Canola Margarine	1 Tbsp	100	11	100	0	0	0	100	0	0	0	0	2 fat

Earth Balance

Avocado Oil Spread	1 Tbsp	100	11	100	3	0	105	0	0	0	2 fat
Olive Oil & Omega-3 Spreads	1 Tbsp	80	9	80	2.5	0	75–80	0	0	0	2 fat
Organic Coconut Spread	1 Tbsp	100	11	100	5	0	70	0	0	0	2 fat
Organic Roasted Garlic & Herbs Spread	1 Tbsp	100	11	100	3.5	0	120	0	0	0	2 fat
Organic Sweet Cinnamon Spread	1 Tbsp	90	9	80	2.5	0	35	3	3	0	2 fat
Organic Whipped Spread	1 Tbsp	80	9	80	2.5	0	100	0	0	0	2 fat
Soy Free Buttery Spread	1 Tbsp	100	11	100	3	0	105–110	0	0	0	2 fat

Fleischmanns Margarine

Light Spread	1 Tbsp	40	4.5	40	0.5	0	65	0	0	0	1 fat
Original Tub	1 Tbsp	60	7	60	1	0	35	0	0	0	2 fat
Original Tub with Olive Oil	1 Tbsp	60	6.5	60	1	0	45	0	0	0	1 fat

BUTTER, MARGARINE, SOUR CREAM

	Serving	Calories	Fat (g)	Cal. from Fat	Sat. Fat (g)	Trans Fat (g)	Chol. (mg)	Sod. (mg)	Carb. (g)	Sugar (g)	Fiber (g)	Prot. (g)	Servings/Exchanges
Gold 'n Soft													
Light Spread 39% Olive Oil	1 Tbsp	50	5	50	1.5	0	0	120	0	0	0	0	1 fat
Regular Spread 60% Olive Oil	1 Tbsp	80	8	70	2	0	0	90	0	0	0	0	2 fat
Regular Spread 70% Olive Oil	1 Tbsp	90	10	90	2.5	0	0	90	0	0	0	0	2 fat
I Can't Believe It's Not Butter													
Light Spread	1 Tbsp	40	4	40	1	0	0	80	0	0	0	0	1 fat
Olive Oil Spread	1 Tbsp	60	6	2	0	0	0	90	0	0	0	0	1 fat
Original Spread	1 Tbsp	60	6	60	2	0	0	90	0	0	0	0	1 fat
Regular Stick	1 Tbsp	100	11	100	3.5	0	0	95	0	0	0	0	2 fat
Spray Original	5 sprays	0	0	0	0	0	0	0	0	0	0	0	free

Imperial

Regular Stick	1 Tbsp	70	7	70	2.5	0	0	105	0	0	0	0	2 fat
Regular Tub	1 Tbsp	40	4	40	1	0	0	90	0	0	0	0	1 fat

Land O'Lakes

Butter with Olive Oil & Sea Salt	1 Tbsp	100	11	100	6	0	25	90	0	0	0	0	2 fat
Cinnamon Sugar Butter Spread	1 Tbsp	70	6	60	2.5	0	10	30	4	4	0	0	1 fat
European Style Premium Salted Butter	1 Tbsp	110	12	110	8	0	30	65	0	0	0	0	2 fat
Fresh Buttery Taste Soft Spread	1 Tbsp	70	8	70	2	0	0	80	0	0	0	0	2 fat
Fresh Buttery Taste Stick Spread	1 Tbsp	90	10	90	2	2	0	95	0	0	0	0	2 fat
Garlic & Herb Butter Tub	1 Tbsp	70	8	70	3	0	10	100	0	0	0	0	2 fat
Honey Butter Tub	1 Tbsp	70	6	60	2.5	0	10	50	4	4	0	0	1 fat
Light Butter Stick	1 Tbsp	50	6	50	3.5	0	15	100	0	0	0	0	1 fat
Margarine Soft Tub	1 Tbsp	100	11	100	3	0	0	105	0	0	0	0	2 fat

BUTTER, MARGARINE, SOUR CREAM

	Serving	Calories	Fat (g)	Cal. from Fat	Sat. Fat (g)	Trans Fat (g)	Chol. (mg)	Sod. (mg)	Carb. (g)	Sugar (g)	Fiber (g)	Prot. (g)	Servings/Exchanges
Margarine Stick	1 Tbsp	100	11	100	5	0	0	100	0	0	0	0	2 fat
Salted Butter Stick	1 Tbsp	100	11	100	7	0	30	90	0	0	0	0	2 fat
Spreadable Butter with Canola Oil	1 Tbsp	100	11	100	4	0	15	85	0	0	0	0	2 fat
Spreadable Light Butter with Canola Oil	1 Tbsp	50	5	50	2	0	5	90	0	0	0	0	1 fat
Unsalted Butter Stick	1 Tbsp	100	11	100	7	0	30	0	0	0	0	0	2 fat
Whipped Salted Butter Tub 45% Less Fat	1 Tbsp	50	6	50	3.5	0	15	50	0	0	0	0	1 fat
Parkay													
Light Spread	1 Tbsp	45	5	45	1	0	0	130	0	0	0	0	1 fat
Original Spread	1 Tbsp	70	7	70	1.5	0	0	80	0	0	0	0	2 fat
Original Stick	1 Tbsp	80	9	80	1.5	1.5	0	130	0	0	0	0	2 fat
Squeeze	1 Tbsp	70	8	70	1.5	0	0	110	0	0	0	0	2 fat

Promise

Activ	1 Tbsp	45	5	45	0.5	0	<5	85	0	0	0	1 fat
Light Spread	1 Tbsp	45	5	45	1	0	0	85	0	0	0	1 fat
Regular Spread	1 Tbsp	80	8	80	1.5	0	0	85	0	0	0	2 fat

Shedd's Spread Country Crock

Calcium Plus Vitamin D Spread	1 Tbsp	45	4.5	40	1	0	0	100	<1	0	0	1 fat
Churn Style Spread	1 Tbsp	50	6	50	1.5	0	0	100	0	0	0	1 fat
Honey Spread	1 Tbsp	70	6	50	1.5	0	0	45	3	3	0	1 fat
Light Spread Tub	1 Tbsp	35	4	35	1	0	0	90	0	0	0	1 fat
Original Spread Tub	1 Tbsp	50	6	50	1.5	0	0	100	0	0	0	1 fat
Spreadable Butter with Canola Oil	1 Tbsp	100	11	100	4.5	0	15	105	0	0	0	2 fat
Spreadable Sticks	1 Tbsp	80	8	80	2.5	0	NA	95	0	0	0	2 fat

Smart Balance

Buttery Burst Spray	5 sprays	0	0	0	0	0	0	0	0	0	0	free

BUTTER, MARGARINE, SOUR CREAM

	Serving	Calories	Fat (g)	Cal. from Fat	Sat. Fat (g)	Trans Fat (g)	Chol. (mg)	Sod. (mg)	Carb. (g)	Sugar (g)	Fiber (g)	Prot. (g)	Servings/Exchanges
Butter & Canola Oil Blend	1 Tbsp	100	11	100	4	0	0	85	0	0	0	0	2 fat
Butter/Canola Oil/EVOO Blend	1 Tbsp	100	11	100	4	0	0	85	0	0	0	0	2 fat
Extra Virgin Olive Oil Buttery Spread	1 Tbsp	70	8	70	2	0	0	70	0	0	0	0	2 fat
Extra Virgin Olive Oil Light Buttery Spread	1 Tbsp	50	5	50	1.5	0	0	70	0	0	0	0	1 fat
Light Butter & Canola Oil Spread	1 Tbsp	50	5	50	2	0	0	90	0	0	0	0	1 fat
Light Spread with Flax Seed Oil	1 Tbsp	50	5	50	1.5	0	0	90	0	0	0	0	1 fat
Low Sodium Buttery Spread	1 Tbsp	70	8	70	2	0	0	30	0	0	0	0	2 fat
Omega-3 Buttery Spread	1 Tbsp	80	9	80	2.5	0	0	85	0	0	0	0	2 fat
Omega-3 Light Buttery Spread	1 Tbsp	50	5	50	1.5	0	0	80	0	0	0	0	1 fat

Organic Buttery Spread	1 Tbsp	80	9	80	2.5	0	0	100	0	0	0	0	2 fat
Original Buttery Spread	1 Tbsp	90	10	90	2.5	0	0	90	0	0	0	0	2 fat

SOUR CREAM

Breakstone's/Knudsen

Sour Cream	2 Tbsp	60	6	50	3.5	0	20	10	1	1	0	<1	1 fat
Sour Cream, Fat Free	2 Tbsp	30	0	0	0	0	<5	25	5	2	0	1	free
Sour Cream, Reduced Fat	2 Tbsp	40	3	30	2	0	15	20	2	2	0	1	1 fat

Daisy

Sour Cream	2 Tbsp	60	5	45	3.5	0	20	15	1	1	0	1	1 fat
Sour Cream, Light	2 Tbsp	40	2.5	25	2	0	10	25	2	2	0	2	1/2 fat

Follow Your Heart

Vegan Sour Cream Substitute	2 Tbsp	50	5	45	1.5	0	0	25	3	0	2	0	1 fat

CANDY & SWEETS

	Serving	Calories	Fat (g)	Cal. from Fat	Sat. Fat (g)	Trans Fat (g)	Chol. (mg)	Sod. (mg)	Carb. (g)	Sugar (g)	Fiber (g)	Prot. (g)	Servings/Exchanges
Almond Roca	1 piece	49	2	20	1	0	1	20	7	6	0	1	1/2 carb
Almonds, Chocolate-Coated	1/4 cup	244	19	190	4	0	3	16	13	8	3	7	1 carb, 1 med-fat protein, 2 fat
Almonds, Sugar-Coated	1/4 cup	231	9	90	1	0	0	6	33	30	1	5	2 carb, 2 fat
Butterscotch	5 pieces	117	1	10	1	0	3	117	27	24	0	0	2 carb
Candies, Chocolate Covered, Caramel with Nuts (Turtles)	3 pieces	197	9	80	2	0	0	66	25	17	2	4	1 1/2 carb, 2 fat
Candy Corn	1/4 cup	187	0	0	0	0	0	6	47	44	0	0	3 carb
Caramels	3 pieces	80	2	20	1	0	1	51	16	14	0	1	1 carb
Chewing Gum	1 piece	14	0	0	0	0	0	0	4	3	0	0	free
Chewing Gum, Sugar-Free	1 piece	5	0	0	0	0	0	0	2	0	0	0	free

Chocolate Covered Fondant Candy (Junior Mints)	1/4 cup	190	5	45	3	0	0	14	42	37	1	1	3 carb, 1 fat
Divinity, Fudge	1-inch cube	48	1	10	0	0	0	8	10	10	0	1	1/2 carb
Fruit Leather	1 oz	102	1	10	0	0	0	102	24	15	0	0	1 1/2 carb
Fudge, Chocolate	1-inch cube	90	2	20	1	0	3	10	17	16	0	1	1 carb
Fudge, Vanilla	1-inch cube	84	1	10	1	0	3	10	18	16	0	0	1 carb
Gumdrops, Sugar-Free	10 small	82	0	0	0	0	0	4	44	36	0	0	3 carb
Gummy Bears	10 small	88	0	0	0	0	0	10	22	12	0	0	1 1/2 carb
Hard Candy, All Flavors	14 pieces	127	0	0	0	0	0	12	32	20	0	0	2 carb
Jellybeans	10	40	0	0	0	0	0	3	10	8	0	0	1/2 carb
Lollipops	1	24	0	0	0	0	0	2	6	4	0	0	1/2 carb

CANDY & SWEETS

	Serving	Calories	Fat (g)	Cal. from Fat	Sat. Fat (g)	Trans Fat (g)	Chol. (mg)	Sod. (mg)	Carb. (g)	Sugar (g)	Fiber (g)	Prot. (g)	Servings/Exchanges
Peanut Brittle, Home-made	1 piece	63	2	20	1	0	2	58	9	6	0	1	1/2 carb
Peanuts, Milk Chocolate–Coated	1/4 cup	193	12	120	5	0	3	15	19	11	2	5	1 carb, 2 fat
Peanuts, Yogurt-Covered	1/4 cup	230	16	160	7	0	0	24	18	13	2	6	1 carb, 3 fat
Praline	2 oz	222	6	60	1	0	1	179	44	39	1	1	3 carb, 1 fat
Raisins, Milk Chocolate-Covered	1/4 cup	185	7	65	5	0	1	17	30	17	1	2	2 carb, 1 fat
Raisins, Yogurt-Covered	1/4 cup	188	6	60	5	0	0	21	35	29	1	2	2 carb, 1 fat
Taffy	1 oz	112	2	20	2	0	0	21	23	16	0	0	1 1/2 carb
Toffee	3 pieces	81	2	20	1	0	0	1	16	11	0	1	1 carb
Truffles	3 pieces	191	13	130	8	0	22	32	17	15	1	2	1 carb, 3 fat
BRANDS													
DeMet's													
Turtles, Minis	1 oz (4 pieces)	140	8	70	3.5	0	5	30	16	14	1	2	1 carb, 2 fat

Turtles, Original Pecan	2 pieces	170	10	90	4	0	5	35	19	16	1	2	1 carb, 2 fat
Hershey's													
5th Avenue Bar	2-oz bar	260	12	110	5	0	0	120	38	29	1	4	2 1/2 carb, 2 fat
Almond Joy	1.6-oz bar	220	12	110	8	0	0	50	26	20	2	2	2 1/2 carb, 2 fat
Brookside Dark Chocolate Açai & Blueberry Flavors	16 pieces	170	8	70	5	0	0	55	28	23	1	1	2 carb, 2 fat
Cadbury Caramel Egg	1 piece	170	8	70	4.5	0	5	45	22	15	0	2	1 1/2 carb, 2 fat
Cadbury Creme Egg	1 piece	150	6	50	4	0	5	15	24	20	0	2	1 1/2 carb, 1 fat
Cadbury Premium Milk Chocolate	7 blocks	200	11	100	7	0	10	40	23	22	1	3	1 1/2 carb, 2 fat
Chocolate Kisses	1.55-oz pkg	210	13	110	8	0	10	35	26	24	1	3	1 1/2 carb, 3 fat
Cookies & Creme Kisses	10 pieces	220	11	100	7	0	5	90	27	20	0	3	2 carb, 2 fat
Dagoba Organic Dark Chocolate	1/2 bar	190	14	130	9	0	0	0	22	16	3	3	1 1/2 carb, 3 fat

CANDY & SWEETS

	Serving	Calories	Fat (g)	Cal. from Fat	Sat. Fat (g)	Trans Fat (g)	Chol. (mg)	Sod. (mg)	Carb. (g)	Sugar (g)	Fiber (g)	Prot. (g)	Servings/Exchanges
Dagoba Organic Milk Chocolate	1/2 bar	210	14	130	9	0	5	20	23	22	1	2	1 1/2 carb, 3 fat
Good & Plenty	33 pieces	140	0	0	0	0	0	100	36	25	0	<1	2 1/2 carb
Heath Toffee Bar	1.4-oz bar	210	13	110	7	0	10	140	24	24	1	1	1 1/2 carb, 3 fat
Hershey's Milk Chocolate Bar	1 bar	220	13	110	8	0	10	35	25	24	1	3	1 1/2 carb, 3 fat
Hershey's Milk Chocolate with Almonds	1 bar	210	14	120	7	0	10	25	21	19	2	4	1 1/2 carb, 3 fat
Hershey's Milk Chocolate with Almonds King Size	1 bar	380	24	220	12	0	15	50	39	36	3	7	2 1/2 carb, 5 fat
Hershey's Milk Chocolate King Size	1 bar	370	22	200	14	0	20	55	43	40	2	5	3 carb, 4 fat
Hershey's Nuggets	4 pieces	210	13	110	8	0	10	30	24	23	1	3	1 1/2 carb, 3 fat

Hershey's Symphony	1 bar	220	14	120	8	0	10	65	23	22	1	4	1 1/2 carb, 3 fat
Icebreakers Mints	1 mint	5	0	0	0	0	0	0	1	0	0	0	free
Jolly Rancher Candy	3 pieces	70	0	0	0	0	0	10	17	11	0	0	1 carb
Kit Kat Bar	1.5-oz bar	210	11	100	7	0	5	30	27	21	1	3	2 carb, 2 fat
Kit Kat Minis	9 pieces	210	11	100	7	0	5	30	27	22	1	3	2 carb, 2 fat
Lancaster Caramel Soft Crémes	7 pieces	190	7	60	5	0	5	160	30	24	0	1	2 carb, 1 fat
Milk Duds	13	170	6	50	3.5	0	0	100	29	21	0	1	2 carb, 1 fat
Mounds	1 pkg	240	13	120	10	0	0	55	28	20	3	2	2 carb, 3 fat
Mr. Goodbar	1.75-oz bar	260	17	150	7	0	5	50	26	23	2	5	1 1/2 carb, 3 fat
Pay Day	2.08-oz bar	240	13	110	2	0	0	120	27	21	2	7	2 carb, 3 fat
Pelon Peloneta Tamarind with Mango	1 lollipop	80	0	0	0	0	0	270	20	15	0	0	1 carb

CANDY & SWEETS

	Serving	Calories	Fat (g)	Cal. from Fat	Sat. Fat (g)	Trans Fat (g)	Chol. (mg)	Sod. (mg)	Carb. (g)	Sugar (g)	Fiber (g)	Prot. (g)	Servings/Exchanges
Reese's Crunchy Peanut Butter Cups	1.5 oz (2 cups)	220	13	110	4.5	0	5	115	22	20	2	5	1 1/2 carb, 3 fat
Reese's Fast Break	3.5-oz bar	230	11	100	4	0	0	170	31	27	1	4	2 carb, 2 fat
Reese's NutRageous	1.82-oz bar	240	14	140	4.5	0	5	65	26	21	2	5	1 1/2 carb, 3 fat
Reese's Peanut Butter Cups	1.5 oz (2 cups)	210	13	110	4.5	0	5	150	24	21	1	5	1 1/2 carb, 3 fat
Reese's Pieces	51 pieces	200	9	80	8	0	0	45	25	21	1	4	1 1/2 carb, 2 fat
Reese's Sticks	1.5-oz bar	220	13	110	6	0	5	135	24	18	2	4	1 1/2 carb, 3 fat
Rolo Caramels	1.7-oz pkg	220	10	80	7	0	5	75	33	30	0	2	2 carb, 2 fat
Skor Bar	1.4-oz bar	200	12	110	7	0	20	130	25	24	1	1	1 1/2 carb, 2 fat

Sugar Free Special Dark	5 pieces	160	13	110	8	0	<5	10	24	0	4	2	1 1/2 carb, 3 fat
TAKE5	1.5-oz bar	210	11	100	5	0	5	160	26	18	2	4	1 1/2 carb, 2 fat
Twizzlers Filled Twists	2 pieces	140	1.5	15	1.5	0	0	80	30	20	0	1	2 carb
Twizzlers, Strawberry	4 pieces	160	0.5	5	0	0	0	95	36	19	0	1	2 1/2 carb
Whatchamacallit Bar	1.6 oz	230	12	110	10	0	5	100	28	21	1	3	2 carb, 2 fat
Whoppers Chocolate Malted Milk Balls	18 pieces	190	7	60	7	0	0	95	31	24	0	1	2 carb, 1 fat
York Minis	10 minis	150	3.5	30	2.5	0	0	10	31	25	1	1	2 carb, 1 fat
York Peppermint Pattie	1 pattie	150	3	25	1.5	0	0	10	32	26	1	1	2 carb, 1 fat
York Sugar Free Peppermint Patties	3 pieces	120	8	60	4.5	0	0	5	24	0	2	1	1 1/2 carb, 2 fat
Zagnut	1.75-oz bar	220	9	80	3.5	0	0	100	35	25	1	3	2 carb, 2 fat

CANDY & SWEETS

	Serving	Calories	Fat (g)	Cal. from Fat	Sat. Fat (g)	Trans Fat (g)	Chol. (mg)	Sod. (mg)	Carb. (g)	Sugar (g)	Fiber (g)	Prot. (g)	Servings/Exchanges
Zero	1.85-oz bar	230	8	70	5	0	0	115	37	31	1	3	2 1/2 carb, 2 fat
Just Born													
Hot Tamales	20 pieces	140	0	0	0	0	0	25	36	25	0	0	2 1/2 carb
Mike and Ike	23 pieces	140	0	0	0	0	0	60	34	23	0	0	2 carb
M&M Mars													
3 Musketeers Bar	1 bar	240	7	70	5	0	5	90	42	36	1	1	3 carb, 1 fat
Dove Bar	1 bar	220	13	120	8	0	15	25	24	22	1	2	1 1/2 carb, 3 fat
M&M's, Chocolate	1.7 oz	240	10	90	6	0	5	30	34	30	1	2	2 carb, 2 fat
M&M's, Peanut	1.75 oz	250	13	120	5	0	5	25	30	25	2	5	2 carb, 3 fat
Milky Way Bar	2.05-oz bar	240	9	80	7	0	10	75	37	31	1	2	2 1/2 carb, 2 fat
Munch Bar	1 bar	220	15	130	3.5	0	10	140	17	13	2	6	1 carb, 3 fat

Skittles	1 bag	230	2.5	20	0	0		15	52	42	0	0	3 1/2 carb
Snickers Almond 2toGo	1 bar	230	10	90	3.5	0	5	100	30	25	1	3	2 carb, 2 fat
Snickers Bar	2.07-oz bar	250	12	110	4.5	0	5	120	33	27	1	4	2 carb, 2 fat
Snickers PB Squared	2 squares	250	14	120	5	0	5	150	29	23	1	5	2 carb, 3 fat
Starburst Fruit Chews	9 pieces	130	0	0	0	0	0	40	31	22	0	2	2 carb
Twix Caramel Cookie Bar	2-oz bar	250	12	110	7	0	5	100	34	24	1	2	2 carb, 2 fat
Nestlé													
100 Grand Bar	1.5-oz bar	190	8	70	5	0	10	90	30	22	0	1	2 carb, 2 fat
Baby Ruth Bar	2 bars (1.3 oz)	170	8	70	4.5	0	0	82	24	20	<1	2	1 1/2 carb, 2 fat
Butterfinger Bar	2 bars (1.3 oz)	170	7	60	3.5	0	0	75	27	17	<1	2	2 carb, 1 fat
Butterfinger Bites	8 pieces	180	7	70	4	0	0	80	29	18	<1	2	2 carb, 1 fat

CANDY & SWEETS

	Serving	Calories	Fat (g)	Cal. from Fat	Sat. Fat (g)	Trans Fat (g)	Chol. (mg)	Sod. (mg)	Carb. (g)	Sugar (g)	Fiber (g)	Prot. (g)	Servings/Exchanges
Crunch Bar	1.4-oz bar	190	9	80	6	0	<5	55	26	21	<1	2	1 1/2 carb, 2 fat
Goobers Chocolate-Covered Peanuts	1/4 cup	220	13	130	5	0	<5	10	22	18	2	5	1 1/2 carb, 3 fat
Raisinets	1/4 cup	190	8	70	5	0	5	5	31	27	2	2	2 carb, 2 fat
Pearson's													
Bit-O-Honey Chews	6 pieces	150	3	25	2	0	0	120	32	19	0	1	2 carb, 1 fat
Bun Bar, Maple	3 pieces	210	10	90	4.5	0	0	60	26	23	1	3	1 1/2 carb, 2 fat
Mint Patties	5 pieces	150	2.5	25	1.5	0	0	70	31	27	<1	<1	2 carb
Nut Goodies, Maple	3 pieces	210	10	90	4.5	0	0	60	26	23	1	3	1 1/2 carb, 2 fat
Salted Nut Roll	3 pieces	200	10	90	2	0	0	140	23	17	<1	7	1 1/2 carb, 2 fat

Russell Stover

Food	Serving	Cal	Total Fat (g)	Fat Cal	Sat Fat (g)	Trans Fat (g)	Chol (mg)	Sodium (mg)	Carb (g)	Sugars (g)	Fiber (g)	Protein (g)	Exchanges/Choices
Chocolate Covered Coconut, Sugar Free	3 pieces	170	10	90	7	0	0	60	28	0	2	2	2 carb, 2 fat
Mint Patties, Sugar Free	3 pieces	180	12	110	8	0	<5	20	26	0	2	2	1 1/2 carb, 2 fat
Peanut Butter Cups, Sugar Free	2 pieces	160	12	110	6	0	0	95	17	0	1	4	1 carb, 2 fat
Pecan Delights, Sugar Free	3 pieces	160	12	110	6	0	0	35	23	0	2	2	1 1/2 carb, 2 fat

SkinnyMe Chocolate

Food	Serving	Cal	Total Fat (g)	Fat Cal	Sat Fat (g)	Trans Fat (g)	Chol (mg)	Sodium (mg)	Carb (g)	Sugars (g)	Fiber (g)	Protein (g)	Exchanges/Choices
Bold Dark Chocolate Squares	1 square	45	4	35	2.5	0	0	0	6	0	3	1	1/2 carb, 1 fat

Storck

Food	Serving	Cal	Total Fat (g)	Fat Cal	Sat Fat (g)	Trans Fat (g)	Chol (mg)	Sodium (mg)	Carb (g)	Sugars (g)	Fiber (g)	Protein (g)	Exchanges/Choices
Swedish Fish	19 pieces	140	0	0	0	0	0	30	36	29	0	0	2 1/2 carb

Tootsie

Food	Serving	Cal	Total Fat (g)	Fat Cal	Sat Fat (g)	Trans Fat (g)	Chol (mg)	Sodium (mg)	Carb (g)	Sugars (g)	Fiber (g)	Protein (g)	Exchanges/Choices
Andes Crème de Menthe	40 g	220	14	130	13	0	0	25	23	22	1	2	1 1/2 carb, 3 fat
Dots	11 pieces	130	0	0	0	0	0	15	33	21	0	0	2 carb

CANDY & SWEETS

	Serving	Calories	Fat (g)	Cal. from Fat	Sat. Fat (g)	Trans Fat (g)	Chol. (mg)	Sod. (mg)	Carb. (g)	Sugar (g)	Fiber (g)	Prot. (g)	Servings/Exchanges
Junior Mints	16 pieces	170	3	30	2.5	0	0	30	35	32	1	1	2 carb, 1 fat
Sugar Babies	10 pieces	160	1.5	15	0	0	0	40	38	30	0	0	2 1/2 carb
Tootsie Roll	13 pieces	140	3	30	0.5	1	0	15	28	19	0	1	2 carb, 1 fat
Werther's													
Caramel Hard Candies	3 pieces	70	1	10	0.5	0	<5	60	14	10	0	0	1 carb
Caramel Hard Candies, Sugar Free	5 pieces	40	1.5	15	1	0	<5	65	14	0	0	0	1 carb
Chewy Caramel	6 pieces	170	5	45	3	0	5	95	28	16	0	1	2 carb, 1 fat

CHEESE, COTTAGE CHEESE, CREAM CHEESE

	Serving	Calories	Fat (g)	Cal. from Fat	Sat. Fat (g)	Trans Fat (g)	Chol. (mg)	Sod. (mg)	Carb. (g)	Sugar (g)	Fiber (g)	Prot. (g)	Servings/Exchanges
American	1 slice	71	6	50	3	0	17	275	2	1	0	4	1 med-fat protein
American, Fat-Free	1 slice	31	0	0	0	0	2	321	3	2	0	5	1 lean protein
American, Low-Fat	1 slice	38	1	10	1	0	7	300	1	0	0	5	1 lean protein
Blue or Roquefort	1 oz	100	8	70	5	0	21	325	1	0	0	6	1 med-fat protein
Brick	1 oz	105	8	70	5	0	27	159	1	0	0	7	1 med-fat protein, 1 fat
Brie	1 oz	95	8	70	5	0	28	178	0	0	0	6	1 med-fat protein
Camembert	1 oz	85	7	65	4	0	20	239	0	0	0	6	1 med-fat protein
Cheddar	1 oz	114	9	80	6	0	30	176	0	0	0	7	1 med-fat protein, 1 fat
Cheddar/Colby, Low-Fat	1 oz	40	2	20	1	0	6	174	1	0	0	7	1 lean protein
Cheddar/Colby, Reduced-Fat	1 oz	65	4	35	3	0	13	167	0	0	0	6	1 med-fat protein
Cheese Spread	2 Tbsp	82	6	55	4	0	15	457	2	2	0	5	1 med-fat protein
Cottage Cheese, 1% Milkfat, Low-Fat	1/2 cup	97	3	25	1	0	11	373	4	4	0	13	2 lean protein

CHEESE, COTTAGE CHEESE, CREAM CHEESE

	Serving	Calories	Fat (g)	Cal. from Fat	Sat. Fat (g)	Trans Fat (g)	Chol. (mg)	Sod. (mg)	Carb. (g)	Sugar (g)	Fiber (g)	Prot. (g)	Servings/Exchanges
Cottage Cheese, Creamed	1/2 cup	103	5	45	2	0	18	382	4	3	0	12	2 lean protein
Cottage Cheese, Nonfat	1/2 cup	52	0	0	0	0	5	270	5	1	0	7	1 lean protein
Cream Cheese	1 oz	97	10	90	5	0	31	103	1	1	0	2	2 fat
Cream Cheese, Fat-Free	1 oz	30	0	0	0	0	3	199	2	2	0	4	1 lean protein
Cream Cheese, Light	1 oz	57	4	35	3	0	15	102	2	2	0	2	1 fat
Cream Cheese, Whipped	1 oz	68	7	60	4	0	22	73	1	1	0	1	1 fat
Edam	1 oz	101	8	70	5	0	27	231	0	0	0	7	1 med-fat protein, 1 fat
Feta	1 oz	75	6	55	4	0	25	260	1	1	0	4	1 med-fat protein
Fontina	1 oz	110	9	80	5	0	33	227	0	0	0	7	1 med-fat protein, 1 fat
Goat Cheese	1 oz	102	8	70	6	0	22	122	0	0	0	7	1 med-fat protein, 1 fat
Gouda	1 oz	101	8	70	5	0	27	231	0	0	0	7	1 med-fat protein, 1 fat
Gruyere	1 oz	117	9	80	5	0	31	202	0	0	0	8	1 med-fat protein, 1 fat
Limburger	1 oz	93	8	70	5	0	26	227	0	0	0	6	1 med-fat protein, 1 fat
Monterey Jack	1 oz	106	9	80	5	0	25	170	0	0	0	7	1 med-fat protein, 1 fat

Food	Serving											Exchanges
Monterey Jack, Low-Fat	1 oz	89	6	55	4	0	18	221	0	0	8	1 med-fat protein
Mozzarella, Fat-Free	1 oz	40	0	0	0	0	5	211	1	0	9	1 lean protein
Mozzarella, Part-Skim	1 oz	86	6	50	3	0	15	185	1	0	7	1 med-fat protein
Mozzarella, Whole Milk	1 oz	85	6	55	4	0	22	178	1	0	6	1 med-fat protein
Muenster	1 oz	104	9	80	5	0	27	178	0	0	7	1 med-fat protein, 1 fat
Parmesan, Grated	2 Tbsp	43	3	30	2	0	9	153	0	0	4	1 lean protein
Port du Salut	1 oz	100	8	70	5	0	35	151	0	0	7	1 med-fat protein, 1 fat
Provolone	1 oz	100	8	70	5	0	20	248	1	0	7	1 med-fat protein, 1 fat
Queso Anejo (Aged Mexican Cheese)	1 oz	106	8	70	5	0	30	321	1	1	6	1 med-fat protein, 1 fat
Queso Fresco	1 oz	85	7	60	4	0	20	213	1	1	5	1 med-fat protein
Ricotta, Part-Skim	1/4 cup	85	5	45	3	0	19	77	3	0	7	1 med-fat protein
Ricotta, Whole Milk	1/4 cup	107	8	70	5	0	31	52	2	0	7	1 med-fat protein, 1 fat
String Cheese, Part-Skim	1	85	6	50	3	0	15	183	1	0	7	1 med-fat protein
Swiss	1 oz	108	8	70	5	0	26	20	2	0	8	1 med-fat protein, 1 fat
Swiss, Low-Fat	1 oz	51	1	10	1	0	10	56	1	0	8	1 lean protein

CHEESE, COTTAGE CHEESE, CREAM CHEESE

	Serving	Calories	Fat (g)	Cal. from Fat	Sat. Fat (g)	Trans Fat (g)	Chol. (mg)	Sod. (mg)	Carb. (g)	Sugar (g)	Fiber (g)	Prot. (g)	Servings/Exchanges
BRANDS													
Alpine Lace													
American, Reduced Fat	1 oz	90	6	50	4	0	20	300	2	2	0	6	1 med-fat protein
Cheddar, Reduced Fat	1 oz	70	6	50	3.5	0	15	150	0	0	0	6	1 med-fat protein
Muenster, Reduced Sodium	1 oz	100	9	80	5	0	20	135	0	0	0	7	1 med-fat protein, 1 fat
Provolone, Reduced Fat	1 oz	80	6	50	3.5	0	15	160	1	0	0	7	1 med-fat protein
Swiss, Reduced Fat	1 oz	90	6	50	3.5	0	20	115	1	1	0	8	1 med-fat protein
Athenos													
Blue Cheese	1 oz	100	8	70	5	0	20	380	1	0	1	6	1 med-fat protein, 1 fat
Fat Free Feta	1 oz	30	0	0	0	0	5	430	1	0	0	7	1 lean protein
Gorgonzola	1 oz	100	8	70	5	0	20	380	1	0	1	6	1 med-fat protein, 1 fat
Traditional Feta	1 oz	70	7	50	3.5	0	20	330	1	0	1	5	1 med-fat protein

Babybel

Gouda or White Cheddar	1 piece	70	6	50	4	0	20	140–160	0	0	4–5	1 med-fat protein
Mini Babybel Light	1 piece	50	3	25	2	0	10	160	0	0	6	1 lean protein
Mozzarella Style	1 piece	50	3.5	30	2.5	0	15	160	0	0	6	1 lean protein

Breakstone's

Cottage Cheese, 2% Milkfat Low-Fat, Small Curd	1/2 cup	90	2.5	15	1.5	0	15	340	5	0	10	1 lean protein
Cottage Cheese, 4% Milkfat, Large Curd	1/2 cup	110	5	45	3	0	25	340	6	5	11	1/2 carb, 1 lean protein
Cottage Cheese, 4% Milkfat, Small Curd	1/2 cup	120	5	45	3	0	25	340	6	5	11	1/2 carb, 1 lean protein
Cottage Cheese, Small Curd, Fat Free	1/2 cup	80	0	0	0	0	10	320	8	6	11	2 lean protein
Ricotta	1/4 cup	110	8	70	5	0	25	65	2	2	7	1 med-fat protein, 1 fat

Horizon Organic

American Singles	1 single	60	5	45	3	0	15	230	2	1	3	1 fat

CHEESE, COTTAGE CHEESE, CREAM CHEESE

	Serving	Calories	Fat (g)	Cal. from Fat	Sat. Fat (g)	Trans Fat (g)	Chol. (mg)	Sod. (mg)	Carb. (g)	Sugar (g)	Fiber (g)	Prot. (g)	Servings/Exchanges
Cheddar Cheese Slices	1 slice	80	7	60	4	0	20	135	0	0	0	5	1 med-fat protein
Cottage Cheese, Low Fat	1/2 cup	100	2.5	25	1.5	0	10	390	4	4	0	14	2 lean protein
Cottage Cheese, Regular	1/2 cup	120	5	45	3	0	20	400	4	4	0	14	2 lean protein
Monterey Jack Shreds	1/4 cup	100	8	70	4.5	0	25	170	0	0	0	6	1 med-fat protein, 1 fat
Knudsen													
Cottage Cheese, 2% Milkfat, Small Curd	1/2 cup	90	2.5	20	1.5	0	15	420	6	4	0	11	2 lean protein
Cottage Cheese, Nonfat	1/2 cup	80	0	0	0	0	3	390	8	6	0	10	1/2 carb, 1 lean protein
Cottage Cheese & Pineapple, Low fat	1/2 cup	110	2	15	1	0	3	340	12	5	0	8	1 carb, 1 lean protein
Creamed Cottage Cheese, 4% Milkfat, Small Curd	1/2 cup	110	5	45	3	0	25	410	6	4	0	11	2 lean protein
Kraft													
American, BIG Slice	1 slice	90	8	70	4.5	0	7	160	0	0	0	5	1 med-fat protein, 1 fat

Cheddar, Natural, BIG Slice	1 slice	90	8	70	5	0	8	140	0	0	0	5	1 med-fat protein, 1 fat
Cheddar, Shredded	1/4 cup	110	9	90	6	0	25	170	1	0	<1	6	1 med-fat protein, 1 fat
Cheez Whiz Cheese Dip	2 Tbsp	80	5	45	1	0	5	410	5	3	0	3	1 med-fat protein
Chipotle String Cheese	1	70	4.5	40	3	0	5	200	0	0	0	6	1 med-fat protein
Colby Jack, Natural, BIG Slice	1 slice	90	7	60	4.5	0	8	150	0	0	0	5	1 med-fat protein
Colby & Monterey Jack, Shredded	1/4 cup	110	8	80	5	0	25	180	1	0	<1	6	1 med-fat protein, 1 fat
Cracker Barrel Aged Reserved Cheddar	1 oz	110	10	90	6	0	30	180	0	0	0	6	1 med-fat protein, 1 fat
Cracker Barrel Cheddar Cheese Sticks, 2% Sharp Cheddar	1	60	4.5	40	2.5	0	15	180	<1	0	0	5	1 med-fat protein
Cracker Barrel Cheddar Cheese Sticks, Sharp Cheddar	1	90	7	70	4.5	0	20	130	0	0	0	5	1 med-fat protein, 1 fat
Cream Cheese, Chive & Onion	2 Tbsp	80	7	70	4.5	0	7	150	1	1	0	2	1 fat

CHEESE, COTTAGE CHEESE, CREAM CHEESE

	Serving	Calories	Fat (g)	Cal. from Fat	Sat. Fat (g)	Trans Fat (g)	Chol. (mg)	Sod. (mg)	Carb. (g)	Sugar (g)	Fiber (g)	Prot. (g)	Servings/Exchanges
Cream Cheese, Philadelphia Soft, Black Cherry	2 Tbsp	70	4.5	40	2.5	0	5	100	5	2	0	2	1 fat
Cream Cheese, Philadelphia Soft, Bacon	2 Tbsp	70	5	50	3	0	7	220	2	1	0	2	1 fat
Cream Cheese, Philadelphia Soft, Original	2 Tbsp	80	7	70	4.5	0	7	125	1	1	0	2	1 fat
Cream Cheese, Philadelphia Soft, Original 1/3 Less Fat	2 Tbsp	70	5	45	3.5	0	7	120	1	1	0	2	1 fat
Cream Cheese, Philadelphia Soft, Original Fat-Free	2 Tbsp	30	0	0	0	0	1	200	1	1	0	4	1 lean protein
Cream Cheese, Philadelphia Soft, Peach	2 Tbsp	70	4	40	2.5	0	5	95	5	2	0	2	1 fat
Cream Cheese, Philadelphia Soft, Strawberry	2 Tbsp	80	6	60	4	0	7	105	5	2	0	1	1 fat

Cream Cheese, Philadelphia Soft, Strawberry 1/3 Less Fat	2 Tbsp	70	4.5	40	3	0	5	115	6	2	0	2	1/2 carb, 1 fat
Cream Cheese, Philadelphia, Whipped	2 Tbsp	50	4.5	40	3	0	15	90	2	1	0	1	1 fat
DiGiorno Parmesan, Grated	2 Tbsp	20	1.5	10	1	0	1	75	0	0	0	2	free
Havarti, Natural, Sliced	1 slice	80	7	60	4	0	20	135	0	0	0	4	1 med-fat protein, 1 fat
Mexican Style Four Cheese, Shredded	1/4 cup	100	8	70	5	0	25	180	1	0	<1	6	1 med-fat protein, 1 fat
Mexican Style Taco, Finely Shredded	1/4 cup	100	8	70	5	0	25	210	1	0	<1	6	1 med-fat protein, 1 fat
Mozzarella & Cheddar Cheese Twists	1	60	4	35	2.5	0	5	140	0	0	0	6	1 med-fat protein
Mozzarella, Part-Skim, Natural, BIG Slice	1 slice	60	4	35	2.5	0	5	105	0	0	0	5	1 med-fat protein
Mozzarella, Part-Skim, Shredded	1/4 cup	90	6	50	3.5	0	15	150	1	0	<1	6	1 med-fat protein
Mozzarella String Cheese	1	80	6	50	3.5	0	7	190	0	0	0	7	1 med-fat protein

CHEESE, COTTAGE CHEESE, CREAM CHEESE

	Serving	Calories	Fat (g)	Cal. from Fat	Sat. Fat (g)	Trans Fat (g)	Chol. (mg)	Sod. (mg)	Carb. (g)	Sugar (g)	Fiber (g)	Prot. (g)	Servings/Exchanges
Parmesan, Finely Shredded	1/4 cup	110	8	70	4.5	0	25	430	<1	0	0	9	1 med-fat protein, 1 fat
Parmesan, Grated	2 tsp	20	1.5	15	1	0	<5	75	0	0	0	2	free
Pepper Jack, Natural, BIG Slice	1 slice	90	7	70	4.5	0	25	140	0	0	0	5	1 med-fat protein, 1 fat
Singles, 2% Milk American	1 slice	45	2.5	20	1.5	0	10	230	2	2	0	4	1 lean protein
Singles, American Cheese	1 slice	60	4.5	40	2.5	0	5	220	2	1	0	4	1 med-fat protein
Singles, Deli Deluxe American	1 slice	90	7	60	4	0	20	330	<1	0	0	4	1 med-fat protein, 1 fat
Singles, White American	1 slice	60	4.5	40	2.5	0	5	220	2	1	0	4	1 med-fat protein
Swiss, Aged, Natural, BIG Slice	1 slice	90	7	60	4.5	0	8	40	0	0	0	6	1 med-fat protein, 1 fat
Velveeta 2% Processed Cheese Loaf	1 oz	60	3	25	1.5	0	5	390	3	1	0	5	1 lean protein

Food	Serving												Exchanges
Velveeta Cheese Spread, Mexican, Mild or Hot	1 oz	60	4	35	2.5	0	5	400	3	1	0	4	1 med-fat protein
Velveeta Processed Cheese Loaf	1 oz	80	5	50	3.5	0	7	410	2	1	0	4	1 med-fat protein
Velveeta Slices, Original	1 slice	40	2	15	1	0	10	320	3	2	0	3	1/2 med-fat protein
Laughing Cow													
Creamy Spicy Pepper Jack	1 wedge	35	1.5	15	1	0	5	180	1	1	0	2	free
Creamy Swiss, Light	1 wedge	35	1.5	15	1	0	5	180	1	1	0	2	free
Creamy Swiss, Original	1 wedge	50	4	35	2.5	0	10	190	1	1	0	2	1 fat
Lifetime													
Cheddar, Fat-Free	1 oz	40	0	0	0	0	3	220	1	1	0	9	1 lean protein
Cheddar, with Plant Sterol	1 oz	47	1.7	15	0.5	0	3.5	200	1	<1	1	7	1 lean protein
President													
Brie	1 oz	100	9	80	4	0	20	120	0	0	0	4	1 med-fat protein, 1 fat

CHEESE, COTTAGE CHEESE, CREAM CHEESE

	Serving	Calories	Fat (g)	Cal. from Fat	Sat. Fat (g)	Trans Fat (g)	Chol. (mg)	Sod. (mg)	Carb. (g)	Sugar (g)	Fiber (g)	Prot. (g)	Servings/Exchanges
Pub Cheese, Sharp Cheddar, Spreadable	2 Tbsp	80	7	60	4.5	0	25	150	1	1	0	2	2 fat
Rondelé, Artichoke & Garlic, Spreadable Cheese	2 Tbsp	70	6	60	4	0	25	160	2	1	0	1	1 fat
Sargento Bistro Blends													
4 Cheese Italian, Shredded, Reduced Fat	1/4 cup	80	4.5	45	3	0	15	210	1	0	0	8	1 med-fat protein
Cheddar, Medium, Reduced Fat, Sliced	1 slice	60	4	35	2.5	0	15	125	0	0	0	6	1 med-fat protein
Cheddar, Sharp, Sliced	1 slice	80	7	60	4	0	20	130	0	0	0	5	1 med-fat protein
Mozzarella Natural Light String Cheese	1 piece	50	2.5	25	1.5	0	10	160	1	0	0	6	1 lean protein
Mozzarella Natural String Cheese	1 piece	80	6	50	3.5	0	15	210	1	0	0	8	1 med-fat protein
Swiss, Sliced	1 slice	70	5	45	3	0	15	35	1	0	0	5	1 med-fat protein

Food	Serving	Calories	Fat (g)	Cal. from Fat	Sat. Fat (g)	Trans Fat (g)	Chol. (mg)	Sodium (mg)	Carb. (g)	Fiber (g)	Sugar (g)	Protein (g)	Exchanges/Choices
Swiss, Ultra Thin Sliced	3 slices	120	9	80	5	0	30	65	1	0	0	9	1 med-fat protein, 1 fat
Shamrock Farms													
Cottage Cheese, Fat Free	1/2 cup	80	0	0	0	0	5	410	6	5	0	13	1/2 carb, 2 lean protein
Cottage Cheese, Lowfat 2%	1/2 cup	100	2	20	1.5	0	15	440	5	4	0	13	2 lean protein
Cottage Cheese, Traditional	1/2 cup	110	4.5	40	3.5	0	20	370	5	3	0	13	2 lean protein
Wisconsin Kaukauna													
Port Wine Spreadable Cheese with Almonds	2 Tbsp	100	7	60	3	0	15	180	5	4	0	5	1 med-fat protein, 1 fat
Spreadable Cheddar	2 Tbsp	80	6	50	3.5	0	15	160	3	3	0	4	1 med-fat protein

COMBINATION FOODS, ENTRÉES, SALADS

	Serving	Calories	Fat (g)	Cal. from Fat	Sat. Fat (g)	Trans Fat (g)	Chol. (mg)	Sod. (mg)	Carb. (g)	Sugar (g)	Fiber (g)	Prot. (g)	Servings/Exchanges
Beef Burgundy	1 cup	337	12	110	3	NA	102	725	10	3	1	36	1 carb, 5 lean protein
Beef with Macaroni & Cheese Sauce	1 cup	335	13	120	5	NA	59	982	30	4	1	30	2 carb, 3 med-fat protein
Beef Stroganoff & Noodles	1 cup	328	18	170	6	NA	74	812	22	2	2	20	1 1/2 carb, 2 med-fat protein, 1 fat
Burrito, Bean	1 medium	483	14	130	4	NA	2	1088	72	3	12	17	5 carb, 2 fat
Burrito, Beef	1 medium	574	34	310	16	NA	98	1150	36	4	2	31	2 1/2 carb, 3 med-fat protein, 3 fat
Cabbage Rolls, Beef & Rice	8 oz	115	5	45	2	NA	39	358	9	4	1	9	1/2 carb, 1 med-fat protein
Chicken à la King (from Frozen)	1 cup	428	21	200	7	NA	121	1071	40	4	1	19	2 1/2 carb, 2 med-fat protein, 2 fat
Chicken Tetrazzini	1 cup	335	14	130	5	NA	52	711	29	1	2	20	2 carb, 2 med-fat protein

Food	Serving											Exchanges
Chicken or Turkey Casserole with Noodles & White Sauce	1 cup	307	10	90	3	NA	83	710	32	5	22	2 carb, 2 med-fat protein
Chili Con Carne, with Beans & Rice	1 cup	285	6	50	2	NA	23	1030	44	4	13	3 carb, 1 med-fat protein
Chili Con Carne, without Beans	1 cup	300	18	160	6	NA	53	1044	15	3	19	1 carb, 2 med-fat protein, 1 fat
Chilies Rellenos, Cheese Filled	1	309	24	220	10	NA	164	442	9	3	15	1/2 carb, 2 med-fat protein, 3 fat
Chimichanga, Beef & Bean	1	304	14	130	4	NA	15	736	34	4	11	2 carb, 1 med-fat protein, 1 fat
Chop Suey & Noodles, Beef	1 cup	282	10	90	2	NA	48	715	25	4	24	1 1/2 carb, 3 lean protein, 1 fat
Chop Suey, Shrimp, with Noodles	1 cup	255	8	70	1	NA	143	1296	26	4	20	2 carb, 2 lean protein
Chow Mein, Beef, No Noodles	1 cup	180	6	50	2	NA	55	557	8	4	24	1/2 carb, 3 lean protein
Chow Mein, Shrimp, with Noodles	1 cup	152	4	35	1	NA	161	1219	9	4	19	1/2 carb, 2 lean protein
Corndog	1	302	15	135	4	NA	41	710	34	10	9	2 carb, 3 fat

COMBINATION FOODS, ENTRÉES, SALADS

	Serving	Calories	Fat (g)	Cal. from Fat	Sat. Fat (g)	Trans Fat (g)	Chol. (mg)	Sod. (mg)	Carb. (g)	Sugar (g)	Fiber (g)	Prot. (g)	Servings/Exchanges
Corned Beef Hash, Canned	1 cup	361	23	210	10	NA	70	906	20	1	2	19	1 carb, 2 med-fat protein, 1 fat
Curry, Beef	1 cup	248	14	130	4	NA	45	203	16	3	4	15	1 carb, 2 med-fat protein, 1 fat
Eggplant Parmesan	1 cup	313	22	200	8	NA	55	699	16	6	4	14	1 carb, 2 med-fat protein, 2 fat
Enchilada, Beans & Cheese	1	172	7	65	2	NA	8	444	22	3	5	6	1 1/2 carb, 1 fat
Enchilada, Beef & Cheese	1	154	8	70	3	NA	27	352	13	3	2	10	1 carb, 1 med-fat protein
Fajita, Chicken	1	355	14	130	4	NA	74	805	33	6	3	23	2 carb, 2 med-fat protein
Goulash, Beef, with Noodles	1 cup	354	13	120	4	NA	92	413	27	2	2	31	2 carb, 4 lean protein, 1 fat
Lasagna, with Beef	1 cup	355	13	120	6	NA	43	995	40	9	4	19	2 1/2 carb, 2 med-fat protein, 1/2 fat

Lasagna, Meatless	1 cup	325	13	120	5	NA	33	710	35	11	4	16	2 carb, 1 med-fat protein, 1 fat
Macaroni & Cheese	1 cup	336	15	135	3	NA	6	602	41	6	2	9	2 1/2 carb, 3 fat
Meat Loaf, Beef & Pork with Sauce	1 slice	206	10	90	3	NA	82	596	9	3	1	19	1/2 carb, 2 med-fat protein
Meat Tortellini	1 cup	363	14	130	5	NA	215	789	33	0	1	24	2 carb, 3 lean protein, 1 fat
Moo Goo Gai Pan	1 cup	160	5	45	1	NA	37	233	14	5	3	16	1 carb, 2 lean protein
Pepper, Stuffed Green Bell with Meat & Rice	1	261	17	155	5	NA	70	481	15	3	2	12	1 carb, 1 lean protein, 3 fat
Pizza, Cheese, Thin Crust	1/8 of 12-inch	223	10	9	5	NA	21	549	23	3	2	10	1 1/2 carb, 1 med-fat protein, 1 fat
Pizza, Meat, Thin Crust	1/8 of 12-inch	311	17	155	7	NA	45	766	23	3	2	17	1 1/2 carb, 2 med-fat protein, 1 fat
Pot Pie, Chicken or Turkey	8 oz	449	26	235	9	NA	39	924	43	5	2	11	3 carb, 5 fat
Quesadilla	1	483	24	215	11	NA	48	906	47	4	2	19	3 carb, 1 med-fat protein, 3 fat

COMBINATION FOODS, ENTRÉES, SALADS

	Serving	Calories	Fat (g)	Cal. from Fat	Sat. Fat (g)	Trans Fat (g)	Chol. (mg)	Sod. (mg)	Carb. (g)	Sugar (g)	Fiber (g)	Prot. (g)	Servings/Exchanges
Quiche Lorraine	1/8 pie	739	58	520	30	NA	298	1062	24	4	1	30	1 1/2 carb, 4 med-fat protein, 7 fat
Ravioli, Cheese with Tomato Sauce	1 cup	245	6	50	3	NA	25	615	38	9	3	10	2 1/2 carb, 1 fat
Salad, Bean, Kidney with Dressing	1/2 cup	177	8	70	1	NA	0	181	22	5	6	6	1 1/2 carb, 1 fat
Salad, Caesar	2 cups	367	31	280	6	NA	86	559	14	3	3	11	1 carb, 1 med-fat protein, 5 fat
Salad, Egg	1/2 cup	285	26	235	5	NA	341	421	1	1	0	11	2 med-fat protein, 3 fat
Salad, Potato, German Style	1/2 cup	91	3	25	1	NA	4	156	14	1	1	2	1 carb
Salad, Shrimp	1/2 cup	181	15	135	2	NA	121	632	1	1	0	10	1 med-fat protein, 2 fat
Salad, Tuna	1/2 cup	202	16	145	3	NA	28	446	3	2	2	11	2 med-fat protein, 1 fat
Salad, Waldorf	1 cup	236	19	170	3	NA	7	118	17	12	3	2	1 carb, 4 fat
Salmon Patty, Fried in Oil	1	264	16	145	3	NA	53	608	14	1	1	16	1 carb, 2 med-fat protein, 1 fat

Food	Amount												Exchanges
Shepherd's Pie, Beef	1 cup	265	8	70	2	NA	29	714	34	3	3	15	2 carb, 1 med-fat protein
Sloppy Joe, Beef, on Bun	1	432	12	110	4	NA	43	1317	61	30	2	19	4 carb, 1 med-fat protein, 1 fat
Soufflé, Cheese	1 cup	194	15	135	9	NA	137	309	6	2	0	9	1/2 carb, 1 med-fat protein, 2 fat
Soufflé, Spinach	1 cup	126	9	80	4	NA	99	171	7	3	1	6	1/2 carb, 1 med-fat protein, 1 fat
Spaghetti with Meatballs	1 cup	332	11	100	3	NA	25	662	43	6	4	14	3 carb, 1 med-fat protein, 1 fat
Sukiyaki	1 cup	151	6	50	2	NA	109	554	7	4	1	18	1/2 carb, 2 lean protein
Swedish Meatballs with Cream Sauce	1 cup	381	21	189	8	NA	153	1255	17	7	1	30	1 carb, 4 med-fat protein
Sweet & Sour Pork with Rice	1 cup	449	17	155	3	NA	85	798	49	19	2	25	3 carb, 2 med-fat protein, 1 fat
Taco, Beef with Cheese, Lettuce, Tomato	1	276	13	120	5	NA	38	722	25	1	2	14	1 1/2 carb, 1 med-fat protein, 1 fat
Tamale, with Beef	1	122	6	50	2	NA	14	331	11	0	2	5	1 carb, 1 fat

COMBINATION FOODS, ENTRÉES, SALADS

	Serving	Calories	Fat (g)	Cal. from Fat	Sat. Fat (g)	Trans Fat (g)	Chol. (mg)	Sod. (mg)	Carb. (g)	Sugar (g)	Fiber (g)	Prot. (g)	Servings/Exchanges
Tamale, Plain, Meatless	1	134	5	45	2	NA	12	199	19	5	2	3	1 carb, 1 fat
Tostada, Bean & Cheese	1	173	8	70	3	NA	7	334	21	1	4	6	1 1/2 carb, 1 fat
Tuna-Noodle Casserole	1 cup	390	17	155	3	NA	34	833	32	3	2	27	2 carb, 3 med-fat protein
Turkey-Noodle Casserole	1 cup	307	10	90	3	NA	83	710	32	5	1	22	2 carb, 2 lean protein, 1 fat
Veal Parmigiana	1 cup	410	24	220	9	NA	159	228	17	4	2	31	1 carb, 4 med-fat protein, 1 fat
BRANDS													
Armour LunchMakers													
Bologna Cracker Crunchers	1 pkg	250	14	130	5	0	30	630	21	7	<1	8	1 1/2 carb, 3 fat
Nachos	1 pkg	210	9	80	1.5	0	0	550	30	13	2	2	2 carb, 2 fat
Pepperoni Pizza	1 pkg	220	10	90	5	0	15	390	35	8	<1	8	2 carb, 2 fat
Turkey Cracker Crunchers	1 pkg	210	10	90	3.5	0	20	620	22	7	<1	8	1 1/2 carb, 2 fat

Betty Crocker

Food	Serving												
Bowl Appetite Herb Chicken Flavored Vegetable Rice	1 bowl	250	3	25	1	0	5	780	51	2	2	6	3 1/2 carb
Bowl Appetite Pasta Alfredo	1 bowl	350	9	80	3	2.5	10	860	55	7	2	11	3 1/2 carb, 1 fat
Bowl Appetite Three Cheese Rotini	1 bowl	340	7	60	2.5	2	10	1010	59	7	2	10	4 carb, 1 fat
Chicken Helper, Cheesy Enchilada (as Packaged)	1/3 cup	170	1	10	0	0	0	550	38	3	1	3	2 1/2 carb
Chicken Helper, Chicken Fried Rice (as Packaged)	1/8 cup	110	0	0	0	0	0	450	24	1	1	3	1 1/2 carb
Chicken Helper, Creamy Chicken & Noodles (as Packaged)	1/3 cup	100	0.5	5	0	0	0	560	20	1	1	3	1 carb
Chicken Helper, Fettuccine Alfredo (as Packaged)	1/3 cup	140	1.5	0.5	0	0	0	560	28	3	1	4	2 carb

COMBINATION FOODS, ENTRÉES, SALADS

	Serving	Calories	Fat (g)	Cal. from Fat	Sat. Fat (g)	Trans Fat (g)	Chol. (mg)	Sod. (mg)	Carb. (g)	Sugar (g)	Fiber (g)	Prot. (g)	Servings/Exchanges
Hamburger Helper, Bacon Cheeseburger (as Packaged)	1/3 cup	100	1	10	0	0	0	660	21	1	1	3	1 1/2 carb
Hamburger Helper, Beef Pasta (as Packaged)	1/3 cup	100	0.5	5	0	0	0	540	21	1	1	4	1 1/2 carb
Hamburger Helper, Cheddar Cheese Melt (as Packaged)	1/2 cup	100	0.5	5	0	0	0	600	20	1	1	3	1 carb
Hamburger Helper, Cheeseburger Macaroni (as Packaged)	1/4 cup	110	0.5	5	0	0	0	740	24	2	1	3	1 1/2 carb
Hamburger Helper, Double Cheesy Quesadilla (as Packaged)	1/8 cup	90	1	10	0	0	0	570	20	2	0	2	1 carb
Hamburger Helper, Lasagna (as Packaged)	1/2 cup	130	0.5	5	0	0	0	670	27	4	1	3	2 carb

Food	Serving												
Hamburger Helper, Philly Cheesesteak (as Packaged)	1/2 cup	130	2	20	1	0	0	520	25	2	1	3	1 1/2 carb
Hamburger Helper, Sloppy Joe (as Packaged)	1/3 cup	130	1	10	0	0	0	610	28	5	1	4	2 carb
Hamburger Helper, Spaghetti (as Packaged)	1/2 cup	130	1	10	0	0	0	580	28	5	1	3	2 carb
Hamburger Helper, Tomato Basil Penne (as Packaged)	1/3 cup	150	0.5	5	0	0	0	600	32	5	1	3	2 carb
Tuna Helper, Creamy Broccoli (as Packaged)	1/3 cup	130	1	10	0	0	0	520	25	2	1	5	1 1/2 carb
Tuna Helper, Fettuccine Alfredo (as Packaged)	1/2 cup	120	1	10	0	0	0	360	23	2	1	4	1 1/2 carb
Tuna Helper, Tetrazzini (as Packaged)	1/2 cup	140	1	10	0	0	0	460	28	2	1	5	2 carb
Tuna Helper, Tuna Melt (as Packaged)	1/3 cup	130	1	10	0	0	0	610	26	1	1	3	1 1/2 carb

COMBINATION FOODS, ENTRÉES, SALADS

	Serving	Calories	Fat (g)	Cal. from Fat	Sat. Fat (g)	Trans Fat (g)	Chol. (mg)	Sod. (mg)	Carb. (g)	Sugar (g)	Fiber (g)	Prot. (g)	Servings/Exchanges
Ultimate Helper, Cheddar Broccoli (as Packaged)	1/3 cup	160	4.5	40	1.5	0	0	580	25	4	1	5	1 1/2 carb, 1 fat
Ultimate Helper, Creamy Stroganoff (as Packaged)	1/3 cup	140	3.5	35	1	0	0	550	24	2	1	4	1 1/2 carb
Ultimate Helper, Southwest Chipotle Chicken (as Packaged)	1/8 cup	120	0.5	5	0	0	0	400	26	3	1	3	1 1/2 carb
Campbell's SpaghettiOs													
SpaghettiOs Original	1 cup	170	1	10	0.5	0	5	600	35	11	3	5	2 carb
SpaghettiOs with Meatballs	1 cup	230	7	60	2.5	0	35	600	31	10	3	11	2 carb, 1 med-fat protein
SpaghettiOs with Sliced Franks	1 cup	210	6	50	2	0	20	600	29	11	3	9	2 carb, 1 fat
Chef Boyardee													
Beefaroni	1 cup	250	10	90	4	0	15	730	30	6	3	9	2 carb, 2 fat

Food	Serving	Cal	Fat (g)	Cal from Fat	Sat Fat (g)	Trans Fat (g)	Chol (mg)	Sodium (mg)	Carb (g)	Fiber (g)	Sugar (g)	Protein (g)	Exchanges/Choices
Beef Ravioli	1 cup	230	7	60	2.5	0	10	870	34	5	3	7	2 carb, 1 fat
BIG BOWL Beefaroni	1 container	500	18	140	7	0	30	1460	68	12	6	18	4 1/2 carb, 1 med-fat protein, 2 fat
BIG BOWL Beef Ravioli	1 container	500	18	140	7	0	30	1440	68	12	6	18	4 1/2 carb, 1 med-fat protein, 2 fat
Healthy Choice													
Café Steamers, Beef & Broccoli	1 pkg	270	6	60	2	0	40	580	34	6	3	20	2 carb, 2 lean protein
Café Steamers, Chicken & Broccoli Alfredo	1 pkg	190	6	60	2.5	0	85	600	8	2	4	27	1/2 carb, 4 lean protein
Café Steamers, Chicken Pasta Primavera	1 pkg	220	2.5	25	0.5	0	40	390	29	8	5	20	2 carb, 2 lean protein
Café Steamers, Meatball Marinara	1 pkg	280	6	50	2	0	35	500	39	8	6	18	2 1/2 carb, 1 lean protein
Café Steamers, Pumpkin Squash Ravioli	1 pkg	260	6	50	2	0	<5	520	44	9	6	8	3 carb, 1 fat
Complete Meals, Classic Meatloaf	1 pkg	280	5	50	2	0	30	550	42	13	6	15	3 carb, 1 lean protein

COMBINATION FOODS, ENTRÉES, SALADS

	Serving	Calories	Fat (g)	Cal. from Fat	Sat. Fat (g)	Trans Fat (g)	Chol. (mg)	Sod. (mg)	Carb. (g)	Sugar (g)	Fiber (g)	Prot. (g)	Servings/Exchanges
Complete Meals, Country Fried Chicken	1 pkg	340	8	70	2	0	25	600	52	16	5	15	3 1/2 carb, 1 lean protein, 1/2 fat
Complete Meals, Four Cheese Tortellini	1 pkg	300	6	60	3	0	20	560	45	9	9	15	3 carb, 1 lean protein
Complete Meals, Pot Roast	1 pkg	260	7	60	2.5	0	45	570	32	14	4	18	2 carb, 2 lean protein
Hormel Compleats Microwave Meals													
Beef Pot Roast	1 tray	200	5	45	2	0	35	1270	22	3	2	16	1 1/2 carb, 2 lean protein
Beef Stew	1 tray	190	7	60	3	0	35	1120	21	2	2	11	1 1/2 carb, 1 lean protein, 1 fat
Chicken Alfredo	1 tray	320	16	150	4	0	40	950	29	0	3	16	2 carb, 1 med-fat protein, 2 fat
Chicken & Dumplings	1 tray	170	4	40	1.5	0	30	690	25	2	1	8	1 1/2 carb, 1 fat
Chicken & Noodles	1 tray	180	6	50	3	0	50	880	20	3	1	12	1 carb, 1 med-fat protein

Food	Serving												Exchanges/Choices
Chili with Beans	1 tray	270	8	70	3.5	0	25	990	33	8	8	17	2 carb, 2 lean protein
Meatloaf & Gravy with Mashed Potatoes	1 tray	280	12	110	5	1	40	720	27	1	3	14	2 carb, 1 med-fat protein, 1 fat
Turkey & Dressing	1 tray	290	9	80	3	0	40	990	31	4	2	20	2 carb, 2 lean protein, 1 fat
Lean Cuisine													
Chicken Fettuccini	1 pkg	280	5	45	2	0	30	600	43	3	3	16	3 carb, 1 lean protein
Meatloaf & Mashed Potatoes	1 pkg	240	7	60	3	0	45	540	25	4	3	20	1 1/2 carb, 2 lean protein
Sesame Chicken	1 pkg	330	9	80	1	0	25	650	48	15	3	14	3 carb, 1 med-fat protein
Spicy Beef & Bean Enchilada	1 pkg	300	6	50	2	0	15	680	50	9	5	11	3 carb, 1 fat
Marie Callender's													
Grilled Chicken Alfredo Bake	1 pkg	480	21	190	8	0.5	60	900	45	4	6	28	3 carb, 3 med-fat protein
Spaghetti & Meatballs	1 pkg	420	13	120	4.5	0	35	600	52	4	8	23	3 1/2 carb, 2 med-fat protein

COMBINATION FOODS, ENTRÉES, SALADS

	Serving	Calories	Fat (g)	Cal. from Fat	Sat. Fat (g)	Trans Fat (g)	Chol. (mg)	Sod. (mg)	Carb. (g)	Sugar (g)	Fiber (g)	Prot. (g)	Servings/Exchanges
Steak & Roasted Potatoes	1 pkg	350	11	100	4	0	45	930	40	4	6	22	2 1/2 carb, 2 med-fat protein
Sweet & Sour Chicken	1 pkg	560	13	120	2	0	15	500	93	33	5	16	6 carb, 2 fat
Weight Watchers Smart Ones													
Apple & Cinnamon Oatmeal	1 cup	180	2	20	0.5	0	<5	170	35	14	5	5	2 carb
Broccoli & Cheddar Roasted Potatoes	1 pkg	190	8	70	5	0	20	640	21	2	4	10	1 1/2 carb, 1 lean protein, 1 fat
Chicken Fajita	1 pkg	260	5	45	1.5	0	30	550	39	4	4	16	2 1/2 carb, 1 lean protein
English Muffin Sandwich, Egg & Cheese	1 pkg	210	5	45	3	0	10	480	28	2	2	13	2 carb, 1 lean protein
Lasagna Florentine	1 pkg	310	9	80	4.5	0	25	520	45	8	6	12	3 carb, 1 fat
Pepperoni Pizza Minis	1 tray	280	7	60	2.5	0	10	460	42	6	6	12	3 carb, 1 fat
Pulled Pork & Black Beans	1 pkg	230	4	35	1.5	0	40	480	30	12	7	19	2 carb, 2 lean protein
Three Cheese Ziti Marinara with Meatballs	1 pkg	320	10	90	4.5	0	25	690	43	3	6	14	3 carb, 1 med-fat protein

COOKING OILS, FATS

OILS

	Serving	Calories	Fat (g)	Cal. from Fat	Sat. Fat (g)	Trans Fat (g)	Chol. (mg)	Sod. (mg)	Carb. (g)	Sugar (g)	Fiber (g)	Prot. (g)	Servings/Exchanges
Avocado Oil, Chosen Foods	1 tsp	43	4.5	43	<1	0	0	0	0	0	0	0	1 fat
Canola Oil	1 tsp	40	5	40	0	0	0	0	0	0	0	0	1 fat
Coconut Oil	1 tsp	39	5	39	4	0	0	0	0	0	0	0	1 fat
Cod Liver/Fish Oil, Carlson	1 tsp	40	4.5	40	1	0	15	0	0	0	0	0	1 fat
Corn Oil	1 tsp	41	5	41	1	0	0	0	0	0	0	0	1 fat
Cottonseed Oil	1 tsp	40	5	40	1	0	0	0	0	0	0	0	1 fat
Flaxseed Oil	1 tsp	40	5	40	0	0	0	0	0	0	0	0	1 fat
Grapeseed Oil	1 tsp	40	4.5	40	<1	0	0	0	0	0	0	0	1 fat
Hazelnut Oil	1 tsp	40	4.5	40	<1	0	0	0	0	0	0	0	1 fat
Olive Oil	1 tsp	40	5	40	1	0	0	0	0	0	0	0	1 fat
Palm Oil, Red, Nutiva	1 tsp	43	4.5	40	2	0	0	0	0	0	0	0	1 fat

COOKING OILS, FATS

	Serving	Calories	Fat (g)	Cal. from Fat	Sat. Fat (g)	Trans Fat (g)	Chol. (mg)	Sod. (mg)	Carb. (g)	Sugar (g)	Fiber (g)	Prot. (g)	Servings/Exchanges
Peanut Oil	1 tsp	40	5	40	1	0	0	0	0	0	0	0	1 fat
Safflower Oil	1 tsp	40	5	40	0	0	0	0	0	0	0	0	1 fat
Sardine/Fish Oil	1 tsp	41	4.5	40	1	0	0	32	0	0	0	0	1 fat
Sesame Oil	1 tsp	40	5	40	1	0	0	0	0	0	0	0	1 fat
Soybean Oil	1 tsp	40	5	40	1	0	0	0	0	0	0	0	1 fat
Soybean & Canola Oil	1 tsp	40	5	40	1	0	0	0	0	0	0	0	1 fat
Sunflower Oil	1 tsp	40	5	40	0	0	0	0	0	0	0	0	1 fat
FATS													
Chitterlings, Cooked	1/4 cup	72	6	50	3	0	86	107	0	0	0	4	1 high-fat protein
Lard	1 tsp	39	4	35	2	0	4	0	0	0	0	0	1 fat
Salt Pork, Cooked	1-inch cube	113	12	110	4	0	13	306	0	0	0	1	2 fat
Shortening	1 Tbsp	113	13	120	3	0	0	1	0	0	0	0	3 fat

DESSERT, CAKE, PIE, CHEESECAKE, COOKIES, BROWNIES

	Serving	Calories	Fat (g)	Cal. from Fat	Sat. Fat (g)	Trans Fat (g)	Chol. (mg)	Sod. (mg)	Carb. (g)	Sugar (g)	Fiber (g)	Prot. (g)	Servings/Exchanges
Angel Food Cake	1/10 cake	146	0	0	0	0	0	291	33	17	0	3	2 carb
Apple Turnover	1	285	15	140	4	0	0	267	36	13	1	3	2 1/2 carb, 3 fat
Brownie	2-inch square	138	6	50	1	0	6	97	22	12	1	2	1 1/2 carb, 1 fat
Cake, Chocolate with Chocolate Icing	1/12 cake	387	13	120	3	0	33	481	69	52	2	4	4 1/2 carb, 3 fat
Cake, Pound, No Icing	1/10 of loaf	321	13	120	4	0	60	343	49	30	1	5	3 carb, 3 fat
Cake, Unfrosted	1/10 cake	154	7	60	2	0	1	213	22	13	0	2	1 1/2 carb, 1 fat
Cake, White with Vanilla Icing	1/12 cake	392	10	90	2	0	0	376	74	61	1	3	5 carb, 2 fat
Cake, Yellow with Chocolate Icing	1/12 cake	382	11	100	2	0	34	398	70	53	1	3	4 1/2 carb, 2 fat

DESSERT, CAKE, PIE, CHEESECAKE, COOKIES, BROWNIES

	Serving	Calories	Fat (g)	Cal. from Fat	Sat. Fat (g)	Trans Fat (g)	Chol. (mg)	Sod. (mg)	Carb. (g)	Sugar (g)	Fiber (g)	Prot. (g)	Servings/Exchanges
Cheesecake	1/12 cake	411	29	260	13	0	70	561	33	28	1	7	2 carb, 6 fat
Cobbler, Apple	1/2 cup	212	5	45	1	0	2	215	40	25	1	3	2 1/2 carb, 1 fat
Cookies, Chocolate Chip	1 (2-inch) cookie	69	4	35	2	0	8	39	8	6	0	1	1/2 carb, 1 fat
Cookies, Fortune	1	30	0	0	0	0	0	2	7	4	0	0	1/2 carb
Cookies, Gingersnaps	3 medium	150	4	35	1	0	0	180	28	7	1	2	2 carb, 1 fat
Cookies, Lady Fingers	4	121	3	25	1	0	73	49	20	8	0	4	1 carb, 1 fat
Cookies, Macaroons	1 (2-inch) cookie	97	3	30	3	0	0	59	17	17	0	1	1 carb, 1 fat
Cookies, Oatmeal	1 medium	59	2	20	1	0	0	50	9	3	0	1	1/2 carb
Cookies, Peanut Butter	1 medium	76	4	35	1	0	0	81	9	5	0	2	1/2 carb, 1 fat

	Serving												
Cookies, Sandwich with Creme Filling	2	106	4	35	1	0	0	77	16	9	0	1	1 carb, 1 fat
Cookies, Shortbread	1 (2-inch) cookie	75	4	35	1	0	3	79	10	2	0	1	1/2 carb, 1 fat
Cookies, Soft Raisin	1	64	2	20	1	0	0	67	11	8	0	1	1 carb
Cookies, Sugar	1 medium	76	3	30	1	0	8	48	11	6	0	1	1 carb, 1 fat
Cookies, Sugar-Free	3	141	7	65	2	0	0	1	20	1	2	2	1 carb, 1 fat
Cookies, Vanilla Wafers	5	88	3	30	1	0	10	78	15	8	0	1	1 carb, 1 fat
Crisp, Apple	1/2 cup	193	4	35	1	0	0	209	38	24	2	2	3 1/2 carb, 1 fat
Cupcake, Frosted	1	160	6	60	2	0	0	133	24	15	1	1	1 1/2 carb, 1 fat
Pie, Fruit, 2-Crust	1/8 pie	356	17	150	6	0	0	302	51	23	2	3	3 1/2 carb, 3 fat
Pie, Pumpkin or Custard	1/8 pie	374	15	135	3	0	40	368	54	29	3	6	3 1/2 carb, 3 fat

CAKE/PIE/CHEESECAKE

Betty Crocker

	Serving												
Angel Food Mix	1/12 pkg	140	0	0	0	0	0	320	32	23	0	3	2 carb

DESSERT, CAKE, PIE, CHEESECAKE, COOKIES, BROWNIES

	Serving	Calories	Fat (g)	Cal. from Fat	Sat. Fat (g)	Trans Fat (g)	Chol. (mg)	Sod. (mg)	Carb. (g)	Sugar (g)	Fiber (g)	Prot. (g)	Servings/Exchanges
Brownie Mix, Chocolate Fudge	1/20 pkg	100	1	10	0	0	0	80	23	15	1	1	1 1/2 carb
Brownie Mix, Low-Fat Fudge	1/18 pkg	130	2	20	1	0	0	110	27	19	1	1	2 carb
Cake Mix, Super Moist Chocolate Fudge	1/10 pkg	160	1.5	15	1	0	0	380	35	18	1	2	2 carb
Cake Mix, Super Moist French Vanilla	1/10 pkg	160	1.5	15	1	0	0	310	35	19	1	1	2 carb
Frosting, Rich & Creamy Chocolate	2 Tbsp	130	5	45	2.5	0	0	95	21	17	1	0	1 1/2 carb, 1 fat
Frosting, Whipped Cream Cheese	2 Tbsp	110	6	50	3	0	0	45	14	13	0	0	1 carb, 1 fat
Lemon Supreme Bars	1/16 pkg	130	3.5	35	1.5	1	0	80	24	17	0	1	1 1/2 carb, 1 fat
Pound Cake Mix	1/8 pkg	220	2.5	25	1.5	0.5	0	200	48	27	1	2	3 carb

Claim Jumper

Chocolate Motherlode 6-Layer Cake	1/10 cake	277	NA	NA	5.4	NA	28	147	34	NA	1	2.7	2 carb, 1 fat
Original Carrot Cake	1/6 cake	321	NA	NA	6.7	NA	50	157	30	NA	1	3	2 carb, 1 fat

Duncan Hines

Pie Filling, Cherry, No Sugar Added	1/3 cup	35	0	0	0	0	0	10	8	4	0	0	1/2 carb
Pie Filling, Country Cherry	1/3 cup	90	0	0	0	0	0	17	22	18	1	0	1 1/2 carb
Pie Filling, More Fruit, Apple	1/3 cup	90	0	0	0	0	0	27	23	20	0	0	1 1/2 carb
Pie Filling, More Fruit, Blueberry	1/3 cup	90	0	0	0	0	0	12	22	18	1.5	0	1 1/2 carb
Pie Filling, More Fruit, Cherry	1/3 cup	90	0	0	0	0	0	22	21	16	0	0	1 1/2 carb
Pie Filling, More Fruit, Peach	1/3 cup	90	0	0	0	0	0	16	21	14	0	0	1 1/2 carb

DESSERT, CAKE, PIE, CHEESECAKE, COOKIES, BROWNIES

	Serving	Calories	Fat (g)	Cal. from Fat	Sat. Fat (g)	Trans Fat (g)	Chol. (mg)	Sod. (mg)	Carb. (g)	Sugar (g)	Fiber (g)	Prot. (g)	Servings/Exchanges
Pie Filling, Premium Strawberry	1/3 cup	100	0	0	0	0	0	15	24	10	0	0	1 1/2 carb
Whipped Chocolate	3 Tbsp	140	7	60	2	2	0	70	21	17	1	1	1 1/2 carb, 1 fat
Whipped Vanilla Frosting	3 Tbsp	150	7	60	2.5	2	0	60	22	20	0	0	1 1/2 carb, 1 fat
Edwards													
Cheesecake (Single)	1 slice	290	20	180	10	0.5	70	200	24	15	<1	4	1 1/2 carb, 4 fat
Cookies & Crème	1/6 pie	470	28	250	20	2	10	310	52	35	2	5	3 1/2 carb, 6 fat
Georgia Pecan Pie	1/8 pie	470	25	230	7	0	80	260	59	23	2	4	4 carb, 5 fat
Hershey's Crème Pie	1/6 pie	450	27	240	17	0	10	320	48	34	1	5	3 carb, 5 fat
Key Lime Pie	1/8 pie	450	22	200	16	0	50	310	57	46	<1	6	4 carb, 4 fat
Lemon Meringue Pie (Single)	1 slice	250	7	60	3.5	0	35	210	41	33	<1	5	2 1/2 carb, 1 fat
Triple Coconut Crème Pie	1/8 pie	240	9	80	5	0	0	260	37	25	1	2	2 1/2 carb, 2 fat
Turtle Pie (Single)	1 slice	290	16	150	9	0	5	210	34	23	1	3	2 carb, 3 fat

Entenmann's

Item	Serving												
All Butter Loaf Cake	1/6 cake	190	8	70	4.5	0	60	230	28	16	0	2	2 carb, 2 fat
Cherry Crumb Loaf Cake	1/8 cake	180	8	70	2	0	35	220	27	16	0	2	2 carb, 2 fat
Deluxe French Cheesecake	1/6 cake	390	24	220	12	0	40	400	39	25	<1	6	2 1/2 carb, 5 fat
Fudge Chocolate Cake	1/8 cake	240	10	90	3.5	0	25	190	37	28	2	2	2 1/2 carb, 2 fat
Glazed Cinnamon Bundt Cake	1/6 cake	360	16	140	5	0	50	290	53	38	<1	3	3 1/2 carb, 3 fat
Lemon Crunch Cake	1/9 cake	330	14	130	4	0	45	300	49	35	<1	3	3 carb, 3 fat
Louisana Crunch Cake	1/9 cake	330	14	130	4	0	45	300	49	35	<1	3	3 carb, 3 fat
Marshmallow Devil's Food Iced Cake	1/8 cake	260	13	120	5	0	25	200	36	28	<1	2	2 1/2 carb, 3 fat

Hostess

Item	Serving												
Ding Dongs	2	330	17	150	12	0	5	290	43	33	1	2	3 carb, 3 fat

DESSERT, CAKE, PIE, CHEESECAKE, COOKIES, BROWNIES

	Serving	Calories	Fat (g)	Cal. from Fat	Sat. Fat (g)	Trans Fat (g)	Chol. (mg)	Sod. (mg)	Carb. (g)	Sugar (g)	Fiber (g)	Prot. (g)	Servings/Exchanges
Ho Hos	3	360	16	140	12	0	5	190	54	43	1	2	3 1/2 carb, 3 fat
Twinkies	2	260	8	80	3.5	0	35	350	43	29	0	2	3 carb, 2 fat
Marie Callender's													
Apple Crumb Cobbler	1/8 pie	330	14	130	3	3	0	180	47	26	2	3	3 carb, 3 fat
Banana Cream Pie	1/10 pie	310	17	150	9	1.5	30	190	37	22	1	3	2 1/2 carb, 3 fat
Cherry Crunch Pie	1/10 pie	360	14	130	3	3	0	200	57	35	2	2	4 carb, 3 fat
Chocolate Satin Pie	1/6 pie	580	38	340	18	4	30	330	54	33	3	5	3 1/2 carb, 7 fat
Coconut Cream Pie	1/9 pie	350	19	170	11	2	25	190	41	21	1	3	3 carb, 4 fat
Dutch Apple Pie	1/10 pie	340	14	130	3	3	0	180	51	28	2	2	3 1/2 carb, 3 fat
I Love Chocolate Cream Pie	1/8 pie	350	17	150	9	2	30	190	45	34	2	4	3 carb, 3 fat
Lattice Apple Pie	1/10 pie	340	16	140	3.5	3	0	150	46	23	2	3	3 carb, 3 fat

Lattice Peach Pie	1/10 pie	370	18	160	3.5	3.5	0	170	48	21	2	3	3 carb, 4 fat
Lemon Meringue Pie	1/10 pie	320	10	90	2.5	2	30	200	55	34	1	2	3 1/2 carb, 2 fat
Peach Cobbler	1/8 cobbler	320	17	150	3.5	3.5	0	160	41	16	2	2	3 carb, 3 fat
Razzleberry Pie	1/9 pie	370	19	170	4	3.5	0	150	46	16	4	3	3 carb, 4 fat
Turtle Pie	1/6 pie	570	35	320	15	4	30	350	59	31	3	5	4 carb, 7 fat
Pepperidge Farm													
Apple Turnover	1	260	13	110	7	0	0	230	31	11	1	4	2 carb, 3 fat
Cherry Turnover	1	260	13	110	7	0	0	230	31	10	1	4	2 carb, 3 fat
Chocolate Fudge 3-Layer Cake	1/8 cake	240	13	120	7	0	20	140	32	22	1	2	2 carb, 3 fat
Coconut 3-Layer Cake	1/8 cake	250	12	110	7	0	20	130	34	23	<1	2	2 carb, 2 fat
German Chocolate Cake	1/8 cake	240	12	110	7	0	20	160	31	21	<1	2	2 carb, 2 fat
Red Velvet 3-Layer Cake	1/8 cake	240	13	120	7	0	25	130	30	20	0	2	2 carb, 3 fat

DESSERT, CAKE, PIE, CHEESECAKE, COOKIES, BROWNIES

	Serving	Calories	Fat (g)	Cal. from Fat	Sat. Fat (g)	Trans Fat (g)	Chol. (mg)	Sod. (mg)	Carb. (g)	Sugar (g)	Fiber (g)	Prot. (g)	Servings/Exchanges
Pillsbury													
Pie Crust, Refrigerated	1/8 crust	100	6	50	2.5	0	5	130	12	0	0	1	1 carb, 1 fat
Sara Lee													
Apple Pie	1/8 pie	320	16	140	7	0	0	410	41	18	0	3	3 carb, 3 fat
Blueberry Pound Cake	1/4 cake	230	8	70	3	0	15	300	38	22	<1	3	2 1/2 carb, 2 fat
Cherry Pie	1/8 pie	330	16	150	7	0	0	350	43	15	0	3	3 carb, 3 fat
Chocolate New York Style Cheesecake	1/6 cake	500	29	260	14	1	100	450	55	39	3	7	3 1/2 carb, 6 fat
Original Cream Cheese-cake	1/4 cake	340	18	160	8	3	75	260	38	27	<1	8	2 1/2 carb, 4 fat
Original Cream Cheese-cake, Strawberry	1/4 cake	330	12	110	4.5	2.5	50	260	51	35	2	6	3 1/2 carb, 2 fat
Pound Cake	1/4 cake	140	16	140	9	9	119	229	35	20	<1	4	2 1/2 carb, 3 fat

Weight Watchers Smart Ones

Food	Serving												
Chocolate Chip Cookie Dough Sundae	1	140	3	30	1	0	5	60	26	16	0	2	1 1/2 carb, 1 fat
Mixed Berry Smoothie	1 cup	120	0.5	5	0	0	<5	70	25	18	4	6	1 1/2 carb
Peanut Butter Cup Sundae	1	130	3	25	1.5	0	<5	55	23	13	<1	2	1 1/2 carb, 1 fat
Strawberry Shortcake	1	120	4	35	2	0	25	210	19	12	<1	2	1 carb, 1 fat

COOKIES/BROWNIES

Archway

Food	Serving												
Cashew Nougat	3	160	10	90	4	0	0	55	18	10	0	2	1 carb, 2 fat
Chocolate Chip	1	140	7	60	3.5	0	5	85	21	11	<1	1	1 1/2 carb, 1 fat
Coconut Macaroon	2	160	7	60	6	0	0	65	24	19	<1	1	1 1/2 carb, 1 fat
Frosty Lemon	1	110	4.5	40	1.5	0	0	80	17	9	0	1	1 carb, 1 fat
Ginger Snap	5	150	5	45	1	0	0	105	24	10	<1	1	1 1/2 carb, 1 fat
Iced Oatmeal	1	140	4	35	1.5	0	0	95	24	14	<1	1	1 1/2 carb, 1 fat
Oatmeal	1	150	5	45	2	0	5	100	24	11	<1	2	1 1/2 carb, 1 fat
Windmill	2	200	8	70	3	0	0	180	30	13	1	3	2 carb, 2 fat

DESSERT, CAKE, PIE, CHEESECAKE, COOKIES, BROWNIES

	Serving	Calories	Fat (g)	Cal. from Fat	Sat. Fat (g)	Trans Fat (g)	Chol. (mg)	Sod. (mg)	Carb. (g)	Sugar (g)	Fiber (g)	Prot. (g)	Servings/Exchanges
Duncan Hines													
Chewy Fudge Brownies	1/20 pkg	180	8	70	1.5	0	20	105	24	16	1	2	1 1/2 carb, 2 fat
El Mexicano													
Animalitos	1/4 cup	130	1	10	0.5	0	0	85	28	2	<1	3	2 carb
Candelas	6	135	5.5	50	1.8	0.7	0	100	19	2	<1	2	1 carb, 1 fat
Cremi Nieves	5	140	7	60	3.5	0	0	25	20	12	0	1	1 carb, 1 fat
Rico Coco	5	140	4	40	1.3	0.8	0	160	22	2	<1	3	1 1/2 carb, 1 fat
Famous Amos													
Chocolate Chip	4	150	7	60	3	0	<5	105	20	9	<1	1	1 carb, 1 fat
Chocolate Chip & Pecans	4	150	8	70	3	0	0	105	18	9	<1	2	1 carb, 2 fat
Fifty50													
Butter	4	190	9	80	6	0	30	50	24	9	<1	2	1 1/2 carb, 2 fat
Chocolate Chip	4	170	9	80	2.5	0	0	35	22	7	1	2	1 1/2 carb, 2 fat

Coconut	4	170	8	80	2	0	0	45	23	8	1	2	1 1/2 carb, 2 fat
Hearty Oatmeal	4	160	7	60	1.5	0	0	60	24	9	1	2	1 1/2 carb, 1 fat

Gamesa

Chokis	3	140	6	60	4	0	0	130	21	11	1	2	1 1/2 carb, 1 fat
Sandwich Créme Cookies, Chocolate	3	160	6	60	3.5	0	0	130	23	11	1	2	1 1/2 carb, 1 fat
Sandwich Créme Cookies, Limon/Lime	3	140	5	45	2.5	0	0	150	23	10	1	2	1 1/2 carb, 1 fat
Vanilla Wafers	3	170	8	80	6.5	0	0	25	23	14	0	1	1 1/2 carb, 2 fat

Girl Scout

Do-Si-Dos	3	160	7	70	2	0	0	100	22	11	1	3	1 1/2 carb, 1 fat
Rah-Rah Raisins	2	120	5	45	2	0	0	135	17	7	<1	1	1 carb, 1 fat
Samoas	2	140	8	70	5	0	0	60	18	10	1	1	1 carb, 2 fat
Savannah Smiles	5	140	5	45	1.5	0	0	125	23	10	0	1	1 1/2 carb, 1 fat
Tagalongs	2	140	9	80	5	0	0	95	13	8	<1	2	1 carb, 2 fat
Thin Mints	4	160	8	70	5	0	0	125	22	10	<1	1	1 1/2 carb, 2 fat
Toffee-tastic	2	140	7	70	4	0	0	90	19	7	0	0	1 carb, 1 fat

DESSERT, CAKE, PIE, CHEESECAKE, COOKIES, BROWNIES

	Serving	Calories	Fat (g)	Cal. from Fat	Sat. Fat (g)	Trans Fat (g)	Chol. (mg)	Sod. (mg)	Carb. (g)	Sugar (g)	Fiber (g)	Prot. (g)	Servings/Exchanges
Trefoils	5	170	7	60	2.5	0	0	110	22	7	0	2	1 1/2 carb, 1 fat
Kashi													
Chocolate Almond Butter	1	130	5	45	1	0	0	80	19	7	3	3	1 carb, 1 fat
Oatmeal Dark Chocolate	1	130	5	45	1	0	0	65	20	8	4	2	1 carb, 1 fat
Oatmeal Raisin Flax	1	120	4.5	40	0	0	0	70	20	7	4	2	1 carb, 1 fat
Keebler													
Chips Deluxe	2	160	8	80	3.5	0	<5	105	19	9	<1	2	1 carb, 2 fat
Chips Deluxe Chocolate Lovers	2	170	9	80	4	0	<5	120	20	11	<1	2	1 carb, 2 fat
Chips Deluxe Coconut	2	160	9	80	4	0	0	90	18	9	1	2	1 carb, 2 fat
Chips Deluxe with Peanut Butter Cups	2	170	9	80	4	0	0	90	19	10	<1	2	1 carb, 2 fat
Chips Deluxe Soft 'N Chewy	2	140	6	60	2.5	0	0	110	21	9	<1	1	1 1/2 carb, 1 fat
E.L. Fudge Original	2	180	7	70	2.5	0	<5	100	25	12	<1	2	1 1/2 carb, 1 fat

E.L. Fudge Double Stuffed Sandwich	2	180	9	80	3.5	0	<5	95	24	13	1	2	1 1/2 carb, 2 fat
Fudge Shoppe Deluxe Grahams	3	140	7	60	4.5	0	0	70	18	10	<1	1	1 carb, 1 fat
Fudge Shoppe Fudge Sticks	3	150	8	70	5	0	0	40	20	15	<1	<1	1 carb, 2 fat
Fudge Shoppe Fudge Stripes	2	140	6	60	4	0	0	75	19	9	<1	1	1 carb, 1 fat
Fudge Shoppe Grasshopper	4	140	7	60	5	0	0	75	20	12	<1	1	1 carb, 1 fat
Sandies Dark Chocolate Almond	2	170	10	90	3.5	0	0	95	19	8	<1	2	1 carb, 2 fat
Sandies Pecan Shortbread	2	170	10	90	3	0	<5	110	18	7	<1	2	1 carb, 2 fat
Sandies Simply Shortbread	2	160	9	80	4	0	10	90	19	7	0	2	1 carb, 2 fat
Soft Batch Chocolate Chip	2	150	7	60	3	0	0	115	21	12	<1	1	1 1/2 carb, 1 fat
Soft Batch Country Style Oatmeal with Raisins	2	140	6	50	2	0	0	100	19	8	<1	2	1 carb, 1 fat

DESSERT, CAKE, PIE, CHEESECAKE, COOKIES, BROWNIES

	Serving	Calories	Fat (g)	Cal. from Fat	Sat. Fat (g)	Trans Fat (g)	Chol. (mg)	Sod. (mg)	Carb. (g)	Sugar (g)	Fiber (g)	Prot. (g)	Servings/Exchanges
Vienna Fingers Crème Filled	2	150	6	50	2	0	0	95	23	10	<1	1	1 1/2 carb, 1 fat
Vienna Fingers Reduced Fat	2	140	4.5	40	1.5	0	0	115	24	12	<1	1	1 1/2 carb, 1 fat
Mother's													
Chocolate Chip Minis	4	150	7	60	2.5	0	10	160	20	10	<1	2	1 carb, 1 fat
Circus Animals	7	150	7	70	7	0	0	55	21	13	0	1	1 1/2 carb, 1 fat
Coconut Cocadas	5	160	8	70	3.5	1.5	<5	140	21	13	1	2	1 1/2 carb, 2 fat
Double Fudge Sandwich	2	190	8	80	3	0	0	100	27	13	1	2	2 carb, 2 fat
English Tea Sandwich	2	190	8	80	3	0	0	100	28	13	0	2	2 carb, 2 fat
Iced Oatmeal	4	150	6	50	2	0	0	160	23	12	<1	1	1 1/2 carb, 1 fat
Taffy Sandwich	2	190	9	80	4.5	0	0	125	28	16	<1	1	2 carb, 2 fat
Vanilla Crème	2	190	8	80	3	0	0	110	28	13	0	2	2 carb, 2 fat
Murray Sugar Free													
Chocolate Chip	3	150	9	80	3.5	0	<5	135	20	0	2	2	1 carb, 2 fat

Chocolate Sandwich	3	130	7	60	2.5	0	0	95	19	0	1	1	1 carb, 1 fat
Creme Sandwich	3	130	6	60	2	0	0	55	20	0	<1	1	1 carb, 1 fat
Dark Fudge Dipped Wafers	4	120	7	60	2.5	0	0	30	19	0	5	1	1 carb, 1 fat
Oatmeal	3	140	7	70	2.5	0	0	130	21	0	3	2	1 1/2 carb, 1 fat
Peanut Butter	3	150	9	80	2.5	0	<5	130	16	0	1	3	1 carb, 2 fat
Shortbread	8	130	5	50	1.5	0	0	140	22	0	2	2	1 1/2 carb, 1 fat
Vanilla Wafers	4	130	8	70	2.5	0	0	20	19	0	4	<1	1 carb, 2 fat
Little Debbie													
Boston Crème Rolls	1	270	12	110	5	0	15	140	40	26	0	1	2 1/2 carb, 2 fat
Chocolate Marshmallow Pies	1	180	7	60	4	0	0	105	28	15	0	2	2 carb, 1 fat
Fancy Cakes	2	300	14	130	8	0	0	130	46	32	0	1	3 carb, 3 fat
Fudge Brownies	1	280	12	110	5	0	10	150	40	21	1	3	2 1/2 carb, 2 fat
Oatmeal Crème Pie	1	170	7	60	3	0	0	150	26	12	<1	1	1 1/2 carb, 1 fat
Nabisco													
Barnum's Animals	14	120	3.5	30	0.5	0	0	85	23	7	1	2	1 1/2 carb, 1 fat

DESSERT, CAKE, PIE, CHEESECAKE, COOKIES, BROWNIES

	Serving	Calories	Fat (g)	Cal. from Fat	Sat. Fat (g)	Trans Fat (g)	Chol. (mg)	Sod. (mg)	Carb. (g)	Sugar (g)	Fiber (g)	Prot. (g)	Servings/Exchanges
Chips Ahoy! Chewy Chocolate Chip	2	140	6	60	3	0	0	95	21	12	1	1	1 1/2 carb, 1 fat
Chips Ahoy! Chewy Chocolate Chip & Oatmeal	2	140	6	50	3	0	0	170	20	9	1	2	1 carb, 1 fat
Chips Ahoy! Chunky Chocolate	1	80	4	35	1.5	0	0	55	10	5	0	1	1/2 carb, 1 fat
Chips Ahoy! Chunky White Fudge	1	80	4	35	1.5	0	0	55	11	6	0	1	1 carb, 1 fat
Chips Ahoy! Original Chocolate Chip	3	160	8	70	2.5	0	0	NA	22	11	1	1	1 1/2 carb, 2 fat
Chips Ahoy! Reese's Peanut Butter	3	160	9	80	4.5	0	0	85	18	9	1	2	1 carb, 2 fat
Lorna Doone Shortbread	6	210	10	90	2	0	0	220	28	8	1	2	2 carb, 2 fat
Mallomars	2	120	5	45	3	0	0	40	18	2	1	1	1 carb, 1 fat
Newtons, Fig	2	110	2	20	0	0	0	110	22	12	2	1	1 1/2 carb

Food	Amount											Exchanges
Newtons, Fig 100% Whole Grain	2	100	1.5	15	0	0	105	21	12	3	1	1 1/2 carb
Newtons, Fig Fat Free	2	100	0	0	0	0	95	24	13	2	1	1 1/2 carb
Newtons Fruit Thins Cranberry Citrus Oat	3	140	5	45	1	0	95	22	7	1	2	1 1/2 carb, 1 fat
Nilla Wafers, Mini	1 oz	140	6	50	1.5	5	115	21	11	0	1	1 1/2 carb, 1 fat
Nilla Wafers, Original	1 oz	140	6	50	1.5	5	115	21	11	0	1	1 1/2 carb, 1 fat
Nilla Wafers, Reduced Fat	1 oz	120	1.5	15	0	0	NA	24	12	0	1	1 1/2 carb
Nutter Butter	1 oz	160	9	80	2.5	0	85	18	8	1	4	1 carb, 2 fat
Nutter Butter Bites	1 oz	140	6	50	1.5	0	120	21	9	1	2	1 1/2 carb, 1 fat
Oreo, Double Stuf Chocolate	2	140	7	60	2	0	90	21	13	1	1	1 1/2 carb, 1 fat
Oreo, Fudge Crèmes	3	180	9	80	5	0	70	24	19	1	1	1 1/2 carb, 2 fat
Oreo, Golden Original	3	160	7	60	2	0	NA	25	12	0	1	1 1/2 carb, 1 fat
Oreo Minis	9	130	6	50	2	0	140	21	11	1	1	1 1/2 carb, 1 fat
Oreo, Original	4	160	7	60	2	0	170	28	13	1	1	2 carb, 1 fat
Oreo Thins, Chocolate	4	140	6	50	2	0	95	21	12	1	1	1 1/2 carb, 1 fat

DESSERT, CAKE, PIE, CHEESECAKE, COOKIES, BROWNIES

	Serving	Calories	Fat (g)	Cal. from Fat	Sat. Fat (g)	Trans Fat (g)	Chol. (mg)	Sod. (mg)	Carb. (g)	Sugar (g)	Fiber (g)	Prot. (g)	Servings/Exchanges
Teddy Grahams Chocolate	24	130	4	35	0.5	0	0	115	22	8	2	2	1 1/2 carb, 1 fat
Teddy Grahams Honey	24	130	4	35	0.5	0	0	100	23	8	2	2	1 1/2 carb, 1 fat
Pepperidge Farm													
Bordeaux	4	130	5	50	3.5	0	10	95	19	12	<1	2	1 carb, 1 fat
Brussels	3	150	7	60	4	0	5	65	20	11	1	2	1 carb, 1 fat
Chessmen	3	120	5	45	3	0	20	80	18	5	<1	2	1 carb, 1 fat
Dessert Shop, Chocolate Brownie Cookie, Soft Baked	1	140	6	50	3	0	10	90	21	11	1	2	1 1/2 carb, 1 fat
Dessert Shop, S'Mores, Soft Baked	1	140	6	60	3	0	10	70	19	10	0	2	1 carb, 1 fat
Geneva	3	160	9	80	4	0	0	95	19	8	1	2	1 carb, 2 fat
Gingerman	4	130	3.5	35	1.5	0	10	90	22	13	<1	1	1 1/2 carb, 1 fat
Maui Milk Chocolate Coconut Almond	1	130	7	60	4	0	10	60	16	9	<1	1	1 carb, 1 fat

Milano, Dark Chocolate	3	180	9	80	4	0	5	60	22	11	1	2	1 1/2 carb, 2 fat
Milano Melts, Boston Cream Pie	2	150	8	70	2.5	0	0	45	18	12	<1	1	1 carb, 2 fat
Milano, Raspberry	2	130	7	60	4.5	0	<5	40	16	8	<1	1	1 carb, 1 fat
Milano Slices, Toffee Cookies	3	150	7	70	3.5	0	<5	75	19	10	<1	1	1 carb, 1 fat
Nantucket Dark Chocolate	1	130	6	50	3	0	10	75	18	9	<1	1	1 carb, 1 fat
Sausalito Milk Chocolate Macadamia	1	130	7	60	3.5	0	10	75	17	9	0	1	1 carb, 1 fat
Shortbread	2	130	6	60	4	0	20	105	17	6	<1	1	1 carb, 1 fat
Soft Baked Montauk Milk Chocolate	1	140	6	50	3	0	10	75	22	10	0	1	1 1/2 carb, 1 fat
Soft Baked Mystic Sugar	1	140	5	45	2	0	10	100	22	9	1	2	1 1/2 carb, 1 fat
Soft Baked Santa Cruz Oatmeal Raisin	1	130	4.5	40	1.5	0	<5	90	23	13	2	2	1 1/2 carb, 1 fat
Tahiti	2	170	10	90	6	0	5	40	17	8	2	2	1 carb, 2 fat

DESSERT, CAKE, PIE, CHEESECAKE, COOKIES, BROWNIES

	Serving	Calories	Fat (g)	Cal. from Fat	Sat. Fat (g)	Trans Fat (g)	Chol. (mg)	Sod. (mg)	Carb. (g)	Sugar (g)	Fiber (g)	Prot. (g)	Servings/Exchanges
Pillsbury													
Milk Chocolate Chip Cookies	1 1/2-inch ball of dough	130	6	50	2.5	0	5	90	18	11	1	1	1 carb, 1 fat
Peanut Butter Cookies	1 1/2-inch ball of dough	120	5	45	1.5	0	5	130	17	10	0	1	1 carb, 1 fat
Sugar Cookies	1/2-inch slice	120	5	45	1.5	0	5	95	18	11	0	1	1 carb, 1 fat
SnackWell's													
Cookie Cakes, Chocolate Mint, Fat Free	1	60	0	0	0	0	0	30	14	9	0	1	1 carb
Cookie Cakes, Devil's Food, Fat Free	1	50	0	0	0	0	0	25	12	7	0	1	1 carb

Crème Sandwich	1 pack	210	6	50	2	0	0	250	38	20	1	2	2 1/2 carb, 1 fat
Dark Chocolate Mocha Biscuit Thins, Whole Grain	1 pack	200	8	70	1	0	15	210	26	8	3	6	1 1/2 carb, 2 fat
French Vanilla Latte Biscuit Thins, Whole Grain	1 pack	210	8	80	1	0	15	220	26	8	3	6	1 1/2 carb, 2 fat
Mini Fudge Dipped Pretzels	1 pack	100	3.5	35	3	0	0	160	16	7	<1	1	1 carb, 1 fat

DIPS, SPREADS, SALSA

	Serving	Calories	Fat (g)	Cal. from Fat	Sat. Fat (g)	Trans Fat (g)	Chol. (mg)	Sod. (mg)	Carb. (g)	Sugar (g)	Fiber (g)	Prot. (g)	Servings/Exchanges
Alouette													
Le Bon Dip, All Varieties	2 Tbsp	45–50	2.5–3	25	1.5–2	0	10	120–150	2–3	1	0–1	2	1 fat
Soft Spreadable Cheese, All Varieties	2 Tbsp	60–80	5–8	50–70	3.5–4.5	0	15–25	105–160	1–2	<1	0	1	1 fat
Athenos													
Hummus, All Varieties	2 Tbsp	45–60	3–4.5	35–40	0–0.5	0	0	90–170	4–5	0	1–2	1–2	1 fat
Dean's													
French Onion, Ranch, Sriracha, Bacon & Horseradish, Creamy Dill, and Veggie Flavors	2 Tbsp	50–60	4–5	40–45	2–3	0	0	170–300	2–3	2	0	1	1 fat
Guacamole Flavored Dips, All	2 Tbsp	80–90	9	80	2.5	0	<5	170–180	2	1	0	1	2 fat
Skinny Dip Light French Onion	2 Tbsp	35	2	15	1	0	10	210	3	2	0	1	1/2 fat

Fritos

French Onion Dip	2 Tbsp	60	5	45	0.5	0	<5	240	3	1	<1	<1	1 fat
Hot Bean Dip	2 Tbsp	35	1	10	0	0	0	230	5	0	2	2	free
Jalapeño Cheddar Flavor Cheese Dip	2 Tbsp	40	2.5	25	0	0	0	220	3	<1	0	<1	1/2 fat
Original Flavor Bean Dip	2 Tbsp	35	1	10	0	0	0	190	5	0	2	2	free

Guiltless Gourmet

Mild or Spicy Black Bean Dip	2 Tbsp	40	0	0	0	0	0	125	7	0	2	2	1/2 carb

Herdez

Salsa Casera	2 tsp	10	0	0	0	0	0	220	2	1	0	0	free
Salsa Verde	2 tsp	10	0	0	0	0	0	310	1	0	0	0	free

Kaukauna/Wisconsin

Port Wine Cheese Spread	2 Tbsp	100	7	60	3	0	15	180	5	4	0	5	1 med-fat protein, 1 fat
Sharp Cheddar Log	2 Tbsp	100	7	60	3.5	0	20	180	4	4	0	5	1 med-fat protein, 1 fat
Sharp & Swiss Log	2 Tbsp	100	7	60	3.5	0	20	180	4	4	0	5	1 med-fat protein, 1 fat
Spreadable Cheddar	2 Tbsp	80	6	50	3.5	0	15	160	3	3	0	4	1 med-fat protein

DIPS, SPREADS, SALSA

	Serving	Calories	Fat (g)	Cal. from Fat	Sat. Fat (g)	Trans Fat (g)	Chol. (mg)	Sod. (mg)	Carb. (g)	Sugar (g)	Fiber (g)	Prot. (g)	Servings/Exchanges
Kraft													
Bacon & Cheddar Dip	2 Tbsp	60	4.5	40	3	0	1	180	1	1	0	1	1 fat
Cheez Whiz Spread	2 Tbsp	90	7	60	4	0	0	540	13	2	0	5	1 carb, 1 fat
Creamy Ranch Dip	2 Tbsp	60	4.5	40	3	0	0	280	1	1	0	1	1 fat
French Onion Dip	2 Tbsp	60	4.5	40	3	0	0	210	1	1	0	1	1 fat
Green Onion Dip	2 Tbsp	60	4.5	40	3	0	0	170	1	1	0	1	1 fat
Old English Sharp Cheddar Spread	2 Tbsp	90	8	70	4.5	0	8	520	0	0	0	5	1 med-fat protein, 1 fat
Pimento Spread	2 Tbsp	80	6	60	4	0	7	160	2	1	0	2	1 fat
Pineapple Cheese Spread	2 Tbsp	70	5	45	3.5	0	7	105	4	1	0	2	1 fat
Roka Blue Cheese Spread	2 Tbsp	80	7	60	4	0	8	340	1	2	0	3	1 fat
La Victoria													
Salsa (All Varieties)	1 oz	10–15	0	0	0	0	0	110–260	2–3	1–1	0–1	0	free

Litehouse

Caramel Dip	2 Tbsp	130	4.5	40	4	0	0	65	21	16	0	1	1 1/2 carb, 1 fat
Caramel Dip, Low Fat	2 Tbsp	100	2	15	2	0	0	80	23	12	3	1	1 1/2 carb
Chipotle Ranch Greek Yogurt Dip	2 Tbsp	60	5	45	0	0	5	300	2	1	0	2	1 fat
Chocolate Dip	1.4 oz	100	1.5	15	0	0	0	45	25	16	4	0	1 1/2 carb
Cream Cheese Dip	2 Tbsp	90	4.5	40	2	0	10	120	11	10	0	1	1 carb, 1 fat
Cucumber Dill Greek Yogurt Dip	2 Tbsp	50	4	40	0	0	5	150	3	1	0	2	1 fat
Dilly Dip	2 Tbsp	150	16	140	2	0	15	200	1	1	0	1	3 fat
Garden Ranch Dip	2 Tbsp	120	13	110	1.5	0	15	170	1	1	0	0	3 fat
Lite Ranch Dip	2 Tbsp	50	3	30	0	0	0	220	5	1	0	0	1 fat
Salsa, Medium	2 Tbsp	10	0	0	0	0	0	210	2	2	0	0	free
Vanilla Almond Greek Yogurt Dip	2 Tbsp	60	1.5	10	0	0	0	10	11	8	0	1	1 carb

Maria's Dip

Creamy Dill	2 Tbsp	100	10	90	3	0	15	140	2	1	0	1	2 fat

DIPS, SPREADS, SALSA

	Serving	Calories	Fat (g)	Cal. from Fat	Sat. Fat (g)	Trans Fat (g)	Chol. (mg)	Sod. (mg)	Carb. (g)	Sugar (g)	Fiber (g)	Prot. (g)	Servings/Exchanges
Guacamole Dip	2 Tbsp	40	3	30	1.5	0	5	140	3	1	1	1	1 fat
Honey Vanilla Cream	2 Tbsp	60	4	40	2.5	0	15	20	5	4	0	1	1 fat
Lite Buttermilk Ranch	2 Tbsp	60	5	45	1.5	0	10	230	3	2	0	1	1 fat
Roasted French Onion	2 Tbsp	100	10	90	3	0	15	220	2	1	0	1	2 fat
Spinach Parmesan	2 Tbsp	90	9	80	3	0	15	200	2	1	0	2	2 fat
Newman's Own													
Black Bean & Corn Salsa	2 Tbsp	20	0	0	0	0	0	140	5	1	2	1	free
Hot Salsa	2 Tbsp	10	0	0	0	0	0	150	3	1	<1	0	free
Mango Salsa	2 Tbsp	25	0	0	0	0	0	200	6	5	<1	0	1/2 carb
Tequila Lime Salsa	2 Tbsp	15	0	0	0	0	0	170	3	2	<1	0	free
Old El Paso													
Cheese 'n Salsa	2 Tbsp	40	3	25	1	0	0	210	3	0	0	<1	1 fat
Thick n' Chunky Salsa	2 Tbsp	10	0	0	0	0	0	200	2	1	0	0	free

Ortega

	Serving												
Black Bean & Corn Salsa	2 Tbsp	15	0	0	0	0	0	180	3	1	1	1	free
Guacamole Style Dip	2 Tbsp	45	3	25	0	0	0	190	4	1	0	1	1 fat
Thick & Chunky Salsa	2 Tbsp	10	0	0	0	0	0	170	2	<1	0	0	free

Pace

	Serving												
Chunky Salsa	2 Tbsp	10	0	0	0	0	0	230	<1	2	0	0	free
Fire Roasted Tomato & Corn	2 Tbsp	10	0	0	0	0	0	110	2	1	1	0	free
Mango & Habanero Fire Salsa	2 Tbsp	10	0	0	0	0	0	140	2	1	<1	0	free
Salsa Con Queso	2 Tbsp	40	3	25	1	0	5	270	3	1	0	0	1 fat

Rojos Salsa

	Serving												
Homestyle Salsa	2 Tbsp	5	0	0	0	0	0	115	2	0	0	0	free

Rondelé

	Serving												
Chipotle & Tomato Spreadable Cheese	2 Tbsp	70	6	50	4	0	25	140	1	1	0	1	1 fat

DIPS, SPREADS, SALSA

	Serving	Calories	Fat (g)	Cal. from Fat	Sat. Fat (g)	Trans Fat (g)	Chol. (mg)	Sod. (mg)	Carb. (g)	Sugar (g)	Fiber (g)	Prot. (g)	Servings/Exchanges
Garlic & Herb Spreadable Cheese	2 Tbsp	70	7	60	4.5	0	30	135	1	0	0	2	1 fat
Lite Garlic & Herbs Spreadable Cheese	2 Tbsp	45	3.5	30	2	0	15	135	2	0	0	2	1 fat
Ruffles													
Creamy Buffalo	2 Tbsp	50	5	45	0	0	<5	230	1	0	0	<1	1 fat
T. Marzetti													
Blue Cheese Veggie Dip	2 Tbsp	150	15	140	3	0	15	210	1	1	0	1	3 fat
Chocolate Fruit Dip	2 Tbsp	110	1	10	0	0	0	85	25	16	1	1	1 1/2 carb
Cream Cheese Fruit Dip	2 Tbsp	70	3	30	2	0	15	85	10	8	0	0	1/2 carb, 1 fat
Dill Veggie Dip	2 Tbsp	110	12	110	3	0	20	180	2	1	0	1	2 fat
Fat Free Ranch Veggie Dip	2 Tbsp	30	0	0	0	0	0	270	6	2	0	1	1/2 carb
French Onion Veggie Dip	2 Tbsp	120	11	100	3	0	20	180	3	1	0	1	2 fat

Greek Yogurt Dip, Roasted Red Pepper	2 Tbsp	60	4.5	45	1.5	0	15	190	2	1	0	2	1 fat
Hummus Veggie Dip & Spread	2 Tbsp	60	4.5	40	0	0	0	140	3	0	1	1	1 fat
Light Caramel Apple Dip	2 Tbsp	120	1.5	15	1	0	5	80	27	16	1	1	2 carb
Light French Vanilla Yogurt Dip	2 Tbsp	45	0	0	0	0	0	50	10	10	0	1	1/2 carb
Light Ranch Veggie Dip	2 Tbsp	60	5	45	1	0	5	200	4	2	0	1	1 fat
Ranch Veggie Dip	2 Tbsp	110	12	100	3	0	20	200	2	1	0	1	2 fat
Spinach Veggie Dip	2 Tbsp	110	12	110	3	0	20	220	2	1	0	1	2 fat
Tostitos													
Chunky Salsa	2 Tbsp	10	0	0	0	0	0	250	2	2	<1	0	free
Creamy Spinach Dip	2 Tbsp	50	4	35	0	0	0	200	2	<1	<1	<1	1 fat
Salsa Con Queso	2 Tbsp	40	2.5	25	1	0	<5	280	5	<1	<1	<1	1 fat

EGGS, EGG DISHES, EGG PRODUCTS

	Serving	Calories	Fat (g)	Cal. from Fat	Sat. Fat (g)	Trans Fat (g)	Chol. (mg)	Sod. (mg)	Carb. (g)	Sugar (g)	Fiber (g)	Prot. (g)	Servings/Exchanges
1-Egg Omelet, Plain	1	82	5	45	2	0	221	161	1	1	0	7	1 med-fat protein
1-Egg Omelet, Spanish	1	114	6	50	2	0	247	183	6	4	1	9	1/2 carb, 1 med-fat protein
1-Egg Omelet with Cheese	1	136	10	90	4	0	240	364	2	2	0	10	1 med-fat protein, 1 fat
1-Egg Omelet with Chorizo	1	192	15	135	5	0	219	464	2	1	0	13	2 med-fat protein, 1 fat
1-Egg Omelet with Ham & Cheese	1	150	11	100	4	0	217	474	2	2	0	12	2 med-fat protein
1-Egg Omelet with Mushroom	1	109	8	70	2	0	188	212	2	1	0	7	1 med-fat protein
1-Egg Omelet with Potatoes & Onions	1	132	6	50	2	0	233	370	12	3	1	8	1 carb, 1 med-fat protein
1-Egg Omelet with Sausage	1	182	14	120	4	0	252	380	1	0	0	13	2 med-fat protein, 1 fat
1-Egg White Omelet, Plain	1	27	1	10	0	0	1	111	1	1	0	4	1 lean protein

Food	Serving												Exchange
Deviled Egg	1/2 egg & filling	61	5	45	1	0	106	133	0	0		4	1 med-fat protein
Egg, Boiled/Cooked	1 extra large	89	6	55	2	0	245	161	1	1		7	1 med-fat protein
Egg, Boiled/Cooked	1 jumbo	100	7	65	2	0	274	181	1	1		8	1 med-fat protein
Egg, Boiled/Cooked	1 large	77	5	45	2	0	211	139	1	1		6	1 med-fat protein
Egg, Boiled/Cooked	1 medium	68	5	45	1	0	186	122	0	0		6	1 med-fat protein
Egg, Boiled/Cooked	1 small	57	4	35	1	0	156	103	0	0		5	1 med-fat protein
Egg, Fried in Margarine	1 large	92	7	65	2	0	207	174	0	0		6	1 high-fat protein
Egg, Scrambled, Cooked with Margarine	1	92	7	65	2	0	207	174	0	0		6	1 high-fat protein
Egg Substitute, Cooked with Nonstick Spray	1/2 cup	39	0	0	0	0	0	234	2	2		8	1 lean protein
Egg Whites	2	32	0	0	0	0	0	211	0	0		7	1 lean protein
Soufflé, Cheese	1 cup	194	15	135	9	0	137	309	6	2		9	1 med-fat protein, 2 fat
Soufflé, Spinach	1 cup	126	9	80	4	0	99	171	7	3	1	6	1 med-fat protein, 1 fat

EGGS, EGG DISHES, EGG PRODUCTS

	Serving	Calories	Fat (g)	Cal. from Fat	Sat. Fat (g)	Trans Fat (g)	Chol. (mg)	Sod. (mg)	Carb. (g)	Sugar (g)	Fiber (g)	Prot. (g)	Servings/Exchanges
BRANDS													
Conagra													
Egg Beaters, 100% Egg Whites	3 Tbsp	10	0	0	0	0	0	75	1	0	0	5	1 lean protein
Egg Beaters, Original	3 Tbsp	25	0	0	0	0	0	90	<1	0	0	5	1 lean protein
Egg Beaters. Southwestern	3 Tbsp	20	0	0	0	0	0	125	<1	0	0	4	1 lean protein
Crystal Farms													
All Whites	3 Tbsp	25	0	0	0	0	0	75	0	0	0	5	1 lean protein
Better'n Eggs	1/4 cup	30	0	0	0	0	0	120	1	0	0	6	1 lean protein

ETHNIC FOODS

	Serving	Calories	Fat (g)	Cal. from Fat	Sat. Fat (g)	Trans Fat (g)	Chol. (mg)	Sod. (mg)	Carb. (g)	Sugar (g)	Fiber (g)	Prot. (g)	Servings/Exchanges
ALASKA NATIVE													
Beach Asparagus	1 cup	15	<1	0	NA	0	0	23	2	NA	NA	1	free
Caribou, Cooked	1 oz	47	1	10	0	0	31	63	0	0	0	8	1 lean protein
Dried Fish/King Salmon	1 oz	113	4	35	1	0	41	66	0	0	0	18	3 lean protein
Fiddlehead Fern, Raw	1 cup	34	<1	0	NA	0	0	84	5	NA	NA	3	1 vegetable
Gumboots/Leathery Chiton	2 oz	47	<1	0	NA	0	NA	NA	0	NA	0	10	1 lean protein
Halibut, Cooked	1 oz	31	0	0	0	0	16	115	0	0	0	6	1 lean protein
Herring Eggs, Plain	1/2 cup	48	<1	0	NA	0	NA	52	4	NA	0	8	1 lean protein
Highbush Cranberries	1 1/4 cups	58	0	0	0	0	0	3	15	5	6	0	1 carb
Hooligan, Smoked	1 oz	86	7	65	NA	0	NA	NA	0	NA	0	6	1 high-fat protein
Huckleberries	1 cup	83	0	0	0	0	0	1	21	14	3	1	1 1/2 carb
Moose, Cooked	1 oz	38	0	0	0	0	22	65	0	0	0	8	1 lean protein

ETHNIC FOODS

	Serving	Calories	Fat (g)	Cal. from Fat	Sat. Fat (g)	Trans Fat (g)	Chol. (mg)	Sod. (mg)	Carb. (g)	Sugar (g)	Fiber (g)	Prot. (g)	Servings/Exchanges
Muktuk with Skin and Fat	1 x 1 x 2 inches	138	12	110	NA	0	NA	NA	0	NA	0	8	1 med-fat protein, 1 fat
Muskrat, Cooked	1 oz	67	3	25	0	0	34	27	0	NA	0	9	1 lean protein
Pike, Cooked	1 oz	38	1	10	0	0	13	98	0	0	0	6	1 lean protein
Pilot Bread	3	71	0	0	0	0	0	0	15	0	1	2	1 carb
Salmonberries	1 1/2 cups	55	<1	0	NA	0	0	52	13	NA	NA	1	1 carb
Salmon, Sockeye, Cooked	1 oz	41	1	10	0	0	18	115	0	0	0	7	1 lean protein
Seal Meat, Raw	1 oz	41	<1	0	<1	0	NA	NA	0	NA	0	9	1 lean protein
Seal Oil	1 tsp	45	5	45	<1	0	8	NA	0	NA	0	0	1 fat
Seaweed, Dried Black	1 cup	45	1	0	0	0	0	86	8	0	1	5	1/2 carb, 1 lean protein
Sour Dock, Cooked	1/2 cup	19	<1	0	NA	0	0	NA	4	NA	NA	1	1 vegetable
Venison, Cooked	1 oz	54	1	10	0	0	32	76	0	0	0	10	1 lean protein
Walrus, Raw	1 oz	56	4	35	<1	0	22	NA	0	NA	0	5	1 lean protein

Food	Serving											Exchanges/Choices
Whale, Bonehead, Raw	1 oz	37	<1	0	0	NA	17	0	NA	0	7	1 lean protein
Willow Greens, Cooked	1/2 cup	28	<1	NA	0	0	NA	6	NA	NA	2	1/2 carb
CAJUN & CREOLE												
Alligator, Cooked	1 oz	42	0.5	<1	0	19	22	0	NA	0	9	1 lean protein
Beef Tasso	1 oz	47	1	0.5	0	12	NA	0	NA	0	8	1 lean protein
Café au Lait	8 oz	76	4	3	0	17	59	6	NA	0	4	1/2 carb, 1 fat
Couche-Couche, No Fat Added	1/2 cup	82	<1	NA	0	0	4	17	NA	1	3	1 carb
Cracklins	1/4 cup	106	8	3	0	23	383	0	0	0	8	1 med-fat protein, 1 fat
Crawfish, Cooked	2 oz	46	0.5	<1	0	81	107	0	NA	0	10	1 lean protein
Cushaw Squash	1/2 cup	41	0.5	<1	0	0	2	9	NA	3	1	1/2 carb
Dewberries/Blackberries	3/4 cup	60	<1	0	0	0	0	15	NA	6	<1	1 carb
Dove, Cooked	1	235	14	4	0	129	243	0	0	0	7	1 med-fat protein, 2 fat
Frog Legs, Steamed	1 oz	26	0	0	0	18	110	0	0	0	6	1 lean protein
Goat, Baked or Roasted	1 oz	40	1	0	0	21	116	0	0	0	8	1 lean protein
Guinea, Flesh Only, Cooked	3 oz	94	2	0.5	0	63	59	0	0	0	18	3 lean protein
Hogshead Cheese	1/4 cup	77	6	2	0	29	455	0	NA	0	6	1 med-fat protein

ETHNIC FOODS

	Serving	Calories	Fat (g)	Cal. from Fat	Sat. Fat (g)	Trans Fat (g)	Chol. (mg)	Sod. (mg)	Carb. (g)	Sugar (g)	Fiber (g)	Prot. (g)	Servings/Exchanges
Kumquats	5	67	1	10	0	0	0	10	15	9	6	2	1 carb
Lamb, Cooked	1 oz	89	6	55	3	0	28	113	0	0	0	7	1 med-fat protein
Mirliton/Chayote, Cooked	1/2 cup	19	0.5	5	0	0	0	1	4	1.5	2	<1	1 vegetable
Muscadines (Scuppernongs)	17	60	0.5	5	0	0	0	2	15	NA	<1	<1	1 carb
Passionfruit (Maypops)	3	52	0	0	0	0	0	15	13	6	6	1	1 carb
Peas, Crowder, Purple Hull	1/2 cup	99	0.5	5	<1	0	0	3	18	2.8	5.6	7	1 carb
Persimmons (Japanese)	1	118	0	0	0	0	0	2	31	21	6	1	2 carb
Pickled Pigs Feet	1 foot	122	9	80	3	0	72	823	0	0	0	10	1 med-fat protein, 1 fat
Pork Sausage, Cooked	1 oz	95	8	70	3	0	24	210	0	0	0	5	1 med-fat protein, 1 fat
Pumpkin, Cooked	1/2 cup	25	0	0	0	0	0	1	6	1	1	1	1/2 carb
Remoulade Sauce	1 Tbsp	52	6	50	2	0	7	54	<1	NA	0	<1	1 fat
Salt Pork or Fatback	1-inch cube	113	12	110	4	0	13	306	0	0	0	1	2 fat
Satsuma/Mandarin	2 small	62	0	0	0	0	0	1	16	NA	1	<1	1 carb

Shrimp, Dried	1/2 cup	48	1	0	0	121	419	0	0	10	1 lean protein
Smoked Beef Sausage	1 oz	92	8	3	15	319	1	1	0	3	2 fat
Smoked Pork Sausage	1 (4-inch link)	209	19	6	41	562	0	1	0	8	1 med-fat protein, 3 fat
Tongue, Beef, Cooked	1 oz	79	6	2	37	108	0	0	0	5	1 med-fat protein
Tripe, Cooked	2 oz	50	2	1	71	247	0	0	0	7	1 lean protein
Turtle, Cooked	3 oz	76	0.5	<1	42	58	0	0	0	17	2 lean protein
CHINESE AMERICAN											
Amaranth/Chinese Spinach, Cooked	1/2 cup	14	<1	0	0	14	3	NA	NA	1	1 vegetable
Amaranth/Chinese Spinach, Raw	1 cup	6	<1	0	0	6	1	NA	NA	<1	1 vegetable
Arrowheads/Fresh Corn, Large	1	25	<1	NA	NA	6	5	NA	NA	1	1 vegetable
Baby Corn, Canned	1/2 cup	13	<1	0	0	730	2	NA	NA	2	1 vegetable
Bamboo Shoots, Canned	1/2 cup	17	0	0	0	145	2	2	<1	2	1 vegetable
Beef Jerky	1 oz	116	7	3	14	590	3	2.5	<1	9	1 med-fat protein

ETHNIC FOODS

	Serving	Calories	Fat (g)	Cal. from Fat	Sat. Fat (g)	Trans Fat (g)	Chol. (mg)	Sod. (mg)	Carb. (g)	Sugar (g)	Fiber (g)	Prot. (g)	Servings/Exchanges
Beef Tongue	1 oz	79	6	55	2	0	37	108	0	0	0	5	1 med-fat protein
Bitter Melon/Bitter Gourd/Balsam-Pear Pods	1 cup	24	0	0	0	0	0	7	5	2	2	1	1 vegetable
Bok Choy/Chinese Cabbage/Pak Choi	1 cup, raw	9	0	0	0	0	0	46	2	1	1	1	1 vegetable
Carambola/Star Fruit, Medium	2	56	1	10	0	0	0	4	12	7	5	2	1 carb
Cellophane/Mung Bean Noodles, Cooked	1 cup	160	0	0	0	0	0	10	39	0	0	0	2 1/2 carb
Cha Shu Bun, Frozen, Steamed	2	360	13	115	5	0	20	410	50	NA	1	8	2 carb, 3 fat
Chayote, Raw	1 cup	25	0	0	0	0	0	3	6	2	2	1	1/2 carb
Chinese Banana	1 small	45	0	0	0	0	0	1	11	6	1	1	1 carb
Chinese Celery, Raw	1 cup	26	<1	0	0	0	0	116	5	NA	0	2	1 vegetable

Food	Serving	Calories											Exchanges/Choices
Chinese Eggplant, Purple, Cooked	1/2 cup	17	<1	0	NA	0	0	NA	4	NA	2	<1	1 vegetable
Chinese Eggplant, White, Cooked	1/2 cup	20	<1	0	NA	0	0	NA	5	NA	2	<1	1 vegetable
Chinese Sausage	1 oz	100	8	70	3	NA	NA	246	2	NA	NA	6	1 high-fat protein
Chinese/Black Mushrooms, Medium, Dried	2	21	<1	0	0	0	0	1	5	NA	<1	<1	1 vegetable
Chinese/Peking/Pe-Tsai/Napa Cabbage, Raw	1 cup	12	<1	0	0	0	0	1	3	NA	<1	<1	1 vegetable
Choy Sum/Chinese Flowering Cabbage	1 cup	9	NA	NA	NA	0	0	NA	2	NA	NA	1	1 vegetable
Coconut Milk	1 Tbsp	35	4	<1	35	3	0	2	1	1	0	0	1 fat
Coriander, Raw	1 cup	4	<1	0	0	0	0	7	<1	<1	<1	<1	free
Dried Mung Beans/Green Beans, Cooked	1/2 cup	112	0	0	0	0	0	15	20	2	5	8	1 carb, 1 lean protein
Dried Red Beans, Cooked	1/3 cup	99	<1	0	0	0	0	6	19	NA	1	6	1 carb, 1 lean protein
Garland Chrysanthemum, Raw	1 cup	4	0	0	NA	0	NA	13	1	NA	NA	<1	free

ETHNIC FOODS

	Serving	Calories	Fat (g)	Cal. from Fat	Sat. Fat (g)	Trans Fat (g)	Chol. (mg)	Sod. (mg)	Carb. (g)	Sugar (g)	Fiber (g)	Prot. (g)	Servings/Exchanges
Ginger Root, Raw	1/4 cup	19	0	0	0	0	0	3	4	0	0	0	free
Gingko Seeds, Canned	1/2 cup	86	1	10	<1	0	0	238	17	NA	7	2	1 carb
Guava, Medium	1/2 cup	56	1	0	0	0	0	2	12	7	4	2	1 carb
Hairy Melon/Hairy Cucumber, Raw	1 cup	22	NA	NA	NA	0	NA	NA	5	NA	2	1	1 vegetable
Kumquat, Medium	5	67	1	10	0	0	0	10	15	6	6	2	1 carb
Leeks, Raw	1 cup	0	0	0	0	0	0	18	13	3	2	1	1 carb
Litchi/Lychee, Canned	1/2 cup	119	0	0	0	0	0	1	30	29	1	1	2 carb
Litchi/Lychee, Raw	1 cup	125	1	10	0	0	0	1	31	29	2	2	2 carb
Longan, Canned	3/4 cup	68	<1	0	NA	0	0	54	18	NA	NA	<1	1 carb
Longan, Raw	30	58	<1	0	0	0	0	0	15	NA	1	1	1 carb
Lotus Root	1 cup	79	0	0	0	0	0	54	19	1	4	2	1 carb
Luffa (Chinese Okra), Cooked	1 cup	39	0	0	0	0	0	11	8	4	4	3	1 carb
Mango, Small	1	124	1	10	0	0	0	2	31	28	3	2	2 carb

Food	Serving												Exchange
Moon Cake, Plain Lotus Seed Paste	1 small	169	2	20	0	0	22	44	34	18	1	3	2 carb
Mung Bean Sprouts, Seed Attached, Raw	1 cup	21	0	0	0	0	0	4	4	3	1	2	1 vegetable
Mustard Greens, Cooked	1/2 cup	21	0	0	0	0	0	22	3	0	3	3	1 1/2 carb
Oriental Radish/Daikon, Cooked	1 cup	28	0	0	0	0	0	31	6	4	2	1	1/2 carb
Papaya, Medium	1 large	163	1	10	0	0	0	30	41	30	6	2	3 carb
Peapods/Sugar Peas, Cooked	1/2 cup	34	0	0	0	0	0	3	6	3	2	3	1/2 carb
Pepper, Chili, Raw	1 cup	60	0	0	0	0	0	12	14	8	2	3	1 carb
Persimmon	1	118	0	0	0	0	0	2	31	21	6	1	2 carb
Pummelo	3/4 cup	58	<1	0	NA	0	0	1	14	NA	<1	1	1 carb
Rice Noodles, Fresh	1/2 cup	86	0	0	0	0	0	3	19	0	1	1	1 carb
Rice Vermicelli, Cooked	1/2 cup	56	0	0	0	0	0	NA	13	NA	NA	1	1 carb
Salted Duck Egg	1	146	11	100	3	0	698	345	1	1	0	10	1 med-fat protein, 1 fat
Scallop, Dried, Large	1	44	<1	0	NA	0	0	NA	1	NA	NA	9	1 lean protein
Sesame Paste	1 Tbsp	95	9	80	1	0	0	18	3	0	1	3	2 fat

ETHNIC FOODS

	Serving	Calories	Fat (g)	Cal. from Fat	Sat. Fat (g)	Trans Fat (g)	Chol. (mg)	Sod. (mg)	Carb. (g)	Sugar (g)	Fiber (g)	Prot. (g)	Servings/Exchanges
Sesame Seeds, Whole, Dried	1 Tbsp	53	5	45	1	0	0	4	2	0	2	2	1 fat
Shrimp, Dried	1/2 cup	48	1	10	0	0	121	419	0	0	0	10	1 lean protein
Soybean Milk, Unsweetened	1 cup	108	4	35	1	0	0	115	12	8	0	6	1 carb, 1 lean protein
Soybean Sprouts, Raw	1 cup	21	0	0	0	0	0	4	4	3	1	2	1 vegetable
Soybeans, Cooked	1/2 cup	155	8	70	1	0	0	1	9	3	5	15	1/2 carb, 2 lean protein, 1 fat
Squid, Raw	2 oz	52	<1	0	<1	0	132	26	2	NA	0	9	1 lean protein
Straw Mushrooms, Canned	1/2 cup	20	<1	0	NA	0	0	172	4	NA	NA	2	1 vegetable
Sweet Rice Dough Ball	3	220	10	90	6	NA	0	0	29	NA	1	3	2 carb, 2 fat
Taro, Cooked	1/2 cup	95	0	0	0	0	0	314	22	0	3	1	1 1/2 carb
Tofu/Soybean Curd	4 oz (1/2 cup)	78	5	45	1	NA	0	13	2	1	1	10	1 med-fat protein

Tripe, Beef, Raw	2 oz	56	2	20	1	0	54	26	0	NA	0	8	1 lean protein
Turnip, Raw	1 cup	36	0	0	0	0	0	87	8	5	2	1	1/2 carb
Water Chestnuts, Chinese	1/2 cup	40	0	0	0	0	0	6	10	2	2	1	1 carb
Watercress, Raw	1 cup	4	0	0	0	0	0	14	0	0	0	1	free
Winter Melon/Wax Gourd/Chinese Preserving Melon	1 cup	25	0	0	0	0	0	592	5	2	2	1	1 vegetable
Won Ton, Meatless	5	181	11	100	2	0	17	441	13	3	1	8	1 carb, 1 med-fat protein, 1 fat
Yardlong Beans, Cooked	1/2 cup	24	<1	0	0	0	0	2	5	NA	NA	1	1 vegetable
Yardlong Beans, Raw	1 cup	43	<1	0	<1	0	0	4	8	NA	NA	3	1 vegetable
FILIPINO AMERICAN													
Bamboo Shoots, Canned	1/2 cup	17	0	0	0	0	0	145	2	2	<1	2	1 vegetable
Banana, Native, Small	1	46	<1	0	<1	0	0	0	12	NA	<1	<1	1 carb
Banana Sauce	1 tsp	11	NA	NA	NA	0	0	NA	3	NA	0	0	free
Banana Squash, Cooked	1/2 cup	24	<1	0	<1	0	0	2	6	NA	1	<1	1 vegetable

ETHNIC FOODS

	Serving	Calories	Fat (g)	Cal. from Fat	Sat. Fat (g)	Trans Fat (g)	Chol. (mg)	Sod. (mg)	Carb. (g)	Sugar (g)	Fiber (g)	Prot. (g)	Servings/Exchanges
Beef Shank, Lean, Cooked	1 oz	57	2	20	<1	0	22	18	0	NA	0	10	1 lean protein
Beef Tongue	1 oz	79	6	55	2	0	37	108	0	0	0	5	1 med-fat protein
Bitter Melon, Cooked	1 cup	24	0	0	0	0	0	7	5	2	2	1	1 vegetable
Bottle Gourd, Cooked	1/2 cup	9	<1	0	NA	0	0	NA	2	NA	<1	<1	free
Cassava Tuber, Cooked	1 cup	213	0	0	0	0	0	18	51	2	2	2	3 1/2 carb
Ceylon Moss Bar, Dried	1/4	8	0	0	0	0	0	3	2	NA	<1	<1	free
Chayote, Cooked	1/2 cup	19	<1	0	0	0	0	1	4	NA	<1	<1	1 vegetable
Chicken Gizzard, Raw	1 oz	25	0	0	0	0	61	9	0	0	0	5	1 lean protein
Chinese Celery, Raw	1 cup	32	2	20	NA	0	NA	48	5	NA	<1	3	1 vegetable
Chinese Sausage	1 oz	100	8	70	3	NA	30	249	2	NA	NA	6	1 med-fat protein, 1 fat
Chinese Spinach, Raw	1 cup	7	<1	0	<1	0	0	5	1	NA	NA	<1	free
Clam, Cooked	3 or 1 oz	48	1	10	0	0	17	430	2	0	0	8	1 lean protein
Coconut Milk	1 Tbsp	35	4	35	3	0	0	2	1	1	0	0	1 fat

Corned Beef, Canned	1 oz	71	4	35	2	0	24	254	0	0	0	8	1 med-fat protein
Cracklings, Crushed	2 Tbsp	42	3	25	<1	0	9	3	0	1	0	4	1 fat
Fish Sauce	1 Tbsp	6	0	0	0	0	0	1320	1	1	0	1	free
Guava, Raw	1 1/2	61	<1	0	<1	0	0	3	14	NA	7	1	1 carb
Horseradish Leaves, Cooked	1/2 cup	13	<1	0	NA	0	0	2	2	NA	NA	1	1 vegetable
Indian Sardines, Dried	1 oz	115	7	60	1	0	44	65	0	0	0	13	2 lean protein, 1 fat
Jicama, Raw	1 cup	49	0	0	0	0	0	5	11	2	6	1	1 carb
Long-Jawed Anchovy, Dried	2 Tbsp	64	1	10	NA	0	NA	26	0	NA	0	12	1 lean protein
Mung Bean Noodles, Cooked	1 cup	224	1	10	0	0	0	30	40	4	11	15	1 carb, 2 lean protein
Mung Beans, Cooked	1/4 cup	83	4	35	1	0	0	111	9	1	4	3	1/2 carb, 1 fat
Native Sausage, Raw	1 oz	167	17	155	NA	NA	NA	NA	<1	NA	0	3	3 fat
Oriental Radish/Daikon, Cooked	1 cup	28	0	0	0	0	0	31	6	4	2	1	1/2 carb
Oyster, Cooked, Medium	3 oz	86	3	25	1	0	67	428	5	1	0	10	1 lean protein
Papaya, Unripe, Cooked	1/2 cup	20	<1	0	NA	0	0	3	5	NA	<1	1	1 vegetable

ETHNIC FOODS

	Serving	Calories	Fat (g)	Cal. from Fat	Sat. Fat (g)	Trans Fat (g)	Chol. (mg)	Sod. (mg)	Carb. (g)	Sugar (g)	Fiber (g)	Prot. (g)	Servings/Exchanges
Papaya, Yellow, Raw, Cubed	1 cup	54	<1	0	<1	0	0	4	14	NA	2	<1	1 carb
Peapods, Cooked	1/2 cup	34	0	0	0	0	0	3	6	3	1	3	1/2 carb
Plantain, Cooked, Sliced	1/2 cup	89	0	0	0	0	0	4	24	11	2	1	1 1/2 carb
Pummelo	3/4 cup	62	<1	0	NA	0	0	0	15	NA	2	1	1 carb
Rice Noodles, Fresh	1/2 cup	86	0	0	0	0	0	3	19	0	1	1	1 carb
Sausage, Simulated	1 oz	72	5	45	<1	NA	0	251	3	NA	0	5	1 med-fat protein
Sesame Seeds, Whole, Dried	1 Tbsp	53	5	45	1	0	0	4	2	0	2	2	1 fat
Shrimp, Fermented, Small	1 Tbsp	12	<1	0	<1	0	0	734	0	NA	<1	3	free
Spanish Sausage	1 oz	125	11	100	4	NA	30	367	NA	NA	0	7	1 med-fat protein, 1 fat
Swamp Cabbage, Cooked	1/2 cup	9	<1	0	NA	0	0	63	<1	NA	<1	1	free
Taro, Cooked	1/2 cup	95	0	0	0	0	0	314	22	0	3	1	1 1/2 carb

Food	Serving												Exchanges
Tofu/Soybean Curd	4 oz (1/2 cup)	78	5	45	1	NA	0	13	2	1	1	10	1 med-fat protein
Watermelon Seeds, Dried	1 Tbsp	38	3	25	<1	0	0	6	1	NA	<1	2	1 fat
Yardlong Beans, Cooked	1/2 cup	24	<1	0	<1	0	0	2	5	NA	NA	1	1 vegetable
HMONG													
Asian Pear	1	51	<1	0	0	0	0	0	13	NA	4	<1	1 carb
Bamboo Shoots, Canned	1/2 cup	17	0	0	0	0	0	145	2	2	<1	2	1 vegetable
Beef Tallow	1 tsp	39	4	35	2	NA	5	0	0	NA	0	0	1 fat
Bitter Melon, Raw	1 cup	16	<1	0	0	0	0	5	3	NA	3	<1	1 vegetable
Cellophane/Mung Bean Noodles, Cooked	1 cup	160	0	0	0	0	0	10	39	0	0	0	2 1/2 carb
Chicken Fat	1 tsp	39	4	35	1	0	4	0	0	NA	0	0	1 fat
Chitterlings, Boiled	1/4 cup	72	6	50	3	0	86	107	6	3	2	3	1 fat
Coconut Cream, Canned	1 Tbsp	66	3	30	3	0	0	7	10	10	0	0	1/2 carb, 1 fat
Coconut Milk	1 Tbsp	35	4	35	3	0	0	2	1	1	0	0	1 fat
Coconut Milk, Raw	1 Tbsp	35	4	35	3	0	0	2	<1	NA	<1	<1	1 fat
Coconut, Raw	2 Tbsp	35	3	25	3	0	0	2	2	NA	<1	<1	1 fat

ETHNIC FOODS

	Serving	Calories	Fat (g)	Cal. from Fat	Sat. Fat (g)	Trans Fat (g)	Chol. (mg)	Sod. (mg)	Carb. (g)	Sugar (g)	Fiber (g)	Prot. (g)	Servings/Exchanges
Condensed Milk, Sweetened	2 Tbsp	123	3	25	2	0	13	49	21	21	0	3	1 1/2 carb
Coriander/Chinese Parsley, Raw	1 cup	3	<1	0	0	0	0	4	<1	NA	<1	<1	free
Cucuzzi Squash, Cooked	1/2 cup	23	<1	0	0	0	0	14	5	NA	1	<1	1 vegetable
Fish Sauce	1 Tbsp	6	0	0	0	0	0	1320	1	1	0	1	free
Guava, Medium	1	37	1	10	0	0	0	1	8	5	3	1	1/2 carb
Jackfruit	1/2 cup	78	<1	0	0	0	0	2	20	NA	1	1	1 carb
Leeks, Cooked	1/2 cup	16	<1	0	0	0	0	6	4	NA	NA	<1	1 vegetable
Luffa (Chinese Okra), Cooked	1 cup	39	0	0	0	0	0	11	8	4	4	3	1 carb
Mango, Small	1	124	1	10	0	0	0	2	31	28	3	2	2 carb
Mung Bean Sprouts, Cooked	1/2 cup	13	<1	0	0	0	0	6	3	NA	<1	1	1 vegetable
Mustard Greens, Cooked	1/2 cup	21	0	0	0	0	0	22	3	0	3	3	1 1/2 carb

Food	Serving												Exchanges/Choices
Papaya, Medium	1 large	163	1	10	0	0	0	30			6	2	3 carb
Peapods, Cooked	1/2 cup	34	0	0	0	0	0	3		3	1	3	1/2 carb
Peas, Podded, Raw	1/2 cup	26	<1	0	0	0	0	3		NA	2	2	1 vegetable
Pheasant, No Skin, Raw	1 breast	302	15	135	5	0	113	260	0	0	0	41	6 lean protein, fat
Pig's Feet	1 foot	205	14	120	4	0	92	344	0	0	0	19	3 med-fat protein
Pork, Ground	1 oz	84	6	55	2	0	26	112	0	0	0	7	1 med-fat protein
Pork Lard	1 tsp	39	4	35	2	NA	4	0	0	0	0	0	1 fat
Pumpkin Blossom, Cooked	1 cup	20	<1	0	0	0	0	8	4	NA	1	2	free
Pumpkin, Cooked	1/2 cup	42	0	0	0	0	0	191	10	4	4	1	1/2 carb
Rice Noodles, Fresh	1/2 cup	86	0	0	0	0	0	3	19	0	1	1	1 carb
Squirrel, Roasted	1/2 cup	120	3	25	0	0	84	197	0	0	0	21	3 lean protein
Tofu/Soybean Curd	4 oz (1/2 cup)	78	5	45	1	NA	0	13	2	1	1	10	1 med-fat protein
Venison, Cooked	1 oz	54	1	10	0	0	32	76	0	0	0	10	1 lean protein
Vinespinach, Raw	1 cup	11	<1	0	0	0	0	13	2	NA	0	1	free
Yardlong Beans, Cooked	1/2 cup	102	<1	0	0	0	0	4	18	NA	NA	7	1 carb, 1 lean protein

ETHNIC FOODS

	Serving	Calories	Fat (g)	Cal. from Fat	Sat. Fat (g)	Trans Fat (g)	Chol. (mg)	Sod. (mg)	Carb. (g)	Sugar (g)	Fiber (g)	Prot. (g)	Servings/Exchanges
INDIAN & PAKISTANI													
Aviyal	1/2 cup	81	2	20	1	0	NA	412	14	NA	NA	2	1 carb
Brinjal, Cooked	1/2 cup	13	0	0	0	0	0	1	3	NA	1	0	1 vegetable
Chai Masala	1/2 cup	14	0	0	0	0	0	0	3	NA	NA	1	free
Chicken Tikka	3 (1-inch) pieces	54	2	20	<1	0	23	156	0	NA	0	9	1 lean protein
Coconut, Fresh Shredded	3 Tbsp	53	5	45	4	0	0	3	2	NA	1	1	1 fat
Coriander, Fresh	1/2 cup	2	0	0	0	0	0	2	0	NA	<1	0	free
Cucumber Raita	1/2 cup	21	0	0	0	0	0	22	3	NA	NA	1	1 vegetable
Dhansak	1/2 cup	104	4	35	0.5	0	NA	137	15	NA	NA	4	1 carb, 1 fat
Dhokla, Khaman	1-inch square	104	5	45	0	0	NA	539	12	NA	NA	5	1 carb, 1 fat
Ghee	1 tsp	45	5	45	3	0	20	0	0	NA	0	0	1 fat
Ginger, Fresh	1/4 cup	17	<1	0	0	0	0	3	4	NA	0.5	0	free

Food	Serving												
Green Plantain, Cooked	1/3 cup	60	<1	0	0	0	0	3	16	NA	1	0	1 carb
Guava, Medium, Raw	1 1/2	61	<1	0	<1	0	0	3	14	NA	7	1	1 carb
Idli	1 (3-inch) idli	70	0	0	0	0	0	12	12	NA	NA	2	1 carb
Jheera Pani	1/2 cup	16	0.5	5	0.5	0	NA	104	3	NA	NA	1	free
Karela, Cooked	1/2 cup	12	0	0	0	0	0	4	3	NA	1	1	1 vegetable
Lassi	1 cup	90	0	0	0	0	4	128	13	NA	0	10	1 carb
Mango, Small, Raw	1/2	68	<1	0	0	0	0	2	18	NA	2	1	1 carb
Matki Usal	1/2 cup	104	6	55	4	0	0	192	10	NA	NA	3	1 carb, 1 fat
Mung Bean Sprouts, Cooked	1/2 cup	13	<1	0	0	0	0	6	3	NA	0.5	1	1/2 carb
Mung Dhal, Cooked	1/2 cup	107	<1	0	<1	0	0	2	19	NA	8	7	1 carb, 1 lean protein
Naan	1/4 of 8 x 2-inch naan	75	2	20	<1	0	9	90	13	NA	<1	2	1 carb
Okra, Cooked	1/2 cup	34	<1	0	0	0	0	3	8	NA	3	2	1/2 carb
Paneer	1 oz	103	3	25	2	0	NA	246	12	NA	0	8	1 carb

ETHNIC FOODS

	Serving	Calories	Fat (g)	Cal. from Fat	Sat. Fat (g)	Trans Fat (g)	Chol. (mg)	Sod. (mg)	Carb. (g)	Sugar (g)	Fiber (g)	Prot. (g)	Servings/Exchanges
Pesarattu	1 (9-inch) pesarattu	127	5	45	1	0	NA	372	14	NA	NA	5	1 carb, 1 fat
Phulka/Chappathi	1 (6-inch)	68	<1	0	<1	0	0	179	15	NA	2	3	1 carb
Poha	1/2 cup	140	6	55	1	0	NA	405	18	NA	NA	2	1 carb, 1 fat
Puri	1 (5-inch) puri	128	7	65	<1	0	0	1	16	NA	2	3	1 carb, 1 fat
Rasam	1 cup	22	1	10	<1	0	NA	255	2	NA	NA	1	free
Sambar	1/2 cup	88	1	10	0	0	NA	263	16	NA	NA	5	1 carb, 1 fat
Tandoori Chicken	1 oz	75	4	35	1	0	NA	152	2	NA	NA	8	1 med-fat protein
Tomato, Dhal	1/2 cup	132	3	25	2	0	NA	262	18	NA	NA	7	1 carb, 1 lean protein
Toor Dhal, Cooked	1/2 cup	103	<1	0	<1	0	0	4	20	NA	5	6	1 carb, 1 lean protein
JEWISH													
Bagel	1/2	78	<1	0	<1	0	0	151	15	NA	<1	3	1 carb

Food	Serving												Exchanges
Beef Brisket	1 oz	52	2	20	<1	0	16	28	1	NA	0	6	1 lean protein
Beef Tongue	1 oz	80	6	55	3	0	30	17	<1	NA	0	6	1 med-fat protein
Bialy	1/2	69	0	0	0	0	0	167	16	NA	1	7	1 carb
Blintzes	2.25 oz	80	2	20	<1	0	118	135	13	NA	0	6	1 carb
Borscht	1/2 cup	26	<1	0	<1	0	0	473	5	NA	1	2	1 vegetable
Bourekas	1/2 pie	114	11	100	5	0	45	191	15	NA	<1	5	1 carb, 2 fat
Bulgur, Cooked	1/2 cup	76	<1	0	0	0	0	5	17	NA	4	3	1 carb
Bulke Roll	1/2 roll	78	<1	0	NA	0	0	137	15	NA	<1	4	1 carb
Challah	1 oz	81	2	20	<1	0	15	139	14	NA	<1	3	1 carb
Chicken Liver	1 oz	45	2	20	<1	0	179	15	<1	NA	0	7	1 lean protein
Chickpeas	1/2 cup	135	2	20	<1	0	0	6	23	NA	6	7	1 1/2 carb, 1 lean protein
Corned Beef	1 oz	71	5	45	2	NA	28	321	<1	NA	0	5	1 med-fat protein
Couscous	1/2 cup	88	<1	0	0	0	0	4	18	NA	1	3	1 carb
Cream Cheese	1 Tbsp	51	5	45	3	0	16	43	<1	NA	0	1	1 fat
Farfel	1/2 cup	73	<1	0	0	0	0	0	15	NA	<1	2	1 carb
Flanken, Raw	1 oz	51	3	25	1	0	15	20	0	NA	0	6	1 lean protein

ETHNIC FOODS

	Serving	Calories	Fat (g)	Cal. from Fat	Sat. Fat (g)	Trans Fat (g)	Chol. (mg)	Sod. (mg)	Carb. (g)	Sugar (g)	Fiber (g)	Prot. (g)	Servings/Exchanges
Gefilte Fish	2 pieces	71	2	20	<1	0	25	440	6	NA	0	8	1/2 carb, 1 lean protein
Herring in Wine Sauce	1/4 cup	90	4	35	1	0	25	420	7	NA	0	5	1/2 carb, 1 med-fat protein
Herring, Pickled	1 oz	74	5	45	<1	0	4	247	3	NA	0	4	1 med-fat protein
Horseradish, Root	1 Tbsp	7	<1	0	0	0	0	47	2	NA	<1	<1	free
Kasha, Cooked	1/2 cup	77	<1	0	<1	0	0	3	17	NA	2	3	1 carb
Kasha, Dry	2 Tbsp	71	<1	0	<1	0	0	2	15	NA	2	2	1 carb
Kichlach	2–3	106	4	35	<1	0	42	13	15	NA	<1	3	1 carb, 1 fat
Knishes	1 1/2 oz	114	5	45	<1	0	35	162	15	NA	1	3	1 carb, 1 fat
Kreplach	2 oz	128	4	35	1	0	62	70	13	NA	<1	10	1 carb, 1 lean protein
Kugel	1/2 cup	113	2	20	<1	0	31	277	17	NA	<1	7	1 carb
Lekach	1 oz	84	2	20	<1	0	13	43	16	NA	<1	1	1 carb
Lentils, Cooked	1/2 cup	115	<1	0	0	0	0	2	20	NA	8	9	1 carb, 1 lean protein
Lox	1 oz	33	1	10	<1	0	7	567	0	NA	0	5	1 lean protein

Matzoh	3/4 oz	84	<1	0	0	0	0	0	18	NA	<1	2	1 carb
Matzoh Ball	3 balls	212	13	115	4	0	127	678	16	NA	<1	6	1 carb, 2 1/2 fat
Matzoh Meal	2 Tbsp	65	<1	0	0	0	0	0	14	NA	<1	2	1 carb
Pastrami	1 oz	99	8	70	3	NA	26	348	<1	0	0	5	1 high-fat protein
Pickles, Dill, Large	1 1/2	36	<1	0	<1	0	0	2596	8	NA	2	1	1 vegetable
Potato Flour	2 Tbsp	71	<1	0	<1	0	0	11	14	NA	1	1	1 carb
Potato Pancakes, Medium	1	124	7	65	1	0	13	232	13	NA	<1	3	1 carb, 1 fat
Pumpernickel Bread	1 oz	71	<1	0	<1	0	0	190	14	NA	2	3	1 carb
Rye Bread	1 oz	73	<1	0	<1	0	0	187	14	NA	2	2	1 carb
Sablefish	1 oz	73	6	55	1	0	18	209	0	NA	0	5	1 med-fat protein
Salmon, Canned	1 oz	39	2	20	<1	0	16	157	0	NA	0	6	1 lean protein
Sardines, Medium, Canned in Oil, Drained	2	60	3	25	<1	0	41	145	0	NA	0	7	1 lean protein
Schmaltz	1 tsp	38	4	35	1	0	4	0	0	NA	0	0	1 fat
Smelt	1 oz	35	<1	0	<1	0	26	22	0	NA	0	6	1 lean protein
Sour Cream	2 Tbsp	52	5	45	3	0	11	13	<1	NA	0	<1	1 fat

ETHNIC FOODS

	Serving	Calories	Fat (g)	Cal. from Fat	Sat. Fat (g)	Trans Fat (g)	Chol. (mg)	Sod. (mg)	Carb. (g)	Sugar (g)	Fiber (g)	Prot. (g)	Servings/Exchanges
Split Peas, Cooked	1/2 cup	116	<1	0	0	0	0	2	21	NA	8	8	1 1/2 carb, 1 lean protein
Tzimmes	1/4 cup	88	<1	0	0	0	0	118	21	NA	2	1	1 1/2 carb
Whitefish, Smoked	1 oz	31	<1	0	<1	0	9	289	0	NA	0	7	1 lean protein
MEXICAN AMERICAN													
Avocado, Medium	1/8	40	4	35	<1	0	0	3	2	NA	<1	<1	1 fat
Bolillo, Large	1/4	82	<1	0	<1	0	0	183	16	NA	<1	3	1 carb
Chayote, Boiled, Drained	1/2 cup	19	<1	0	0	0	0	1	4	NA	2	<1	1 vegetable
Chorizo	1 oz	129	11	100	4	NA	25	351	<1	NA	0	7	1 med-fat protein, 1 fat
Corn Tortilla, 6-inch	1	58	<1	0	<1	0	0	42	12	NA	1	2	1 carb
Corn Tortilla, Fat Added, 6-inch	1	102	6	55	<1	NA	0	42	12	NA	1	2	1 carb, 1 fat
Flour Tortilla, 6-inch	1	104	2	20	<1	0	0	153	18	NA	1	3	1 carb
Flour Tortilla, Fat Added, 6-inch	1	148	7	65	1	NA	0	153	18	NA	1	3	1 carb, 1 fat

Frijoles Cocidos	1/2 cup	117	<1	0	0	0	2	22	NA	7	7	1 carb, 1 lean protein
Frijoles Refritos, Fat Added	1/2 cup	161	5	45	<1	0	378	22	NA	7	7	1 carb, 1 med-fat protein
Jicama, Raw	1 cup	49	<1	0	0	0	5	12	NA	6	<1	1 carb
Mango, Small, Raw	1/2	68	<1	0	0	0	2	18	NA	2	<1	1 carb
Menudo	1 cup	170	9	65	4	NA	950	1	NA	NA	20	3 lean protein
Nopales, Cooked	1/2 cup	11	0	0	0	0	15	3	NA	2	1	1 vegetable
Nopales, Raw	1 cup	14	<1	0	0	0	19	3	NA	2	1	1 vegetable
Pan Dulce, 5-inch	1	458	21	190	NA	NA	389	59	NA	NA	8	4 carb, 3 fat
Papaya, Raw, Cubed	1 cup	55	<1	0	0	0	4	14	NA	3	<1	1 carb
Peppers, Hot Green Chili, Chopped, Raw	1 cup	60	<1	0	0	0	11	14	NA	2	3	1 carb
Queso Anejo	1 oz	106	9	80	5	30	321	1	NA	0	6	1 med-fat protein, 1 fat
Queso Asadero	1 oz	101	8	70	5	30	186	<1	NA	0	6	1 med-fat protein, 1 fat
Queso Chihuahua	1 oz	106	8	70	5	30	175	2	NA	0	6	1 med-fat protein, 1 fat
Queso Fresco	1 oz	83	7	65	4	NA	200	NA	NA	0	6	1 med-fat protein
Salsa De Chile	1/4 cup	14	<1	0	0	0	166	3	NA	1	<1	free

ETHNIC FOODS

	Serving	Calories	Fat (g)	Cal. from Fat	Sat. Fat (g)	Trans Fat (g)	Chol. (mg)	Sod. (mg)	Carb. (g)	Sugar (g)	Fiber (g)	Prot. (g)	Servings/Exchanges
Taco Shell, 6-inch	2	122	6	55	<1	0	0	95	16	NA	2	2	1 carb, 1 fat
Verdolagas, Cooked	1/2 cup	10	<1	0	0	0	0	26	2	NA	1	<1	1 vegetable
NAVAJO													
Blue Corn Mush	3/4 cup	94	<1	0	NA	0	0	32	21	NA	NA	3	1 carb
Corn Hominy, Steamed	1/2 cup	70	1	10	<1	0	0	18	13	NA	3	2	1 carb
Four Tortilla, 8-inch	1/4	87	<1	0	NA	0	0	211	19	NA	1	3	1 carb
Mutton, Lean and with Fat, Cooked	1 oz	96	9	80	NA	0	NA	NA	0	NA	0	4	1 med-fat protein, 1 fat
Mutton, Lean, Cooked	1 oz	55	3	25	1	0	21	10	0	NA	0	8	1 lean protein
Piñon Nuts, In Shell	1 Tbsp or 25	60	6	55	<1	0	0	7	<1	NA	1	1	1 fat
PLAINS INDIAN													
Beans, Dried, Cooked	1/2 cup	117	<1	0	<1	0	0	1	22	NA	7	7	1 1/2 carb, 1 lean protein
Beef Fat, Raw	1 tsp	38	4	35	2	0	5	0	0	NA	0	0	1 fat

Food	Serving											Exchange
Biscuit Mix, Dry	1/4 cup	129	5	45	1	0	19	383	19	NA	<1	2	1 carb, 1 fat
Buffalo/Bison	1 oz	40	<1	0	<1	0	23	16	0	NA	0	8	1 lean protein
Chicken with Skin, Fried	1 oz	76	4	35	1	0	26	24	<1	NA	0	8	1 med-fat protein
Commodity Meat, Luncheon	1 oz	97	9	80	NA	NA	NA	420	1	NA	NA	3	1 med-fat protein, 1 fat
Cracklings	1/3 oz	57	5	45	2	0	9	18	0	NA	0	2	1 fat
Dry Meat	1 oz	47	1	10	<1	0	12	984	<1	NA	0	8	1 lean protein
Eggs, Dried Powdered	3 Tbsp	81	7	65	2	0	351	12	0	NA	0	4	1 med-fat protein
Elk, Roasted	1 oz	41	<1	0	<1	0	0	17	0	NA	0	9	1 lean protein
Huckleberries	1 cup	56	<1	0	NA	0	NA	15	13	NA	NA	<1	1 carb
Indian Corn, Dried	1/4 cup	132	2	20	NA	0	NA	37	26	NA	<1	4	2 carb
Kidney, Raw	1 oz	30	<1	0	<1	0	81	51	<1	NA	0	5	1 lean protein
Lemon, Raw, Peeled	1	17	<1	0	NA	0	0	1	5	NA	0	<1	free
Liver, Beef	1 oz	46	1	10	<1	0	110	20	1	NA	0	7	1 lean protein
Pheasant, Skinless	1 oz	38	1	10	<1	0	0	10	0	NA	0	7	1 lean protein
Pilot Bread	1 (4-inch) piece	104	2	20	NA	0	NA	142	18	NA	NA	2	1 carb

ETHNIC FOODS

	Serving	Calories	Fat (g)	Cal. from Fat	Sat. Fat (g)	Trans Fat (g)	Chol. (mg)	Sod. (mg)	Carb. (g)	Sugar (g)	Fiber (g)	Prot. (g)	Servings/Exchanges
Potatoes, Fried	1/2 cup	163	11	100	4	0	NA	19	17	NA	2	2	1 carb, 2 fat
Short Ribs	1 oz	83	5	45	2	0	0	16	0	NA	0	9	1 med-fat protein
Sweetbreads, Breaded, Fried	1 oz	108	8	70	3	NA	NA	126	1	NA	0	7	1 high-fat protein
Venison	1 oz	45	<1	0	<1	0	32	15	0	NA	0	9	1 lean protein
White Fish, Dry Heat Cooked	1 oz	49	2	20	<1	0	22	19	0	NA	0	7	1 lean protein
Wild Rice, Zizania Aquatica	1/2 cup	82	<1	0	0	0	0	3	17	NA	<1	3	1 carb
SOUTHERN & SOUL													
Fatback, Raw	1/4 oz	58	6	55	2	0	4	1	0	NA	0	0	1 fat
Ham Hock	1 oz	90	7	65	2	0	18	383	2	NA	0	6	1 high-fat protein
Hog Jowl	1 oz	54	5	55	2	0	9	7	0	NA	0	2	1 fat
Hog Maw	1 oz	45	3	25	NA	0	55	15	0	NA	0	5	1 lean protein
Hominy	3/4 cup	86	1	10	<1	0	0	252	17	NA	3	2	1 carb

Food	Serving												Exchange
Kale, Cooked	1/2 cup	21	0	0	0	0	0	15	4	NA	1	1	1 vegetable
Lard	1 tsp	38	4	40	2	0	4	0	0	NA	0	0	1 fat
Muscadines	17	60	0.5	5	0	NA	0	2	15	NA	1	<1	1 carb
Opossum	1 oz	63	3	25	NA	0	23	27	0	NA	0	9	1 lean protein
Oxtail	1 oz	72	4	35	1	0	30	20	0	NA	0	9	1 med-fat protein
Pig Ear	1 oz or 1/4 ear	47	3	25	NA	0	26	48	0	NA	0	5	1 lean protein
Pig Foot	1/2 foot	68	4	35	2	0	35	58	0	NA	0	7	1 med-fat protein
Pig Tail	1 oz or 1/3 tail	113	10	90	4	0	37	48	0	NA	0	5	1 high-fat protein
Poke Salad, Cooked	1/2 cup	16	0	0	0	0	0	NA	3	NA	1	2	1 vegetable
Pork Brains	1 oz	39	3	25	0.5	0	727	26	0	NA	0	4	1 lean protein
Pork Cracklings	1 Tbsp	57	5	45	2	0	9	18	0	NA	0	7	1 fat
Pork Neck Bones	1 oz	66	4	35	2	0	24	20	0	NA	0	7	1 med-fat protein
Pork Skin (Rind), Fried	1 cup	68	4	35	2	0	17	231	0	NA	0	8	1 med-fat protein
Pork Tongue	1 oz or 1/3 tongue	77	5	45	2	0	42	31	0	NA	0	7	1 med-fat protein

ETHNIC FOODS

	Serving	Calories	Fat (g)	Cal. from Fat	Sat. Fat (g)	Trans Fat (g)	Chol. (mg)	Sod. (mg)	Carb. (g)	Sugar (g)	Fiber (g)	Prot. (g)	Servings/Exchanges
Souse Meat (Head-cheese)	1 oz	60	5	45	1	0	23	357	0	NA	0	5	1 med-fat protein
Succotash	1/2 cup	79	1	10	0	0	0	38	17	NA	5	4	1 carb
Tripe	2 oz	56	2	20	1	0	54	26	0	NA	0	8	1 lean protein

FAST FOOD

ARBY'S

Roast Beef Sandwiches

	Serving	Calories	Fat (g)	Cal. from Fat	Sat. Fat (g)	Trans Fat (g)	Chol. (mg)	Sod. (mg)	Carb. (g)	Sugar (g)	Fiber (g)	Prot. (g)	Servings/Exchanges
Beef 'n Cheddar Classic	1 (7 oz)	450	20	180	6	1	60	1310	45	9	2	24	3 carb, 2 med-fat protein, 2 fat
Beef 'n Cheddar Mid	1 (9 oz)	560	27	240	9	1.5	95	1760	45	9	2	34	3 carb, 4 med-fat protein, 1 fat
French Dip & Swiss/ Au Jus	1	540	23	210	11	1	100	2560	50	3	2	34	3 carb, 4 med-fat protein, 1 fat
Roast Beef Classic	1 (5.5 oz)	360	14	130	5	1	60	970	35	6	1	23	2 carb, 2 med-fat protein, 1 fat
Roast Beef Max	1 (9.5 oz)	560	27	240	11	2	135	1860	35	6	1	45	2 carb, 5 med-fat protein
Roast Beef Mid	1 (7.5 oz)	460	21	180	8	1.5	95	1420	35	6	1	34	2 carb, 4 med-fat protein

FAST FOOD

	Serving	Calories	Fat (g)	Cal. from Fat	Sat. Fat (g)	Trans Fat (g)	Chol. (mg)	Sod. (mg)	Carb. (g)	Sugar (g)	Fiber (g)	Prot. (g)	Servings/Exchanges
Ultimate Angus													
Angus Philly	1	590	27	250	8	0.5	95	2130	48	5	3	38	3 carb, 4 med-fat protein, 1 fat
Angus Three Cheese & Bacon	1	630	30	270	11	0.5	120	2220	45	4	2	47	3 carb, 5 med-fat protein, 1 fat
Roast Turkey													
Grand Turkey Club	1	480	24	210	8	0	70	1610	37	8	5	31	3 1/2 carb, 3 med-fat protein, 2 fat
Reuben	1	640	30	270	8	0	55	1610	62	7	4	32	4 carb, 3 med-fat protein, 3 fat
Market Fresh Sandwiches													
Roast Turkey Ranch & Bacon	1	800	35	310	9	0.5	100	2250	76	18	5	48	5 carb, 5 med-fat protein, 2 fat
Roast Turkey Ranch & Bacon Wrap	1	580	32	290	9	0.5	100	2030	38	6	7	43	2 1/2 carb, 5 med-fat protein, 1 fat
Roast Turkey & Swiss	1	700	28	250	7	0	75	1760	77	18	5	39	5 carb, 3 med-fat protein, 3 fat

Roast Turkey & Swiss Wrap	1	490	25	230	7	0.5	75	1540	38	6	7	35	2 1/2 carb, 4 med-fat protein, 1 fat
Market Fresh Salads													
Chopped Farmhouse Salad, Crispy Chicken	1	420	23	210	8	0	70	1020	24	4	4	30	1 1/2 carb, 3 med-fat protein, 2 fat
Chopped Farmhouse Salad, Roast Turkey	1	230	13	120	7	0	60	780	8	4	3	23	1/2 carb, 3 med-fat protein
Chopped Side Salad	1	70	5	45	3	0	15	105	4	2	1	5	1 med-fat protein
Salad Dressing													
Balsamic Vinaigrette Dressing	1 (1.5 oz)	130	12	110	2	0	0	470	5	5	0	0	1 fat
Buttermilk Ranch Dressing	1 (1.5 oz)	210	22	200	3.5	0	10	310	2	1	0	0	4 fat
Dijon Honey Mustard Dressing	1 (1.5 oz)	180	16	150	2.5	0	15	230	8	7	0	0	1/2 carb, 3 fat
Light Italian Dressing	1 (1.5 oz)	20	1	5	0	0	0	750	3	2	0	0	free
Prime-Cut Chicken													
Chicken Bacon & Swiss, Crispy	1	600	29	260	7	0	80	1430	49	9	3	36	3 carb, 4 med-fat protein, 2 fat

FAST FOOD

	Serving	Calories	Fat (g)	Cal. from Fat	Sat. Fat (g)	Trans Fat (g)	Chol. (mg)	Sod. (mg)	Carb. (g)	Sugar (g)	Fiber (g)	Prot. (g)	Servings/Exchanges
Crispy Chicken Sand-wich	1	540	27	240	4.5	0	55	990	48	8	3	27	3 carb, 3 med-fat protein, 2 fat
Prime-Cut Chicken Tenders	3	350	17	150	2.5	0	45	970	25	0	2	25	1 1/2 carb, 3 med-fat protein
Prime-Cut Chicken Tenders	5	590	28	250	4	0	75	1610	42	0	4	42	3 carb, 5 med-fat protein, 1 fat
Sauces													
Bronco Berry Sauce	1 (1 oz)	60	0	0	0	0	0	20	14	14	0	0	1 carb
Buffalo Dipping Sauce	1 (1 oz)	10	1	10	0	0	0	720	1	0	0	0	free
Honey Mustard Dipping Sauce	1 (1 oz)	140	13	120	2	0	10	130	5	4	0	0	3 fat
Marinara Sauce	1 (1 oz)	25	0.5	5	0	0	0	140	4	2	1	1	free
Ranch Dipping Sauce	1 (1 oz)	100	11	100	2.5	0	20	190	1	1	0	1	2 fat
Tangy BBQ Sauce	1 (1 oz)	45	0	0	0	0	0	350	11	8	0	0	1 carb

Sides

Chopped Side Salad	1	70	5	45	3	0	15	105	4	2	1	5	1 med-fat protein
Curly Fries, Large	1 (7.2 oz)	630	35	310	5	0	0	1420	74	0	8	7	5 carb, 7 fat
Curly Fries, Medium	1 (6.1 oz)	540	29	260	4	0	0	1200	62	0	7	6	4 carb, 6 fat
Curly Fries, Small	1 (4.6 oz)	400	22	200	3	0	0	900	47	0	5	5	3 carb, 4 fat
Potato Cakes	2	230	14	120	2	0	0	460	25	0	3	2	1 1/2 carb, 3 fat
Potato Cakes	4	460	27	240	4.5	0	0	930	50	0	5	3	3 1/2 carb, 5 fat
Steakhouse Onion Rings	5	410	20	180	3	0	0	1690	51	6	3	6	3 1/2 carb, 5 fat

Snack 'N Save

Apple Slices	1	35	0	0	0	0	0	0	9	6	1	0	1 fruit
Crispy Onion Mighty Minis, Roast Beef	2	550	30	270	7	1	55	1260	47	6	2	23	3 carb, 2 med-fat protein, 4 fat
Curly Fries, Snack	1 (2.8 oz)	240	13	120	2	0	0	540	28	0	3	3	2 carb, 3 fat
Jalapeño Bites	5	280	16	140	6	0	25	600	31	3	2	5	2 carb, 3 fat

FAST FOOD

	Serving	Calories	Fat (g)	Cal. from Fat	Sat. Fat (g)	Trans Fat (g)	Chol. (mg)	Sod. (mg)	Carb. (g)	Sugar (g)	Fiber (g)	Prot. (g)	Servings/Exchanges
Jalapeno Bites	8	460	25	230	10	0.5	45	970	49	4	4	8	3 carb, 5 fat
Jr. Bacon Cheddar Melt	1	280	12	110	4	6	40	890	25	4	1	17	1 1/2 carb, 2 med-fat protein
Jr. Ham & Cheese Melt	1	210	6	60	1.5	0	25	900	25	4	1	14	1 1/2 carb, 1 med-fat protein
Jr. Roast Beef	1	210	8	70	2.5	0	30	530	22	4	1	13	1 1/2 carb, 1 med-fat protein, 1 fat
Mozzarella Sticks	4	420	21	190	9	0.5	50	1690	35	4	2	21	2 carb, 2 med-fat protein, 2 fat
Mozzarella Sticks	6	620	32	290	13	1	75	2530	52	6	3	32	3 1/2 carb, 3 med-fat protein, 3 fat
Original Mighty Minis, Roast Beef	2	380	14	130	4.5	0.5	50	980	40	5	2	22	2 1/2 carb, 2 med-fat protein, 1 fat
Desserts													
Apple Turnover	1	430	18	160	18	9	0	210	64	39	2	4	4 carb, 4 fat

Cherry Turnover	1	390	13	120	6	0	0	200	64	40	2	4	4 carb, 3 fat
Chocolate Turnover	1	520	26	230	12	0	0	280	69	39	3	5	4 1/2 carb, 5 fat
Molten Lava Cake	1	340	14	120	4	0	25	280	53	35	2	4	3 1/2 carb, 3 fat
Vanilla Shake, Large	22 oz	470	15	130	10	0	50	390	75	61	0	14	5 carb, 3 fat
Vanilla Shake, Medium	16 oz	380	12	110	8	0	40	310	60	49	0	11	4 carb, 2 fat
Vanilla Shake, Small	12 oz	250	8	70	5	0	25	210	40	33	0	8	4 carb, 2 fat

BOSTON MARKET

Individual Meals

Meatloaf, Large	1	730	45	410	19	3	215	1640	38	5	10	42	2 1/2 carb, 5 med-fat protein, 4 fat
Meatloaf, Regular	1	480	30	270	13	2	145	1090	25	3	6	28	1 1/2 carb, 3 med-fat protein, 3 fat
Parmesan Tuscan Chicken, Half Chicken	1	800	47	420	13	0	355	2000	7	2	1	85	1/2 carb, 12 lean protein
Parmesan Tuscan Chicken, Quarter Dark	1	390	27	240	7	0	180	980	3	1	1	34	5 med-fat protein
Parmesan Tuscan Chicken, Quarter White	1	400	20	180	5	0	175	1020	4	1	1	51	7 lean protein

FAST FOOD

	Serving	Calories	Fat (g)	Cal. from Fat	Sat. Fat (g)	Trans Fat (g)	Chol. (mg)	Sod. (mg)	Carb. (g)	Sugar (g)	Fiber (g)	Prot. (g)	Servings/Exchanges
Parmesan Tuscan Chicken, Three Piece Dark	1	510	32	290	8	0	300	1730	4	1	1	52	7 med-fat protein
Pastry Top Chicken Pot Pie	1	800	45	410	23	0	100	1280	60	7	5	33	4 carb, 3 med-fat protein, 6 fat
Pastry Top Turkey Pot Pie	1	820	49	450	22	0	95	1450	61	7	5	27	4 carb, 2 med-fat protein, 8 fat
Roast Beef Brisket, Large	1	400	23	210	6	0	165	990	1	1	0	48	7 lean protein
Roast Beef Brisket, Regular	1	230	13	120	3.5	0	95	570	0	1	0	28	4 lean protein
Rotisserie Chicken, Half Chicken	1	640	33	290	10	0	340	1380	2	1	0	84	12 lean protein
Rotisserie Chicken, Quarter Dark (1 Thigh & 1 Drumstick)	1	310	20	180	6	0	175	670	1	1	0	33	5 lean protein

Item													Exchanges/Choices
Rotisserie Chicken, Quarter White	1	320	13	110	4	0	165	710	1	1	0	51	7 lean protein
Rotisserie Chicken, Quarter White, Skinless	1	220	2.5	20	1	0	145	700	1	0	0	49	7 lean protein
Rotisserie Chicken, Three Piece Dark (Thigh & 2 Drumsticks)	1	390	22	190	6	0	290	1270	1	1	0	51	7 lean protein
Rotisserie Chicken, Three Piece Dark, Skinless (Thigh & 2 Drumsticks)	1	280	12	110	3.5	0	200	630	1	1	0	41	6 lean protein
Rotisserie Chicken, Three Piece Dark (2 Thighs & Drumstick)	1	540	36	320	11	0	280	1080	1	1	0	53	7 med-fat protein
Rotisserie Chicken, Three Piece Dark, Skinless (2 Thighs & Drumstick)	1	340	17	150	5	0	220	720	1	1	0	47	7 lean protein
St. Louis Style BBQ Ribs, 1/2 Rack	1	1180	74	660	29		215	3150	67	58	2	65	4 1/2 carb, 7 med-fat protein, 8 fat

FAST FOOD

	Serving	Calories	Fat (g)	Cal. from Fat	Sat. Fat (g)	Trans Fat (g)	Chol. (mg)	Sod. (mg)	Carb. (g)	Sugar (g)	Fiber (g)	Prot. (g)	Servings/Exchanges
St. Louis Style BBQ Ribs, 1/4 Rack	1	590	37	330	14	0	105	1580	33	29	1	32	2 carb, 4 med-fat protein, 3 fat
Turkey Breast, Large	1	280	12	110	0	0	115	990	2	0	0	39	5 lean protein
Turkey Breast, Regular	1	200	9	80	0	0	80	710	1	0	0	28	4 lean protein
Homestyle Sides													
Bacon Mac & Cheese	1	360	22	200	13	0	70	870	24	3	1	15	1 1/2 carb, 2 med-fat protein, 2 fat
Caesar Side Salad	1	210	18	160	4	0	15	490	8	2	0	4	2 vegetable, 4 fat
Cinnamon Apples	1	240	3.5	30	0.5	0	0	270	55	49	4	0	3 1/2 carb, 1 fat
Creamed Spinach	1	260	21	180	12	1	60	530	11	2	4	9	2 vegetable, 4 fat
Fresh Steamed Vegetables	1	80	5	45	0	0	0	160	8	3	3	2	2 vegetable, 1 fat
Fresh Vegetable Stuffing	1	220	10	90	1	0	<5	640	28	4	2	4	2 carb, 2 fat
Garlic Dill New Potatoes	1	100	2	20	0.5	0	0	80	20	1	2	2	1 carb
Garlicky Lemon Spinach	1	110	9	80	5	0	20	510	7	1	3	4	1 vegetable, 2 fat

Green Beans	1	90	6	50	2	0	0	200	9	2	4	2	2 vegetable, 1 fat
Loaded Mashed Potatoes	1	310	16	140	9	0	40	840	31	3	3	9	2 carb, 3 fat
Macaroni & Cheese	1	280	11	100	7	0	30	1050	33	5	2	10	2 carb, 1 med-fat protein, 1 fat
Mashed Potatoes	1	240	10	90	5	0	25	540	32	2	3	5	2 carb, 2 fat
Squash Casserole	1	260	17	150	7	0	35	1050	18	8	2	10	1 carb, 1 med-fat protein, 2 fat
Sweet Corn	1	120	2.5	20	0	0	0	55	25	7	1	4	1 1/2 carb, 1 fat
Sweet Potato Casserole	1	450	13	110	3.5	0	10	220	83	59	4	3	5 1/2 carb, 3 fat
Sandwiches													
All-White Chicken Salad	1	970	65	580	10	0	80	1670	63	7	4	29	4 carb, 2 med-fat protein, 11 fat
Meatloaf Carver	1	910	39	350	18	0	170	2340	92	11	10	44	6 carb, 4 med-fat protein, 4 fat
Mediterranean Chicken Carver	1	650	24	210	6	0	75	1590	65	7	4	40	4 carb, 4 med-fat protein, 1 fat
Pulled BBQ Chicken	1	620	14	120	6	0	100	1890	84	24	4	39	5 1/2 carb, 3 med-fat protein

FAST FOOD

	Serving	Calories	Fat (g)	Cal. from Fat	Sat. Fat (g)	Trans Fat (g)	Chol. (mg)	Sod. (mg)	Carb. (g)	Sugar (g)	Fiber (g)	Prot. (g)	Servings/Exchanges
Roast Beef Brisket Dip Carver	1	820	44	400	12	0	135	1590	58	3	4	45	4 carb, 5 med-fat protein, 4 fat
Roasted Turkey Carver	1	850	46	410	9	0	105	1710	62	5	4	39	4 carb, 4 med-fat protein, 5 fat
Rotisserie Chicken Carver	1	750	34	310	8	0	100	1690	62	6	4	43	4 carb, 4 med-fat protein, 3 fat
Salad Bowls & Soups													
Caesar Salad, Entrée	1	440	29	260	6	0	80	1070	16	6	2	34	3 vegetable, 4 med-fat protein, 2 fat
Chicken Noodle Soup	1	230	8	70	2	0	85	1300	22	2	2	20	1 1/2 carb, 2 med-fat protein
Chicken Tortilla Soup	1	440	24	220	5	0	80	2940	39	5	3	23	2 1/2 carb, 2 med-fat protein, 3 fat
Mediterranean Salad, Entrée	1	550	39	350	11	0	100	1290	14	8	3	39	3 vegetable, 5 med-fat protein, 3 fat
Southwest Sante Fe Salad, Entrée	1	530	30	270	7	0	80	880	30	8	4	36	1 carb, 3 vegetable, 4 med-fat protein, 2 fat

Desserts

	Serving												Exchanges
Apple Pie, Slice	1	430	21	190	9	0	0	460	59	28	2	3	4 carb, 4 fat
Chocolate Brownie, Single	1	530	26	230	5	0	85	290	74	49	3	6	5 carb, 5 fat
Chocolate Cake, Slice	1	580	32	290	11	0	45	360	67	47	3	5	4 1/2 carb, 6 fat
Chocolate Chunk Cookie, Single	1	370	18	160	9	0	30	210	53	32	2	4	3 1/2 carb, 4 fat
Cornbread	1	160	3	30	1.5	0	15	230	30	12	1	2	2 carb, 1 fat
Pecan Pie, Slice	1	640	36	320	11	0	115	340	74	46	2	7	5 carb, 7 fat

Sauces

	Serving												Exchanges
Au Jus	1	20	0	5	0	0	0	730	4	2	0	0	free
Beef Gravy	1	10	0	0	0	0	0	130	2	0	0	0	free
Cranberry Walnut Relish	1	140	2	20	0	0	0	0	30	27	2	1	2 carb
Honey Habanero	1	70	0	0	0	0	0	200	17	15	0	0	1 carb
Poultry Gravy	1	10	0	0	0	0	0	85	2	0	0	0	free
Sweet Thai Chili Gravy	1	60	1	10	0	0	0	210	13	13	1	0	1 carb
Zesty Barbecue	1	40	0	0	0	0	0	240	11	9	0	0	1 carb

FAST FOOD

BURGER KING

Whopper Sandwiches

	Serving	Calories	Fat (g)	Cal. from Fat	Sat. Fat (g)	Trans Fat (g)	Chol. (mg)	Sod. (mg)	Carb. (g)	Sugar (g)	Fiber (g)	Prot. (g)	Servings/Exchanges
Angry Whopper	1	840	51	460	17	1.5	95	1610	58	16	2	29	4 carb, 2 med-fat protein, 8 fat
BBQ Bacon Whopper	1	790	48	440	16	2	95	1380	53	15	2	29	3 1/2 carb, 3 med-fat protein, 7 fat
Double Whopper	1	900	56	510	19	3	115	980	50	12	2	35	3 carb, 4 med-fat protein, 7 fat
Double Whopper with Cheese	1	1070	70	630	28	3.5	155	1780	52	14	2	44	3 1/2 carb, 5 med-fat protein, 9 fat
Triple Whopper	1	1160	75	670	27	4	170	1050	50	12	2	49	3 carb, 6 med-fat protein, 9 fat
Whopper	1	650	37	340	11	1.5	60	910	50	12	2	22	3 carb, 2 med-fat protein, 5 fat
Whopper with Cheese	1	730	44	400	15	2	85	1260	51	13	2	26	3 1/2 carb, 2 med-fat protein, 7 fat

Food	Serving												Exchanges/Choices
Whopper Jr.	1	300	16	150	4.5	0.5	25	460	27	7	1	9	2 carb, 1 med-fat protein, 2 fat
Whopper Jr. with Cheese	1	350	21	190	7	1	40	640	28	7	1	12	2 carb, 1 med-fat protein, 3 fat
Flame Broiled Burgers													
Bacon Cheeseburger	1	290	13	120	6	0.5	40	680	27	7	1	12	2 carb, 1 med-fat protein, 2 fat
Bacon Cheeseburger Deluxe	1	290	14	120	6	0.5	40	720	28	7	1	12	2 carb, 1 med-fat protein, 2 fat
Bacon Double Cheeseburger	1	390	21	190	9	1	65	790	27	7	1	17	2 carb, 2 med-fat protein, 2 fat
Big King	1	530	31	280	11	1.5	75	790	38	8	2	19	2 1/2 carb, 2 med-fat protein, 4 fat
Cheeseburger	1	270	12	110	5	0.5	35	630	27	7	1	11	2 carb, 1 med-fat protein, 1 fat
Double Cheeseburger	1	360	19	170	8	1	60	670	27	7	1	16	2 carb, 1 med-fat protein, 3 fat
Double Hamburger	1	320	15	140	6	1	45	450	26	6	1	14	2 carb, 1 med-fat protein, 2 fat

FAST FOOD

	Serving	Calories	Fat (g)	Cal. from Fat	Sat. Fat (g)	Trans Fat (g)	Chol. (mg)	Sod. (mg)	Carb. (g)	Sugar (g)	Fiber (g)	Prot. (g)	Servings/Exchanges
Extra Long BBQ Cheese-burger	1	590	28	250	11	1.5	70	1080	62	14	4	22	4 carb, 1 med-fat protein, 5 fat
Hamburger	1	230	9	80	3	0	25	460	26	6	1	9	2 carb, 1 med-fat protein, 1 fat
King Jr. Cheeseburger	1	310	17	150	6	0.5	40	580	26	5	1	11	2 carb, 1 med-fat protein, 2 fat
Chicken, Fish, Ribs, and Veggie Burgers													
BBQ Rib Sandwich	1	450	28	250	9	0	70	930	29	9	1	19	2 carb, 2 med-fat protein, 4 fat
Big Fish Deluxe	1	580	31	280	6	0.5	40	1650	57	8	2	20	4 carb, 1 med-fat protein, 5 fat
Big Fish Sandwich	1	530	27	250	4.5	0	30	1360	54	7	2	17	3 1/2 carb, 1 med-fat protein, 4 fat
BK Veggie Burger	1	390	16	140	2.5	0	5	900	44	9	5	21	3 carb, 1 med-fat protein, 2 fat
Buffalo Chicken Strips, 3 Pieces	1 order	380	20	180	3.5	0	55	1820	27	0	3	22	2 carb, 2 med-fat protein, 2 fat

Item	Amount	Cal.	Fat Cal.	Fat (g)	Sat. Fat (g)	Trans Fat (g)	Chol. (mg)	Sod. (mg)	Carb. (g)	Fiber (g)	Pro. (g)	Choices/Exchanges
Buffalo Chicken Strips, 5 Piece	1 order	620	33	300	5	0.5	90	2920	45	1	4	37 — 3 carb, 4 med-fat protein, 3 fat
Chicken Big King	1	710	42	380	9	0.5	65	1660	60	9	3	23 — 4 carb, 2 med-fat protein, 6 fat
Chicken Nuggets, 4 Piece	1 order	190	11	100	2	0	20	360	13	0	2	8 — 1 carb, 1 med-fat protein, 1 fat
Chicken Nuggets, 6 Piece	1 order	280	17	150	3	0	30	540	20	0	3	13 — 1 carb, 1 med-fat protein, 2 fat
Chicken Nuggets, 10 Piece	1 order	470	29	260	5	0	50	890	34	0	5	21 — 2 carb, 2 med-fat protein, 4 fat
Chicken Nuggets, 20 Piece	1 order	950	57	510	11	0	100	1790	67	0	9	42 — 4 1/2 carb, 4 med-fat protein, 7 fat
Crispy Chicken Jr.	1	430	28	250	4.5	0	30	760	34	4	2	12 — 2 carb, 1 med-fat protein, 5 fat
Home-Style Chicken Strips, 3 Piece	1 order	340	17	150	2.5	0	55	1130	26	0	3	22 — 2 carb, 2 med-fat protein, 1 fat
Home-Style Chicken Strips, 5 Piece	1 order	570	28	250	4.5	0.5	90	1890	44	0	4	36 — 3 carb, 4 med-fat protein, 2 fat
Honey BBQ Chicken Strips, 3 Piece	1 order	410	17	150	3	0	55	1400	42	13	3	22 — 3 carb, 1 med-fat protein, 2 fat

FAST FOOD

	Serving	Calories	Fat (g)	Cal. from Fat	Sat. Fat (g)	Trans Fat (g)	Chol. (mg)	Sod. (mg)	Carb. (g)	Sugar (g)	Fiber (g)	Prot. (g)	Servings/Exchanges
Honey BBQ Chicken Strips, 5 Piece	1 order	690	28	250	4.5	0.5	90	1940	72	25	4	37	5 carb, 3 med-fat protein, 3 fat
Original Chicken Sandwich	1	640	36	320	6	0	70	1140	53	7	3	29	3 1/2 carb, 2 med-fat protein, 5 fat
Spicy Crispy Chicken Jr.	1	410	25	220	4.5	0	35	850	35	5	2	12	2 carb, 1 med-fat protein, 4 fat
Spicy Original Chicken Sandwich	1	640	38	340	6	0.5	55	1310	57	7	3	23	4 carb, 2 med-fat protein, 6 fat
Tendercrisp Chicken Sandwich	1	640	36	330	6	0	70	1270	52	8	4	28	3 1/2 carb, 3 med-fat protein, 4 fat
Tendergrill Chicken Sandwich	1	410	16	140	2.5	0	75	830	38	6	2	31	2 1/2 carb, 3 med-fat protein
Sauces													
Barbeque Dipping Sauce	1 (1 oz)	40	0	0	0	0	0	310	11	10	0	0	1 carb
Buffalo Dipping Sauce	1 (1 oz)	80	8	70	1.5	0	5	360	2	1	0	0	2 fat

	Amount												Exchanges
Honey Mustard Dipping Sauce	1 (1 oz)	90	6	60	1	0	10	170	8	7	0	0	1/2 carb, 1 fat
Ranch Dipping Sauce	1 (1 oz)	140	15	140	2.5	0	10	230	1	1	0	1	3 fat
Sweet & Sour Dipping Sauce	1 (1 oz)	45	0	0	0	0	0	55	11	10	0	0	1 carb

BK Garden Fresh Salads & Sides

	Amount												Exchanges
Apple Slices	1	30	0	0	0	0	0	0	7	6	1	0	1 fruit
Chicken Apple & Cranberry Garden Fresh Salad Wrap, Crispy	1	490	24	210	6	0	35	990	53	18	4	16	3 1/2 carb, 1 med-fat protein, 4 fat
Chicken Apple & Cranberry Garden Fresh Salad Wrap, Grilled	1	400	16	140	4.5	0	45	730	48	20	5	19	3 carb, 2 med-fat protein, 1 fat
Chicken Apple & Cranberry Garden Fresh Salad with Tendercrisp & Dressing	1	680	42	370	9	0	75	1010	53	36	4	24	3 1/2 carb, 2 med-fat protein, 6 fat

FAST FOOD

	Serving	Calories	Fat (g)	Cal. from Fat	Sat. Fat (g)	Trans Fat (g)	Chol. (mg)	Sod. (mg)	Carb. (g)	Sugar (g)	Fiber (g)	Prot. (g)	Servings/Exchanges
Chicken Apple & Cranberry Garden Fresh Salad with Tendergrill & Dressing	1	480	26	230	7	0	95	480	34	34	4	28	2 carb, 3 med-fat protein, 3 fat
Chicken BLT Garden Fresh Salad Wrap, Crispy	1	470	26	230	7	0	45	1270	42	4	4	19	3 carb, 1 med-fat protein, 4 fat
Chicken BLT Garden Fresh Salad Wrap, Grilled	1	380	19	170	6	0	60	1030	33	3	4	22	2 carb, 2 med-fat protein, 2 fat
Chicken BLT Garden Fresh Salad with Tendercrisp & Dressing	1	640	45	410	11	0.5	95	1610	30	8	4	28	2 carb, 3 med-fat protein, 6 fat
Chicken BLT Garden Fresh Salad with Tendergrill & Dressing	1	440	29	260	8	0	115	1080	11	5	3	33	1 carb, 4 med-fat protein, 2 fat

Item	Amount	Calories	Fat (g)	Cal. from Fat	Sat. Fat (g)	Trans Fat (g)	Chol. (mg)	Sodium (mg)	Carb (g)	Fiber (g)	Sugar (g)	Protein (g)	Exchanges
Chicken Caesar Garden Fresh Salad Wrap, Crispy	1	440	24	210	4.5	0	35	1220	42	4	4	18	3 carb, 1 med-fat protein, 4 fat
Chicken Caesar Garden Fresh Salad Wrap, Grilled	1	340	16	140	3.5	0	45	960	33	3	4	21	2 carb, 2 med-fat protein, 1 fat
Chicken Caesar Garden Fresh Salad with Tendercrisp & Dressing	1	650	43	390	7	0	75	1670	39	8	4	30	2 1/2 carb, 3 med-fat protein, 6 fat
Chicken Caesar Garden Fresh Salad with Tendergrill & Dressing	1	450	27	250	4.5	0	95	1150	20	6	3	35	1 carb, 5 med-fat protein
French Fries, Large (Salted)	1 (6.8 oz)	500	22	200	3.5	0	0	710	72	0	5	5	5 carb, 4 fat
French Fries, Medium (Salted)	1 (5.5 oz)	410	18	160	3	0	0	570	58	0	4	4	4 carb, 4 fat
French Fries, Small (Salted)	1 (4.6 oz)	340	15	130	2.5	0	0	480	49	0	4	4	3 carb, 3 fat
French Fries, Value (Salted)	1 (3.2 oz)	240	10	90	1.5	0	0	330	34	0	3	2	2 carb, 2 fat

FAST FOOD

	Serving	Calories	Fat (g)	Cal. from Fat	Sat. Fat (g)	Trans Fat (g)	Chol. (mg)	Sod. (mg)	Carb. (g)	Sugar (g)	Fiber (g)	Prot. (g)	Servings/Exchanges
Home-Style Caesar Croutons, 1 Packet	1	60	2	20	0	0	10	160	9	1	0	2	1/2 carb
Honey Mustard Crispy Chicken Wrap	1	380	20	180	6	0	35	900	35	6	2	15	2 carb, 1 med-fat protein, 3 fat
Honey Mustard Grilled Chicken Wrap	1	330	16	150	5	0	55	700	26	6	1	19	2 carb, 2 med-fat protein, 1 fat
Ken's Apple Cider Vinaigrette	1 (1.8-oz) packet	210	18	160	2.5	0	10	115	10	7	0	0	1/2 carb, 4 fat
Ken's Avocado Ranch Dressing	1 (1.8-oz) packet	170	17	150	3	0	15	420	4	3	0	1	3 fat
Ken's Citrus Caesar Dressing	1 (1.8-oz) packet	180	18	160	3.5	0	5	460	4	2	0	2	4 fat
Ken's Honey Mustard Dressing	1 (1.8-oz) packet	220	18	160	2.5	0	15	270	13	12	1	1	1 carb, 4 fat
Ken's Lite Honey Balsamic	1 (1.8-oz) packet	120	7	70	1	0	0	220	14	11	0	0	1 carb, 1 fat

Item	Amount												Exchanges
Mozzarella Sticks, 4 Piece	1	280	15	140	5	0	35	650	24	2	2	11	1 1/2 carb, 3 fat
Onion Rings, Large	1 (5.1 oz)	500	25	230	4.5	0	0	1310	64	7	5	5	4 carb, 5 fat
Onion Rings, Medium	1 (4.2 oz)	410	21	190	3.5	0	0	1080	53	5	4	4	3 1/2 carb, 4 fat
Onion Rings, Small	1 (3.3 oz)	320	16	150	3	0	0	840	41	4	3	3	2 1/2 carb, 3 fat
Onion Rings, Value	1 (1.5 oz)	150	8	70	1.5	0	0	400	19	2	1	1	1 carb, 2 fat
Ranch Crispy Chicken Wrap	1	360	20	180	6	0.5	40	970	30	1	2	15	2 carb, 1 med-fat protein, 3 fat
Ranch Grilled Chicken Wrap	1	310	16	150	5	0	55	770	21	1	1	19	1 1/2 carb, 2 med-fat protein, 1 fat
Side Caesar Salad & Dressing	1	290	22	200	3.5	0	20	710	17	5	2	8	1 carb, 1 med-fat protein, 3 fat
Side Garden Salad & Avocado Ranch Dressing	1	240	22	200	5	0	30	540	6	2	2	6	1/2 carb, 1 med-fat protein, 3 fat

FAST FOOD

Breakfast

	Serving	Calories	Fat (g)	Cal. from Fat	Sat. Fat (g)	Trans Fat (g)	Chol. (mg)	Sod. (mg)	Carb. (g)	Sugar (g)	Fiber (g)	Prot. (g)	Servings/Exchanges
Bacon, Egg & Cheese Biscuit	1	450	27	240	16	0.5	170	1490	33	4	1	16	2 carb, 1 med-fat protein, 4 fat
BK Breakfast Muffin Sandwich, Bacon, Egg & Cheese	1	300	14	120	5	0	175	990	27	3	2	15	2 carb, 1 med-fat protein, 2 fat
BK Breakfast Muffin Sandwich, Egg & Cheese	1	260	11	100	4	0	170	830	27	3	2	13	2 carb, 1 med-fat protein, 1 fat
BK Breakfast Muffin Sandwich, Ham, Egg & Cheese	1	310	13	120	4.5	0	185	1290	29	4	2	18	2 carb, 2 med-fat protein, 1 fat
BK Breakfast Muffin Sandwich, Sausage & Cheese	1	390	23	210	9	0	55	1130	27	2	2	17	2 carb, 2 med-fat protein, 3 fat

Item	Amount	Cal.											Exchanges
BK Breakfast Muffin Sandwich, Sausage, Egg & Cheese	1	430	26	230	8	0	200	1140	28	3	2	20	2 carb, 2 med-fat protein, 3 fat
BK Ultimate Breakfast Platter	1	1420	79	710	29	1	460	3020	139	41	5	36	9 carb, 1 med-fat protein, 15 fat
Cinnabon Roll	1	300	11	100	5	0	5	280	45	20	2	6	3 carb, 2 fat
Country Ham & Egg Biscuit	1	440	26	230	15	0.5	190	1980	33	4	1	18	2 carb, 2 med-fat protein, 3 fat
Croissan'wich, Bacon, Egg & Cheese	1	370	21	190	9	0	165	770	31	6	1	13	2 carb, 1 med-fat protein, 3 fat
Croissan'wich, Egg & Cheese	1	330	18	160	8	0	155	620	31	5	1	11	2 carb, 4 fat
Croissan'wich, Ham, Egg & Cheese	1	390	20	180	8	0	175	1080	33	7	1	17	2 carb, 2 med-fat protein, 2 fat
Croissan'wich, Sausage & Cheese	1	420	27	240	11	0	45	710	31	4	1	14	2 carb, 1 med-fat protein, 4 fat
Croissand'wich, Sausage, Egg & Cheese	1	500	33	290	12	0	190	930	32	5	1	19	2 carb, 2 med-fat protein, 5 fat

FAST FOOD

	Serving	Calories	Fat (g)	Cal. from Fat	Sat. Fat (g)	Trans Fat (g)	Chol. (mg)	Sod. (mg)	Carb. (g)	Sugar (g)	Fiber (g)	Prot. (g)	Servings/Exchanges
Double Croissan'wich with Bacon, Egg & Cheese	1	440	27	240	12	0.5	190	1070	32	6	1	17	2 carb, 2 med-fat protein, 3 fat
Double Croissan'wich with Ham, Bacon, Egg & Cheese	1	470	27	240	12	0.5	205	1430	34	7	1	21	2 carb, 2 med-fat protein, 3 fat
Double Croissan'wich with Ham, Egg & Cheese	1	480	26	230	11	0	205	1720	36	9	1	25	2 1/2 carb, 3 med-fat protein, 2 fat
Double Croissan'wich with Ham, Sausage, Egg & Cheese	1	600	39	350	15	0.5	230	1580	35	7	1	27	2 carb, 3 med-fat protein, 5 fat
Double Croissan'wich with Sausage, Bacon, Egg & Cheese	1	580	39	350	15	0.5	215	1250	33	6	1	23	2 carb, 2 med-fat protein, 6 fat
Double Croissan'wich with Sausage, Egg & Cheese	1	790	57	510	21	1	380	1630	35	7	1	34	2 carb, 4 med-fat protein, 7 fat

French Toast Sticks, 3 Piece	1 order	230	11	100	2	0	0	260	29	8	1	3	2 carb, 2 fat
French Toast Sticks, 5 Piece	1 order	380	18	160	3	0	0	430	49	13	2	5	3 carb, 4 fat
Ham, Egg & Cheese Biscuit	1	430	23	210	15	0.5	175	1630	35	6	1	18	2 carb, 2 med-fat protein, 3 fat
Hash Browns, Large	1 (8 oz)	670	44	390	9	0	0	1080	65	0	9	5	4 carb, 9 fat
Hash Browns, Medium	1 (6 oz)	500	33	290	7	0	0	810	48	0	7	4	3 carb, 7 fat
Hash Browns, Small	1 (3 oz)	250	16	150	3.5	0	0	410	24	0	3	2	1 1/2 carb, 3 fat
Pancakes (3) & 1 oz Breakfast Syrup	1	490	16	140	4	0	45	710	82	36	1	5	5 1/2 carb, 3 fat
Pancake & Sausage Platter	1	660	31	270	8	0	80	1020	83	36	1	13	5 1/2 carb, 6 fat
Quaker Oatmeal Maple & Brown Sugar	1	270	3.5	35	1.5	0	5	270	55	32	5	5	3 1/2 carb, 1 fat
Quaker Oatmeal Original	1	140	3.5	30	1	0	5	100	23	1	3	5	1 1/2 carb, 1 fat
Sausage Biscuit	1	420	27	240	15	0.5	35	1090	32	3	1	13	2 carb, 1 med-fat protein, 4 fat

FAST FOOD

	Serving	Calories	Fat (g)	Cal. from Fat	Sat. Fat (g)	Trans Fat (g)	Chol. (mg)	Sod. (mg)	Carb. (g)	Sugar (g)	Fiber (g)	Prot. (g)	Servings/Exchanges
Sausage Breakfast Burrito	1	310	19	170	7	0	145	820	22	2	1	14	1 1/2 carb, 4 fat
Sausage, Egg & Cheese Biscuit	1	550	36	320	19	0.5	190	1480	34	4	1	20	2 carb, 2 med-fat protein, 5 fat
Southwestern Breakfast Burrito	1	600	38	340	13	0	210	1660	43	4	4	23	3 carb, 2 med-fat protein, 6 fat
Desserts													
Brownie Sundae	1	530	17	150	10	0	55	390	89	70	2	10	6 carb, 3 fat
Caramel Sundae	1	280	6	50	3.5	0	20	250	52	37	0	5	3 1/2 carb, 1 fat
Chocolate Chip Cookies (2)	1	330	15	140	8	0	20	250	47	29	1	3	3 carb, 3 fat
Chocolate Fudge Sundae	1	280	7	60	5	0	15	220	50	43	1	6	3 carb, 1 fat
Dutch Apple Pie	1	340	14	130	6	0	0	310	51	25	1	3	3 1/2 carb, 3 fat
Hershey's Sundae Pie	1	310	19	170	12	0	10	220	32	22	1	3	2 carb, 4 fat
Oatmeal Raisin Cookies (2)	1	310	13	120	8	0	20	260	46	26	3	4	3 carb, 3 fat

Item	Serving	Cal.										Exchanges
Oreo Sundae	1	440	12	110	7	0	25	390	77	57	1	8	5 carb, 2 fat
Soft Serve Cone	1	160	4	35	2.5	0	15	130	27	20	0	4	2 carb, 1 fat
Soft Serve Cup	1	140	4	35	2.5	0	15	125	23	19	0	4	1 1/2 carb, 1 fat
Strawberry Sundae	1	190	4	35	2.5	0	15	125	35	31	0	4	3 carb, 1 fat
White Chocolate Macadamia Nut Cookies (2)	1	340	18	160	8	0	20	240	44	28	0	4	3 carb, 4 fat
Beverages												
Caramel Frappe	12 oz	410	19	170	11	0	5	230	58	39	0	3	4 carb, 4 fat
Chocolate Milk Shake	12 oz	580	17	150	13	0.5	40	310	97	83	0	10	6 1/2 carb, 3 fat
Mocha Frappe	12 oz	410	19	170	11	0	5	230	58	39	0	3	4 carb, 4 fat
Smoothie: Strawberry Banana	12 oz	200	0	5	0	0	0	20	48	40	2	1	3 carb
Strawberry Milk Shake	12 oz	500	16	140	12	0.5	40	320	79	67	0	10	5 carb, 3 fat
Vanilla Milk Shake	12 oz	550	16	140	12	0.5	40	310	91	81	0	10	6 carb, 3 fat

FAST FOOD

CARL'S JR.

Charbroiled Burgers

	Serving	Calories	Fat (g)	Cal. from Fat	Sat. Fat (g)	Trans Fat (g)	Chol. (mg)	Sod. (mg)	Carb. (g)	Sugar (g)	Fiber (g)	Prot. (g)	Servings/Exchanges
Big Hamburger	1	480	18	160	8	0.5	50	870	56	13	3	25	3 1/2 carb, 2 med-fat protein, 2 fat
Double Western Bacon Cheeseburger	1	990	53	480	24	2	140	1820	75	16	4	52	5 carb, 6 med-fat protein, 5 fat
Famous Star with Cheese	1	670	37	330	13	1	75	1210	57	13	3	28	4 carb, 2 med-fat protein, 5 fat
Kid's Cheeseburger	1	330	15	140	7	0.5	40	810	34	7	1	14	2 carb, 1 med-fat protein, 2 fat
Kid's Hamburger	1	270	10	90	3.5	0.5	25	540	33	7	1	11	2 carb, 1 med-fat protein, 1 fat
Super Star with Cheese	1	930	56	510	23	2	140	1540	59	14	3	48	4 carb, 5 med-fat protein, 6 fat
Teriyaki Burger	1	630	29	260	11	1	70	1060	65	20	3	28	4 carb, 2 med-fat protein, 4 fat

The Big Carl	1	920	58	520	23	2	140	1380	56	12	3	47	3 1/2 carb, 5 med-fat protein, 7 fat
The Guacamole Bacon Thickburger	1	1090	75	680	24	2.5	135	1970	57	14	4	47	4 carb, 5 med-fat protein, 10 fat
The Jalapeño Thickburger	1	980	65	590	21	2.5	130	1870	55	13	3	43	3 1/2 carb, 5 med-fat protein, 8 fat
The Low Carb Thickburger	1	550	41	370	18	2	120	1370	9	6	1	38	1/2 carb, 5 med-fat protein, 3 fat
The Original Six Dollar Thickburger	1	940	58	520	21	2.5	125	1880	62	20	3	44	4 carb, 5 med-fat protein, 7 fat
The Western Bacon Thickburger	1	980	55	490	21	2	125	2210	74	17	3	49	5 carb, 5 med-fat protein, 6 fat
Western Bacon Cheeseburger	1	730	34	310	14	1	75	1500	74	16	4	33	5 carb, 3 med-fat protein, 4 fat
Charbroiled Turkey Burgers												
Guacamole Turkey Burger	1	480	19	170	6	0	85	1000	44	9	3	32	3 carb, 3 med-fat protein, 1 fat
Jalapeño Turkey Burger	1	500	22	200	6	0	90	1150	43	9	3	31	3 carb, 3 med-fat protein, 1 fat

FAST FOOD

	Serving	Calories	Fat (g)	Cal. from Fat	Sat. Fat (g)	Trans Fat (g)	Chol. (mg)	Sod. (mg)	Carb. (g)	Sugar (g)	Fiber (g)	Prot. (g)	Servings/Exchanges
Teriyaki Turkey Burger	1	480	14	130	5	0	85	1120	56	19	3	32	3 1/2 carb, 3 med-fat protein
Turkey Burger	1	490	22	200	4.5	0	80	960	45	10	3	29	3 carb, 3 med-fat protein, 1 fat
Chicken & Other Choices													
Bacon Swiss Crispy Chicken Sandwich	1	860	49	440	11	0.5	105	2540	67	12	4	41	4 1/2 carb, 4 med-fat protein, 6 fat
Big Chicken Fillet Sandwich	1	760	41	370	7	0	85	2050	64	11	4	35	4 carb, 3 med-fat protein, 5 fat
Charbroiled Atlantic Cod Fish Sandwich	1	390	11	100	2	0	35	780	52	9	3	20	3 1/2 carb, 1 med-fat protein, 1 fat
Charbroiled BBQ Chicken Sandwich	1	390	7	70	1.5	0	60	990	50	13	3	30	3 carb, 3 lean protein
Charbroiled Chicken Club Sandwich	1	580	28	260	8	0	90	1290	46	11	2	36	3 carb, 4 med-fat protein, 2 fat
Charbroiled Santa Fe Chicken Sandwich	1	560	27	250	7	0	85	1290	46	10	3	33	3 carb, 3 med-fat protein, 2 fat

	Amount	Cal.	Fat (g)	Fat Cal.	Sat. Fat (g)	Trans Fat (g)	Chol. (mg)	Sod. (mg)	Carb. (g)	Fiber (g)	Sugar (g)	Prot. (g)	Choices/Exchanges
Chicken Stars, 4 Pieces	1 order	170	10	90	2	0	20	360	12	0	1	8	1 carb, 1 med-fat protein, 1 fat
Chicken Stars, 6 Pieces	1 order	260	16	140	3.5	0	30	540	18	0	2	12	1 carb, 1 med-fat protein, 2 fat
Chicken Stars, 9 Pieces	1 order	390	23	210	5	0	45	810	26	0	3	18	2 carb, 2 med-fat protein, 3 fat
Hand-Breaded Chicken Tenders, 3 Pieces	1 order	260	13	110	2.5	0	70	770	13	0	2	25	1 carb, 3 med-fat protein
Hand-Breaded Chicken Tenders, 5 Pieces	1 order	440	21	190	4.5	0	115	1290	21	0	3	41	1 1/2 carb, 5 med-fat protein
Kid's Hand-Breaded Chicken Tenders, 2 Pieces	1 order	180	9	80	2	0	45	520	9	0	1	16	1/2 carb, 2 med-fat protein
Spicy Chicken Sandwich	1	460	24	220	4.5	0	30	1360	47	5	4	14	3 carb, 1 med-fat protein, 4 fat
Sides													
Chili Cheese Fries	1 order	810	46	410	14	1.5	55	2050	80	2	9	21	5 carb, 1 med-fat protein, 8 fat
CrissCut Fries	1 order	450	29	260	5	0	0	900	42	0	4	5	3 carb, 6 fat

FAST FOOD

	Serving	Calories	Fat (g)	Cal. from Fat	Sat. Fat (g)	Trans Fat (g)	Chol. (mg)	Sod. (mg)	Carb. (g)	Sugar (g)	Fiber (g)	Prot. (g)	Servings/Exchanges
Fried Zucchini	1 order	330	18	160	3	0	0	610	36	7	2	6	2 1/2 carb, 4 fat
Natural-Cut Fries, Kids	1 (3 oz)	240	12	100	2	0	0	480	31	0	3	3	2 carb, 2 fat
Natural-Cut Fries, Large	1 (5.6 oz)	460	22	200	4	0	0	920	59	0	6	5	4 carb, 4 fat
Natural-Cut Fries, Medium	1 (5.3 oz)	430	21	190	4	0	0	860	55	0	5	5	3 1/2 carb, 4 fat
Natural-Cut Fries, Small	1 (3.7 oz)	300	15	130	2.5	0	0	600	39	0	4	3	2 1/2 carb, 3 fat
Onion Rings	1 order	530	28	250	4.5	0	0	590	61	6	3	8	4 carb, 6 fat
Sweet Potato Fries, Large	1 (6.4 oz)	540	26	230	4.5	0	5	900	71	29	9	5	4 1/2 carb, 5 fat
Sweet Potato Fries, Medium	1 (6.1 oz)	510	25	220	4	0	5	860	68	27	9	5	4 1/2 carb, 5 fat
Sweet Potato Fries, Small	1 (4.2 oz)	360	17	160	3	0	0	590	47	19	6	3	3 carb, 3 fat
Salads (No Dressing)													
Crispy Chicken Salad	1	350	16	140	4.5	0	60	810	29	7	5	24	2 carb, 3 med-fat protein

Garden Side Salad	1	110	4.5	40	1.5	0	5	230	14	3	2	4	1 carb, 1 fat
Original Grilled Chicken Salad	1	280	12	110	4.5	0	40	880	26	8	4	18	2 carb, 2 med-fat protein
Salad Dressing & Dipping Sauces													
Blue Cheese Dressing	1 (2 oz)	320	34	310	7	0	20	410	1	1	0	2	7 fat
Buttermilk Ranch Dipping Sauce	1 (0.9 oz)	100	10	90	1.5	0	10	220	2	2	0	0	2 fat
Honey Mustard Dipping Sauce	1 (0.9 oz)	120	12	110	2	0	10	130	4	3	0	0	2 fat
House Dressing	1 (2 oz)	220	22	200	3.5	0	20	440	3	2	0	1	4 fat
Low Fat Balsamic Vinaigrette Dressing	1 (2 oz)	35	1.5	15	0	0	0	480	5	3	0	0	free
Sweet & Bold BBQ Dipping Sauce	1 (0.9 oz)	50	0	0	0	0	0	190	13	5	0	0	1 carb
Breakfast													
Bacon Bacon Biscuit	1	530	32	290	12	6	210	1550	39	4	3	22	2 1/2 carb, 2 med-fat protein, 4 fat
Bacon & Egg Burrito	1	570	34	310	18	0	375	1000	38	1	1	26	2 1/2 carb, 3 med-fat protein, 4 fat

FAST FOOD

	Serving	Calories	Fat (g)	Cal. from Fat	Sat. Fat (g)	Trans Fat (g)	Chol. (mg)	Sod. (mg)	Carb. (g)	Sugar (g)	Fiber (g)	Prot. (g)	Servings/Exchanges
Bacon, Egg & Cheese Biscuit	1	480	30	270	12	6	190	1180	38	3	3	15	2 1/2 carb, 1 med-fat protein, 5 fat
Big Country Breakfast Burrito	1	720	43	390	18	0.5	370	1390	55	1	3	25	3 1/2 carb, 2 med-fat protein, 7 fat
Biscuit 'N' Gravy	1	460	26	230	7	7	10	1390	49	2	3	9	3 carb, 5 fat
Breakfast Burger	1	800	43	390	18	1	245	1380	68	13	4	37	4 1/2 carb, 3 med-fat protein, 6 fat
Hash Brown Nuggets, Large	1 (6.2 oz)	560	37	330	7	0	0	710	52	0	5	5	3 1/2 carb, 7 fat
Hash Brown Nuggets, Medium	1 (4.3 oz)	390	26	230	4.5	0	0	490	36	0	4	3	2 1/2 carb, 5 fat
Hash Brown Nuggets, Small	1 (3.9 oz)	350	23	210	4	0	0	440	32	0	3	3	2 carb, 5 fat
Loaded Breakfast Burrito	1	770	48	430	22	0	395	1420	53	2	3	31	3 1/2 carb, 3 med-fat protein, 7 fat
Loaded Omelet Biscuit	1	560	37	330	15	6	210	1370	38	3	3	19	2 1/2 carb, 2 med-fat protein, 5 fat

Made From Scratch Biscuit	1	300	15	130	4	6	0	780	36	2	3	5	2 1/2 carb, 3 fat
Monster Biscuit	1	810	60	540	25	6	400	1850	40	4	3	29	2 1/2 carb, 3 med-fat protein, 9 fat
Sausage, Egg & Cheese Biscuit	1	620	44	390	17	6	215	1430	38	3	3	19	2 1/2 carb, 2 med-fat protein, 7 fat
Sourdough Breakfast Sandwich	1	470	24	220	12	0.5	215	1340	40	4	1	28	2 1/2 carb, 3 med-fat protein, 2 fat
Steak & Egg Burrito	1	650	36	330	20	0	415	1730	44	3	2	35	3 carb, 4 med-fat protein, 3 fat
Strawberry Biscuit	1	390	15	130	4	6	0	800	60	24	3	5	4 carb, 3 fat
Desserts													
Chocolate Cake	1	300	12	110	3	0	30	350	48	36	1	3	3 carb, 2 fat
Chocolate Chip Cookie	1	370	19	170	10	0	30	350	48	27	2	3	3 carb, 4 fat
Strawberry Swirl Cheesecake	1	290	16	140	9	0	55	230	32	21	0	6	2 carb, 3 fat
Hand-Scooped Ice Cream Shakes & Malts													
Chocolate Malt	14.8 oz	770	37	330	25	1.5	105	350	99	70	1	14	6 1/2 carb, 7 fat

FAST FOOD

	Serving	Calories	Fat (g)	Cal. from Fat	Sat. Fat (g)	Trans Fat (g)	Chol. (mg)	Sod. (mg)	Carb. (g)	Sugar (g)	Fiber (g)	Prot. (g)	Servings/Exchanges
Chocolate Shake	14.2 oz	700	36	330	25	1.5	105	300	84	59	1	12	5 1/2 carb, 7 fat
Oreo Cookie Malt	14.8 oz	790	41	370	26	1.5	110	390	94	64	1	15	6 carb, 8 fat
Oreo Cookie Shake	14.2 oz	720	40	360	26	1.5	105	340	79	53	1	13	5 carb, 8 fat
Strawberry Malt	14.8 oz	770	37	330	25	1.5	105	290	98	75	0	13	6 carb, 7 fat
Strawberry Shake	14.2 oz	700	36	320	24	1.5	105	250	83	63	0	12	5 1/2 carb, 7 fat
Vanilla Malt	14.8 oz	780	37	330	25	1.5	105	290	100	76	0	13	6 1/2 carb, 7 fat
Vanilla Shake	14.2 oz	710	36	320	24	1.5	105	240	86	65	0	12	5 1/2 carb, 7 fat
CHIPOTLE													
Ingredients													
Barbacoa	4 oz	165	7	63	2.5	0	65	530	2	0	1	24	3 lean protein
Black Beans	4 oz	120	1	9	0	0	0	260	22	1	12	7	1 1/2 carb
Brown Rice	4 oz	200	7	63	0	0	0	165	32	0.5	2.5	3.5	2 carb, 1 fat
Carnitas	4 oz	220	13	117	6	0	65	500	0.5	0	0	26	4 lean protein
Cheese	1 oz	100	7.5	68	5	0	30	190	1	0	0	6	1 high-fat protein

Chicken	4 oz	180	7	63	3	0	125	310	0	0	0.5	32	5 lean protein
Chips	4 oz	570	27	243	3.5	0	0	420	73	4	8	8	5 carb, 5 fat
Crispy Corn Tortillas	2	140	2	50	2	0	0	20	20	0	4	2	1 carb, 1 fat
Fajita Veggies	2.5 oz	20	0.5	5	0	0	0	170	4	2	1	1	free
Fresh Tomato Salsa	3.5 oz	20	0	0	0	0	0	500	4	3	0.5	1	free
Guacamole	3.5 oz	200	19	171	3	0	0	330	7	1	5	2	1/2 carb, 4 fat
Pinto Beans	4 oz	115	1	9	0	0	0	300	21	1	10	6	1 1/2 carb
Roasted Chili-Corn Salsa	3.5 oz	80	1.5	14	0	0	0	330	16	4	3	3	1 carb
Romaine Lettuce	1 oz	5	0	0	0	0	0	0	1	0	1	0	free
Sofritas	4 oz	145	10	90	1.5	0	0	555	9	4.5	3.5	8	1/2 carb, 1 med-fat protein, 1 fat
Soft Corn Tortilla	2	140	1	10	0	0	0	50	28	0	4	2	2 carb
Soft Flour Tortilla	2	170	5	50	2	0	0	380	26	0	1	4	2 carb, 1 fat
Sour Cream	2 oz	115	9.5	86	7	0	40	30	1	2	0	2	2 fat
Steak	4 oz	190	6.5	59	2	0	65	320	2	1	0	30	4 lean protein
Tomatillo-Green Chili Salsa	2 oz	20	0	0	0	0	0	250	4	2	1	0.5	free

FAST FOOD

	Serving	Calories	Fat (g)	Cal. from Fat	Sat. Fat (g)	Trans Fat (g)	Chol. (mg)	Sod. (mg)	Carb. (g)	Sugar (g)	Fiber (g)	Prot. (g)	Servings/Exchanges
Tomatillo-Red Chili Salsa	2 oz	25	1	9	0	0	0	500	4	1	2	1	1 vegetable
Vinaigrette	2 oz	270	25	225	4.5	0	10	850	18	12	2	0.5	1 carb, 5 fat
White Rice	4 oz	185	4	36	0	0	0	375	34	0	1	3.5	2 carb, 1 fat
CHURCH'S CHICKEN													
Big Tex Tender Sandwich	1	740	37	333	8	0	60	1652	63	8	0	29	4 carb, 2 med-fat protein, 5 fat
Boneless Wing, with Sauce	1	90–100	5	45	1	0	10	240–440	16–20	7–10	1	6	1 carb, 1 fat
Chicken Fried Steak	1	470	28	252	7	1	65	1620	36	4	1	21	2 1/2 carb, 2 med-fat protein, 3 fat
Chicken Sandwich with Cheese	1	500	26	234	7	0	50	1460	48	5	3	19	3 carb, 1 med-fat protein, 4 fat
Double Chicken & Cheese Sandwich	1	690	30	270	7.5	0	40	1313	38	4	1	16	2 1/2 carb, 1 med-fat protein, 4 1/2 fat

	Serving												Exchanges
Fish Fillet	1 fillet	190	10	90	4	0	25	380	14	4	1	8	1 carb, 1 med-fat protein, 1 fat
Livers	6 livers	840	42	378	9	0	570	1200	54	0	0	48	3 1/2 carb, 5 med-fat protein, 3 fat
Original Breast	1	200	11	99	3	0	80	440	3	0	1	22	3 med-fat protein
Original Chicken Sandwich	1	401	22	198	3–5	0	20	893	36	4	1	12	2 1/2 carb, 1 med-fat protein, 3 fat
Original Leg	1	110	6	54	1.5	0	55	280	3	0	0	10	1 med-fat protein
Original Thigh	1	330	23	207	6	0	110	680	8	0	1	21	1/2 carb, 3 med-fat protein, 1 1/2 fat
Original Wing	1	300	18	162	5	0	120	540	7	0	3	27	1/2 carb, 4 med-fat protein
Spicy Breast	1	320	20	180	5	0	75	760	12	0	2	21	1 carb, 3 med-fat protein, 1 fat
Spicy Leg	1	180	11	99	3	0	65	470	8	0	1	12	1/2 carb 1 med-fat protein, 1 fat
Spicy Tender Strips	1	140	7	63	2	0	25	480	7	0	4	11	1/2 carb, 1 med-fat protein

FAST FOOD

	Serving	Calories	Fat (g)	Cal. from Fat	Sat. Fat (g)	Trans Fat (g)	Chol. (mg)	Sod. (mg)	Carb. (g)	Sugar (g)	Fiber (g)	Prot. (g)	Servings/Exchanges
Spicy Thigh	1	480	35	315	9	0	135	1040	20	0	2	22	1 carb, 3 med-fat protein, 4 fat
Spicy Wing	1	430	27	243	7	0	125	1020	17	0	2	29	1 carb, 4 med-fat protein, 1 fat
Tender Strips	1	120	6	54	1.5	0	35	440	6	0	0	12	1/2 carb, 1 med-fat protein
Small Sides													
Baked Macaroni & Cheese	1	260	8	72	4	0	10	1240	24	2	2	9	1 1/2 carb, 1 med-fat protein
Cajun Rice	1	290	17	153	5	0	70	1037	27	2	2	3	2 carb, 3 fat
Cole Slaw	1	150	10	90	2	0	5	170	15	7	2	1	1 carb, 2 fat
Corn	1	140	3	27	0	0	0	15	24	2	9	4	1 1/2 carb
French Fries	1	140	6	54	1	0	0	320	19	0	1	1	1 carb, 1 fat
Honey-Butter Biscuit	1	240	15	135	7	0	4	540	28	4	1	3	2 carb, 3 fat
Jalapeño Cheese Bombers	4 bombers	190	7	63	4	0	20	770	24	1	1	7	1 1/2 carb, 1 fat

Mashed Potatoes & Gravy	1	110	2	18	0.5	0	0	780	21	3	2	3	1 1/2 carb
Okra	1	170	11	99	3	0	0	340	17	2	2	2	1 carb, 2 fat
Sweet Corn Nuggets	8 nuggets	240	7	63	1	0	0	520	40	2	2	4	2 1/2 carb, 1 fat
Dessert													
Apple Pie	1	260	10	90	3	0	5	250	40	15	1	2	2 1/2 carb, 1 1/2 fat
CINNABON													
Caramel Pecan Minibon Roll	1	450	22	200	8	0	30	390	60	32	2	6	4 carb, 4 fat
Caramel Pecanbon	1	1080	51	460	20	0	65	950	146	75	3	14	10 carb, 8 fat
Churro	1	280	11	102	2	0	0	375	39	8	1	5	2 1/2 carb, 2 fat
Cinnabon Classic Roll	1	880	37	330	17	0	55	820	127	58	2	13	8 1/2 carb, 6 fat
Cinnabon Stix	5 stix	400	21	190	9	0	20	440	46	16	1	6	3 carb, 4 fat
Classic Bites	6 bites	650	24	220	12	0	35	570	95	48	1	8	6 carb, 4 fat
Minibon Roll	1	350	15	130	7	0	25	330	51	23	1	5	3 1/2 carb, 2 fat

FAST FOOD

CULVER'S

ButterBurgers

	Serving	Calories	Fat (g)	Cal. from Fat	Sat. Fat (g)	Trans Fat (g)	Chol. (mg)	Sod. (mg)	Carb. (g)	Sugar (g)	Fiber (g)	Prot. (g)	Servings/Exchanges
Cheddar Bacon, Double	1	760	48	435	21.5	1	155	1090	39	6	1	48	2 1/2 carb, 6 med-fat protein, 3 fat
Cheddar Bacon, Single	1	510	28	260	12	0.5	85	850	39	6	1	29	2 1/2 carb, 3 med-fat protein, 2 fat
Cheddar Bacon, Triple	1	1010	68	610	31	1.5	225	1330	39	6	1	67	2 1/2 carb, 8 1/2 med-fat protein, 5 fat
Cheddar, Double	1	720	46	405	20.5	1	145	950	39	6	1	44	2 1/2 carb, 5 med-fat protein, 4 fat
Cheddar, Single	1	470	26	230	11	0.5	75	710	39	6	1	25	2 1/2 carb, 2 1/2 med-fat protein, 2 fat
Cheddar, Triple	1	970	66	580	30	1.5	215	1190	39	6	1	63	2 1/2 carb, 8 med-fat protein, 5 fat
Cheese, Double	1	700	44	385	18.5	1	135	950	41	8	1	40	2 1/2 carb, 5 med-fat protein, 3 fat

Item												Exchanges/Choices
Cheese, Single	1	460	24	220	10	0.5	70	710	40	7	1	23	2 1/2 carb, 2 med-fat protein, 2 fat
Cheese, Triple	1	940	62	550	27	1.5	200	1190	42	9	1	57	3 carb, 7 med-fat protein, 5 fat
Mushroom & Swiss, Double	1	760	48	421	18.5	1	145	840	41	6	1	46	2 1/2 carb, 5 1/2 med-fat protein, 4 fat
Mushroom & Swiss, Single	1	490	26	238	10	0.5	75	655	40	7	1	26	2 1/2 carb, 3 med-fat protein, 2 fat
Mushroom & Swiss, Triple	1	1030	68	604	27	1.5	215	1025	42	6	1	66	3 carb, 8 med-fat protein, 5 fat
Pepper Grinder Pub Burger, Double	1	940	64	565	24.5	1	170	990	45	5	1	51	3 carb, 6 med-fat protein, 6 fat
Pepper Grinder Pub Burger, Single	1	770	51	450	19.5	0.5	120	890	45	5	1	37	3 carb, 4 med-fat protein, 6 fat
Pepper Grinder Pub Burger, Triple	1	1110	77	680	29.5	1.5	220	1090	45	5	1	65	3 carb, 8 med-fat protein, 7 fat
Sourdough Melt, Double	1	710	46	402	21	1	150	950	36	2	1	44	2 1/2 carb, 5 med-fat protein, 4 fat
Sourdough Melt, Single	1	460	26	226	11.5	0.5	80	710	36	2	1	25	2 1/2 carb, 2 1/2 med-fat protein, 2 fat

FAST FOOD

	Serving	Calories	Fat (g)	Cal. from Fat	Sat. Fat (g)	Trans Fat (g)	Chol. (mg)	Sod. (mg)	Carb. (g)	Sugar (g)	Fiber (g)	Prot. (g)	Servings/Exchanges
Sourdough Melt, Triple	1	970	66	576	30.5	1.5	220	1190	36	2	1	63	2 1/2 carb, 8 med-fat protein, 5 fat
Swiss, Double	1	720	44	385	18.5	1	145	740	39	6	1	46	2 1/2 carb, 5 1/2 med-fat protein, 3 fat
Swiss, Single	1	470	24	220	10	0.5	75	605	39	6	1	26	2 1/2 carb, 3 med-fat protein, 1 fat
Swiss, Triple	1	970	62	550	27	1.5	215	875	39	6	1	66	3 carb, 8 med-fat protein, 4 fat
The Culver's Bacon Deluxe, Double	1	850	58	515	21.5	1	155	1320	43	8	1	44	3 carb, 5 med-fat protein, 6 fat
The Culver's Bacon Deluxe, Single	1	610	38	350	13	0.5	90	1080	42	8	1	27	3 carb, 3 med-fat protein, 4 fat
The Culver's Bacon Deluxe, Triple	1	1090	76	680	30	1.5	220	1560	44	10	1	61	3 carb, 7 1/2 med-fat protein, 7 fat
The Culver's Deluxe, Double	1	810	54	485	20.5	1	145	1180	43	8	1	40	3 carb, 4 1/2 med-fat protein, 6 fat

The Culver's Deluxe, Single	1	570	36	320	12	0.5	80	940	42	8	1	23	3 carb, 2 med-fat protein, 5 fat
The Culver's Deluxe, Triple	1	1050	74	650	29	1.5	210	1420	44	10	1	57	3 carb, 7 med-fat protein, 7 fat
The Original, Double	1	560	32	285	11.5	1	105	670	39	6	1	34	2 1/2 carb, 4 med-fat protein, 2 fat
The Original, Single	1	390	18	170	6.5	0.5	55	570	39	6	1	20	2 1/2 carb, 2 med-fat protein, 1 fat
The Original, Triple	1	730	44	400	16.5	1.5	155	770	39	6	1	48	2 1/2 carb, 6 med-fat protein, 2 fat
Wisconsin Swiss Melt, Double	1	730	44	382	19	1	150	860	38	2	4	46	2 1/2 carb, 5 1/2 med-fat protein, 3 fat
Wisconsin Swiss Melt, Single	1	480	24	216	10.5	0.5	80	725	38	2	4	26	2 1/2 carb, 3 med-fat protein, 1 fat
Wisconsin Swiss Melt, Triple	1	990	62	546	27.5	1.5	220	995	38	2	4	66	2 1/2 carb, 8 med-fat protein, 3 1/2 fat

Sandwiches & Favorites

Beef Pot Roast Sandwich	1	410	14	145	6.5	1	140	830	41	8	1	31	2 1/2 carb, 3 med-fat protein

FAST FOOD

	Serving	Calories	Fat (g)	Cal. from Fat	Sat. Fat (g)	Trans Fat (g)	Chol. (mg)	Sod. (mg)	Carb. (g)	Sugar (g)	Fiber (g)	Prot. (g)	Servings/Exchanges
Buffalo Chicken Tenders, 4 Piece	1 order	460	22	190	3	0	100	1820	32	0	2	34	2 carb, 4 med-fat protein
Chicken Tenders, 4 Piece	1 order	540	24	220	3	0	100	1840	42	0	2	40	3 carb, 4 1/2 med-fat protein
Crispy Chicken Sandwich	1	460	16	145	2.5	0	55	1200	57	6	1	25	4 carb, 2 med-fat protein
Grilled Chicken Sandwich	1	390	8	65	2.5	0	110	1190	39	5	1	41	2 1/2 carb, 5 lean protein
Grilled Reuben Melt	1	670	34	302	13.5	0	105	1880	49	7	4	37	3 carb, 4 med-fat protein, 2 fat
North Atlantic Cod Filet Sandwich	1	600	34	300	7.5	0	102	865	48	7	1	26	3 carb, 2 1/2 med-fat protein, 4 fat
Pork Tenderloin Sandwich	1	630	26	245	4.5	0	45	990	73	6	3	18	5 carb, 2 fat
Concrete Mixers													
Chocolate Oreo Concrete Mini Mixer	1	430	21	188	11.2	0.6	119	225	57	44	2	8	4 carb, 3 fat

Chocolate Oreo Concrete Mixer, Regular	1	880	43	385	23	1.2	245	458	116	90	4	16	7 1/2 carb, 7 fat
Chocolate Oreo Concrete Mixer, Short	1	680	34	301	18.7	1	207	331	88	70	3	13	6 carb, 6 fat
Chocolate Oreo Concrete Mixer, Tall	1	1270	62	555	33	1.7	350	665	167	129	5	23	11 carb, 10 fat
Vanilla & M&Ms Concrete Mini Mixer	1	510	27	252	17	0.8	135	121	57	50	1	8	4 carb, 5 fat
Vanilla & M&Ms Concrete Mixer, Regular	1	1050	57	520	35	1.8	280	250	117	102	2	17	8 carb, 10 fat
Vanilla & M&Ms Concrete Mixer, Short	1	790	44	405	27.1	1.5	236	197	85	74	1	13	5 1/2 carb, 8 fat
Vanilla & M&Ms Concrete Mixer, Tall	1	1520	82	750	50.5	2.5	400	360	170	149	3	24	11 carb, 14 fat
Dinners													
Beef Pot Roast Dinner	1	750	31	296	14.2	1	181	2260	80	13	6	37	5 carb, 3 med-fat protein, 2 fat
Butterfly Jumbo Shrimp Dinner, 10 Piece	1	1310	67	612	6.5	0	125	3130	150	44	7	30	10 carb, 11 fat

FAST FOOD

	Serving	Calories	Fat (g)	Cal. from Fat	Sat. Fat (g)	Trans Fat (g)	Chol. (mg)	Sod. (mg)	Carb. (g)	Sugar (g)	Fiber (g)	Prot. (g)	Servings/Exchanges
Butterfly Jumbo Shrimp Dinner, 6 Piece	1	1090	55	500	6.5	0	85	2410	130	44	7	22	8 1/2 carb, 9 fat
Chopped Steak Dinner	1	810	47	424	18.2	1	141	1950	61	10	5	37	4 carb, 4 med-fat protein, 5 fat
Fresh Fried Chicken Dinner, 2 Piece (Breast, Wing)	1	890	38	334	11	0	293	2550	60	10	5	78	4 carb, 9 1/2 lean protein, 3 fat
Fresh Fried Chicken Dinner, 2 Piece (Leg, Thigh)	1	770	38	334	11	0	253	2250	60	10	5	49	4 carb, 5 med-fat protein, 2 fat
Fresh Fried Chicken Dinner, 4 Piece	1	1250	59	514	15	0	503	3300	64	10	5	118	4 carb, 15 lean protein, 5 fat
Fresh Fried Chicken Value Basket, 2 Piece (Breast, Wing)	1	840	35	310	6	0	250	1580	57	22	4	75	4 carb, 9 lean protein, 3 fat

Item	Serving												Exchanges/Choices
Fresh Fried Chicken Value Basket, 2 Piece (Leg, Thigh)	1	720	35	310	6	0	210	1280	57	22	4	46	4 carb, 5 med-fat protein, 1 fat
North Atlantic Cod Dinner, 2 Piece	1	1480	100	892	14.5	0.5	175	1690	107	41	6	42	7 carb, 3 med-fat protein, 16 fat
North Atlantic Cod Dinner, 3 Piece	1	1680	112	994	15.5	0.5	234	1876	115	42	6	58	7 1/2 carb, 5 med-fat protein, 16 fat
Fresh Fried Chicken													
Fresh Fried Chicken, 4 Piece	1 order	840	42	360	8	0	460	1800	8	0	0	109	1/2 carb, 15 lean protein, 2 fat
Fresh Fried Chicken, 8 Piece	1 order	1680	84	720	16	0	920	3600	16	0	0	218	1 carb, 31 lean protein, 4 fat
Fresh Fried Chicken, 12 Piece	1 order	2520	126	1080	24	0	1380	5400	24	0	0	327	1 1/2 carb, 46 lean protein, 6 fat
Fresh Fried Chicken, 16 Piece	1 order	3360	168	1440	32	0	1840	7200	32	0	0	436	2 carb, 62 lean protein, 8 fat
Fresh Fried Chicken, 20 Piece	1 order	4200	210	1800	40	0	2300	9000	40	0	0	545	2 1/2 carb, 77 lean protein, 11 fat

FAST FOOD

	Serving	Calories	Fat (g)	Cal. from Fat	Sat. Fat (g)	Trans Fat (g)	Chol. (mg)	Sod. (mg)	Carb. (g)	Sugar (g)	Fiber (g)	Prot. (g)	Servings/Exchanges
Sides													
Chili Cheddar Fries	1 order (10.9 oz)	670	32	280	8.5	0	40	1340	78	31	7	20	5 carb, 1 med-fat protein, 4 fat
Cole Slaw	1 (4 oz)	210	17	150	2.5	0	10	240	15	12	2	0	1 carb, 3 fat
Cole Slaw, Large	1 (12 oz)	630	51	450	7.5	0	30	720	45	36	6	0	3 carb, 10 fat
Crinkle Cut Fries, Large	1 (6.3 oz)	460	18	160	2	0	0	680	68	29	5	7	4 1/2 carb, 3 fat
Crinkle Cut Fries, Medium	1 (4.9 oz)	360	14	130	2	0	0	530	53	22	4	6	3 1/2 carb, 2 fat
Crinkle Cut Fries, Small	1 (3.2 oz)	240	9	80	1	0	0	350	35	15	3	4	2 carb, 1 fat
Dinner Roll	1 (1.4 oz)	110	2	20	0	0	5	170	20	3	0	3	1 carb
Green Beans	1 (4.9 oz)	130	9	82	5	0	26	950	11	4	3	2	1/2 carb, 2 fat
Green Beans, Large	1 (15.9 oz)	420	29	265	16.1	0	84	3068	37	13	11	6	2 1/2 carb, 5 fat
Mashed Potatoes & Gravy	1 (7 oz)	140	2	21	0	0	2	350	25	3	2	4	1 1/2 carb

Food	Amount												Exchanges
Mashed Potatoes & Gravy, Large	1 (21.6 oz)	430	9	92	0	0	12	1348	71	8	5	10	4 1/2 carb, 1 fat
Onion Rings	1 order (4.2 oz)	400	22	200	2.5	0	0	530	44	3	3	6	3 carb, 4 fat
Sweet Potato Fries, Crinkle Cut, Family Size	1 (19.9 oz)	1590	70	630	7	0	0	2530	229	90	24	12	15 carb, 11 fat
Sweet Potato Fries, Crinkle Cut, Large	1 (6.4 oz)	510	22	200	2	0	0	810	74	29	8	4	5 carb, 3 fat
Sweet Potato Fries, Crinkle Cut, Regular	1 (5 oz)	400	18	160	2	0	0	630	57	22	6	3	4 carb, 3 fat
Sweet Potato Fries, Crinkle Cut, Small	1 (3.2 oz)	260	11	100	1	0	0	410	37	15	4	2	2 1/2 carb, 2 fat
Wisconsin Cheese Curds	1 order (5.3 oz)	510	25	230	12	0.7	55	1230	51	4	0	20	3 1/2 carb, 1 med-fat protein, 3 fat
Sundaes													
Banana Split, 2 Scoop	1	1060	60	545	26.6	1.2	222	365	122	92	8	15	8 carb, 10 fat
Banana Split, 3 Scoop	1	1350	73	650	34	0.2	285	500	166	126	8	20	11 carb, 12 fat
Caramel Cashew, 1 Scoop	1	600	33	305	14.6	0.7	120	290	68	45	1	10	4 1/2 carb, 6 fat

FAST FOOD

	Serving	Calories	Fat (g)	Cal. from Fat	Sat. Fat (g)	Trans Fat (g)	Chol. (mg)	Sod. (mg)	Carb. (g)	Sugar (g)	Fiber (g)	Prot. (g)	Servings/Exchanges
Caramel Cashew, 2 Scoop	1	1000	51	470	26.6	1.2	230	470	122	85	1	16	8 carb, 9 fat
Caramel Cashew, 3 Scoop	1	1150	61	550	31.6	0.2	290	510	138	98	1	19	9 carb, 10 fat
Fudge Pecan Sundae, 1 Scoop	1	640	43	395	16.5	0.7	115	280	58	48	2	10	4 carb, 8 fat
Fudge Pecan Sundae, 2 Scoop	1	1040	64	580	31.2	1.2	220	450	107	91	2	16	7 carb, 11 fat
Fudge Pecan Sundae, 3 Scoop	1	1190	74	660	36.2	0.2	280	490	123	104	2	20	8 carb, 13 fat
Turtle Sundae, 1 Scoop	1	640	42	385	15.1	0.7	118	285	60	46	2	9	4 carb, 8 fat
Turtle Sundae, 2 Scoop	1	1040	62	560	28.5	1.2	225	460	112	88	2	16	7 1/2 carb, 11 fat
Turtle Sundae, 3 Scoop	1	1190	72	640	33.5	0.2	285	500	128	101	2	18	8 1/2 carb, 13 fat
Soups													
Baja Chicken Enchilada	1	300	18	160	8	0	65	1300	25	6	6	12	1 1/2 carb, 1 med-fat protein, 2 fat
Bean with Ham	1	160	2	20	0.5	0	5	1270	28	3	7	7	2 carb

Item													Exchanges/Choices
Boston Clam Chowder	1	260	11	100	4	0	30	1530	27	8	1	12	2 carb, 1 med-fat protein, 1 fat
Broccoli Cheese	1	220	12	100	5.5	0	31	1160	17	9	1	10	1 carb, 1 med-fat protein, 1 fat
Cauliflower Cheese	1	270	15	130	6	0	26	1320	25	15	1	10	1 1/2 carb, 1 med-fat protein, 2 fat
Cheesy Chicken Tortilla	1	150	6	50	3	0	27	1450	16	4	1	8	1 carb, 1 med-fat protein
Chicken & Dumpling	1	240	12	110	3	0	50	1290	23	5	1	9	1 1/2 carb, 1 med-fat protein, 1 fat
Chicken Noodle	1	110	2	20	0.5	0	30	1110	14	1	1	7	1 carb, 1 lean protein
George's Chili	1	300	14	120	4.5	0	45	1470	27	6	6	18	2 carb, 2 med-fat protein
George's Chili Supreme	1	400	22	204	6.8	0	75	1516	28	7	6	20	2 carb, 2 med-fat protein, 2 fat
Oven-Roasted Turkey Noodle	1	170	5	40	2	0	43	1280	21	1	0	11	1 1/2 carb, 1 med-fat protein
Potato Au Gratin	1	330	20	170	10	0	45	1180	28	9	1	10	2 carb, 1 med-fat protein, 3 fat

FAST FOOD

	Serving	Calories	Fat (g)	Cal. from Fat	Sat. Fat (g)	Trans Fat (g)	Chol. (mg)	Sod. (mg)	Carb. (g)	Sugar (g)	Fiber (g)	Prot. (g)	Servings/Exchanges
Potato with Bacon	1	240	10	80	4	0	25	1140	28	9	2	9	2 carb, 2 fat
Stuffed Green Pepper	1	140	2	20	1	0	10	1170	24	6	1	5	1 1/2 carb
Tomato Florentine	1	110	1	10	0.5	0	0	1280	22	7	2	4	1 1/2 carb
Vegetable Beef	1	160	4	50	2	0	20	1280	22	4	2	8	1 1/2 carb, 1/2 med-fat protein
Wild & Brown Rice with Chicken	1	270	14	120	5	0	38	1220	26	9	1	10	1 1/2 carb, 1 med-fat protein, 1 1/2 fat
Wisconsin Cheese	1	320	20	180	9	0	37	1090	27	16	0	9	2 carb, 4 fat
Cones and Dishes													
Chocolate, Cake Cone, 1 Scoop	1	300	14	124	8.2	0.5	96	127	39	29	1	6	2 1/2 carb, 2 fat
Chocolate, Cake Cone, 2 Scoop	1	560	27	241	16	0.9	187	237	72	56	3	11	5 carb, 4 fat
Chocolate, Cake Cone, 3 Scoop	1	700	34	304	20.2	1.1	236	297	89	71	3	14	6 carb, 6 fat
Chocolate, Dish, 1 Scoop	1	280	14	130	9	0.5	95	120	35	29	1	6	2 carb, 2 fat

Item													
Chocolate, Dish, 2 Scoop	1	540	28	250	17	1	185	220	68	57	2	11	4 1/2 carb, 5 fat
Chocolate, Dish, 3 Scoop	1	680	35	310	21	1	235	280	85	71	3	14	5 1/2 carb, 6 fat
Chocolate, Waffle Cone, 1 Scoop	1	380	16	155	9.5	0.5	100	120	53	37	1	7	3 1/2 carb, 2 1/2 fat
Chocolate, Waffle Cone, 2 Scoop	1	640	30	275	17.5	1	190	220	86	65	2	12	5 1/2 carb, 5 fat
Chocolate, Waffle Cone, 3 Scoop	1	78	38	335	21.5	1	240	280	103	79	3	15	7 carb, 6 fat
Mini Scoop Chocolate, Cake Cone	1	210	11	101	6.7	0.4	67	60	23	16	0	3	1 1/2 carb, 2 fat
Plain Cake Cone	1	25	0	0	0	0	0	10	5	0	0	0	free
Plain Waffle Cone	1	100	2	25	0.5	0	5	0	18	8	0	1	1 carb
Vanilla, Cake Cone, 1 Scoop	1	330	18	166	11.1	0.7	111	93	35	26	0	6	2 carb, 3 fat
Vanilla, Cake Cone, 2 Scoop	1	610	35	319	21.3	1.3	213	170	64	51	0	11	4 carb, 6 fat
Vanilla, Cake Cone, 3 Scoop	1	760	43	401	26.7	1.7	267	210	78	63	0	13	5 carb, 8 fat
Vanilla, Dish, 1 Scoop	1	310	18	170	11	0.5	115	80	31	27	0	5	2 carb, 3 fat

FAST FOOD

	Serving	Calories	Fat (g)	Cal. from Fat	Sat. Fat (g)	Trans Fat (g)	Chol. (mg)	Sod. (mg)	Carb. (g)	Sugar (g)	Fiber (g)	Prot. (g)	Servings/Exchanges
Vanilla, Dish, 2 Scoop	1	590	35	320	22	1	220	160	59	52	0	10	4 carb, 6 fat
Vanilla, Dish, 3 Scoop	1	740	45	400	27	0	280	200	75	65	0	13	5 carb, 8 fat
Vanilla, Waffle Cone, 1 Scoop	1	410	20	195	11.5	0.5	120	80	49	35	0	6	3 carb, 3 fat
Vanilla, Waffle Cone, 2 Scoop	1	690	38	345	22.5	1	225	160	77	60	0	11	5 carb, 7 fat
Vanilla, Waffle Cone, 3 Scoop	1	840	48	425	27.5	0	285	200	93	73	0	14	6 carb, 8 fat
Kids' Meals													
Applesauce	1	0	0	0	0	0	0	0	0	0	0	0	1 fruit
Buffalo Chicken Tenders, 2 Pieces	1	230	11	95	1.5	0	50	910	16	0	1	17	1 carb, 2 med-fat protein
Chicken Tenders, 2 Pieces	1	270	12	110	1.5	0	50	920	21	0	1	20	1 1/2 carb, 2 med-fat protein
Corn Dog	1	230	14	130	4	0	15	500	17	6	0	7	1 carb, 1 med-fat protein, 2 fat

													Exchanges/Choices
Grilled Cheese on Sourdough	1	350	18	152	9	0	40	670	38	4	1	12	2 1/2 carb, 1 med-fat protein, 2 fat
Hand Crafted Beverages													
Chocolate Malt, Regular	1	880	30	356	22	1	240	320	120	94	0	14	8 carb, 4 fat
Chocolate Shake, Regular	1	820	38	350	22	1	240	280	108	84	0	13	7 carb, 6 fat
Culver's Root Beer Float, Regular	1	440	18	169	11.3	0.7	113	149	66	61	0	6	4 1/2 carb, 3 fat
Lemon Ice Cooler, Regular	1	420	0	0	0	0	0	10	105	95	0	0	7 carb
Lemon Ice Smoothie, Regular	1	230	0	0	0	0	0	0	56	50	0	0	3 1/2 carb
Mint Chip Shake, Regular	1	850	45	414	28	1	240	290	102	89	1	14	7 carb, 8 fat
Mint Shake, Regular	1	840	38	350	22	1	240	390	114	98	0	13	7 1/2 carb, 6 fat
Pumpkin Spice Shake, Regular	1	710	38	350	22	1	240	265	82	72	0	14	5 1/2 carb, 6 1/2 fat
Raspberry Malt, Regular	1	780	39	356	22	1	240	230	96	84	2	14	6 1/2 carb, 6 1/2 fat
Raspberry Shake, Regular	1	720	38	350	22	1	240	190	84	74	2	13	5 1/2 carb, 6 1/2 fat

FAST FOOD

	Serving	Calories	Fat (g)	Cal. from Fat	Sat. Fat (g)	Trans Fat (g)	Chol. (mg)	Sod. (mg)	Carb. (g)	Sugar (g)	Fiber (g)	Prot. (g)	Servings/Exchanges
Strawberry Malt, Regular	1	770	38	347	21.7	1.2	232	210	96	88	0	13	6 1/2 carb, 6 fat
Strawberry Shake, Regular	1	730	38	350	22	1	240	190	86	80	0	13	5 1/2 carb, 6 1/2 fat
Vanilla Malt, Regular	1	790	45	406	26	0	270	260	85	76	0	15	5 1/2 carb, 8 fat
Vanilla Shake, Regular	1	730	44	400	26	0	270	220	73	66	0	14	5 carb, 8 fat
Lemon Ice													
Lemon Ice, 1 Scoop	1	200	0	0	0	0	0	0	49	42	0	0	3 carb
Lemon Ice, 2 Scoop	1	270	0	0	0	0	0	0	67	58	0	0	4 1/2 carb
Lemon Ice, 3 Scoop	1	360	0	0	0	0	0	0	88	78	0	0	6 carb
DAIRY QUEEN													
Burgers													
1/2 lb Cheese GrillBurger	1	770	46	410	20	1.5	140	1410	43	10	2	45	3 carb, 5 med-fat protein, 3 fat
1/2 lb FlameThrower GrillBurger	1	950	66	600	25	2	155	1540	39	7	2	49	2 1/2 carb, 6 med-fat protein, 1 fat

Item													Exchanges/Choices
1/4 lb Bacon Cheese GrillBurger	1	620	36	320	14	1	100	1320	41	9	1	34	2 1/2 carb, 4 med-fat protein, 3 fat
1/4 lb Cheese GrillBurger	1	520	28	250	11	1	75	1100	43	10	2	25	3 carb, 2 med-fat protein, 3 fat
1/4 lb Mushroom Swiss GrillBurger	1	560	33	300	12	1	80	890	39	5	1	27	2 1/2 carb, 3 med-fat protein, 3 fat
Original Cheeseburger	1	380	19	170	8	1	90	930	34	8	1	21	2 carb, 2 med-fat protein, 1 fat
Original Double Cheeseburger	1	580	34	310	16	1.5	150	1240	35	9	1	37	2 carb, 4 1/2 med-fat protein, 2 fat
Hot Dogs													
Chili Cheese Dog	1	390	25	230	11	1	55	1000	25	4	1	16	1 1/2 carb, 2 med-fat protein, 3 fat
Hot Dog	1	300	18	160	8	1	35	750	23	4	1	11	1 1/2 carb, 1 med-fat protein, 2 fat
Sandwiches/Baskets													
Chicken Bacon Ranch	1	500	21	190	7	0	55	1590	45	3	3	29	3 carb, 3 med-fat protein, 1 fat
Chicken Mozzarella	1	630	26	240	9	0	70	1500	63	3	9	34	4 carb, 3 med-fat protein, 1 fat

FAST FOOD

	Serving	Calories	Fat (g)	Cal. from Fat	Sat. Fat (g)	Trans Fat (g)	Chol. (mg)	Sod. (mg)	Carb. (g)	Sugar (g)	Fiber (g)	Prot. (g)	Servings/Exchanges
Chicken Strip Basket with Country Gravy	4 pieces	1020	52	470	9	0.5	80	2570	101	4	17	37	7 carb, 2 med-fat protein, 7 fat
Turkey BLT	1	530	24	220	7	0	60	1590	46	3	3	29	3 carb, 3 med-fat protein, 2 fat
Fresh Choice Salads & Wraps													
Grilled Chicken BLT Salad	1	380	19	170	9	0	100	1540	11	6	3	42	1/2 carb, 6 lean protein, 1 fat
Grilled Chicken Garden Greens Salad	1	150	2	20	0.5	0	40	730	10	6	3	23	1/2 carb, 3 lean protein
Grilled Chicken Sandwich	1	390	14	130	2.5	0	35	920	44	3	2	20	3 carb, 2 med-fat protein
Grilled Chicken Wrap	1	290	15	140	4	0	30	790	24	1	2	16	1 1/2 carb, 2 med-fat protein, 1 fat
Side Items													
French Fries, Regular	1 (5 oz)	380	17	150	2.5	0	0	790	54	0	4	4	3 1/2 carb, 3 fat
Onion Rings	1 (4 oz)	360	16	140	2.5	0	0	840	48	3	2	6	3 carb, 3 fat

Side Salad	1 (4 oz)	25	0	0	0	0	0	15	5	3	2	1	1 vegetable
Breakfast													
Biscuits & Gravy	1	720	410	46	16	1.5	15	2240	64	4	2	12	4 carb, 8 fat
Buttermilk Pancake Platter	1	260	45	5	1.5	0	45	530	46	8	3	7	3 carb
Country Platter	1	780	410	46	16	2	340	1710	69	3	4	21	4 1/2 carb, 1 med-fat protein, 7 fat
Sausage Biscuit Sandwich	1	410	240	27	9	0	195	990	25	1	1	16	1 1/2 carb, 2 med-fat protein, 3 fat
Ultimate Breakfast Burrito, Sausage	1	620	300	33	11	1.5	205	1120	57	2	6	24	4 carb, 2 med-fat protein, 4 fat
Ultimate Hashbrown Platter	1	670	390	43	14	2.5	370	1050	45	2	5	24	3 carb, 2 med-fat protein, 6 fat
Cones													
Dipped Cone, Chocolate, Large	1	650	270	30	24	1	45	220	85	61	1	13	5 1/2 carb, 5 fat
Dipped Cone, Chocolate, Medium	1	470	200	22	17	0.5	30	150	61	43	1	9	4 carb, 4 fat

FAST FOOD

	Serving	Calories	Fat (g)	Cal. from Fat	Sat. Fat (g)	Trans Fat (g)	Chol. (mg)	Sod. (mg)	Carb. (g)	Sugar (g)	Fiber (g)	Prot. (g)	Servings/Exchanges
Dipped Cone, Chocolate, Small	1	330	15	130	12	0	25	110	42	30	0.5	6	3 carb, 2 fat
Vanilla Cone, Kids'	1	170	4.5	45	3	0	15	75	28	18	0	4	2 carb, 1/2 fat
Vanilla Cone, Large	1	470	14	120	9	1	45	200	74	52	0	12	5 carb, 2 fat
Vanilla Cone, Medium	1	330	10	90	6	0.5	30	140	53	36	0	8	3 1/2 carb, 1 fat
Vanilla Cone, Small	1	230	7	60	4.5	0	25	100	37	26	0	6	2 1/2 carb, 1 fat
Malts, Shakes, & Arctic Rush													
Arctic Rush, All Flavors, Large	1	370	0	0	0	0	0	55	92	92	0	0	6 carb
Arctic Rush, All Flavors, Small	1	220	0	0	0	0	0	30	54	54	0	0	3 1/2 carb
Chocolate Malt, Large	1	1020	28	250	20	1	75	460	171	147	2	23	11 1/2 carb, 3 fat
Chocolate Malt, Medium	1	790	23	210	17	1	60	350	130	112	1	17	8 1/2 carb, 3 fat
Chocolate Malt, Small	1	590	19	170	14	0.5	50	260	92	79	0.5	14	6 carb, 3 fat
Chocolate Shake, Large	1	940	28	250	20	1	75	390	153	133	2	21	10 carb, 4 fat

Item	Serving												Exchanges
Chocolate Shake, Medium	1	720	23	200	17	1	60	300	115	101	1	16	7 1/2 carb, 3 fat
Chocolate Shake, Small	1	550	19	170	14	0.5	45	220	82	71	0.5	13	5 1/2 carb, 3 fat

Moolatte Frozen Blended Coffee

Item	Serving												Exchanges
Cappuccino Moolatte, Medium	1 (16.5 oz)	570	19	170	15	0.5	45	220	90	79	0	10	6 carb, 3 fat
Caramel Moolatte, Medium	1 (17 oz)	650	19	170	15	0.5	45	280	110	88	0	11	7 carb, 2 fat
Mocha Moolatte, Medium	1 (17.2 oz)	690	27	240	17	0.5	40	260	104	91	1	11	7 carb, 4 fat

Sundaes

Item	Serving												Exchanges
Chocolate Sundae, Large	1	570	14	130	9	1	45	240	98	84	1	12	6 1/2 carb, 1 1/2 fat
Chocolate Sundae, Medium	1	400	10	90	7	0.5	35	170	70	60	1	8	4 1/2 carb, 1 fat
Chocolate Sundae, Small	1	280	7	60	4.5	0	25	115	48	41	0.5	6	3 carb, 1 fat

Royal Treats

Item	Serving												Exchanges
Banana Split	1	530	13	120	10	0.5	30	160	96	74	4	9	6 1/2 carb, 1 fat
Peanut Buster Parfait	1	710	31	280	18	1	35	350	95	69	3	16	6 carb, 5 fat

FAST FOOD

	Serving	Calories	Fat (g)	Cal. from Fat	Sat. Fat (g)	Trans Fat (g)	Chol. (mg)	Sod. (mg)	Carb. (g)	Sugar (g)	Fiber (g)	Prot. (g)	Servings/Exchanges
Novelties													
Buster Bar Treat	1	470	30	270	18	0	15	220	46	37	3	10	3 carb, 5 fat
Cherry Starkiss Bar	1	80	0	0	0	0	0	5	21	17	0	0	1 1/2 carb
Chocolate Dilly Bar	1	220	12	110	10	0	15	80	26	21	1	3	1 1/2 carb, 2 fat
Dilly Bar, No Sugar Added	1	200	13	120	10	0	15	55	23	5	5	3	1 1/2 carb, 2 fat
DQ Sandwich	1	190	5	50	3	0	10	140	31	18	1	4	2 carb, 1 fat
Fudge Bar	1	50	0	0	0	0	0	40	13	4	6	4	1 carb
Vanilla Orange Bar	1	60	0	0	0	0	45	18	6	2	4	2	1/2 carb
Blizzard Treats													
Oreo Blizzard Cake (8 inch)	1/8 cake	560	25	220	17	0	30	330	77	59	1	9	5 carb, 4 fat
Oreo Cookies Blizzard, Large	1	1150	43	390	19	1	75	970	169	123	2	22	11 carb, 6 fat

Oreo Cookies Blizzard, Medium	1	790	30	270	13	1	50	690	117	84	2	15	8 carb, 4 fat
Oreo Cookies Blizzard, Small	1	620	23	210	11	0.5	45	500	92	67	1	12	6 carb, 3 fat
Peanut Butter Cookie Dough Smash, Large	1	1500	69	620	34	1.5	110	910	194	138	5	28	13 carb, 11 fat
Peanut Butter Cookie Dough Smash, Medium	1	1140	52	470	26	1	85	680	150	107	4	22	10 carb, 8 fat
Peanut Butter Cookie Dough Smash, Small	1	820	35	320	19	1	65	470	110	81	2	16	7 carb, 6 fat

DOMINO'S

Hand Tossed Pizza, Large

Cheese	1/8 pizza	256	9	78	3.8	0	18	530	34	3	1.8	10	2 carb, 1 med-fat protein
Ham	1/8 pizza	271	10	84	4	0	24	700	34	3	1.8	12	2 carb, 1 med-fat protein, 1 fat
Italian Sausage	1/8 pizza	319	14	126	5.8	0	28	714	37	4	1.8	14	2 1/2 carb, 1 med-fat protein, 1 fat

FAST FOOD

	Serving	Calories	Fat (g)	Cal. from Fat	Sat. Fat (g)	Trans Fat (g)	Chol. (mg)	Sod. (mg)	Carb. (g)	Sugar (g)	Fiber (g)	Prot. (g)	Servings/Exchanges
Pepperoni	1/8 pizza	296	12	109	5	0	26	701	34	3	1.8	12	2 carb, 1 med-fat protein, 1 fat
Handmade Pan Pizza, Regular Cheese, Large													
Cheese	1/8 pizza	288	14	128	8	0	27	471	28	1.5	1	10	2 carb, 1 med-fat protein, 1 fat
Ham	1/8 pizza	285	14	123	7.6	0	27	553	28	1.5	1	11	2 carb, 1 med-fat protein, 1 fat
Italian Sausage	1/8 pizza	318	17	152	8.8	0	30	554	29	2	1	11	2 carb, 1 med-fat protein, 2 fat
Pepperoni	1/8 pizza	304	16	142	8.4	0	29	553	28	1.6	1	11	2 carb, 1 med-fat protein, 2 fat
Thin Crust, Large													
Cheese	1/8 pizza	194	9	84	3.8	0	19	350	20	2.6	1.6	7	1 carb, 1 med-fat protein, 1 fat
Ham	1/8 pizza	209	10	90	4	0	25	520	20	2.6	1.6	9	1 carb, 1 med-fat protein, 1 fat

	Serving	Cal.	Fat					Sod.					Exchanges
Italian Sausage	1/8 pizza	257	14	132	5.8	0	29	534	21	3.4	1.6	9	1 1/2 carb, 1 med-fat protein, 1 1/2 fat
Pepperoni	1/8 pizza	234	13	115	5	0	27	521	20	2.7	1.6	9	1 carb, 1 med-fat protein, 1 fat
Bread Bowl Pasta													
Chicken Alfredo	1/2 bowl	700	26	230	11	0.5	50	1040	94	4.5	3	26	6 carb, 1 med-fat protein, 3 fat
Italian Sausage Marinara	1/2 bowl	735	27	235	10	0.5	33	1385	99	10	4.5	26	6 1/2 carb, 1 med-fat protein, 3 fat
Pasta Primavera	1/2 bowl	670	25	220	11	0.5	33	885	94	4.5	3.5	20	6 carb, 4 fat
Oven Baked Sandwiches													
Buffalo Chicken	1	830	41	370	16	1	115	2690	74	5	3	42	5 carb, 4 med-fat protein, 3 fat
Chicken Bacon Ranch	1	870	45	400	16	1	125	2380	72	4	2	45	5 carb, 4 med-fat protein, 4 fat
Chicken Parm	1	750	30	270	16	1	120	2200	73	4	3	47	5 carb, 5 med-fat protein
Salads (No Dressing)													
Chicken Apple Pecan	1	190	6	50	2	0	35	390	20	14	4	15	1 carb, 2 lean protein

FAST FOOD

	Serving	Calories	Fat (g)	Cal. from Fat	Sat. Fat (g)	Trans Fat (g)	Chol. (mg)	Sod. (mg)	Carb. (g)	Sugar (g)	Fiber (g)	Prot. (g)	Servings/Exchanges
Classic Garden Salad	1	120	7	60	4	0	20	160	8	5	3	7	1/2 carb, 1 med-fat protein
Side Items													
BBQ Buffalo Wings	2 pieces	123	7	58	1.8	0	43	680	8	5.5	0.5	9	1/2 carb, 1 med-fat protein
Blue Cheese Dipping Cup	1 (1.5 oz)	240	25	230	4.5	0	20	310	2	2	0	1	5 fat
Breadsticks	2 pieces	218	13	113	2.5	0	0	195	22	1	1	4	1 1/2 carb, 2 fat
Cheese Stuffed Cheesy Bread	2 pieces	278	11	100	6	0	30	480	32	2	1	12	2 carb, 1 med-fat protein, 1 fat
Chocolate Lava Crunch Cakes	1 of 2 cakes	345	17	155	10	0	65	170	47	31	1.5	4	3 carb, 3 fat
Cinna Stix	2 pieces	235	12	110	2.3	0	0	173	27	6	1	4	2 carb, 2 fat
Classic Hot Buffalo Wings	2 pieces	103	7	58	1.8	0	43	680	5	0	0	9	1 med-fat protein
Garlic Dipping Cup	1 (1 oz)	250	28	250	5	0	0	160	0	0	0	0	6 fat

	Amount												
Marbled Cookie Brownie	1 of 9 pieces	192	9	83	4	0	22	122	25	18	0.5	2	1 1/2 carb, 1 1/2 fat
Marinara Dipping Cup	1 (2 oz)	25	0	0	0	0	0	270	5	4	1	1	free
Ranch Dipping Cup	1 (1.5 oz)	200	21	190	3	0	10	340	2	1	0	0	4 fat
Sweet Icing Dipping Cup	1 (1 oz)	250	2.5	25	0.5	0	0	0	57	55	0	0	4 carb

DUNKIN DONUTS

Donuts, Danishes & Other Sweets

	Amount												
Apple Cheese Danish	1	400	19	170	8	0	5	310	53	29	1	5	3 1/2 carb, 3 fat
Apple Crumb Donut	1	320	15	140	7	0	0	350	42	21	1	3	3 carb, 2 fat
Apple Fritter	1	420	19	170	8	0	0	380	58	24	2	6	4 carb, 3 fat
Bavarian Crème Donut	1	270	15	140	7	0	0	350	31	9	1	4	2 carb, 3 fat
Blueberry Crumb Donut	1	410	16	140	8	0	0	340	64	40	1	4	4 carb, 2 fat
Boston Kreme Donut	1	300	16	140	7	0	0	360	37	17	1	3	2 1/2 carb, 3 fat
Brownie	1	440	23	210	5	0	55	250	58	49	1	3	4 carb, 4 fat
Caramel Cheesecake Square	1	360	19	170	10	0	10	360	43	20	1	5	3 carb, 3 fat

FAST FOOD

	Serving	Calories	Fat (g)	Cal. from Fat	Sat. Fat (g)	Trans Fat (g)	Chol. (mg)	Sod. (mg)	Carb. (g)	Sugar (g)	Fiber (g)	Prot. (g)	Servings/Exchanges
Cheese Danish	1	420	21	190	9	0	10	320	52	27	1	5	3 1/2 carb, 3 1/2 fat
Chocolate Chip Coffee Cake	1	230	9	80	2.5	0	25	180	34	20	1	3	2 carb, 2 fat
Chocolate Coconut Donut	1	400	23	210	12	0	0	420	45	22	2	4	3 carb, 4 fat
Chocolate Crème Donut	1	320	19	170	8	0	0	360	35	14	1	4	2 carb, 3 fat
Chocolate Frosted Cake Donut	1	350	19	170	9	0	25	340	40	20	1	4	2 1/2 carb, 3 fat
Cinnamon Stick	1	380	25	220	12	0	30	370	35	13	1	4	2 carb, 5 fat
Coffee Roll	1	390	18	160	7	0	0	410	51	17	2	7	3 1/2 carb, 3 fat
Éclair	1	380	18	160	7	0	0	350	50	22	2	5	3 carb, 3 fat
French Roll	1	260	1.5	10	0	0	0	550	52	2	2	9	3 1/2 carb, 1 fat
Glazed Donut	1	260	14	130	6	0	0	330	31	12	1	3	2 carb, 2 fat
Glazed Old Fashioned Donut	1	340	19	170	8	0	25	320	39	19	1	4	2 1/2 carb, 3 fat

Homestyle Apple Pie	1	280	14	130	5	0	0	240	36	15	1	3	2 1/2 carb, 3 fat
Jelly Donut	1	270	14	130	6	0	0	330	32	15	1	3	2 carb, 3 fat
Strawberry Cheese Danish	1	400	19	170	8	0	0	310	52	26	1	5	3 1/2 carb, 3 fat
Strawberry Dream Swirl Donut	1	370	19	170	8	0	0	360	47	28	1	3	3 carb, 3 fat
Vanilla Frosted Coffee Roll	1	400	19	170	8	0	0	430	52	19	2	7	3 1/2 carb, 3 fat
Munchkins													
Boston Kreme	1	70	4.5	40	2	0	0	85	7	2	0	1	1/2 carb, 1 fat
Coconut	1	80	4.5	40	2.5	5	5	50	10	5	0	1	1/2 carb, 1 fat
Glazed Old Fashioned	1	70	3.5	30	1.5	0	5	50	9	4	0	1	1/2 carb, 1 fat
Powdered	1	60	3.5	30	1.5	0	5	50	7	3	0	1	1/2 carb, 1 fat
Toasted Coconut	1	90	5	45	3	0	5	50	10	6	1	1	1/2 carb, 1 fat
Bagels													
Cinnamon Raisin	1	320	1	10	0	0	0	500	66	14	4	12	4 1/2 carb
Everything	1	340	3	25	0	0	0	630	67	7	5	12	4 1/2 carb

FAST FOOD

	Serving	Calories	Fat (g)	Cal. from Fat	Sat. Fat (g)	Trans Fat (g)	Chol. (mg)	Sod. (mg)	Carb. (g)	Sugar (g)	Fiber (g)	Prot. (g)	Servings/Exchanges
Multigrain	1	350	7	60	0.5	0	0	450	63	8	8	15	4 carb, 1 fat
Plain	1	310	1	5	0	0	0	620	64	7	4	11	4 carb
Cream Cheese													
Plain	1 unit (1.8 oz)	150	15	130	9	0.5	40	250	3	3	0	3	3 fat
Reduced-Fat Plain	1 unit (1.8 oz)	100	8	70	5	0	25	250	5	2	0	4	2 fat
Reduced-Fat Strawberry Cream	1 unit (1.8 oz)	150	10	90	6	0	30	200	15	11	1	2	1 carb, 2 fat
Muffins													
Blueberry	1	460	15	130	3	0	60	450	76	44	2	6	5 carb, 2 fat
Blueberry, Reduced Fat	1	410	10	90	2	0	55	620	75	40	2	7	5 carb, 1 fat
Chocolate Chip	1	550	21	180	6	0	65	470	83	50	2	7	5 1/2 carb, 3 fat
Coffee Cake	1	590	24	220	8	0	65	480	86	51	1	7	5 1/2 carb, 4 fat
Corn	1	460	16	140	3	0	70	770	72	31	1	7	5 carb, 2 fat

Honey Bran Rasin	1	440	13	120	2.5	0	55	410	74	40	4	7	5 carb, 2 fat
Other Bakery Items												
Biscuit	1	320	17	150	10	0	0	740	35	3	1	6	2 carb, 3 fat
Plain Croissant	1	340	18	160	8	0	0	350	37	5	1	6	2 1/2 carb, 3 fat
Pretzel Twist	1	280	2.5	25	1	0	0	1340	54	2	2	10	3 1/2 carb
Breakfast Sandwiches												
Bacon, Egg & Cheese on English Muffin	1	300	12	100	5	0	80	630	32	2	7	16	2 carb, 1 med-fat protein, 1 fat
Bacon, Egg & Cheese on Plain Bagel	1	470	12	110	5	0	80	1140	67	7	4	23	4 1/2 carb, 1 med-fat protein, 1/2 fat
Egg & Cheese on English Muffin	1	240	7	60	3.5	0	70	470	32	2	7	12	2 carb, 1 med-fat protein
Egg & Cheese on Plain Bagel	1	410	7	70	3.5	0	70	980	67	7	4	19	4 1/2 carb, 1 med-fat protein
Ham, Egg & Cheese on English Muffin	1	270	8	70	4	0	80	740	33	2	7	17	2 carb, 1 med-fat protein
Ham, Egg & Cheese on Plain Bagel	1	440	8	70	4	0	80	1260	67	7	4	24	4 1/2 carb, 1 med-fat protein

FAST FOOD

	Serving	Calories	Fat (g)	Cal. from Fat	Sat. Fat (g)	Trans Fat (g)	Chol. (mg)	Sod. (mg)	Carb. (g)	Sugar (g)	Fiber (g)	Prot. (g)	Servings/Exchanges
Sausage, Egg & Cheese on English Muffin	1	450	26	240	11	0	115	970	33	2	7	20	2 carb, 2 med-fat protein, 3 fat
Sausage, Egg & Cheese on Plain Bagel	1	620	26	240	11	0	115	1480	67	7	4	21	4 1/2 carb, 1 med-fat protein, 3 fat
Bakery Sandwiches & Wraps													
Bacon Ancho Chicken Sandwich	1	640	25	220	7	0	65	1620	70	7	3	34	4 1/2 carb, 3 med-fat protein, 1 fat
Chicken Salad on Croissant	1	580	39	350	11	0	45	850	42	7	2	16	3 carb, 1 med-fat protein, 6 fat
Snack n' Go Steak Wrap	1	210	11	100	5	0	35	430	15	3	1	12	1 carb, 1 med-fat protein, 1 fat
Turkey, Bacon, Cheddar Flatbread	1	380	17	160	6	0	60	1060	32	4	3	24	2 carb, 3 med-fat protein
Coffee Drinks													
Caramel Mocha	14 oz	170	0	5	0	0	0	30	39	36	1	2	2 1/2 carb

Item	Amount												Exchanges/Choices
Coffee with Cream & Sugar	14 oz	190	9	80	5	0	30	25	29	26	0	2	2 carb, 1 fat
Coffee with Skim Milk & Splenda	14 oz	30	0	0	0	0	0	30	6	2	0	2	1/2 carb
Mocha Swirl Coffee with Cream	14 oz	260	9	80	6	0	30	45	41	34	2	3	3 carb, 1 fat
Coolatta													
Mango Passion Fruit	16 oz	250	0	0	0	0	0	30	63	61	0	0	4 carb
Mango Passion Fruit Lite	16 oz	90	0	0	0	0	0	20	24	18	0	0	1 1/2 carb
Vanilla Bean	16 oz	420	6	50	3.5	0	20	150	92	87	0	3	6 carb
Vanilla Bean Lite	16 oz	250	0	0	0	0	5	170	59	52	0	5	4 carb
EINSTEIN BROS. BAGELS													
Bagels													
9-Grain	1	300	6	50	0	0	0	470	51	6	8	13	3 1/2 carb, 1/2 fat
Asiago Cheese	1	300	4	35	2	0	10	560	54	5	2	12	3 1/2 carb
Blueberry	1	290	1	10	0	0	0	460	60	10	2	10	4 carb
Chocolate Chip	1	290	3	25	1.5	0	0	460	58	10	2	10	4 carb

FAST FOOD

	Serving	Calories	Fat (g)	Cal. from Fat	Sat. Fat (g)	Trans Fat (g)	Chol. (mg)	Sod. (mg)	Carb. (g)	Sugar (g)	Fiber (g)	Prot. (g)	Servings/Exchanges
Cinnamon Raisin	1	290	1	10	0	0	0	440	61	13	2	10	4 carb
Cinnamon Sugar	1	320	6	50	0.5	0	0	540	59	12	2	9	4 carb
Everything	1	280	2	20	0	0	0	640	54	5	2	10	3 1/2 carb
Gingerbread	1	290	4	35	0	0	0	430	55	7	2	9	3 1/2 carb
Honey Whole Wheat	1	260	3	25	0	0	0	440	50	7	7	12	3 carb
Onion	1	270	1	10	0	0	0	460	59	5	2	9	4 carb
Plain	1	260	1	10	0	0	0	480	55	5	2	9	3 1/2 carb
Poppy	1	280	2.5	25	0	0	0	470	54	5	2	10	3 1/2 carb
Red Velvet	1	300	6	50	1.5	0	0	390	54	10	3	9	3 1/2 carb, 1/2 fat
Sourdough	1	280	3	25	0	0	0	520	53	2	2	11	3 1/2 carb
Gourmet Bagels													
Apple Cinnamon	1	440	8	70	1.5	0	0	600	82	26	2	10	5 1/2 carb, 1/2 fat
French Toast	1	380	7	70	1.5	0	15	450	69	21	2	10	4 1/2 carb, 1/2 fat
Jalapeño Cheddar	1	390	11	100	4	0	20	1160	58	6	3	15	4 carb, 1 fat

Multigrain Roll	1	330	7	60	1	0	0	480	54	8	9	14	3 1/2 carb, 1 fat
Power Protein Bagel	1	350	6	50	1	0	0	290	64	17	4	12	4 carb
Spinach Florentine	1	380	11	100	3.5	0	15	710	58	6	2	15	4 carb, 1 fat

Specialty Bread

Bagel Baguette	1	420	6	50	0	0	0	790	77	8	3	14	5 carb
Ciabatta	1	260	2	20	0	0	0	700	52	0	2	9	3 1/2 carb
Multigrain	2 slices	190	1.5	15	0	0	0	240	41	5	3	8	2 1/2 carb
Tortilla	1	290	7	60	3	0	0	750	50	0	6	9	3 carb, 1 fat

Whipped Cream Cheese Shmear

Apple Cinnamon	1.5 oz	130	10	90	6	0	30	190	11	11	0	2	1/2 carb, 2 fat
Blueberry, Reduced Fat	1.5 oz	150	10	90	7	0	30	100	13	11	0	2	1 carb, 2 fat
Cream Cheese Icing	1.5 oz	130	5	45	3.5	0	15	50	22	20	0	1	1 1/2 carb, 1 fat
Garden Vegetable, Reduced Fat	1.5 oz	130	10	90	7	0	30	210	6	2	0	3	1/2 carb, 2 fat
Garlic Herb, Reduced Fat	1.5 oz	130	10	90	7	0	30	210	6	2	1	3	1/2 carb, 2 fat
Honey Almond, Reduced Fat	1.5 oz	150	10	90	7	0	25	90	13	9	0	2	1 carb, 2 fat

FAST FOOD

	Serving	Calories	Fat (g)	Cal. from Fat	Sat. Fat (g)	Trans Fat (g)	Chol. (mg)	Sod. (mg)	Carb. (g)	Sugar (g)	Fiber (g)	Prot. (g)	Servings/Exchanges
Jalapeño Salsa, Reduced Fat	1.5 oz	130	10	90	7	0	30	220	7	2	1	2	1/2 carb, 2 fat
Plain	1.5 oz	150	14	130	10	0	45	135	2	2	0	2	3 fat
Plain, Reduced Fat	1.5 oz	130	10	90	7	0	30	210	5	2	0	3	2 fat
Smoked Salmon	1.5 oz	130	12	110	8	0	40	300	4	2	0	3	2 fat
Egg Sandwiches, Classic													
Applewood Bacon & Cheddar	1	520	19	170	8	0	340	1160	56	6	2	29	3 1/2 carb, 3 med-fat protein
Ham & Swiss	1	490	15	140	6	0	350	1410	57	7	2	31	4 carb, 3 lean protein, 1 fat
Egg Sandwiches, Signature													
Applewood Bacon & Spinach Florentine	1	890	56	500	17	0.5	400	1870	65	8	4	37	4 carb, 4 med-fat protein, 6 fat
Cinnamon Toast Egg	1	680	30	270	12	0	360	1300	73	22	3	30	5 carb, 2 med-fat protein, 3 fat

Einstein's Club	1	990	50	450	14	1	140	2480	84	12	3	52	5 1/2 carb, 5 med-fat protein, 4 fat
French Toast Egg	1	740	34	300	15	0.5	385	1230	79	21	2	31	5 carb, 2 med-fat protein, 4 fat
Harvest Chicken Salad	1	620	26	230	4	0	60	730	66	15	11	34	4 1/2 carb, 3 med-fat protein, 1 fat
Hummus Veg Out	1	440	12	110	4	0	15	810	72	14	11	19	5 carb, 1 med-fat protein
Nova Lox & Bagel	1	480	17	150	9	0	50	1320	61	9	2	22	4 carb, 1 med-fat protein, 2 fat
Southwest Thintastic, Whole Egg on Plain Thin	1	430	18	160	8	0	220	1030	44	6	2	25	3 carb, 2 med-fat protein, 1 fat
Spinach, Mushroom & Swiss on Plain Bagel	1	490	18	160	7	0	325	1070	58	6	3	26	4 carb, 2 med-fat protein, 1 fat
Tasty Turkey on Asiago Bagel	1	510	15	130	9	0	80	1310	63	9	3	33	4 carb, 3 lean protein, 1 fat
Thintastic Club	1	410	15	140	2.5	0	50	1160	42	8	6	29	3 carb, 3 lean protein, 1 fat

FAST FOOD

	Serving	Calories	Fat (g)	Cal. from Fat	Sat. Fat (g)	Trans Fat (g)	Chol. (mg)	Sod. (mg)	Carb. (g)	Sugar (g)	Fiber (g)	Prot. (g)	Servings/Exchanges
Turkey, Bacon & Avocado	1	700	39	350	7	0	90	1680	60	11	9	34	4 carb, 4 med-fat protein, 3 fat
Turkey & Cheddar	1	690	30	270	7	0.5	70	1670	67	13	3	35	4 1/2 carb, 4 med-fat protein, 1 fat
Low Carb Options													
Chicken Salad, Deli (without Bread)	1 (6.3 oz)	290	19	170	3	0	60	250	11	7	2	19	1/2 carb, 2 1/2 med-fat protein, 1 fat
Tuna Salad, Deli (without Bread)	1 (7.1 oz)	270	21	190	3	0	45	390	5	3	1	17	2 1/2 med-fat protein, 2 fat
Turkey & Cheddar (without Bread)	1 (7.5 oz)	350	25	230	7	0	70	1100	9	2	1	23	1/2 carb, 3 med-fat protein, 2 fat
Hot Sandwiches													
Italian Chicken Panini	1	690	31	280	11	0	100	1690	58	3	9	47	4 carb, 5 med-fat protein
Original Bagel Dog	1	610	32	290	12	1.5	55	1510	57	5	2	22	4 carb, 1 med-fat protein, 5 fat

Pizza Bagel Pepperoni	1	530	23	200	12	0	55	1340	58	7	2	27	4 carb, 2 med-fat protein, 2 fat
Thintastic Chicken Pesto	1	470	17	150	6	0	80	910	45	6	5	37	3 carb, 4 lean protein, 1 fat

Flatbreads & Wraps

BBQ Chicken Flatbread	1	600	21	190	10	0	80	1240	67	19	3	37	4 1/2 carb, 3 med-fat protein
Chicken Caesar Wrap	1	630	28	250	12	0	110	1480	61	6	7	37	4 carb, 4 med-fat protein, 1 fat
Sante Fe Wrap	1	650	32	290	16	0	380	1750	59	4	6	33	4 carb, 3 med-fat protein, 3 fat
White Vegetarian Flatbread	1	520	25	220	11	0	40	1110	56	6	4	21	3 1/2 carb, 1 med-fat protein, 3 fat

Salads

Chicken Caesar	1	340	16	140	4.5	0	75	840	26	6	4	25	1 1/2 carb, 3 med-fat protein
Chicken Club	1	390	25	230	6	0	65	910	17	5	3	23	1 carb, 3 med-fat protein, 2 fat
Strawberry Chicken	1	330	13	110	1.5	0	40	270	37	29	5	18	2 1/2 carb, 1 med-fat protein, 1 fat

FAST FOOD

	Serving	Calories	Fat (g)	Cal. from Fat	Sat. Fat (g)	Trans Fat (g)	Chol. (mg)	Sod. (mg)	Carb. (g)	Sugar (g)	Fiber (g)	Prot. (g)	Servings/Exchanges
Soups (Cup)													
Broccoli Cheddar	8.7 oz	290	21	190	12	0	50	1250	15	7	2	13	1 carb, 1 med-fat protein, 3 fat
Chicken Noodle	8.7 oz	110	3.5	30	0	0	30	970	14	1	1	6	1 carb, 1/2 lean protein
Turkey Chili	8.7 oz	160	4.5	40	1	0	20	930	22	6	5	12	1 1/2 carb, 1 lean protein
HARDEE'S													
Breakfast													
Bacon, Egg & Cheese Biscuit	1	480	27	250	9	NA	220	1350	39	3	4	19	2 1/2 carb, 2 med-fat protein, 3 fat
Biscuit 'n' Gravy	1	460	26	230	7	NA	10	1390	49	2	3	9	3 carb, 5 fat
Chicken Filet Biscuit	1	550	32	290	7	NA	45	1330	47	3	4	20	3 carb, 1 med-fat protein, 5 fat
Cinnamon 'n' Raisin Biscuit	1	340	15	130	3.5	NA	0	680	49	26	1	3	3 carb, 3 fat

Country Ham Biscuit	1	370	19	170	6	NA	35	1610	37	2	3	15	2 1/2 carb, 1 med-fat protein, 2 fat
Country Steak Biscuit	1	510	31	280	9	NA	25	1180	44	2	4	13	3 carb, 1 med-fat protein, 5 fat
Frisco Breakfast Sandwich	1	450	19	170	8	NA	230	1570	45	5	2	24	3 carb, 2 med-fat protein, 1 fat
Ham, Egg & Cheese Biscuit	1	450	24	220	8	NA	220	1440	39	3	3	19	2 1/2 carb, 2 med-fat protein, 2 fat
Hardee Breakfast Platter	1	830	50	450	13	NA	235	2160	68	4	13	24	4 1/2 carb, 1 med-fat protein, 8 fat
Jelly Biscuit	1	430	26	230	6	NA	0	890	45	9	3	5	3 carb, 5 fat
Loaded Breakfast Burrito	1	580	30	270	12	NA	445	1320	46	2	3	30	3 carb, 3 med-fat protein, 2 fat
Loaded Omelet Biscuit	1	490	28	250	10	NA	230	1310	40	3	4	18	2 1/2 carb, 1 med-fat protein, 4 fat
Low Carb Breakfast Bowl	1	660	52	470	20	NA	675	1550	10	2	2	38	1/2 carb, 5 med-fat protein, 5 fat
Made from Scratch Biscuit	1	300	15	130	4	NA	0	780	36	2	3	5	2 1/2 carb, 2 1/2 fat

FAST FOOD

	Serving	Calories	Fat (g)	Cal. from Fat	Sat. Fat (g)	Trans Fat (g)	Chol. (mg)	Sod. (mg)	Carb. (g)	Sugar (g)	Fiber (g)	Prot. (g)	Servings/Exchanges
Monster Biscuit	1	750	50	450	18	NA	275	2320	40	3	4	34	2 1/2 carb, 4 med-fat protein, 5 1/2 fat
Sausage Biscuit	1	490	33	290	10	NA	30	1150	37	3	3	12	2 1/2 carb, 1 med-fat protein, 5 fat
Sausage & Egg Biscuit	1	560	37	330	12	NA	225	1230	39	3	4	17	2 1/2 carb, 1 med-fat protein, 6 fat
Sunrise Croissant with Ham	1	400	23	210	9	NA	225	880	29	4	2	18	2 carb, 2 med-fat protein, 2 fat
Sandwiches													
1/3 lb Bacon Cheese Thickburger	1	900	59	530	18	NA	140	1680	54	13	10	40	3 1/2 carb, 4 med-fat protein, 7 fat
1/3 lb Cheeseburger	1	640	35	310	13	NA	105	1630	55	15	10	31	3 1/2 carb, 3 med-fat protein, 3 fat
1/3 lb Low Carb Thickburger	1	440	35	320	13	NA	110	1180	9	6	9	25	1/2 carb, 3 med-fat protein, 4 fat
1/3 lb Mushroom & Swiss Thickburger	1	690	40	360	15	NA	115	1630	52	11	10	34	3 1/2 carb, 3 med-fat protein, 4 fat

1/3 lb Original Thickburger	1	820	53	480	16	NA	120	1660	56	15	10	32	3 1/2 carb, 3 med-fat protein, 7 fat
1/4 lb Little Thickburger	1	600	42	370	13	NA	90	1250	33	8	2	23	2 carb, 2 med-fat protein, 6 fat
1/4 lb Little Thick Cheeseburger	1	450	25	230	10	NA	75	1210	33	8	2	23	2 carb, 2 med-fat protein, 3 fat
2/3 lb Double Thickburger	1	1140	79	710	27	NA	220	2460	58	17	18	56	4 carb, 6 med-fat protein, 9 fat
2/3 lb Monster Thickburger	1	1340	96	860	34	NA	275	3130	52	14	17	74	3 1/2 carb, 9 med-fat protein, 9 1/2 fat
3 Piece Hand-Breaded Chicken Tenders	1 order	260	13	110	2.5	NA	70	770	13	0	2	25	1 carb, 3 med-fat protein
5 Piece Hand-Breaded Chicken Tenders	1 order	440	21	190	4.5	NA	115	1290	21	0	3	41	1 1/2 carb, 5 med-fat protein
Big Chicken Fillet Sandwich	1	750	42	370	8	NA	85	1490	63	11	3	32	4 carb, 3 med-fat protein, 5 fat
Big Hot Ham 'n' Cheese	1	530	22	200	9	NA	75	2190	50	11	2	32	3 carb, 3 med-fat protein, 1 fat
Charbroiled BBQ Chicken Sandwich	1	340	4	40	1	NA	80	1020	42	16	2	32	3 carb, 3 med-fat protein, 4 fat

FAST FOOD

	Serving	Calories	Fat (g)	Cal. from Fat	Sat. Fat (g)	Trans Fat (g)	Chol. (mg)	Sod. (mg)	Carb. (g)	Sugar (g)	Fiber (g)	Prot. (g)	Servings/Exchanges
Charbroiled Chicken Club Sandwich	1	590	31	280	8	NA	130	1510	35	9	2	42	2 carb, 5 med-fat protein, 1 fat
Hot Ham 'n' Cheese	1	290	11	100	4	NA	35	1150	29	5	1	17	2 carb, 1 med-fat protein, 1 fat
Jumbo Chili Dog	1	370	25	220	8	NA	50	1210	22	3	2	15	1 1/2 carb, 1 med-fat protein, 4 fat
Low Carb Charbroiled Chicken Club	1	380	22	200	7	NA	125	1230	8	6	1	38	1/2 carb, 5 lean protein, 2 fat
Regular Roast Beef Sandwich	1	300	14	120	4.5	NA	40	830	28	5	2	18	2 carb, 2 med-fat protein
Small Cheeseburger	1	330	15	140	4	NA	40	860	32	7	1	16	2 carb, 1 med-fat protein, 2 fat
Small Hamburger	1	280	12	100	3.5	NA	30	630	32	7	1	14	2 carb, 1 med-fat protein, 1 fat
Spicy Chicken Sandwich	1	450	24	210	4.5	NA	30	1290	44	4	3	13	3 carb, 1 med-fat protein, 3 fat

Chicken & Sides

	Serving	Cal	Fat (g)	Cal from Fat	Sat Fat (g)	Trans Fat	Chol (mg)	Sod (mg)	Carb (g)	Fiber (g)	Sugar (g)	Prot (g)	Exchanges/Choices
Beer Battered Onion Rings	1 order (4.3 oz)	410	24	220	4.5	NA	0	470	45	5	3	3	3 carb, 4 fat
Cole Slaw	1 small (4 oz)	270	22	200	5	NA	15	310	17	14	2	1	1 carb, 4 fat
Crispy Curls, Large	1 order	570	28	250	7	NA	0	1420	72	0	6	7	5 carb, 5 fat
Crispy Curls, Medium	1 order	470	23	210	6	NA	0	1180	60	0	5	6	4 carb, 4 fat
Crispy Curls, Small	1 order	360	18	160	4.5	NA	0	910	46	0	4	5	3 carb, 3 fat
Fried Chicken Breast	1	370	15	130	4	NA	75	1190	29	0	0	29	2 carb, 3 med-fat protein
Fried Chicken Leg	1	170	7	60	2	NA	45	570	15	0	0	13	1 carb, 1 med-fat protein
Fried Chicken Thigh	1	330	15	130	4	NA	60	1000	30	0	0	19	2 carb, 2 med-fat protein, 1 fat
Fried Chicken Wing	1	200	8	70	2	NA	30	740	23	0	0	10	1 1/2 carb, 1 med-fat protein
Green Beans	1 order (4.7 oz)	60	3.5	30	1.5	NA	5	680	6	1	2	2	1 vegetable, 1 fat

FAST FOOD

	Serving	Calories	Fat (g)	Cal. from Fat	Sat. Fat (g)	Trans Fat (g)	Chol. (mg)	Sod. (mg)	Carb. (g)	Sugar (g)	Fiber (g)	Prot. (g)	Servings/Exchanges
Mashed Potatoes & Gravy	1 small (5 oz)	80	1	10	0	NA	0	430	15	2	1	1	1 carb
Natural Cut French Fries, Large	1 order	530	26	230	4.5	NA	0	1060	69	1	6	6	4 1/2 carb, 4 fat
Natural Cut French Fries, Medium	1 order	490	24	210	4.5	NA	0	970	63	0	6	5	4 carb, 4 fat
Natural Cut French Fries, Small	1 order	360	18	160	3	NA	0	730	47	0	4	4	3 carb, 3 fat
Peach Cobbler	1 small	320	8	70	2	NA	0	210	61	50	1	1	4 carb, 1 fat
Side Salad, No Dressing	1	120	7	70	4.5	NA	20	160	7	4	2	7	1/2 carb, 1 med-fat protein
IN-N-OUT BURGER													
Cheeseburger with Onion	1	480	27	240	10	0.5	60	1000	39	10	3	22	2 1/2 carb, 2 med-fat protein, 3 fat
Cheeseburger with Onion, Protein Style	1	330	25	220	9	0	60	720	11	7	3	18	1 carb, 2 med-fat protein, 3 fat

	Serving											
Chocolate Shake	15 oz	590	29	260	19	1	15	320	72	65	0	10	5 carb, 5 fat
Double-Double with Onion	1	670	41	370	18	1	120	1440	39	10	3	37	2 1/2 carb, 4 med-fat protein, 4 fat
Double-Double with Onion, Protein Style	1	520	39	350	17	1	120	1160	11	7	3	33	1 carb, 4 med-fat protein, 4 fat
French Fries	1 order	395	18	160	5	0	0	245	54	0	2	7	3 1/2 carb, 3 fat
Hamburger with Onion	1	390	19	170	5	0	40	650	39	10	3	16	2 1/2 carb, 1 med-fat protein, 2 fat
Hamburger with Onion, Protein Style	1	240	17	150	4	0	40	370	11	7	3	13	1 carb, 1 med-fat protein, 2 fat
Strawberry Shake	15 oz	590	27	240	18	1	15	270	81	67	0	8	5 1/2 carb, 4 fat
Vanilla Shake	15 oz	580	31	280	20	1	20	300	67	57	0	10	4 1/2 carb, 5 fat

JACK IN THE BOX

Better For You

	Serving											
Chicken Fajita Pita with Whole Grain (No Salsa)	1	340	12	110	6	0	55	1000	35	3	4	23	2 carb, 2 med-fat protein
Chicken Teriyaki Bowl	1	690	6	50	1	0	40	1910	134	35	5	27	9 carb
Grilled Chicken Salad	1	250	9	90	4.5	0	80	750	13	6	5	30	1 carb, 4 lean protein

FAST FOOD

	Serving	Calories	Fat (g)	Cal. from Fat	Sat. Fat (g)	Trans Fat (g)	Chol. (mg)	Sod. (mg)	Carb. (g)	Sugar (g)	Fiber (g)	Prot. (g)	Servings/Exchanges
Jr. Jack	1	320	15	140	5	0.5	30	610	33	6	2	14	2 carb, 1 med-fat protein, 2 fat
Smoothie, Strawberry	16 oz	270	0	0	0	0	0	70	67	51	1	2	4 1/2 carb
Burgers & More													
Bacon & Swiss Buttery Jack	1	890	59	530	25	2	145	1350	48	11	3	42	3 carb, 5 med-fat protein, 6 fat
Bacon Ultimate Cheeseburger	1	910	56	500	24	3	165	2200	44	7	2	57	3 carb, 7 med-fat protein, 4 fat
Cheeseburger	1	320	14	130	6	1	35	830	32	5	1	16	2 carb, 1 med-fat protein, 1 fat
Hamburger	1	280	11	90	4	0.5	25	620	32	5	1	14	2 carb, 1 med-fat protein, 1 fat
Jr. Bacon Cheeseburger	1	390	21	180	8	1	45	910	32	5	1	19	2 carb, 2 med-fat protein, 2 fat
Jumbo Jack	1	490	23	210	8	1.5	60	910	44	7	3	26	3 carb, 2 med-fat protein, 2 fat

Sirloin Cheeseburger	1	760	43	390	18	2	110	1480	52	14	4	41	3 1/2 carb, 4 med-fat protein, 4 fat
Sirloin Swiss & Grilled Onions	1	740	42	380	17	2	110	1150	52	14	4	42	3 1/2 carb, 4 med-fat protein, 4 fat
Sourdough Jack	1	660	41	360	15	1.5	90	1450	39	7	3	35	2 1/2 carb, 4 med-fat protein, 4 fat
Spicy Sriracha Burger	1	690	46	410	14	1.5	90	1610	38	6	4	33	2 1/2 carb, 4 med-fat protein, 5 fat
Ultimate Cheeseburger	1	820	49	440	21	3	145	1780	44	7	2	50	3 carb, 6 med-fat protein, 3 fat
Chicken & More												
Chicken Fajita Pita with Whole Grain & Salsa	1	350	12	110	6	0	55	1120	36	4	4	24	2 1/2 carb, 2 med-fat protein
Chicken Nuggets	5 pieces	240	17	150	2	0	25	600	13	0	1	9	1 carb, 1 med-fat protein, 2 fat
Chicken Nuggets	10 pieces	480	33	300	4.5	0	50	1210	26	0	2	19	2 carb, 2 med-fat protein, 4 fat
Chicken Sandwich	1	410	21	190	3.5	0	30	880	42	4	2	15	3 carb, 1 med-fat protein, 3 fat

FAST FOOD

	Serving	Calories	Fat (g)	Cal. from Fat	Sat. Fat (g)	Trans Fat (g)	Chol. (mg)	Sod. (mg)	Carb. (g)	Sugar (g)	Fiber (g)	Prot. (g)	Servings/Exchanges
Grilled Sourdough Chicken Club	1	540	26	230	7	0	90	1490	38	6	3	39	2 1/2 carb, 4 med-fat protein, 1 fat
Homestyle Ranch Chicken Club	1	710	33	290	8	0	80	1880	66	12	4	40	4 1/2 carb, 4 med-fat protein, 2 fat
Jack's Spicy Chicken	1	530	20	180	3	0	55	820	61	6	3	28	4 carb, 2 med-fat protein, 1 fat
Something Different													
Bacon Ranch Monster Taco	1	340	24	220	6	0.5	30	660	19	1	1	11	1 carb, 1 med-fat protein, 4 fat
Monster Taco	1	270	17	150	6	0.5	25	630	19	1	2	9	1 carb, 1 med-fat protein, 2 fat
Turkey, Bacon & Cheddar Grilled Sandwich	1	660	31	280	11	0.5	95	2160	53	4	5	41	3 1/2 carb, 4 med-fat protein, 2 1/2 fat
Salads (without Dressing)													
Chicken Club Salad with Crispy Chicken	1	510	28	250	9	0	65	1220	36	4	5	32	2 1/2 carb, 3 med-fat protein, 2 fat

	Serving	Cal.	Fat (g)	Cal. Fat	Sat. Fat (g)	Trans Fat (g)	Chol. (mg)	Sod. (mg)	Carb. (g)	Fiber (g)	Sugar (g)	Pro. (g)	Choices/Exchanges
Chicken Club Salad with Grilled Chicken	1	370	20	180	9	0	105	1060	11	5	4	39	1 carb, 5 lean protein, 2 fat
Southwest Chicken Salad with Crispy Chicken	1	500	23	210	7	0	55	1260	52	5	8	29	3 1/2 carb, 3 med-fat protein, 1 fat
Southwest Chicken Salad with Grilled Chicken	1	350	15	140	6	0	90	1090	27	6	7	35	2 carb, 4 lean protein, 1 fat
Snacks & Sides													
Bacon Cheddar Potato Wedges	1 order	600	41	370	9		30	1250	58	2	5	17	4 carb, 1 med-fat protein, 6 fat
Egg Roll	1 piece	150	7	70	1.5		5	320	15	2	2	5	1 carb, 1 fat
French Fries, Large	1 order	550	25	230	2.5		0	1010	75	1	5	6	5 carb, 4 fat
French Fries, Medium	1 order	430	20	180	2		0	780	58	0	4	5	4 carb, 3 fat
French Fries, Small	1 order	300	14	120	1		0	540	40	0	3	3	2 1/2 carb, 2 fat
Onion Rings	1 order	450	28	250	2		0	620	45	5	3	6	3 carb, 5 fat
Seasoned Curly Fries, Large	1 order	480	28	250	2.5		0	1060	52	0	4	6	3 1/2 carb, 5 fat

FAST FOOD

	Serving	Calories	Fat (g)	Cal. from Fat	Sat. Fat (g)	Trans Fat (g)	Chol. (mg)	Sod. (mg)	Carb. (g)	Sugar (g)	Fiber (g)	Prot. (g)	Servings/Exchanges
Seasoned Curly Fries, Medium	1 order	430	25	220	2	0	0	940	46	0	4	5	3 carb, 4 fat
Seasoned Curly Fries, Small	1 order	280	16	150	1.5	0	0	610	30	0	3	3	2 carb, 3 fat
Stuffed Jalapeños	3 pieces	220	12	110	4.5	0	15	730	21	2	1	6	1 1/2 carb, 2 fat
Taco, Regular	1	170	9	80	3	0	15	360	16	1	2	6	1 carb, 2 fat
Breakfast													
Bacon, Egg & Cheese Biscuit	1	410	25	230	12	0	240	1180	26	3	2	16	2 carb, 1 med-fat protein, 3 fat
Breakfast Jack	1	280	11	100	4.5	0	240	780	30	4	1	16	2 carb, 1 med-fat protein, 1 fat
Extreme Sausage Sandwich	1	640	45	410	17	0.5	305	1330	32	4	1	27	2 carb, 3 med-fat protein, 6 fat
Grande Sausage Breakfast Burrito with Salsa	1	1040	70	630	20	0.5	390	2130	68	5	5	36	4 1/2 carb, 3 med-fat protein, 10 fat
Hash Browns	1 order	190	13	110	1	0	0	350	17	0	2	2	1 carb, 2 fat

Jumbo Breakfast Platter with Bacon	1	540	29	260	6	0	345	1390	47	7	3	23	3 carb, 2 med-fat protein, 3 fat
Loaded Breakfast Sandwich	1	710	47	420	16	0	515	1690	36	4	2	36	2 1/2 carb, 4 med-fat protein, 5 fat
Mini Pancakes	8 pieces	140	15	1.5	0	0	0	350	28	6	1	4	2 carb, 3 fat
Sausage Croissant	1	560	39	350	16	0.5	275	760	32	3	2	19	2 carb, 2 med-fat protein, 5 fat
Sourdough Breakfast Sandwich	1	410	21	190	8	0	250	1010	35	4	2	20	2 carb, 2 med-fat protein, 2 fat
Spicy Chicken Biscuit	1	550	29	260	9	0	50	1110	44	3	2	25	3 carb, 2 med-fat protein, 3 fat
Ultimate Breakfast Sandwich	1	520	25	220	10	0	490	1590	42	5	2	33	3 carb, 3 med-fat protein, 1 fat
Jack's Munchie Meals													
Chick-N-Tater Melt Munchie Meal	1	1760	109	980	28	1.5	120	3460	151	7	13	44	10 carb, 2 med-fat protein, 18 fat
Hella-Peño Burger Munchie Meal	1	1560	81	730	23	2.5	115	3840	153	10	13	52	10 carb, 3 med-fat protein, 11 fat
Loaded Nuggets Munchie Meal	1	1550	98	880	19	1	115	3680	118	4	11	47	8 carb, 4 med-fat protein, 14 fat

FAST FOOD

KFC

Salads (No Dressing)

	Serving	Calories	Fat (g)	Cal. from Fat	Sat. Fat (g)	Trans Fat (g)	Chol. (mg)	Sod. (mg)	Carb. (g)	Sugar (g)	Fiber (g)	Prot. (g)	Servings/Exchanges
Caesar Side Salad	1	40	2	20	1	0	5	90	2	1	1	3	1 vegetable
Crispy Chicken BLT Salad	1	350	18	160	3.5	0	75	990	18	5	5	30	1 carb, 4 med-fat protein
Crispy Chicken Caesar Salad	1	330	17	160	4	0	70	810	16	3	4	29	1 carb, 4 med-fat protein
House Side Salad	1	15	0	0	0	0	0	10	3	2	2	1	1 vegetable
Pot Pie & Bowls													
Chicken Pot Pie	1	790	45	410	37	0	75	1970	66	7	3	29	4 1/2 carb, 3 med-fat protein, 5 fat
KFC Famous Bowl	1	710	31	280	6	1	50	2450	82	2	6	26	5 1/2 carb, 1 med-fat protein, 4 fat
KFC Famous Bowl, Snack Size	1	270	12	110	3	0	25	840	28	1	2	11	2 carb, 1 med-fat protein, 1 fat

Sandwiches

	Amount												Exchanges/Choices
Chicken Littles	1	310	18	160	2.5	0	40	590	23	4	2	14	1 1/2 carb, 1 med-fat protein, 2 fat
Colonel's Original Sandwich	1	500	23	210	3.5	0	65	1150	47	7	3	27	3 carb, 3 med-fat protein, 1 fat
Crispy Twister	1	630	34	300	7	0	80	1300	49	4	5	30	3 carb, 3 med-fat protein, 3 fat
Doublicious	1	580	29	260	6	0	80	1390	47	7	3	32	3 carb, 3 med-fat protein, 2 fat
Honey BBQ Sandwich	1	320	3.5	35	1	0	70	770	47	21	3	24	3 carb, 2 lean protein

Original Recipe Chicken

	Amount												Exchanges/Choices
Breast	1	320	14	120	3	0	145	1140	13	0	2	37	1 carb, 5 lean protein, 1 fat
Breast without Skin or Breading	1	130	2	20	0.5	0	90	520	0	0	0	29	4 lean protein
Drumstick	1	120	7	60	1.5	0	60	380	3	0	0	11	1 med-fat protein
Thigh	1	290	21	190	5	0	100	850	8	0	<1	18	1/2 carb, 2 med-fat protein, 2 fat
Whole Wing	1	140	8	70	1.5	0	50	450	5	0	0	11	1 med-fat protein, 1 fat

FAST FOOD

	Serving	Calories	Fat (g)	Cal. from Fat	Sat. Fat (g)	Trans Fat (g)	Chol. (mg)	Sod. (mg)	Carb. (g)	Sugar (g)	Fiber (g)	Prot. (g)	Servings/Exchanges
Extra Crispy Chicken													
Breast	1	490	29	260	4.5	0	110	1140	20	0	1	35	1 carb, 5 med-fat protein, 1 fat
Drumstick	1	160	10	90	1.5	0	55	390	5	0	0	13	2 med-fat protein
Thigh	1	370	26	240	4.5	1	85	760	15	0	<1	18	1 carb, 2 med-fat protein, 3 fat
Whole Wing	1	210	15	140	2.5	0	60	490	8	0	0	12	1/2 carb, 1 med-fat protein, 2 fat
Kentucky Grilled Chicken													
Breast	1	220	7	60	2	0	135	730	0	0	0	40	6 lean protein
Drumstick	1	90	4	35	1	0	60	290	0	0	0	13	2 lean protein
Thigh	1	170	10	90	3	0	90	530	0	0	0	19	3 lean protein, 1 fat
Whole Wing	1	80	4.5	40	1.5	0	50	250	<1	0	0	10	1 med-fat protein
Hot Wings													
Fiery Buffalo Hot Wings	1 wing	70	4	40	1	0	20	290	5	0	0	4	1 med-fat protein

	Serving	Cal	Total Fat (g)	Cal from Fat	Sat Fat (g)	Trans Fat (g)	Chol (mg)	Sodium (mg)	Total Carb (g)	Sugars (g)	Fiber (g)	Protein (g)	Exchanges
HBBQ Hot Wings	1 wing	80	4	40	1	0	20	270	8	2	0	4	1/2 carb, 1 med-fat protein
Hot Wings	1 wing	70	4	40	1	0	20	160	3	0	0	4	1 med-fat protein
Popcorn Nuggets													
1/2 Family Tray	1 order	700	41	370	5	0	80	2330	46	0	4	37	3 carb, 5 med-fat protein, 3 fat
Family Tray	1 order	1410	83	740	10	0	155	4670	92	0	8	74	6 carb, 8 med-fat protein, 7 fat
Kids	1 order	270	16	140	2	0	30	900	18	0	2	14	1 carb, 1 med-fat protein, 2 fat
Large	1 order	570	33	300	4	0	65	1890	37	0	3	30	2 1/2 carb, 3 med-fat protein, 3 fat
Homestyle Sides (Individual)													
Biscuit	1 (1.9 oz)	180	8	70	6	1.5	0	530	23	2	1	4	1 1/2 carb, 1 fat
Coleslaw	1 order	170	10	90	1.5	0	<5	170	19	15	3	<1	1 carb, 2 fat
Corn on the Cob	1 (2.5 oz)	70	0.5	5	0	0	0	0	16	3	2	2	1 carb
Green Beans	1 order	25	0	0	0	0	0	260	4	<1	2	1	1 vegetable
Kentucky Baked Beans	1 order	230	1.5	15	0	0	20	780	39	16	7	14	2 1/2 carb, 1 lean protein

FAST FOOD

	Serving	Calories	Fat (g)	Cal. from Fat	Sat. Fat (g)	Trans Fat (g)	Chol. (mg)	Sod. (mg)	Carb. (g)	Sugar (g)	Fiber (g)	Prot. (g)	Servings/Exchanges
KFC Cornbread Muffin	1 (1.8 oz)	210	9	80	1.5	0	35	240	28	11	<1	3	2 carb, 1 fat
Macaroni & Cheese	1 order	170	6	60	1.5	0	<5	830	22	2	2	5	1 1/2 carb, 1 fat
Mashed Potatoes	1 order	90	3	25	0.5	0	0	320	15	0	1	2	1 carb
Mashed Potatoes with Gravy	1 order	120	4	35	1	0	0	530	19	0	1	2	1 carb, 1 fat
Potato Wedges	1 order	290	15	140	2.5	0	0	810	35	0	2	4	2 carb, 2 fat
Sweet Kernel Corn	1 order	100	0.5	5	0	0	0	0	21	3	2	3	1 1/2 carb
Go Cups													
Chicken Littles	1 order	600	33	300	5	0	40	1400	58	4	4	18	4 carb, 1 med-fat protein, 5 fat
Extra Crispy Tenders	1 order	540	28	260	4	0	60	1440	46	0	4	26	3 carb, 2 med-fat protein, 3 fat
Fiery Buffalo Hot Wings	1 order	510	28	250	6	0	55	1680	50	0	3	15	3 carb, 1 med-fat protein, 4 fat
HBBQ Hot Wings	1 order	540	28	250	6	0	55	1610	58	6	3	15	4 carb, 5 fat

Hot Wings	1 order	490	27	250	6	0	55	1290	45	0	3	15	3 carb, 1 med-fat protein, 4 fat
KRISPY KREME DOUGHNUTS													
Apple Fritter	1	390	20	180	9	0	0	160	50	28	2	4	3 carb, 3 fat
Chocolate Iced Custard Filled	1	350	22	190	9	0	0	130	35	17	1	4	2 carb, 4 fat
Chocolate Iced Glazed	1	240	12	100	5	0	0	80	32	21	1	3	2 carb, 2 fat
Chocolate Iced with KREME Filling	1	340	17	150	7	0	0	140	42	24	1	4	3 carb, 3 fat
Cinnamon Apple Filled	1	330	19	170	8	0	0	170	36	12	1	5	2 1/2 carb, 3 fat
Cinnamon Bun	1	220	12	110	5	0	0	95	27	13	1	3	2 carb, 2 fat
Cinnamon Twist	1	230	12	110	5	0	0	75	30	17	1	2	2 carb, 2 fat
Glazed Blueberry Cake	1	370	24	220	10	0	20	210	39	10	1	2	2 1/2 carb, 4 fat
Glazed Chocolate Cake	1	330	22	200	9	0	35	330	32	20	0	2	2 carb, 4 fat
Glazed Chocolate Cake Doughnut Holes	4 holes	180	10	90	4	0	15	220	21	11	0	2	1 1/2 carb, 2 fat
Glazed with KREME Filling	1	370	23	200	10	0	0	125	38	22	1	4	2 1/2 carb, 4 fat

FAST FOOD

	Serving	Calories	Fat (g)	Cal. from Fat	Sat. Fat (g)	Trans Fat (g)	Chol. (mg)	Sod. (mg)	Carb. (g)	Sugar (g)	Fiber (g)	Prot. (g)	Servings/Exchanges
Oreo Cookies and Kreme	1	420	22	190	9	0	0	200	53	29	1	5	3 1/2 carb, 4 fat
Original Glazed Doughnut	1	190	11	100	5	0	0	75	21	10	1	2	1 1/2 carb, 2 fat
Powdered Cinnamon Cake	1	250	16	140	6	0	25	340	24	6	1	3	1 1/2 carb, 3 fat
Traditional Cake	1	230	15	140	6	0	25	340	20	3	1	3	1 carb, 3 fat
LONG JOHN SILVER'S													
Alaskan Pollock & Seafood													
Baked Cod	1 piece	160	1	10	0	0	120	390	1	0	0	36	5 lean protein
Baked Shrimp	3 pieces	25	0	0	0	0	45	105	0	0	0	5	1 lean protein
Battered Alaskan Pollock	1 piece	230	14	130	5	0	40	580	14	0	1	12	1 carb, 1 med-fat protein, 2 fat
Battered Alaskan Pollock Tender	1 piece	200	14	130	6	0	25	580	11	0	0	7	1 carb, 1 med-fat protein, 2 fat
Battered Cod	1 piece	280	19	180	8	0	60	640	6	0	0	19	1/2 carb, 2 med-fat protein, 2 fat
Battered Shrimp	3 pieces	130	7	60	3	0	45	350	5	0	0	6	1 med-fat protein

Breaded Clam Strips	1 snack box	280	16	115	6	10	1030	20	5	1	7	1 carb, 1 med-fat protein, 2 fat
Crab Cake	1 cake	280	15	140	6	35	880	26	3	1	10	2 carb, 1 med-fat protein, 2 fat
Popcorn Shrimp	1 snack box	330	12	110	5	70	510	20	0	1	8	1 carb, 1 med-fat protein, 1 fat

Chicken

Chicken Bites	1 piece	60	4	30	2	10	200	4	0	0	2	1 fat
Chicken Tenders	1 piece	170	8	70	3	20	400	11	0	0	8	1 carb, 1 med-fat protein

Sandwiches & Tacos

Baja Chicken Taco	1	530	33	300	11	30	1200	40	1	2	13	2 1/2 carb, 1 med-fat protein, 4 fat
Baja Fish Taco	1	580	39	350	10	45	1330	41	2	2	16	2 1/2 carb, 1 med-fat protein, 5 fat
Ciabatta Jack Chicken Sandwich	1	660	33	300	10	60	1520	57	2	3	26	4 carb, 2 med-fat protein, 4 fat
Ciabatta Jack Fish Sandwich	1	550	30	270	10	50	1300	48	3	2	22	3 carb, 2 med-fat protein, 3 fat

FAST FOOD

	Serving	Calories	Fat (g)	Cal. from Fat	Sat. Fat (g)	Trans Fat (g)	Chol. (mg)	Sod. (mg)	Carb. (g)	Sugar (g)	Fiber (g)	Prot. (g)	Servings/Exchanges
Seafood Salad Sandwich	1	470	27	250	6	0	50	1230	42	5	2	17	3 carb, 1 med-fat protein, 3 fat
Sauces													
Cocktail Sauce	1 dipping cup (1 oz)	25	0	0	0	0	0	330	6	3	0	0	1/2 carb
Tartar Sauce	1 packet	40	4	30	1	0	5	110	2	2	0	0	1 fat
Zesty Tartar Sauce	1 dipping cup (1 oz)	140	15	140	3	0	0	220	1	1	0	0	3 fat
Sides													
Battered Onion Rings	5 pieces	350	26	240	10	0	0	730	25	2	1	2	1 1/2 carb, 5 fat
Breaded Mozzarella Sticks	3 pieces	170	10	90	5	0	15	400	12	1	0	5	1 carb, 2 fat
Cole Slaw	Individual	200	15	130	3	0	20	340	15	10	3	1	1 carb, 3 fat

Corn Cobbette with Butter Oil	1 cobbette	150	10	90	2	0	0	30	14	6	3	3	1 carb, 2 fat
Crumblies	1 oz	150	13	110	5	0	0	360	8	0	0	1	1/2 carb, 2 1/2 fat
Fries	Individual	350	17	150	5	0	0	500	44	0	4	4	3 carb, 3 fat
Hushpuppies	2 pups	160	13	120	5	0	0	390	18	1	1	2	1 carb, 2 fat
Jalapeño Cheddar Bites	5 pieces	240	16	150	7	0	10	630	18	3	1	6	1 carb, 3 fat
Macaroni & Cheese	Individual	150	6	50	3	0	10	490	19	3	1	6	1 carb, 1 fat
Rice	Individual	180	1	10	1	0	0	470	37	1	2	4	2 1/2 carb, 1 1/2 fat
Seafood Salad	Individual	150	10	90	2	0	30	510	8	2	0	7	1/2 carb, 1 med-fat protein, 1 fat
Desserts													
Chocolate Cream Pie	1 slice	280	17	160	10	0	10	230	28	19	1	3	2 carb, 3 fat
Pecan Pie	1 slice	410	21	190	6	0	70	220	52	22	1	4	3 1/2 carb, 3 1/2 fat
Pineapple Cream Pie	1 slice	300	17	150	11	0	10	250	35	25	0	3	2 carb, 3 fat

FAST FOOD

McDONALD'S

Burgers & Sandwiches

	Serving	Calories	Fat (g)	Cal. from Fat	Sat. Fat (g)	Trans Fat (g)	Chol. (mg)	Sod. (mg)	Carb. (g)	Sugar (g)	Fiber (g)	Prot. (g)	Servings/Exchanges
Artisan Grilled Chicken Sandwich	1	360	6	50	1.5	0	75	960	43	10	3	33	3 carb, 3 lean protein
Bacon Buffalo Ranch McChicken	1	440	21	190	5	0	55	1120	41	6	2	20	2 1/2 carb, 2 med-fat protein, 2 fat
Bacon Cheddar McChicken	1	490	25	220	7	0	70	1120	43	6	2	22	3 carb, 2 med-fat protein, 2 fat
Bacon Clubhouse Burger	1	740	41	370	16	1.5	125	1480	51	14	4	40	3 1/2 carb, 4 med-fat protein, 3 1/2 fat
Bacon Clubhouse Crispy Chicken Sandwich	1	750	38	340	10	0.5	90	1720	65	16	4	36	4 carb, 3 med-fat protein, 4 fat
Bacon Clubhouse Grilled Chicken Sandwich	1	610	26	230	8	0	125	1750	50	14	3	45	3 carb, 5 med-fat protein
Big Mac	1	540	28	250	10	1	80	970	47	9	3	25	3 carb, 2 med-fat protein, 3 fat

Item													Exchanges
Cheeseburger	1	300	12	110	6	5	40	680	33	7	2	15	2 carb, 1 med-fat protein, 1 fat
Double Cheeseburger	1	440	22	200	11	1	85	1050	35	7	2	25	2 carb, 3 med-fat protein, 1 fat
Double Quarter Pounder with Cheese	1	780	45	410	21	2.5	175	1310	43	10	3	50	3 carb, 6 med-fat protein, 2 fat
Filet-O-Fish	1	390	19	170	4	0	40	590	39	5	2	15	2 1/2 carb, 1 med-fat protein, 2 fat
Hamburger	1	250	8	70	3	0	30	490	32	6	1	12	2 carb, 1 med-fat protein
McChicken	1	370	17	150	3.5	0	40	650	40	5	2	14	2 1/2 carb, 1 med-fat protein, 2 fat
McDouble	1	390	18	160	8	1	70	850	34	7	2	22	2 carb, 2 med-fat protein, 1 fat
McRib	1	500	26	240	10	0	70	980	44	11	3	22	3 carb, 2 med-fat protein, 3 fat
Quarter Pounder with Cheese	1	540	28	250	13	1.5	100	1110	42	10	3	31	3 carb, 3 med-fat protein, 2 fat

FAST FOOD

	Serving	Calories	Fat (g)	Cal. from Fat	Sat. Fat (g)	Trans Fat (g)	Chol. (mg)	Sod. (mg)	Carb. (g)	Sugar (g)	Fiber (g)	Prot. (g)	Servings/Exchanges
Southern Style Buttermilk Crispy Chicken Sandwich	1	470	21	190	3.5	0	60	810	46	5	2	25	3 carb, 2 med-fat protein, 2 fat
Snack Wraps & Premium Wraps													
Mac Snack Wrap	1	330	19	170	7	1	45	670	26	3	1	14	2 carb, 1 med-fat protein, 2 fat
McWrap Chicken & Bacon (Crispy)	1	640	32	290	9	0.5	80	1550	56	7	4	33	3 1/2 carb, 3 med-fat protein, 3 fat
McWrap Chicken & Bacon (Grilled)	1	500	19	180	8	0.5	115	1570	41	5	3	41	2 1/2 carb, 5 lean protein, 1 fat
McWrap Chicken Sweet Chili (Crispy)	1	540	23	200	4.5	0	50	1260	61	13	4	24	4 carb, 2 med-fat protein, 2 fat
McWrap Chicken Sweet Chili (Grilled)	1	400	10	90	3	0	80	1250	46	11	3	31	3 carb, 3 lean protein
Ranch Snack Wrap (Crispy)	1	360	20	180	5	0	40	810	32	3	1	15	2 carb, 1 med-fat protein, 3 fat

	Amount												Exchanges
Ranch Snack Wrap (Grilled)	1	290	13	120	4.5	0	55	820	25	2	1	19	1 1/2 carb, 2 med-fat protein
Chicken Nuggets & Strips, Sauces													
Chicken McNuggets, 6 Piece	1 order	280	18	160	3	0	13	540	18	0	1	13	1 carb, 1 med-fat protein, 2 fat
Chicken McNuggets, 10 Piece	1 order	470	30	270	5	0	65	900	30	0	2	22	2 carb, 2 med-fat protein, 4 fat
Chicken McNuggets, 20 Piece	1 order	940	59	530	10	0	135	1800	59	0	3	44	4 carb, 5 med-fat protein, 6 fat
Chicken Selects, 3 Piece	1 order	190	12	110	2	0	25	360	12	0	1	9	1 carb, 1 med-fat protein, 1 fat
Honey Mustard Sauce	1 pkg	60	4	35	0.5	0	5	115	6	4	1	5	1/2 carb, 1/2 med-fat protein
Sweet 'N Sour Sauce	1 pkg	50	0	0	0	0	0	150	12	10	0	0	1 carb
Tangy BBQ Sauce	1 pkg	50	0	0	0	0	0	260	12	10	0	0	1 carb
Salads (No Dressing)													
Premium Asian Salad (Crispy Chicken)	1	410	22	200	3	0	45	740	32	12	5	23	2 carb, 2 med-fat protein, 2 fat

FAST FOOD

	Serving	Calories	Fat (g)	Cal. from Fat	Sat. Fat (g)	Trans Fat (g)	Chol. (mg)	Sod. (mg)	Carb. (g)	Sugar (g)	Fiber (g)	Prot. (g)	Servings/Exchanges
Premium Asian Salad (Grilled Chicken)	1	270	9	80	1	0	75	760	18	10	5	32	1 carb, 4 lean protein
Premium Asian Salad (No Chicken)	1	140	7	70	0.5	0	0	20	13	7	5	7	1 carb, 1 med-fat protein
Premium Bacon Ranch Salad (Crispy Chicken)	1	450	26	240	8	0	85	1100	23	6	3	30	1 1/2 carb, 4 med-fat protein, 1 fat
Premium Bacon Ranch Salad (Grilled Chicken)	1	310	14	120	6	0	115	1120	9	3	3	38	1/2 carb, 5 lean protein, 1 fat
Premium Bacon Ranch Salad (No Chicken)	1	190	12	110	6	0	40	530	8	3	3	14	1/2 carb, 2 med-fat protein
Premium Southwest Salad (Crispy Chicken)	1	470	24	210	6	0	60	890	40	11	7	24	2 1/2 carb, 2 med-fat protein, 2 fat
Premium Southwest Salad (Grilled Chicken)	1	330	11	100	4	0	90	920	26	9	6	33	2 carb, 4 lean protein
Premium Southwest Salad (No Chicken)	1	160	7	60	3	0	15	190	18	4	5	8	1 carb, 1 med-fat protein

Salad Dressings

Newman's Own Creamy Southwest	1 pkg (1.5 oz)	120	8	70	1.5	0	20	300	11	3	0	1	1 carb, 2 fat
Newman's Own Low Fat Balsamic Vinaigrette	1 pkg (1.5 oz)	35	1.5	15	0	0	0	300	11	3	0	1	1 carb
Newman's Own Low Fat Family Recipe Italian	1 pkg (1.5 oz)	50	1.5	15	0	0	0	380	8	2	1	0	1/2 carb
Newman's Own Low Fat Sesame Ginger	1 pkg (1.5 oz)	80	2.5	25	0	0	0	400	14	9	1	1	1 carb, 1/2 fat

Fries

Kids Fries	1 order	110	5	50	1	0	0	65	15	0	1	1	1 carb, 1 fat
Large Fries	1 order	510	24	220	3.5	0	0	290	67	0	5	6	4 1/2 carb, 4 fat
Medium Fries	1 order	340	15	140	2.5	0	0	190	44	0	4	4	3 carb, 2 fat
Small Fries	1 order	230	11	100	1.5	0	0	130	30	0	2	2	2 carb, 2 fat

Snacks & Sides

Apple Slices	1 order	15	0	0	0	0	0	0	4	3	0	0	free
Baked Mozzarella Sticks, 3 Piece	1 order	200	10	90	4	0	20	560	18	1	1	9	1 carb, 1 med-fat protein, 1 fat

FAST FOOD

	Serving	Calories	Fat (g)	Cal. from Fat	Sat. Fat (g)	Trans Fat (g)	Chol. (mg)	Sod. (mg)	Carb. (g)	Sugar (g)	Fiber (g)	Prot. (g)	Servings/Exchanges
Cuties	1	40	0	0	0	0	0	0	10	8	1	1	1/2 carb
Fruit 'N Yogurt Parfait	1	150	2	20	1	0	5	80	30	23	1	4	2 carb
Go-GURT Strawberry Low Fat Yogurt Tube	1	50	0.5	5	0	0	5	35	9	6	0	2	1/2 carb
Breakfast													
Bacon, Egg & Cheese Bagel	1	590	29	260	10	0.5	265	1340	56	7	3	27	3 1/2 carb, 2 med-fat protein, 3 fat
Bacon, Egg & Cheese Biscuit with Egg Whites (Large Biscuit)	1	470	25	220	12	0	35	1420	42	4	3	20	3 carb, 2 med-fat protein, 2 fat
Bacon, Egg & Cheese McGriddles with Egg Whites	1	400	15	140	7	0	35	1250	47	16	2	20	3 carb, 2 med-fat protein
Big Breakfast (Large Size Biscuit)	1 order	800	52	470	18	0	555	1680	56	3	4	28	3 1/2 carb, 2 1/2 med-fat protein, 7 fat

Big Breakfast with Egg Whites (Large Size Biscuit)	1 order	690	41	370	14	0	35	1700	55	4	4	26	3 1/2 carb, 2 med-fat protein, 5 1/2 fat
Big Breakfast with Hotcakes (Large Size Biscuit)	1 order	1150	60	540	20	0	575	2260	116	17	7	36	7 1/2 carb, 2 med-fat protein, 8 1/2 fat
Big Breakfast with Hotcakes (Regular Size Biscuit)	1 order	1090	56	510	19	0	575	2150	111	17	6	36	7 1/2 carb, 2 med-fat protein, 8 fat
Cinnamon Melts	1 order	460	19	170	9	0	15	370	66	32	3	6	4 1/2 carb, 3 fat
Egg White Delight	1	250	8	70	3	0	25	770	30	3	4	18	2 carb, 2 lean protein
Fruit & Maple Oatmeal	1	290	4	35	1.5	0	5	160	58	32	5	5	4 carb
Hash Browns	1 order	150	9	80	1.5	0	0	310	15	0	2	1	1 carb, 2 fat
Hotcakes	1 order	350	9	80	2	0	20	590	60	14	3	8	4 carb, 1 fat
Sausage Biscuit (Large Size Biscuit)	1	480	31	280	13	0	30	1190	39	3	3	11	2 1/2 carb, 1/2 med-fat protein, 5 fat
Sausage Biscuit with Egg (Large Size Biscuit)	1	570	37	330	15	0	250	1280	42	3	3	18	3 carb, 1 med-fat protein, 6 fat

FAST FOOD

	Serving	Calories	Fat (g)	Cal. from Fat	Sat. Fat (g)	Trans Fat (g)	Chol. (mg)	Sod. (mg)	Carb. (g)	Sugar (g)	Fiber (g)	Prot. (g)	Servings/Exchanges
Sausage, Egg & Cheese McGriddles with Egg Whites	1	500	25	230	10	0	50	1320	46	15	2	21	3 carb, 2 med-fat protein, 2 fat
Sausage McMuffin	1	370	23	200	8	0	45	780	29	2	4	14	2 carb, 1 med-fat protein, 3 fat
Sausage McMuffin with Egg Whites	1	400	23	210	8	0	50	880	30	2	4	21	2 carb, 2 med-fat protein, 2 fat
Southern Style Chicken Biscuit (Large Size Biscuit)	1	470	24	220	9	0	30	1290	46	4	3	17	3 carb, 1 med-fat protein, 3 fat
Steak & Egg McMuffin	1	430	23	210	9	1	300	960	31	3	4	26	2 carb, 3 med-fat protein, 1 fat
Desserts/Shakes													
Baked Hot Apple Pie	1	250	13	110	7	0	0	170	32	13	4	2	2 carb, 2 fat
Blueberry Pomegranate Smoothie, Large	22 oz	340	1	10	0.5	0	5	65	79	70	5	4	5 carb

Item													
Blueberry Pomegranate Smoothie, Medium	16 oz	260	1	5	0	0	5	50	62	54	4	3	4 carb
Blueberry Pomegranate Smoothie, Small	12 oz	220	0.5	5	0	0	5	40	50	44	3	2	3 carb
Chocolate Chip Cookie	1	160	8	70	3.5	0	10	90	21	15	1	2	1 1/2 carb, 1 fat
Chocolate McCafé Shake, Large	22 oz	850	23	210	15	1	85	380	141	120	2	19	9 1/2 carb, 3 fat
Chocolate McCafé Shake, Medium	16 oz	700	20	180	12	1	75	300	114	97	2	15	7 1/2 carb, 2 1/2 fat
Chocolate McCafé Shake, Small	12 oz	560	16	140	10	1	60	240	91	77	1	12	6 carb, 2 fat
Fried Cherry Pie	1	230	10	90	3.5	0	0	135	33	15	1	2	2 carb, 2 fat
Hot Caramel Sundae	1	340	8	70	5	0	30	150	60	43	0	7	4 carb, 1 fat
Hot Fudge Sundae	1	330	9	80	7	0	25	170	53	48	1	8	3 1/2 carb, 1 fat
Kiddie Cone	1	45	1.5	10	1	0	5	20	7	6	0	1	1/2 carb
McFlurry with M&M's	12 oz	650	23	210	14	0.5	50	180	96	89	1	13	6 1/2 carb, 3 fat
McFlurry with OREO Cookies	12 oz	520	17	150	9	0.5	45	260	80	64	1	12	5 carb, 2 fat

FAST FOOD

	Serving	Calories	Fat (g)	Cal. from Fat	Sat. Fat (g)	Trans Fat (g)	Chol. (mg)	Sod. (mg)	Carb. (g)	Sugar (g)	Fiber (g)	Prot. (g)	Servings/Exchanges
Snack Size McFlurry with M&M's	7.3 oz	430	15	140	10	0	35	120	64	59	1	9	4 carb, 2 fat
Snack Size McFlurry with OREO Cookies	6.7 oz	340	11	100	6	0	30	170	53	43	0	8	3 1/2 carb, 1 1/2 fat
Strawberry & Créme Pie	1	310	17	150	9	0	10	180	36	15	1	4	2 1/2 carb, 3 fat
Strawberry Sundae	1	280	6	60	4	0	25	85	49	45	0	6	3 carb, 1 fat
Vanilla Reduced Fat Ice Cream Cone	1	170	4.5	40	3	0	15	70	27	20	0	5	2 carb, 1/2 fat
McCafé Coffee, Nonfat Milk													
Iced Mocha with Nonfat Milk, Large	22 oz	380	5	45	3	0	20	220	70	62	2	14	4 1/2 carb
Iced Mocha with Nonfat Milk, Medium	16 oz	280	5	45	3	0	20	150	50	43	1	10	3 carb
Iced Mocha with Nonfat Milk, Small	12 oz	240	4.5	40	3	0	20	125	40	34	1	8	2 1/2 carb

Nonfat Caramel Latte, Large	20 oz	310	0.5	0	0	10	180	63	59	1	16	4 carb, 1 lean protein
Nonfat Caramel Latte, Medium	16 oz	250	0	0	0	5	135	51	48	1	12	3 1/2 carb
Nonfat Caramel Latte, Small	12 oz	200	0	0	0	5	110	41	39	1	10	2 1/2 carb
Nonfat French Vanilla Latte, Large	20 oz	300	0.5	0	0	10	180	60	56	1	16	4 carb, 1 lean protein
Nonfat French Vanilla Latte, Medium	16 oz	240	0	0	0	5	140	49	46	1	12	3 carb
Nonfat French Vanilla Latte, Small	12 oz	190	0	0	0	5	115	39	37	1	10	2 1/2 carb
Nonfat Latte, Large	20 oz	170	0.5	0	0	10	180	25	21	1	16	1 1/2 carb, 2 lean protein
Nonfat Latte, Medium	16 oz	130	0	0	0	5	135	19	16	1	12	1 carb, 1 lean protein
Nonfat Latte, Small	12 oz	100	0	0	0	5	110	15	13	1	10	1 carb, 1 lean protein
Nonfat Latte with Sugar Free French Vanilla Syrup, Large	20 oz	220	0.5	0	0	10	240	38	21	2	16	2 1/2 carb, 1 lean protein

FAST FOOD

	Serving	Calories	Fat (g)	Cal. from Fat	Sat. Fat (g)	Trans Fat (g)	Chol. (mg)	Sod. (mg)	Carb. (g)	Sugar (g)	Fiber (g)	Prot. (g)	Servings/Exchanges
Nonfat Latte with Sugar Free French Vanilla Syrup, Medium	16 oz	170	0	0	0	0	5	180	30	16	1	12	2 carb, 1 lean protein
Nonfat Latte with Sugar Free French Vanilla Syrup, Small	12 oz	140	0	0	0	0	5	150	24	13	1	10	1 1/2 carb, 1 lean protein
McCafé Coffee, Whole Milk													
McCafé Caramel Mocha, Large	20 oz	480	17	150	10	0.5	50	270	66	60	1	16	4 1/2 carb, 2 1/2 fat
McCafé Caramel Mocha, Medium	16 oz	390	14	120	8	0	40	220	55	50	1	12	3 1/2 carb, 2 fat
McCafé Caramel Mocha, Small	12 oz	320	11	100	7	0	35	170	45	40	1	10	3 carb, 2 fat
McCafé Frappe Mocha, Large	22 oz	670	26	230	17	1	90	190	97	88	1	11	6 1/2 carb, 4 fat
McCafé Frappe Mocha, Medium	16 oz	540	22	190	14	1	75	160	79	71	1	9	5 carb, 3 fat

Item	Serving	Cal											Exchanges
McCafé Frappe Mocha, Small	12 oz	440	18	160	11	1	60	125	64	57	1	7	4 carb, 3 fat
McCafé Iced Mocha, Large	22 oz	480	16	140	9	0.5	50	220	69	61	2	13	4 1/2 carb, 2 fat
McCafé Iced Mocha, Medium	16 oz	340	12	110	7	0	40	150	49	43	1	9	3 carb, 2 fat
McCafé Iced Mocha, Small	12 oz	290	11	100	6	0	35	125	40	34	1	8	2 1/2 carb, 2 fat
McCafé Latte, Large	20 oz	280	14	120	8	0	40	180	24	20	1	15	1 1/2 carb, 1 med-fat protein, 1 1/2 fat
McCafé Latte, Medium	16 oz	210	10	90	6	0	30	140	18	15	1	11	1 carb, 1 med-fat protein, 1 fat
McCafé Latte, Small	12 oz	170	9	80	5	0	25	115	15	12	1	9	1 carb, 1 med-fat protein, 1 fat
McCafé Mocha, Large	20 oz	500	17	150	10	0.5	50	240	72	63	2	16	5 carb, 2 fat
McCafé Mocha, Medium	16 oz	410	14	120	8	0	40	190	60	53	2	13	4 carb, 2 fat
McCafé Mocha, Small	12 oz	340	11	100	7	0	35	150	49	42	2	10	3 carb, 1 med-fat protein, 1 fat

FAST FOOD

PANDA EXPRESS

Vegetables

	Serving	Calories	Fat (g)	Cal. from Fat	Sat. Fat (g)	Trans Fat (g)	Chol. (mg)	Sod. (mg)	Carb. (g)	Sugar (g)	Fiber (g)	Prot. (g)	Servings/Exchanges
Country Style Bean Curd	1	191	12	113	1.5	0	0	945	14	8	2	7	1 carb, 1 med-fat protein, 1 fat
Eggplant Tofu	1	340	24	210	3.5	0	0	520	23	17	3	7	1 1/2 carb, 4 1/2 fat
Hot Szechuan Tofu	1	140	8	70	1	0	0	580	10	5	2	6	1/2 carb, 1 med-fat protein, 1 fat
Mixed Vegetables (Entrée)	1	35	0	0	0	0	0	280	8	2	3	2	1/2 carb
Chicken													
Asian Chicken	1	340	13	110	3.5	0	195	630	14	10	3	41	1 carb, 5 lean protein
Black Pepper Chicken	1	280	19	165	3	0	52	1140	14	7	1	13	1 carb, 1 med-fat protein, 3 fat
Honey Sesame Chicken Breast	1	420	22	200	4	0	45	480	40	19	2	16	2 1/2 carb, 1 med-fat protein, 3 fat

Item	Amt	Cal.	Fat (g)	Cal. Fat	Sat. Fat (g)	Trans Fat (g)	Chol. (mg)	Sod. (mg)	Carb. (g)	Sugar (g)	Fiber (g)	Prot. (g)	Exchanges/Choices
Kung Pao Chicken	1	290	19	170	3	0	53	970	14	6	2	16	1 carb, 2 med-fat protein, 2 fat
Mushroom Chicken	1	170	9	80	2	0	41	750	11	4	1	12	1 carb, 1 med-fat protein, 1 fat
Orange Chicken	1	380	18	160	3.5	0	80	620	45	19	0	14	3 carb, 1 med-fat protein, 2 fat
String Bean Chicken Breast	1	190	9	80	2	0	34	590	13	4	4	14	1 carb, 2 med-fat protein
SweetFire Chicken Breast	1	380	15	140	3	0	35	320	47	27	1	13	3 carb, 1 med-fat protein, 1 fat
Sweet & Sour Chicken Breast	1	300	12	110	3	0	25	260	40	24	1	10	2 1/2 carb, 2 fat
Teriyaki Chicken	1	300	13	120	4	0	185	530	8	8	0	36	1/2 carb, 4 lean protein
Beef													
Beijing Beef	1	470	26	240	5	0	25	660	46	24	1	13	3 carb, 1 med-fat protein, 4 fat
Broccoli Beef	1	150	7	70	1.5	0	12	520	13	7	2	9	1 carb, 1 med-fat protein

FAST FOOD

	Serving	Calories	Fat (g)	Cal. from Fat	Sat. Fat (g)	Trans Fat (g)	Chol. (mg)	Sod. (mg)	Carb. (g)	Sugar (g)	Fiber (g)	Prot. (g)	Servings/Exchanges
Shanghai Angus Steak	1	310	19	170	4	0	50	830	16	11	1	22	1 carb, 3 med-fat protein, 1 fat
Shrimp													
Crispy Shrimp (Entrée), 6 Piece	1	260	13	120	2	0	60	800	26	2	1	9	2 carb, 2 fat
Honey Walnut Shrimp	1	360	23	200	3.5	0	100	440	35	9	2	13	2 carb, 1 med-fat protein, 3 fat
Sides & Appetizers													
Brown Steamed Rice	1	420	4	35	1	0	0	15	86	1	4	9	5 1/2 carb
Chicken Egg Roll	1 roll	200	10	90	2	0	20	340	20	2	2	6	1 carb, 2 fat
Chicken Potsticker	3 pieces	160	6	60	1.5	0	20	250	20	2	1	6	1 carb, 1 fat
Chow Mein	1	510	22	200	4	0	0	980	65	9	4	13	4 carb, 4 fat
Fried Rice	1	410	9	80	1	0	0	1110	73	6	1	9	5 carb, 1 fat
Vegetable Spring Roll	1 roll	190	8	80	1.5	0	0	520	27	3	2	3	2 carb, 1 fat
White Steamed Rice	1	380	0	0	0	0	0	0	87	0	0	7	6 carb

Soup

Item	Serving	Cal.	Fat (g)	Cal. Fat	Sat. Fat (g)	Trans Fat (g)	Chol. (mg)	Sod. (mg)	Carb. (g)	Sugar (g)	Fiber (g)	Prot. (g)	Choices/Exchanges
Hot & Sour Soup, Cup	1	120	4.5	40	0.5	0	65	880	14	4	1	7	1 carb, 1 lean protein
Hot & Sour Soup, Bowl	1	170	6	60	1	0	90	1260	20	6	1	10	1 carb, 1 med-fat protein

Sauces & Cookies

Item	Serving	Cal.	Fat (g)	Cal. Fat	Sat. Fat (g)	Trans Fat (g)	Chol. (mg)	Sod. (mg)	Carb. (g)	Sugar (g)	Fiber (g)	Prot. (g)	Choices/Exchanges
Fortune Cookies	1 cookie	32	0	2	0	0	0	8	7	3	0	1	1/2 carb
Plum Sauce	1 packet	15	0	0	0	0	0	55	3	3	0	0	free
Sweet & Sour Sauce	1.8 oz	70	0	0	0	0	0	115	21	20	0	0	1 1/2 carb
Teriyaki Sauce	1.8 oz	10	0	0	0	0	0	380	16	14	0	0	1 carb

PANERA BREAD

Breakfast Favorites

Item	Serving	Cal.	Fat (g)	Cal. Fat	Sat. Fat (g)	Trans Fat (g)	Chol. (mg)	Sod. (mg)	Carb. (g)	Sugar (g)	Fiber (g)	Prot. (g)	Choices/Exchanges
Power Almond & Quinoa Oatmeal	1 bowl	290	6	55	1	0	0	220	51	7	9	8	3 1/2 carb, 1/2 fat
Steel Cut Oatmeal with Apple Chips & Pecans	1 1/3 cups	370	15	135	2	0	0	170	53	18	9	6	3 1/2 carb, 2 fat
Strawberry Granola Parfait	1 parfait	310	11	100	4.5	0	10	100	43	30	3	9	3 carb, 2 fat

FAST FOOD

Breakfast Sandwiches

	Serving	Calories	Fat (g)	Cal. from Fat	Sat. Fat (g)	Trans Fat (g)	Chol. (mg)	Sod. (mg)	Carb. (g)	Sugar (g)	Fiber (g)	Prot. (g)	Servings/Exchanges
Avocado, Egg White & Spinach Breakfast Power Sandwich	1 sandwich	400	13	115	6	0	25	650	52	5	5	12	3 1/2 carb, 2 fat
Bacon, Egg & Cheese on Asiago Bagel	1 sandwich	610	28	250	13	0.5	245	1350	55	4	2	34	3 1/2 carb, 3 med-fat protein, 2 fat
Egg & Cheese on Ciabatta	1 sandwich	390	15	135	7	0	205	720	43	2	2	19	3 carb, 1 med-fat protein, 1 fat
Ham, Egg & Cheese Breakfast Power Sandwich	1 sandwich	350	15	135	7	0	220	910	31	3	4	16	2 carb, 1 med-fat protein, 1 fat
Mediterranean Egg White on Ciabatta	1 sandwich	410	15	135	6	0	25	780	48	2	2	12	3 carb, 2 fat
Sausage, Egg & Cheese on Ciabatta	1 sandwich	550	29	260	12	0	250	1050	44	2	2	28	3 carb, 3 med-fat protein, 2 fat
Steak & Egg on Everything Bagel	1 sandwich	550	18	160	8	0	240	1080	60	4	3	33	4 carb, 3 med-fat protein

Turkey Sausage, Egg White & Spinach Breakfast Power Sandwich	1 sandwich	390	10	90	5	0	40	790	50	4	3	16	3 carb, 1 med-fat protein
Soufflés													
Four Cheese	1 soufflé	480	29	260	15	0.5	190	690	37	8	2	16	2 1/2 carb, 1 med-fat protein, 4 fat
Ham & Swiss	1 soufflé	500	30	270	16	0.5	175	790	37	8	2	20	2 1/2 carb, 2 med-fat protein, 3 1/2 fat
Spinach & Artichoke	1 soufflé	540	34	305	19	0.5	165	910	39	9	2	19	2 1/2 carb, 2 med-fat protein, 4 fat
Bagels													
Asiago Cheese Bagel	1 bagel	330	6	55	3.5	0	10	580	55	3	2	13	3 1/2 carb, 1/2 fat
Blueberry Bagel	1 bagel	340	1.5	14	0	0	0	510	68	8	2	11	4 1/2 carb
Chocolate Chip Bagel	1 bagel	380	6	55	3	0	5	480	68	13	3	11	4 1/2 carb
Cinnamon Crunch Bagel	1 bagel	420	6	55	4.5	0	0	440	81	31	2	10	5 1/2 carb
Cranberry Walnut Bagel	1 bagel	340	5	45	0.5	0	0	440	64	13	3	10	4 carb
Everything Bagel	1 bagel	300	2.5	25	0	0	0	640	59	4	2	10	4 carb

FAST FOOD

	Serving	Calories	Fat (g)	Cal. from Fat	Sat. Fat (g)	Trans Fat (g)	Chol. (mg)	Sod. (mg)	Carb. (g)	Sugar (g)	Fiber (g)	Prot. (g)	Servings/Exchanges
Plain Bagel	1 bagel	290	1.5	14	0	0	0	460	59	3	2	10	4 carb
Pumpkin Pie Bagel	1 bagel	380	5	45	3	0	0	410	75	24	4	9	5 carb
Whole Grain Bagel	1 bagel	340	2.5	25	0	0	0	400	67	5	6	13	4 1/2 carb
Cream Cheese Spreads													
Plain Cream Cheese	2-oz cup	190	18	160	11	1	55	210	2	1	0	3	4 fat
Reduced Fat Chive & Onion Cream Cheese	2-oz cup	130	11	100	7	0.5	35	370	4	2	1	5	1 med-fat protein, 2 fat
Reduced Fat Hazelnut Cream Cheese	2-oz cup	140	11	100	6	0.5	35	210	6	6	1	5	1/2 carb, 2 fat
Reduced Fat New York Style Cheesecake Cream Cheese	2-oz cup	160	8	70	5	0	25	240	18	16	1	4	1 carb, 2 fat
Reduced Fat Plain Cream Cheese	2-oz cup	130	12	110	7	0.5	35	230	2	1	1	5	1 med-fat protein, 1 fat
Reduced Fat Wild Blueberry Cream Cheese	2-oz cup	150	10	90	6	0	30	190	11	9	1	4	1 carb, 2 fat

Bakery Pastries & Sweets

Item	Serving												
Bear Claw	1 pastry	570	28	250	13	0.5	70	410	69	32	3	10	4 1/2 carb, 5 fat
Blueberry Muffin with Fresh Blueberries	1 muffin	460	18	160	3	0	60	340	69	40	2	6	4 1/2 carb, 3 fat
Carrot Cake with Walnuts	1 cake	650	26	235	9	0	80	670	98	62	4	8	6 1/2 carb, 4 fat
Cherry Pastry	1 pastry	420	17	155	10	0.5	55	330	60	30	1	7	4 carb, 3 fat
Chocolate Chip Cookie	1 cookie	440	22	225	14	0.5	60	330	58	33	3	5	4 carb, 4 fat
Chocolate Chip Muffie	1 muffie	320	14	125	4	0	35	200	46	27	2	4	3 carb, 2 fat
Chocolate Duet Sandwich Cookie with Walnuts	1 cookie	380	21	190	10	0	40	240	46	32	2	4	3 carb, 4 fat
Chocolate Pastry	1 pastry	410	23	210	14	0.5	55	250	47	18	2	7	3 carb, 4 fat
Cinnamon Crumb Coffee Cake	1 slice	470	25	225	9	0	105	320	53	29	1	6	3 1/2 carb, 4 fat
Cinnamon Roll	1 roll	630	24	215	14	0.5	100	510	91	35	4	13	6 carb, 4 fat
Cobblestone	1 roll	560	12	110	7	0	60	500	103	56	3	11	7 carb, 1 fat
Double Fudge Brownie	1 brownie	500	22	225	10	0	80	240	73	53	4	7	5 carb, 3 fat

FAST FOOD

	Serving	Calories	Fat (g)	Cal. from Fat	Sat. Fat (g)	Trans Fat (g)	Chol. (mg)	Sod. (mg)	Carb. (g)	Sugar (g)	Fiber (g)	Prot. (g)	Servings/Exchanges
French Croissant	1 crois-sant	300	17	155	10	0.5	45	220	32	5	1	6	2 carb, 3 fat
Mini Scones Multi Pack	9 pack	1460	57	515	36	2	210	2360	216	96	6	24	14 1/2 carb, 8 1/2 fat
Oatmeal Raisin Cookie	1 cookie	400	14	125	8	0	50	320	62	32	3	5	4 carb, 2 fat
Orange Mini Scone	1 mini scone	180	7	65	4.5	0	25	270	27	13	1	3	2 carb, 1 fat
Orange Scone	1 scone	540	20	180	13	0.5	75	810	81	38	3	9	5 1/2 carb, 3 fat
Pecan Braid	1 pastry	470	26	235	11	0.5	55	280	53	23	2	8	3 1/2 carb, 5 fat
Petite Chocolate Chipper	1 petite cookie	100	5	45	3	0	15	75	14	8	1	1	1 carb, 1 fat
Pumpkin Muffie	1 muffie	290	11	100	2	0	15	240	45	26	1	3	3 carb, 2 fat
Pumpkin Muffin	1 muffin	590	22	200	4	0	30	480	91	53	2	7	6 carb, 3 fat
Shortbread Cookie	1 cookie	380	23	210	14	1	60	170	40	12	1	4	2 1/2 carb, 4 fat
Wild Blueberry Mini Scone	1 mini scone	160	7	65	4	0	25	300	22	8	1	3	1 1/2 carb, 1 fat

Wild Blueberry Scone	1 scone	470	20	180	12	1	75	900	66	25	2	8	4 1/2 carb, 3 fat
Artisan Breads													
Asiago Cheese Focaccia (Loaf)	1 slice	150	3.5	30	1.5	0	5	240	24	1	1	6	1 1/2 carb
Ciabatta (Loaf)	1 slice	150	2	20	0	0	0	240	27	1	1	5	2 carb
Country (Loaf)	1 slice	140	0.5	5	0	0	0	310	27	0	1	5	2 carb
French (Baguette)	1 slice	150	1	10	0	0	0	370	30	0	1	5	2 carb
Rye (Loaf)	1 slice	140	0.5	5	0	0	0	380	28	0	2	5	2 carb
Sea Salt Focaccia (Loaf)	1 slice	160	2.5	25	0	0	0	340	29	1	1	5	2 carb
Sesame Semolina (Miche)	1 slice	140	1	10	0	0	0	360	30	1	1	5	2 carb
Whole Grain (Loaf)	1 slice	130	1	10	0	0	0	290	27	2	3	6	2 carb
Specialty Breads													
All Natural White (Loaf)	1 slice	150	2.5	25	1	0	5	270	27	1	1	5	2 carb
Asiago Cheese (Loaf)	1 slice	160	4	35	2.5	0	10	320	23	0	1	7	1 1/2 carb, 1/2 fat
Cinnamon Raisin Swirl (Loaf)	1 slice	190	6	55	3	0	30	190	31	12	1	5	2 carb, 1 fat

FAST FOOD

	Serving	Calories	Fat (g)	Cal. from Fat	Sat. Fat (g)	Trans Fat (g)	Chol. (mg)	Sod. (mg)	Carb. (g)	Sugar (g)	Fiber (g)	Prot. (g)	Servings/Exchanges
Cranberry Walnut (Miche)	1 slice	150	1.5	15	0	0	0	270	27	4	2	5	2 carb
Holiday Bread (Loaf)	1 slice	170	4.5	40	2.5	0	25	200	30	14	1	4	2 carb, 1/2 fat
Honey Wheat (Loaf)	1 slice	160	3	25	1.5	0	0	230	29	4	2	4	2 carb
Sourdough (Loaf)	1 slice	140	0.5	5	0	0	0	290	28	0	1	5	2 carb
Sourdough Bread Bowl	1 bowl	660	3	25	0	0	0	1340	131	1	4	23	8 1/2 carb
Tomato Basil (XL Loaf)	1 slice	130	0.5	5	0	0	0	320	27	1	1	5	2 carb
Panini, Flatbread & Sandwiches													
Asiago Steak on Asiago Cheese Demi	1 sandwich	810	38	340	17	1	125	1340	67	4	4	50	4 1/2 carb, 5 med-fat protein, 2 fat
Bacon Turkey Bravo on Tomato Basil	1 sandwich	800	27	245	10	1	100	2910	85	8	4	52	5 1/2 carb, 5 med-fat protein
Chicken, Ham & Swiss Flatbread	1 flatbread	350	17	155	10	0	70	580	31	4	3	15	2 carb, 1 med-fat protein, 2 fat
Classic Grilled Cheese on All-Natural White Bread	1 sandwich	580	19	170	15	0	55	1450	74	6	2	26	5 carb, 2 med-fat protein, 1 fat

	Serving	Cal.	Fat Cal.	Fat (g)	Sat Fat (g)	Trans Fat (g)	Chol. (mg)	Sod. (mg)	Carb. (g)	Fiber (g)	Sugar (g)	Pro. (g)	Exchanges/Choices
Frontega Chicken Panini on Focaccia	1 panini	740	215	24	7	0	85	2150	86	8	5	46	5 1/2 carb, 4 med-fat protein
Italian Combo on Ciabatta	1 sand- wich	1000	370	41	16	1	160	2810	97	8	5	59	6 1/2 carb, 6 med-fat protein, 1 fat
Mediterranean Veggie on Tomato Basil	1 sand- wich	570	110	12	3	0	10	1430	94	10	7	20	6 carb, 1 fat
Napa Almond Chicken Salad on Sesame Semolina	1 sand- wich	690	235	26	4.5	0	70	1150	90	13	5	30	6 carb, 2 med-fat protein, 2 fat
Roasted Turkey, Apple & Cheddar on Cranberry Walnut Miche	1 sand- wich	730	290	32	12	1	110	1260	65	16	6	34	4 carb, 3 med-fat protein, 3 fat
Roasted Turkey & Avocado BLT on Sourdough	1 sand- wich	540	200	22	4	0	65	950	48	3	6	37	3 carb, 4 med-fat protein
Roasted Turkey Cranberry Flatbread	1 flat- bread	300	110	12	4	0	65	470	34	8	3	13	2 carb, 1 med-fat protein, 1 fat
Sierra Turkey on Asiago Cheese Focaccia	1 sand- wich	730	245	27	7	1.5	75	1930	81	4	4	40	5 1/2 carb, 3 med-fat protein, 1 fat

FAST FOOD

	Serving	Calories	Cal. from Fat	Fat (g)	Sat. Fat (g)	Trans Fat (g)	Chol. (mg)	Sod. (mg)	Carb. (g)	Sugar (g)	Fiber (g)	Prot. (g)	Servings/Exchanges
Smoked Ham & Swiss on Rye	1 sandwich	620	160	18	9	0.5	100	2230	67	6	5	45	4 1/2 carb, 4 lean protein, 1 fat
Smoked Turkey Breast on Country	1 sandwich	430	30	3.5	1	1	50	1790	67	5	4	33	4 1/2 carb, 3 lean protein
Southwestern Flatbread	1 flatbread	380	160	18	7	0	50	560	41	9	6	9	2 1/2 carb, 3 fat
Steak & White Cheddar Panini on French Baguette	1 panini	1060	415	46	17	1	130	1810	104	4	5	52	7 carb, 4 med-fat protein, 4 fat
Tomato Mozzarella Flatbread	1 flatbread	330	160	18	9	0	35	460	34	5	4	6	2 carb, 3 fat
Tuna Salad on Honey Wheat	1 sandwich	510	145	16	4	0	35	1100	65	12	5	28	4 carb, 2 med-fat protein
Hand-Tossed Salads													
Ancient Grain, Arugula & Chicken	1 whole salad	420	125	14	3	0	80	300	41	20	6	25	2 1/2 carb, 2 med-fat protein

Asian Sesame Chicken	1 whole salad	400	20	180	3.5	0	80	520	25	5	5	31	1 1/2 carb, 4 med-fat protein
BBQ Chicken	1 whole salad	450	20	180	3.5	0	90	540	37	18	5	31	2 1/2 carb, 3 med-fat protein, 1/2 fat
Caesar	1 whole salad	330	26	325	7	0.5	45	530	15	1	2	9	1 carb, 1 med-fat protein, 4 fat
Chicken Cobb with Avocado	1 whole salad	660	50	450	11	0	295	970	14	3	7	42	1 carb, 6 med-fat protein, 4 fat
Classic	1 whole salad	170	11	100	1.5	0	0	140	18	13	3	2	1 carb, 2 fat
Fuji Apple Chicken	1 whole salad	560	34	305	7	0	95	610	35	22	6	32	2 carb, 4 med-fat protein, 2 fat
Greek	1 whole salad	370	34	305	8	0	25	1140	11	4	4	8	1 carb, 1 med-fat protein, 6 fat
Mediterranean Chicken & Quinoa	1 whole salad	580	38	340	6	0	80	870	31	4	8	25	2 carb, 3 med-fat protein, 4 fat
Power Kale Caesar Salad with Chicken	1 whole salad	650	40	360	16	0.5	165	1290	11	2	2	49	1 carb, 7 med-fat protein, 1 fat
Thai Chicken	1 whole salad	490	19	170	3	0	80	910	42	14	8	41	3 carb, 5 lean protein, 1 fat

FAST FOOD

Broth Bowls & Soups

	Serving	Calories	Fat (g)	Cal. from Fat	Sat. Fat (g)	Trans Fat (g)	Chol. (mg)	Sod. (mg)	Carb. (g)	Sugar (g)	Fiber (g)	Prot. (g)	Servings/Exchanges
All Natural Turkey Chili	1 bowl	320	11	100	2	0	45	1090	35	7	12	17	2 carb, 2 med-fat protein
Baked Potato Soup	1 bowl	340	24	215	13	0	65	1230	27	6	4	7	2 carb, 4 fat
Broccoli Cheddar Soup	1 bowl	330	21	190	14	0.5	75	1390	23	0	8	14	1 1/2 carb, 1 med-fat protein, 3 fat
Lentil Quinoa with Chicken Broth Bowl	1 bowl	390	8	70	1.5	0	65	1390	49	6	10	34	3 carb, 4 lean protein
Low-Fat All Natural Chicken Noodle	1 bowl	170	4	35	2	0	40	1330	20	3	2	14	1 carb, 2 lean protein
Low-Fat Vegetarian Black Bean	1 bowl	230	3.5	30	0.5	0	0	1120	42	2	9	17	3 carb, 1 lean protein
Low-Fat Vegetarian Garden Vegetable with Pesto	1 bowl	140	5	45	0.5	0	0	830	24	5	11	4	1 1/2 carb, 1 fat
New England Clam Chowder	1 bowl	720	62	560	41	1.5	160	1020	31	7	3	9	2 carb, 12 fat

Food	Serving												Exchanges/Choices
Soba Noodle with Edamame Broth Bowl	1 bowl	370	12	110	1	0	0	1340	52	6	7	17	3 1/2 carb, 1 med-fat protein, 1 fat
Vegetarian Creamy Tomato	1 bowl	450	32	290	18	0.5	75	680	33	12	7	8	2 carb, 6 fat
Pastas													
Butternut Squash Ravioli	2 cups (16 oz)	690	25	225	12	0.5	95	1340	92	6	8	23	6 carb, 1 med-fat protein, 3 fat
Mac & Cheese	2 cups (16 oz)	980	61	550	26	1	125	2030	75	12	3	34	5 carb, 3 med-fat protein, 8 fat
Pasta Primavera	2 cups (16 oz)	710	41	370	23	1.5	130	850	68	8	8	17	4 1/2 carb, 7 fat
Tortellini Alfredo	2 cups (16 oz)	680	38	340	22	0	160	1520	65	3	3	21	4 carb, 1 med-fat protein, 6 fat
Coffee & Tea Drinks													
Café Mocha	16 oz	370	13	115	8	0	45	180	53	38	2	12	3 1/2 carb, 2 fat
Cappuccino	16 oz	130	5	45	3	0	20	110	14	12	0	9	1 carb, 1 med-fat protein
Chai Tea Latte	16 oz	240	4.5	40	3	0	20	95	42	40	0	7	3 carb
Iced Café Mocha	20 oz	400	14	125	9	0	50	210	56	42	2	14	3 1/2 carb, 2 fat

FAST FOOD

	Serving	Calories	Fat (g)	Cal. from Fat	Sat. Fat (g)	Trans Fat (g)	Chol. (mg)	Sod. (mg)	Carb. (g)	Sugar (g)	Fiber (g)	Prot. (g)	Servings/Exchanges
Iced Chai Latte	20 oz	190	3.5	30	2.5	0	15	80	34	32	0	6	2 carb
Iced Green Tea	20 oz	160	0	0	0	0	0	10	41	38	0	0	2 1/2 carb
Skinny Café Mocha	16 oz	240	1.5	15	1	0	5	170	46	34	2	11	3 carb
Fruit Smoothies													
Low-Fat Strawberry Banana with Ginseng	16 oz	260	1	10	0.5	0	5	55	59	47	4	5	4 carb
Low-Fat Wild Berry	16 oz	340	1.5	15	1	0	5	105	75	68	2	6	5 carb
Superfruit Power with Ginseng	16 oz	210	0	0	0	0	0	75	34	30	2	14	2 carb, 1 lean protein
PAPA JOHN'S PIZZA													
Original Crust, Large													
BBQ Chicken Bacon	1 slice	340	11	100	4.5	0	40	1020	45	11	2	16	3 carb, 1 med-fat protein, 1 fat
Cheese	1 slice	290	10	90	4.5	0	25	710	38	5	2	11	2 1/2 carb, 1 1/2 fat
Garden Fresh	1 slice	300	9	80	3.5	0	20	680	39	5	2	10	2 1/2 carb, 1 fat

Hawaiian BBQ Chicken	1 slice	360	11	100	4.5	0	40	1040	47	12	2	17	3 carb, 1 med-fat protein, 1 fat
Pepperoni	1 slice	320	13	120	5	0	30	810	36	5	2	12	2 1/2 carb, 1 med-fat protein, 1 fat
Sausage	1 slice	330	14	130	6	0	30	810	38	5	2	12	2 1/2 carb, 1 med-fat protein, 1 fat
Spicy Italian	1 slice	380	18	170	7	0	40	930	38	5	2	14	2 1/2 carb, 1 med-fat protein, 2 fat
Spinach Alfredo	1 slice	280	10	90	5	0	25	640	36	3	1	10	2 1/2 carb, 1 1/2 fat
The Meats	1 slice	380	17	160	7	0	45	1040	39	5	2	15	2 1/2 carb, 1 med-fat protein, 2 fat
The Works	1 slice	360	14	130	5	0	35	890	39	5	2	13	2 1/2 carb, 1 med-fat protein, 1 fat
Tuscan Six Cheese	1 slice	320	12	110	6	0	30	780	38	4	2	14	2 1/2 carb, 1 med-fat protein, 1 fat

Thin Crust, Large

BBQ Chicken Bacon	1 slice	270	12	110	5	0	40	800	27	8	1	13	2 carb, 1 med-fat protein, 1 fat

FAST FOOD

	Serving	Calories	Fat (g)	Cal. from Fat	Sat. Fat (g)	Trans Fat (g)	Chol. (mg)	Sod. (mg)	Carb. (g)	Sugar (g)	Fiber (g)	Prot. (g)	Servings/Exchanges
Cheese	1 slice	210	11	100	4.5	0	25	490	20	2	1	8	1 carb, 1 med-fat protein, 1 fat
Garden Fresh	1 slice	230	10	90	4	0	20	460	21	3	1	8	1 1/2 carb, 2 fat
Hawaiian BBQ Chicken	1 slice	280	12	110	5	0	40	800	29	10	1	13	2 carb, 1 med-fat protein, 1 fat
Pepperoni	1 slice	250	14	130	5	0	30	590	20	2	1	9	1 carb, 1 med-fat protein, 2 fat
Sausage	1 slice	260	16	140	6	0	30	600	20	2	1	9	1 carb, 1 med-fat protein, 2 fat
Spicy Italian	1 slice	310	20	180	7	0	40	710	21	2	1	11	1 1/2 carb, 1 med-fat protein, 3 fat
Spinach Alfredo	1 slice	210	11	100	5	0	25	430	18	1	1	8	1 carb, 1 med-fat protein, 1 fat
The Meats	1 slice	300	19	170	7	0	45	830	21	2	1	13	1 1/2 carb, 1 med-fat protein, 2 1/2 fat
The Works	1 slice	290	15	140	6	0	35	670	21	2	1	11	1 1/2 carb, 1 med-fat protein, 2 fat

	Serving											
Tuscan Six Cheese	1 slice	250	13	120	6	0	30	560	20	2	1	11	1 carb, 1 med-fat protein, 1 fat

Lighter Choice Pizzas, Large

	Serving												
Chicken & Veggie (Original Crust)	1 slice	280	7	60	2	0	15	620	39	5	2	10	2 1/2 carb, 1 fat
Chicken & Veggie (Thin Crust)	1 slice	210	8	70	2.5	0	15	400	21	2	1	8	1 1/2 carb, 1 fat
Grilled Chicken & Canadian Bacon (Original Crust)	1 slice	270	7	60	2.5	0	25	750	38	5	2	13	2 1/2 carb, 1 med-fat protein
Grilled Chicken & Canadian Bacon (Thin Crust)	1 slice	190	8	70	2.5	0	25	530	20	2	1	11	1 carb, 1 med-fat protein
Hawaiian Chicken (Original Crust)	1 slice	260	6	60	2	0	25	650	39	6	2	12	2 1/2 carb, 1 med-fat protein
Hawaiian Chicken (Thin Crust)	1 slice	190	7	70	2.5	0	25	430	21	4	1	10	1 1/2 carb, 1 med-fat protein
Mediterranean Veggie (Original Crust)	1 slice	270	7	60	2	0	10	630	38	5	2	9	2 1/2 carb, 1 fat

FAST FOOD

	Serving	Calories	Fat (g)	Cal. from Fat	Sat. Fat (g)	Trans Fat (g)	Chol. (mg)	Sod. (mg)	Carb. (g)	Sugar (g)	Fiber (g)	Prot. (g)	Servings/Exchanges
Mediterranean Veggie (Thin Crust)	1 slice	200	8	70	2.5	0	10	410	21	2	1	5	1 1/2 carb, 1 fat
Tropical Luau (Original Crust)	1 slice	260	6	60	2.5	0	15	670	39	6	2	10	2 1/2 carb, 1 fat
Tropical Luau (Thin Crust)	1 slice	190	8	70	2.5	0	15	450	21	4	1	7	1 1/2 carb, 1 fat
Sides, Desserts & Extras													
BBQ Wings	2 wings	220	14	130	3.5	0	50	490	5	4	0	17	2 med-fat protein, 1 fat
Breadsticks	2 sticks	300	4.5	40	0.5	0	0	550	55	5	2	8	3 1/2 carb
Cheese Sauce	1 cup (1 oz)	40	3.5	30	1	0	5	160	1	1	0	1	1 fat
Cheese Sticks	4 sticks	360	20	180	8	0	40	1130	51	5	2	16	3 1/2 carb, 1 med-fat protein, 2 fat
Cinnamon Knots	2 knots	370	8	70	2	0	0	390	68	32	2	6	4 1/2 carb, 1 fat
Cinnapie	4 sticks	560	14	130	4	0	0	530	100	48	3	8	6 1/2 carb, 1 1/2 fat

Item	Serving	Cal.	Fat (g)	Cal. Fat	Sat. Fat (g)	Trans Fat (g)	Chol. (mg)	Sod. (mg)	Carb. (g)	Sugar (g)	Fiber (g)	Prot. (g)	Choices/Exchanges
Garlic Dipping Sauce	1 cup (1 oz)	150	17	150	3	0	0	310	0	0	0	0	3 fat
Garlic Knots	2 knots	220	9	80	2	0	0	510	29	2	2	5	2 carb, 1 fat
Garlic Parmesan Breadsticks	2 sticks	350	10	90	2	0	0	720	55	5	5	9	3 1/2 carb, 1 fat
Honey Chipotle Wings	2 wings	230	14	130	3.5	0	50	450	7	5	0	17	1/2 carb, 2 med-fat protein, 1 fat
Papa's Chicken Poppers	5 poppers	180	7	80	1.5	0	40	540	15	1	1	11	1 carb, 1 med-fat protein
Pizza Sauce	1 cup (1 oz)	20	1	10	0	0	0	230	3	1	1	0	free
Spicy Buffalo Wings	2 wings	210	14	130	3.5	0	50	730	3	1	1	17	2 med-fat protein, 1 fat

PEI WEI ASIAN DINER

Wok Classics

Item	Serving	Cal.	Fat (g)	Cal. Fat	Sat. Fat (g)	Trans Fat (g)	Chol. (mg)	Sod. (mg)	Carb. (g)	Sugar (g)	Fiber (g)	Prot. (g)	Choices/Exchanges
Ginger Broccoli with Chicken	1 regular	480	15	135	2.5	NA	95	3530	42	24	4	43	3 carb, 5 lean protein
Ginger Broccoli with Shrimp	1 regular	400	12	110	2	NA	170	3710	41	24	4	31	2 1/2 carb, 3 lean protein, 1 fat

FAST FOOD

	Serving	Calories	Fat (g)	Cal. from Fat	Sat. Fat (g)	Trans Fat (g)	Chol. (mg)	Sod. (mg)	Carb. (g)	Sugar (g)	Fiber (g)	Prot. (g)	Servings/Exchanges
Ginger Broccoli with Steak	1 regular	550	24	215	6.5	NA	30	3860	48	24	6	34	3 carb, 4 med-fat protein
Ginger Broccoli with Vegetables & Tofu	1 regular	550	23	205	4	NA	0	3780	55	34	12	30	3 1/2 carb, 3 med-fat protein, 1 fat
Honey Sriracha with Chicken	1 regular	1170	59	530	3.5	NA	65	1810	114	72	1	34	7 1/2 carb, 2 med-fat protein, 8 fat
Honey Sriracha with Shrimp	1 regular	1130	61	550	3.5	NA	115	2310	112	72	1	21	7 1/2 carb, 11 fat
Honey Sriracha with Steak	1 regular	1170	60	540	11	NA	65	1880	113	72	6	32	7 1/2 carb, 1 med-fat protein, 9 1/2 fat
Honey Sriracha with Vegetables & Tofu	1 regular	1000	48	430	7	NA	0	1950	103	82	11	26	7 carb, 1 med-fat protein, 7 fat
Kung Pao with Chicken	1 regular	830	43	390	7	NA	90	3350	56	33	6	52	3 1/2 carb, 6 med-fat protein, 2 fat
Kung Pao with Shrimp	1 regular	640	37	335	6	NA	75	3620	51	25	12	25	3 1/2 carb, 2 med-fat protein, 5 fat

Kung Pao with Steak	1 regular	990	58	520	11	NA	65	4190	76	28	11	39	5 carb, 3 med-fat protein, 8 fat
Kung Pao with Vegetables & Tofu	1 regular	780	46	415	7	NA	0	3710	58	32	15	31	4 carb, 3 med-fat protein, 5 fat
Lemon Pepper with Chicken	1 regular	590	19	170	3	NA	90	2380	56	46	2	47	3 1/2 carb, 5 lean protein, 1 fat
Lemon Pepper with Shrimp	1 regular	400	13	115	2	NA	75	2650	51	38	8	20	3 1/2 carb, 1 med-fat protein, 1 fat
Lemon Pepper with Steak	1 regular	740	34	305	8	NA	65	2690	73	38	7	34	5 carb, 3 med-fat protein, 3 fat
Lemon Pepper with Vegetables & Tofu	1 regular	570	23	205	3.5	NA	0	2760	63	48	12	28	4 carb, 2 med-fat protein, 2 fat
Mongolian with Chicken	1 regular	480	15	135	2.5	NA	95	3320	44	33	2	41	3 carb, 5 lean protein
Mongolian with Shrimp	1 regular	370	12	110	2	NA	115	3390	43	33	1	21	3 carb, 2 med-fat protein
Mongolian with Steak	1 regular	550	24	215	6.5	NA	30	3650	50	33	3	32	3 carb, 3 med-fat protein, 1 fat
Mongolian with Vegetables & Tofu	1 regular	570	23	210	4	NA	0	3580	59	43	10	28	4 carb, 2 med-fat protein, 2 fat

FAST FOOD

	Serving	Calories	Fat (g)	Cal. from Fat	Sat. Fat (g)	Trans Fat (g)	Chol. (mg)	Sod. (mg)	Carb. (g)	Sugar (g)	Fiber (g)	Prot. (g)	Servings/Exchanges
Orange Peel with Chicken	1 regular	840	39	350	6	NA	90	2800	77	57	6	46	5 carb, 4 med-fat protein, 3 fat
Orange Peel with Shrimp	1 regular	570	22	200	3.5	NA	75	3070	71	49	12	19	4 1/2 carb, 1 med-fat protein, 2 1/2 fat
Orange Peel with Steak	1 regular	980	43	390	9	NA	65	4530	110	64	12	34	7 carb, 2 med-fat protein, 5 fat
Orange Peel with Vegetables & Tofu	1 regular	710	32	290	5	NA	0	3160	78	56	15	26	5 carb, 2 med-fat protein, 3 fat
Pei Wei Spicy with Chicken	1 regular	880	29	260	5	NA	90	1600	112	95	3	44	7 1/2 carb, 3 med-fat protein, 1 fat
Pei Wei Spicy with Shrimp	1 regular	700	23	210	4	NA	75	1870	107	87	9	17	7 carb, 3 fat
Pei Wei Spicy with Steak	1 regular	1120	44	400	9	NA	65	2310	150	108	8	31	10 carb, 7 fat
Pei Wei Spicy with Vegetables & Tofu	1 regular	860	33	300	5	NA	0	1980	119	97	13	25	8 carb, 5 fat
Sesame with Chicken	1 regular	750	30	270	5	NA	90	3590	70	50	2	47	4 1/2 carb, 5 med-fat protein

Food	Amount												Exchanges
Sesame with Shrimp	1 regular	570	23	210	4	NA	75	3770	65	42	8	21	4 carb, 1 med-fat protein, 3 fat
Sesame with Steak	1 regular	890	45	405	9	NA	65	3900	86	42	7	34	5 1/2 carb, 3 med-fat protein, 5 fat
Sesame with Vegetables & Tofu	1 regular	730	33	300	5	NA	0	3890	78	52	13	28	5 carb, 2 med-fat protein, 4 fat
Sweet & Sour with Chicken	1 regular	820	33	300	0	NA	65	1140	96	57	2	32	6 1/2 carb, 2 med-fat protein, 3 fat
Sweet & Sour with Shrimp	1 regular	770	35	315	0	NA	115	1640	93	58	2	19	6 carb, 6 fat
Sweet & Sour with Steak	1 regular	820	34	305	7.5	NA	65	1210	95	58	7	30	6 carb, 2 med-fat protein, 4 fat
Teriyaki with Chicken	1 regular	720	18	160	3	NA	100	3290	98	76	6	46	6 1/2 carb, 4 lean protein, 1 fat
Teriyaki with Shrimp	1 regular	610	14	125	2	NA	205	3660	96	76	6	30	6 1/2 carb, 1 med-fat protein, 1/2 fat
Teriyaki with Steak	1 regular	700	19	170	6	NA	30	3520	99	76	6	37	6 1/2 carb, 2 med-fat protein, 1/2 fat
Teriyaki with Vegetables & Tofu	1 regular	790	28	250	4.5	NA	0	3530	110	84	14	30	7 carb, 1 med-fat protein, 3 fat

FAST FOOD

	Serving	Calories	Fat (g)	Cal. from Fat	Sat. Fat (g)	Trans Fat (g)	Chol. (mg)	Sod. (mg)	Carb. (g)	Sugar (g)	Fiber (g)	Prot. (g)	Servings/Exchanges
Thai Dynamite with Chicken	1 regular	730	38	340	1	NA	65	1930	62	25	2	34	4 carb, 3 med-fat protein, 4 fat
Thai Dynamite with Shrimp	1 regular	690	40	360	1	NA	115	2430	59	25	2	21	4 carb, 1 med-fat protein, 6 fat
Thai Dynamite with Steak	1 regular	750	39	350	8.5	NA	65	2300	65	29	7	33	4 carb, 3 med-fat protein, 4 fat
Thai Dynamite with Vegetables & Tofu	1 regular	560	28	250	4.5	NA	0	2070	51	35	12	26	3 1/2 carb, 2 med-fat protein, 3 fat
Wok Classics (Steamed)													
Honey Sriracha with Steamed Chicken	1 regular	830	31	280	5	NA	95	1590	84	72	1	41	5 1/2 carb, 3 med-fat protein, 2 fat
Honey Sriracha with Steamed Shrimp	1 regular	710	27	245	4	NA	115	1660	83	72	1	21	5 1/2 carb, 1 med-fat protein, 3 fat
Honey Sriracha with Steamed Vegetables & Tofu	1 regular	910	39	350	6	NA	0	1850	99	82	10	28	6 1/2 carb, 1 med-fat protein, 5 1/2 fat

Item	Serving											Exchanges
Kung Pao with Steamed Chicken	1 regular	650	28	4.5	NA	95	3370	47	25	7	48	3 carb, 6 lean protein, 3 fat
Kung Pao with Steamed Shrimp	1 regular	530	25	4	NA	115	3440	46	25	7	28	3 carb, 3 med-fat protein, 1 fat
Kung Pao with Steamed Vegetables & Tofu	1 regular	700	37	6	NA	0	3620	56	32	14	34	3 1/2 carb, 3 med-fat protein, 4 fat
Lemon Pepper with Steamed Chicken	1 regular	400	4.5	1	NA	95	2400	44	38	3	43	3 carb, 5 lean protein
Lemon Pepper with Steamed Shrimp	1 regular	280	1.5	0	NA	115	2470	43	38	3	23	3 carb, 2 lean protein
Lemon Pepper with Steamed Vegetables & Tofu	1 regular	480	13	2.5	NA	0	2660	59	48	11	30	4 carb, 3 lean protein, 1 fat
Orange Peel with Steamed Chicken	1 regular	560	14	2.5	NA	95	2810	65	49	7	43	4 carb, 4 lean protein
Orange Peel with Steamed Shrimp	1 regular	440	11	2	NA	115	2880	63	49	7	22	4 carb, 1 med-fat protein
Orange Peel with Steamed Vegetables & Tofu	1 regular	620	22	4	NA	0	3060	73	56	14	29	5 carb, 2 med-fat protein, 1 fat

FAST FOOD

	Serving	Calories	Fat (g)	Cal. from Fat	Sat. Fat (g)	Trans Fat (g)	Chol. (mg)	Sod. (mg)	Carb. (g)	Sugar (g)	Fiber (g)	Prot. (g)	Servings/Exchanges
Pei Wei Spicy with Steamed Chicken	1 regular	690	15	135	2.5	NA	95	1620	100	87	4	41	6 1/2 carb, 3 lean protein, 1/2 fat
Pei Wei Spicy with Steamed Shrimp	1 regular	570	11	100	2	NA	115	1690	98	87	4	20	6 1/2 carb, 1 fat
Pei Wei Spicy with Steamed Vegetables & Tofu	1 regular	770	23	205	4	NA	0	1880	114	97	12	28	7 1/2 carb, 1 med-fat protein, 2 fat
Sesame with Steamed Chicken	1 regular	550	15	135	2.5	NA	95	3600	58	42	3	44	4 carb, 5 lean protein
Sesame with Steamed Shrimp	1 regular	440	12	110	2	NA	115	3590	57	42	3	24	4 carb, 2 lean protein, 1 fat
Sesame with Steamed Vegetables & Tofu	1 regular	640	24	215	4	NA	0	3790	73	52	11	31	5 carb, 2 med-fat protein, 2 fat
Sweet & Sour with Steamed Chicken	1 regular	470	5	45	1	NA	95	920	66	57	2	40	4 1/2 carb, 4 lean protein
Sweet & Sour with Steamed Shrimp	1 regular	350	1.5	15	0.5	NA	115	990	64	57	2	19	4 carb, 1 lean protein

	Serving											Exchanges
Sweet & Sour with Steamed Vegetables & Tofu	1 regular	550	13	115	2.5	NA	0	1180	80	67	10	27	5 carb, 2 lean protein, 1 fat
Teriyaki with Steamed Chicken	1 regular	630	10	90	2	NA	95	3190	94	76	5	46	6 carb, 4 lean protein
Teriyaki with Steamed Shrimp	1 regular	510	7	65	1	NA	115	3260	92	76	5	26	6 carb, 1 lean protein
Teriyaki with Steamed Vegetables & Tofu	1 regular	700	18	160	3.5	NA	0	3430	105	84	12	33	7 carb, 2 med-fat protein
Thai Dynamite with Steamed Chicken	1 regular	380	10	90	2	NA	95	1710	32	25	3	42	2 carb, 5 lean protein
Thai Dynamite with Steamed Shrimp	1 regular	260	6	55	1	NA	110	1770	30	25	3	20	2 carb, 2 lean protein
Thai Dynamite with Steamed Vegetables & Tofu	1 regular	470	18	160	3.5	NA	0	1970	46	35	11	29	3 carb, 3 med-fat protein
Noodle Bowls													
Blazing Noodles with Chicken	1 regular	600	11	100	2.5	NA	10	1750	71	19	5	13	4 1/2 carb, 1 fat

FAST FOOD

	Serving	Calories	Fat (g)	Cal. from Fat	Sat. Fat (g)	Trans Fat (g)	Chol. (mg)	Sod. (mg)	Carb. (g)	Sugar (g)	Fiber (g)	Prot. (g)	Servings/Exchanges
Blazing Noodles with Shrimp	1 regular	540	8	70	1.5	NA	60	2040	87	24	8	15	6 carb
Blazing Noodles with Steak	1 regular	630	14	125	3.5	NA	15	2170	90	24	7	21	6 carb, 2 fat
Blazing Noodles with Vegetables & Tofu	1 regular	640	14	125	2.5	NA	0	2140	95	29	10	19	6 carb, 2 fat
Lo Mein with Chicken	1 regular	1040	34	305	6	NA	150	2910	123	26	8	62	8 carb, 5 med-fat protein
Lo Mein with Shrimp	1 regular	880	27	245	4.5	NA	240	3230	120	26	7	41	8 carb, 2 med-fat protein, 2 fat
Lo Mein with Steak	1 regular	1000	34	305	8	NA	75	3140	124	26	8	51	8 carb, 4 med-fat protein, 1 fat
Lo Mein with Vegetables & Tofu	1 regular	1080	41	370	6	NA	35	3120	137	26	16	41	9 carb, 2 med-fat protein, 4 fat
Pad Thai with Chicken	1 regular	1510	31	280	6	NA	300	6140	201	65	13	83	13 1/2 carb, 6 lean protein, 1 fat

Pad Thai with Shrimp	1 regular	1370	27	245	4.5	NA	305	6180	199	65	13	56	13 carb, 6 lean protein
Pad Thai with Steak	1 regular	1570	41	370	10	NA	220	6500	207	65	15	71	14 carb, 6 lean protein, 3 fat
Pad Thai with Vegetables & Tofu	1 regular	1550	39	350	7	NA	185	6380	215	65	21	64	14 carb, 6 lean protein, 3 fat
Sushi													
Kung Pao Shrimp Roll	4 rolls	450	21	190	3	NA	40	1630	49	17	5	16	3 carb, 1 med-fat protein, 3 fat
Mango California Roll	4 rolls	170	5	45	1	NA	5	580	26	12	2	5	2 carb, 1 fat
Spicy Tuna Roll	4 rolls	120	1.5	15	0	NA	10	500	19	8	2	7	1 carb, 1 lean protein
Wasabi Crunch Roll	4 rolls	300	16	145	2.5	NA	25	1100	31	13	3	9	2 carb, 3 fat
Lettuce Wraps													
Lettuce Wrap Sauce	2 oz	70	3.5	30	0	NA	0	2700	4	1	1	4	1 med-fat protein
Thai Chicken	1 wrap	540	30	270	7	NA	35	3130	31	15	5	38	2 carb, 5 med-fat protein, 1 fat
Traditional Chicken	1 wrap	720	36	325	7	NA	30	2540	66	21	7	34	4 1/2 carb, 3 med-fat protein, 3 fat

EAST FOOD

	Serving	Calories	Fat (g)	Cal. from Fat	Sat. Fat (g)	Trans Fat (g)	Chol. (mg)	Sod. (mg)	Carb. (g)	Sugar (g)	Fiber (g)	Prot. (g)	Servings/Exchanges
Soups & Salads (No Dressing)													
Asian Chopped Chicken Salad	1 original	470	16	145	3	NA	15	540	37	6	6	46	2 1/2 carb, 5 lean protein, 1 fat
Hot & Sour Soup	1 bowl	180	2.5	25	0.5	NA	25	630	6	1	1	5	1/2 carb, 1/2 med-fat protein
Pei Wei Spicy Chicken Salad	1 original	930	34	305	5	NA	80	1590	120	95	5	41	8 carb, 2 med-fat protein, 3 fat
Thai Mango Chicken Salad	1 regular	560	22	200	6	NA	125	1330	50	28	6	48	3 carb, 6 lean protein, 1 fat
Thai Wonton Soup	1 bowl	160	4.5	40	1	NA	15	2120	22	7	3	9	1 1/2 carb, 1 lean protein
Vietnamese Chicken Salad Rolls	3 rolls	550	19	170	2	NA	5	900	65	14	5	26	4 carb, 2 med-fat protein, 1 fat
Sauces & Dressings													
Lime Vinaigrette Original	1 oz	110	10	90	0.5	NA	0	550	6	6	0	0	1/2 carb, 2 fat

Sesame Ginger Vinaigrette	1 oz	90	9	80	1	NA	0	480	3	3	0	1	2 fat
Sweet Chili Sauce	2 oz	130	0	0	0	NA	0	0	32	26	2	0	2 carb
Thai Peanut Dipping Sauce	2 oz	160	10	90	5	NA	0	290	15	11	1	2	1 carb, 2 fat
Sides & Extras													
Brown Rice	1 small	250	2	20	0	NA	0	0	53	0	4	5	3 1/2 carb
Crab Wontons (No Sauce)	2 wontons	170	10	90	3.5	NA	10	250	13	0	1	6	1 carb, 2 fat
Crispy Potstickers (No Sauce)	2 potstickers	150	8	90	2.5	NA	5	310	12	0	1	7	1 carb, 1 med-fat protein
Egg Noodles	1 small	350	6	55	1	NA	30	630	62	2	2	11	4 carb
Fried Rice	1 small	520	20	180	4	NA	185	2180	68	15	3	12	4 1/2 carb, 3 fat
Pork Egg Roll (No Sauce)	1 roll	170	7	65	1.5	NA	25	550	19	5	2	6	1 carb, 1 1/2 fat
Traditional Edamame	1 small	160	7	65	1	NA	0	500	10	0	5	15	1/2 carb, 2 lean protein, 1/2 fat
Vegetable Spring Roll (No Sauce)	1 roll	120	5	45	1	NA	0	300	13	0	1	3	1 carb, 1 fat
White Rice	1 small	290	0	0	0	NA	0	0	65	1	1	5	4 carb

FAST FOOD

PIZZA HUT

6-Inch Personal Pan Pizza

	Serving	Calories	Fat (g)	Cal. from Fat	Sat. Fat (g)	Trans Fat (g)	Chol. (mg)	Sod. (mg)	Carb. (g)	Sugar (g)	Fiber (g)	Prot. (g)	Servings/Exchanges
7-Alarm Fire	1 pizza	620	27	240	10	0.5	45	1730	71	10	4	24	4 1/2 carb, 1 med-fat protein, 3 1/2 fat
BBQ Lover's	1 pizza	740	36	320	14	0.5	75	1590	74	12	3	30	5 carb, 2 med-fat protein, 4 fat
Cheese	1 pizza	600	25	220	11	0.5	50	1400	69	7	4	26	4 1/2 carb, 2 med-fat protein, 2 fat
Meat Lover's	1 pizza	850	48	430	18	1	100	2170	69	7	4	35	4 1/2 carb, 3 med-fat protein, 6 fat
Pepperoni	1 pizza	620	28	225	11	0.5	55	1590	67	7	4	25	4 1/2 carb, 2 med-fat protein, 3 fat
Pretzel Piggy	1 pizza	640	30	270	10	0.5	45	2130	68	7	4	24	4 1/2 carb, 1 med-fat protein, 4 fat
Supreme	1 pizza	690	34	310	13	1	70	1660	70	8	4	28	4 1/2 carb, 2 med-fat protein, 4 fat

	Serving											Exchanges
Sweet Sriracha Dynamite	1 pizza	600	21	190	8	0	55	1690	77	13	4	28	5 carb, 2 med-fat protein, 1 fat
Veggie Lover's	1 pizza	550	20	180	8	0	35	1290	70	8	5	22	4 1/2 carb, 1 med-fat protein, 2 fat

14-Inch Large Pan Pizza

	Serving											Exchanges
7-Alarm Fire	1 slice (1/8 pizza)	360	17	150	6	0	25	930	37	3	2	13	2 1/2 carb, 1 mec-fat protein, 2 fat
BBQ Lover's	1 slice (1/8 pizza)	410	20	180	7	0	40	830	41	6	1	16	2 1/2 carb, 1 med-fat protein, 2 1/2 fat
Cheese	1 slice (1/8 pizza)	350	17	150	7	0	30	730	36	1	1	14	2 1/2 carb, 1 med-fat protein, 2 fat
Meat Lover's	1 slice (1/8 pizza)	460	27	240	9	0.5	50	1090	36	1	1	18	2 1/2 carb, 1 med-fat protein, 4 fat
Pepperoni	1 slice (1/8 pizza)	370	19	170	7	0	35	870	35	1	1	14	2 carb, 1 med-fat protein, 2 fat

FAST FOOD

	Serving	Calories	Fat (g)	Cal. from Fat	Sat. Fat (g)	Trans Fat (g)	Chol. (mg)	Sod. (mg)	Carb. (g)	Sugar (g)	Fiber (g)	Prot. (g)	Servings/Exchanges
Pretzel Piggy	1 slice (1/8 pizza)	360	19	170	6	0	25	810	36	2	1	13	2 1/2 carb, 1 med-fat protein, 2 fat
Supreme	1 slice (1/8 pizza)	390	20	180	7	0	35	840	37	2	2	15	2 1/2 carb, 1 med-fat protein, 2 1/2 fat
Sweet Sriracha Dynamite	1 slice (1/8 pizza)	350	14	130	5	0	30	920	42	5	1	14	3 carb, 1 med-fat protein, 1 fat
Veggie Lover's	1 slice (1/8 pizza)	320	14	130	5	0	20	670	37	2	2	12	2 1/2 carb, 1 med-fat protein, 1 fat
14-Inch Large Original Stuffed Crust Pizza													
7-Alarm Fire	1 slice (1/8 pizza)	320	14	130	7	0	40	950	36	3	2	14	2 1/2 carb, 1 med-fat protein, 1 fat

	Serving											Choices
BBQ Lover's	1 slice (1/8 pizza)	380	17	160	8	0	50	860	40	6	1	16	2 1/2 carb, 1 med-fat protein, 2 fat
Cheese	1 slice (1/8 pizza)	310	13	120	7	0	35	730	35	2	2	14	2 carb, 1 med-fat protein, 1 fat
Meat Lover's	1 slice (1/8 pizza)	430	24	220	10	0.5	60	1120	35	2	2	19	2 carb, 2 med-fat protein, 2 fat
Pepperoni	1 slice (1/8 pizza)	340	16	140	8	0	45	870	34	2	2	14	2 carb, 1 med-fat protein, 2 fat
Pretzel Piggy	1 slice (1/8 pizza)	330	15	140	7	0	35	830	35	2	2	14	2 carb, 1 med-fat protein, 2 fat
Supreme	1 slice (1/8 pizza)	360	18	160	8	0.5	45	870	36	2	2	15	2 1/2 carb, 1 med-fat protein, 2 fat
Sweet Sriracha Dynamite	1 slice (1/8 pizza)	320	11	100	6	0	40	940	41	6	2	15	2 1/2 carb, 1 med-fat protein, 1 fat

FAST FOOD

	Serving	Calories	Fat (g)	Cal. from Fat	Sat. Fat (g)	Trans Fat (g)	Chol. (mg)	Sod. (mg)	Carb. (g)	Sugar (g)	Fiber (g)	Prot. (g)	Servings/Exchanges
Veggie Lover's	1 slice (1/8 pizza)	300	12	110	6	0	30	700	36	2	2	13	2 1/2 carb, 1 med-fat protein, 1 fat
14-Inch Large Hand Tossed Pizza													
7-Alarm Fire	1 slice (1/8 pizza)	290	11	100	5	0	25	850	35	3	2	12	2 carb, 1 med-fat protein, 1 fat
BBQ Lover's	1 slice (1/8 pizza)	340	15	130	6	0	40	740	39	6	1	15	2 1/2 carb, 1 med-fat protein, 1 1/2 fat
Cheese	1 slice (1/8 pizza)	290	11	100	6	0	30	640	34	1	2	13	2 carb, 1 med-fat protein, 1 fat
Meat Lover's	1 slice (1/8 pizza)	390	21	190	9	0	50	1010	34	1	2	17	2 carb, 2 med-fat protein, 2 fat

Pepperoni	1 slice (1/8 pizza)	300	13	120	6	0	30	750	33	1	2	13	2 carb, 1 med-fat protein, 1 fat
Pretzel Piggy	1 slice (1/8 pizza)	300	13	120	5	0	25	720	34	2	2	12	2 carb, 1 med-fat protein, 1 fat
Supreme	1 slice (1/8 pizza)	330	15	130	6	0	35	750	34	2	2	14	2 carb, 1 med-fat protein, 2 fat
Sweet Sriracha Dynamite	1 slice (1/8 pizza)	280	8	70	4	0	30	840	40	6	2	13	2 1/2 carb, 1 med-fat protein
Veggie Lover's	1 slice (1/8 pizza)	260	9	80	4	0	20	590	35	2	2	11	2 carb, 1 med-fat protein

14-Inch Large Thin N' Crispy Pizza

7-Alarm Fire	1 slice (1/8 pizza)	270	12	100	5	0	25	1060	30	7	2	11	2 carb, 1 med-fat protein, 1 fat

FAST FOOD

	Serving	Calories	Fat (g)	Cal. from Fat	Sat. Fat (g)	Trans Fat (g)	Chol. (mg)	Sod. (mg)	Carb. (g)	Sugar (g)	Fiber (g)	Prot. (g)	Servings/Exchanges
BBQ Lover's	1 slice (1/8 pizza)	330	15	140	7	0	40	890	33	9	1	14	2 carb, 1 med-fat protein, 2 fat
Cheese	1 slice (1/8 pizza)	260	11	100	6	0	30	790	29	5	1	12	2 carb, 1 med-fat protein, 1 fat
Meat Lover's	1 slice (1/8 pizza)	370	22	190	9	0	50	1180	28	5	1	16	2 carb, 1 med-fat protein, 3 fat
Pepperoni	1 slice (1/8 pizza)	280	14	120	6	0	35	940	28	5	1	12	2 carb, 1 med-fat protein, 1 fat
Pretzel Piggy	1 slice (1/8 pizza)	290	14	130	6	0	25	890	28	5	1	11	2 carb, 1 med-fat protein, 1 fat
Supreme	1 slice (1/8 pizza)	300	15	130	6	0	35	910	30	6	2	13	2 carb, 1 med-fat protein, 2 fat

	Serving	Cal											Exchanges
Sweet Sriracha Dynamite	1 slice (1/8 pizza)	260	9	80	4	0	30	1010	35	10	1	12	2 carb, 1 med-fat protein
Veggie Lover's	1 slice (1/8 pizza)	240	9	80	4	0	20	760	30	6	2	10	2 carb, 1 med-fat protein
14-Inch Large Skinny Slice Pizza													
Skinny Beach	1 slice (1/8 pizza)	200	6	50	3	0	20	440	27	2	2	10	2 carb, 1 med-fat protein
Skinny Club	1 slice (1/8 pizza)	230	9	80	4	0	25	540	25	1	1	12	1 1/2 carb, 1 med-fat protein, 1/2 fat
Skinny Italy	1 slice (1/8 pizza)	220	8	70	3.5	0	20	460	28	3	2	9	2 carb, 2 fat
10-Inch Gluten-Free Pizza													
Cheese	1 slice (1/6 pizza)	150	6	50	3	0	15	400	19	3	1	6	1 carb, 1 fat

FAST FOOD

	Serving	Calories	Fat (g)	Cal. from Fat	Sat. Fat (g)	Trans Fat (g)	Chol. (mg)	Sod. (mg)	Carb. (g)	Sugar (g)	Fiber (g)	Prot. (g)	Servings/Exchanges
Pepperoni	1 slice (1/6 pizza)	170	8	70	3	0	20	499	19	3	1	6	1 carb, 2 fat
Tuscani Pastas													
Creamy Chicken Alfredo	1/2 of pan	510	26	240	7	0	40	900	47	3	3	22	3 carb, 2 med-fat protein, 3 fat
Meaty Marinara	1/2 of pan	450	19	170	8	1	45	1000	48	9	3	21	3 carb, 2 med-fat protein, 1 fat
Appetizers/Sides/Sauces													
Baked Boneless Wings	2 wings	100	3	25	0.5	0	15	450	10	0	0	9	1/2 carb, 1 med-fat protein
Baked Hot Wings	2 wings	100	7	60	2	0	55	420	0	0	0	10	1 med-fat protein, 1/2 fat
BBQ Wing Sauce for Baked Boneless Wings	3 oz	170	0	5	0	0	0	8870	40	29	1	1	2 1/2 carb
Breadsticks	1 stick	130	4.5	40	1	0	0	260	19	1	1	4	1 carb, 1 fat

Item	Serving	Cal	Fat	Fat Cal	Sat Fat	Trans Fat	Chol	Sodium	Carb	Fiber	Protein	Choices/Exchanges
Cheese Sticks	1 stick	160	6	60	2.5	0	10	370	20	1	1	7	1 carb, 1 med-fat protein
Marinara Dipping Sauce	3 oz	45	0	0	0	0	0	290	9	6	2	1	1/2 carb
Ranch Dipping Sauce	1.5 oz	220	23	210	3.5	0	10	420	2	1	0	0	5 fat
Waffle Fries	1 side order	660	41	360	8	0	10	440	66	0	7	8	4 1/2 carb, 7 fat
WingStreet													
Buffalo (Bone In)	2 wings	220	12	110	2.5	0	40	820	19	2	1	9	1 carb, 1 med-fat protein, 1 fat
Buffalo (Bone Out)	2 wings	200	9	80	2	0	25	860	18	2	1	10	1 carb, 1 med-fat protein, 1 fat
Honey BBQ (Bone In)	2 wings	250	12	110	2.5	0	40	540	28	12	1	9	2 carb, 2 fat
Honey BBQ (Bone Out)	2 wings	230	9	80	1.5	0	25	570	27	12	1	10	2 carb, 1 med-fat protein
Honey Sriracha (Bone In)	2 wings	200	10	90	2	0	35	590	20	4	1	9	1 carb, 1 med-fat protein, 1 fat
Honey Sriracha (Bone Out)	2 wings	190	9	80	1.5	0	25	620	18	4	1	10	1 carb, 1 med-fat protein, 1 fat

FAST FOOD

	Serving	Calories	Fat (g)	Cal. from Fat	Sat. Fat (g)	Trans Fat (g)	Chol. (mg)	Sod. (mg)	Carb. (g)	Sugar (g)	Fiber (g)	Prot. (g)	Servings/Exchanges
Naked (Bone In)	2 wings	180	12	100	2.5	0	40	300	11	0	1	9	1 carb, 1 med-fat protein, 1 fat
Naked (Bone Out)	2 wings	160	9	80	1.5	0	25	340	11	0	1	10	1 carb, 1 med-fat protein, 1 fat
Desserts													
Cinnamon Sticks	2 pieces	160	4.5	40	0.5	0	0	200	26	8	1	4	2 carb, 1/2 fat
HERSHEY'S Chocolate Dipping Sauce	1.5 oz	120	2	20	1	0	0	65	25	19	1	1	1 1/2 carb
HERSHEY'S Chocolate Dunkers	2 pieces	190	8	70	3	0	0	210	26	9	1	5	2 carb, 1 fat
The Ultimate Chocolate Chip Cookie	1 piece	180	9	80	4.5	0	10	110	24	16	2	2	1 1/2 carb, 1 1/2 fat
White Icing Dipping Sauce	2 oz	170	0	0	0	0	0	5	44	38	0	0	3 carb

QUIZNOS

Breakfast

Egg & Cheddar Biscuit	1 biscuit	420	24	210	12	0	270	1240	38	6	1	15	2 1/2 carb, 1 med-fat protein, 3 fat
Egg & Cheddar Flatbread	1 flat-bread	330	15	130	6	0	275	660	31	5	1	16	2 carb, 1 med-fat protein, 2 fat
Egg & Cheddar Sub	1 sub	370	16	140	6	0	270	760	39	4	1	18	2 1/2 carb, 1 med-fat protein, 2 fat

Deli Classics with Cheese & Dressing

Classic Italian Flatbread	1 flat-bread	480	29	260	9	0.5	50	1360	34	6	4	20	2 carb, 2 med-fat protein, 3 fat
Classic Italian on Ciabatta	1 sand-wich	900	51	460	17	1	105	2600	72	16	3	40	5 carb, 4 med-fat protein, 5 fat
Classic Italian Sub	8-inch sub	900	53	470	18	1	105	2600	67	12	4	41	4 1/2 carb, 4 med-fat protein, 6 fat
Honey Bacon Club Flatbread	1 flat-bread	480	24	220	7	0	50	1320	41	12	4	24	2 1/2 carb, 2 med-fat protein, 2 fat

FAST FOOD

	Serving	Calories	Fat (g)	Cal. from Fat	Sat. Fat (g)	Trans Fat (g)	Chol. (mg)	Sod. (mg)	Carb. (g)	Sugar (g)	Fiber (g)	Prot. (g)	Servings/Exchanges
Honey Bacon Club on Ciabatta	1 sand-wich	860	38	340	13	0.5	90	2460	84	27	3	47	5 1/2 carb, 4 med-fat protein, 2 1/2 fat
Honey Bacon Club Sub	8-inch sub	850	40	360	13	0.5	90	2390	80	24	4	47	5 carb, 5 med-fat protein, 2 fat
Spicy Monterey Flat-bread	1 flat-bread	330	12	110	3.5	0	35	1200	36	8	4	18	2 1/2 carb, 1 med-fat protein, 1 fat
Spicy Monterey on Ciabatta	1 sand-wich	610	19	170	7	0	65	2360	77	20	3	37	5 carb, 3 med-fat protein
Spicy Monterey Sub	8-inch sub	610	21	190	8	0	65	2300	72	16	4	38	5 carb, 3 med-fat protein
The Traditional Flatbread	1 flat-bread	370	18	160	5	0	50	1020	33	4	4	20	2 carb, 2 med-fat protein, 1 fat
The Traditional on Ciabatta	1 sand-wich	710	31	280	11	0	100	2050	71	14	3	40	4 1/2 carb, 4 med-fat protein, 1 fat
The Traditional Sub	8-inch sub	710	33	300	11	0	100	1990	66	11	4	41	4 1/2 carb, 4 med-fat protein, 2 fat

Tuna Flatbread	1 flat-bread	440	23	210	6	0	45	1050	35	4	4	24	2 carb, 3 med-fat protein, 1 fat
Tuna on Ciabatta	1 sand-wich	760	36	320	11	0	70	1820	72	13	3	41	5 carb, 4 med-fat protein, 2 fat
Tuna Sub	8-inch sub	760	37	340	12	0	75	1760	67	10	4	42	4 1/2 carb, 4 med-fat protein, 2 1/2 fat
Veggie Guacamole Flatbread	1 flat-bread	430	26	230	8	0	25	770	35	5	6	14	2 carb, 1 med-fat protein, 4 fat
Veggie Guacamole on Ciabatta	1 sand-wich	770	42	380	14	0.5	50	1440	73	14	6	28	5 carb, 2 med-fat protein, 5 fat
Veggie Guacamole Sub	8-inch sub	760	43	390	15	0.5	50	1370	68	11	7	28	4 1/2 carb, 2 med-fat protein, 6 fat
Salads (No Dressing)													
Açai Vinaigrette Dressing	2 oz	140	11	100	1.5	0	0	280	10	9	0	0	1/2 carb, 2 fat
Apple Harvest Chicken	1 full salad	390	16	140	2.5	0	50	590	41	28	7	22	2 1/2 carb, 2 med-fat protein, 2 fat
Honey Mustard Chicken	1 full salad	290	14	120	5	0	105	1130	7	3	3	35	1/2 carb, 5 lean protein, 1 fat
Honey Mustard Dressing	2 oz	290	26	240	4	0	20	330	12	10	0	1	1 carb, 5 fat

FAST FOOD

	Serving	Calories	Fat (g)	Cal. from Fat	Sat. Fat (g)	Trans Fat (g)	Chol. (mg)	Sod. (mg)	Carb. (g)	Sugar (g)	Fiber (g)	Prot. (g)	Servings/Exchanges
Peppercorn Caesar	1 full salad	190	5	50	1	0	80	870	7	3	2	28	1/2 carb, 4 lean protein
Peppercorn Caesar Dressing	2 oz	310	32	280	6	0	25	550	4	2	0	2	6 fat
Soups (No Crackers)													
Broccoli Cheese	1 regular	155	8.5	75	4.5	0	25	1535	13	2	1	7	1 carb, 1 med-fat protein, 1/2 fat
Broccoli Cheese Bread Bowl	1 bowl	760	27	240	8	0	35	2210	103	4	5	31	7 carb, 1 med-fat protein, 3 fat
Chicken Noodle	1 regular	115	4	35	1	0	25	1465	15	2	1	7	1 carb, 1 lean protein
Chicken Noodle Bread Bowl	1 bowl	650	17	150	2	0	15	2030	103	4	5	25	7 carb, 1 med-fat protein, 1 fat
Clam Chowder	1 regular	255	15.5	135	8	0	35	1395	25	5	1	5	1 1/2 carb, 3 fat
Clam Chowder Bread Bowl	1 bowl	730	23	210	6	0	20	1990	108	6	5	24	7 carb, 3 fat

Crackers	2 crackers	25	0.5	5	0	0	0	75	4	0	0	0	free
Tomato Bisque	1 regular	185	12.5	115	7	0	40	1015	21	9	2	5	1 1/2 carb, 2 fat
Tomato Bisque Bread Bowl	1 bowl	690	22	200	5	0	20	1780	106	8	5	24	7 carb, 3 fat
Desserts													
Chocolate Brownie	1 brownie	310	16	150	3.5	0	15	150	40	24	2	4	2 1/2 carb, 3 fat
Chocolate Chunk Cookie	1 cookie	390	19	170	11	0	55	170	54	31	1	4	3 1/2 carb, 3 fat
Oatmeal Raisin Cookie	1 cookie	360	12	110	7	0	50	200	58	34	3	5	4 carb, 2 fat
RUBIO'S BAJA GRILL													
Burritos													
Ancho Citrus Shrimp Burrito	1	660	31	280	7	NA	115	1880	75	4	8	24	5 carb, 1 med-fat protein, 4 fat
Atlantic Salmon Burrito	1	700	32	290	8	NA	45	1630	74	4	6	33	5 carb, 3 med-fat protein, 2 fat
Baja Grill Burrito, Chicken	1	600	25	220	10	NA	100	1590	52	4	4	46	3 1/2 carb, 5 lean protein, 2 fat

FAST FOOD

	Serving	Calories	Fat (g)	Cal. from Fat	Sat. Fat (g)	Trans Fat (g)	Chol. (mg)	Sod. (mg)	Carb. (g)	Sugar (g)	Fiber (g)	Prot. (g)	Servings/Exchanges
Baja Grill Burrito, Grilled Steak	1	640	28	260	11	NA	100	1490	52	4	4	45	3 1/2 carb, 5 lean protein, 3 fat
Bean & Cheese Burrito	1	710	31	380	16	NA	60	1650	74	3	15	38	5 carb, 3 med-fat protein, 2 fat
Beer-Battered Fish Burrito	1	850	53	480	10	NA	55	1510	68	5	8	26	4 1/2 carb, 2 med-fat protein, 8 fat
Especial Burrito with Veggies	1	820	33	300	8	NA	5	1920	113	8	16	19	7 1/2 carb, 5 fat
Pacific Mahi Mahi Burrito	1	690	31	280	7	NA	50	1740	74	5	5	32	5 carb, 2 med-fat protein, 3 fat
Tacos													
Atlantic Salmon Taco	1	220	10	90	2	NA	25	400	22	2	3	14	1 1/2 carb, 1 med-fat protein, 1 fat
Classic Chicken Taco	1	240	13	120	4	NA	35	370	19	1	2	15	1 carb, 2 med-fat protein
Classic Steak Taco	1	190	7	60	3	NA	30	280	19	1	2	14	1 carb, 2 lean protein

Fish Taco Especial	1	370	25	220	4	NA	35	480	25	2	3	14	1 1/2 carb, 1 med-fat protein, 4 fat
Grilled Gourmet Taco, Chicken	1	320	19	170	7	NA	60	560	19	1	2	21	1 carb, 3 med-fat protein, 1 fat
Grilled Gourmet Taco, Shrimp	1	310	20	180	7	NA	90	700	19	1	2	18	1 carb, 2 med-fat protein, 2 fat
Grilled Gourmet Taco, Steak	1	330	20	180	7	NA	60	520	19	1	2	21	1 carb, 3 med-fat protein, 1 fat
Grilled Gourmet Taco, Veggies	1	280	18	170	6	NA	25	360	23	3	3	11	1 1/2 carb, 1 med-fat protein, 2 fat
Pacific Mahi Mahi Taco	1	220	10	90	2	NA	25	460	22	2	3	14	1 1/2 carb, 1 med-fat protein, 1 fat
Street Taco, Chicken	1	100	3	25	0	NA	25	200	9	1	2	10	1/2 carb, 1 lean protein
Street Taco, Steak	1	120	4	35	1	NA	25	170	10	1	2	10	1/2 carb, 1 med-fat protein
The Original Fish Taco	1	310	20	180	2	NA	25	390	23	1	2	11	1 1/2 carb, 1 med-fat protein, 3 fat

FAST FOOD

	Serving	Calories	Fat (g)	Cal. from Fat	Sat. Fat (g)	Trans Fat (g)	Chol. (mg)	Sod. (mg)	Carb. (g)	Sugar (g)	Fiber (g)	Prot. (g)	Servings/Exchanges
Enchiladas													
Cheese Enchilada Plate with Fire Roasted Sauce	1	800	38	340	17	NA	80	1570	83	3	13	40	5 1/2 carb, 3 med-fat protein, 3 1/2 fat
Chicken Enchilada Plate with Fire Roasted Sauce	1	770	30	270	12	NA	100	1730	84	4	13	50	5 1/2 carb, 5 med-fat protein
Shrimp Enchilada Plate with Verde Sauce	1	810	33	300	12	NA	165	1940	90	8	16	46	6 carb, 4 med-fat protein, 1 fat
Nachos & Quesadillas													
Cheese Nachos	1 order	1110	45	410	22	NA	100	1220	137	6	19	43	9 carb, 2 med-fat protein, 5 fat
Cheese Quesadilla	1	970	50	450	24	NA	100	1370	96	5	6	37	6 1/2 carb, 2 med-fat protein, 7 fat
Chicken Nachos	1 order	1220	46	420	22	NA	160	1640	138	6	19	66	9 carb, 6 med-fat protein, 1 fat

Item	Serving	Calories	Fat Cal	Total Fat	Sat Fat	Chol	Sodium	Carb	Fiber	Sugar	Protein	Exchanges
Chicken Quesadilla	1	1070	51	460	25	NA	160	1790	97	5	6	60	6 1/2 carb, 6 med-fat protein, 3 fat

Kids

Item	Serving	Calories	Fat Cal	Total Fat	Sat Fat	Chol	Sodium	Carb	Fiber	Sugar	Protein	Exchanges
Kids Bean & Cheese Burrito	1	540	22	200	11	NA	35	1210	62	2	10	26	4 carb, 2 med-fat protein, 2 fat
Kids Cheese Quesadilla	1	490	26	230	13	NA	50	940	44	1	0	23	3 carb, 2 med-fat protein, 3 fat
Kids Chicken Bites	1 order	240	11	100	1	NA	35	870	21	0	1	21	1 1/2 carb, 2 med-fat protein
Kids Chicken Quesadilla	1	530	26	240	11	NA	35	1110	45	1	0	32	3 carb, 3 med-fat protein, 2 fat
Kids Chicken Taco	1	150	4	40	2	NA	30	240	16	1	1	14	1 carb, 1 lean protein
Kids Chicken Taquitos	1 order	250	10	90	3	NA	45	380	24	0	2	19	1 1/2 carb, 2 lean protein, 1 fat
Original Fish Taco (No Salsa)	1	300	20	180	2	NA	25	350	22	1	2	10	1 1/2 carb, 1 med-fat protein, 3 fat

Sides

Item	Serving	Calories	Fat Cal	Total Fat	Sat Fat	Chol	Sodium	Carb	Fiber	Sugar	Protein	Exchanges
Black Beans, Large	1 order	380	4	35	1	NA	2	1110	64	3	37	24	4 carb, 2 lean protein

FAST FOOD

	Serving	Calories	Fat (g)	Cal. from Fat	Sat. Fat (g)	Trans Fat (g)	Chol. (mg)	Sod. (mg)	Carb. (g)	Sugar (g)	Fiber (g)	Prot. (g)	Servings/Exchanges
Black Beans, Regular	1 order	130	2	15	1	NA	2	380	22	1	12	8	1 1/2 carb, 1/2 lean protein
Citrus Rice, Large	1 order	400	6	60	1	NA	0	1030	78	1	1	8	5 carb
Citrus Rice, Regular	1 order	150	2	20	0	NA	0	390	29	0	0	3	2 carb
Mexican Rice, Large	1 order	360	5	50	1	NA	0	840	71	3	1	0	4 1/2 carb
Mexican Rice, Regular	1 order	140	2	20	0	NA	0	320	27	1	0	3	2 carb
"No-Fried" Pinto Beans, Large	1 order	370	3	25	1	NA	2	1210	62	2	32	24	4 carb, 2 lean protein
"No-Fried" Pinto Beans, Regular	1 order	130	1	15	1	NA	2	410	21	1	11	8	1 1/2 carb, 1/2 lean protein
Tortilla Chips, Large	1 order	460	5	45	1	NA	0	95	96	2	5	7	6 1/2 carb
Tortilla Chips, Regular	1 order	210	2	20	1	NA	0	45	43	1	2	3	3 carb

SONIC

Burgers & Sandwiches

Grilled Cheese Sandwich	1	410	18	170	7	0	35	1040	45	6	1	14	3 carb, 1 med-fat protein, 2 fat
Jr. Burger	1	330	17	150	6	0.5	35	480	30	3	1	15	2 carb, 1 med-fat protein, 2 fat
Jr. Deluxe Cheeseburger	1	420	25	230	9	0.5	60	830	32	5	1	19	2 carb, 2 med-fat protein, 3 fat
Jr. Double Cheeseburger	1	520	33	300	13	1	90	860	31	4	1	28	2 carb, 3 med-fat protein, 3 fat
Sonic Bacon Cheeseburger with Mayo	1	820	54	490	20	2	140	1260	43	7	2	39	3 carb, 4 med-fat protein, 6 fat
Sonic Burger with Ketchup	1	650	37	340	14	1.5	100	840	46	10	2	31	3 carb, 3 med-fat protein, 4 fat
Sonic Cheeseburger with Ketchup	1	720	43	380	17	1.5	115	1170	47	11	2	35	3 carb, 4 med-fat protein, 4 fat
Super Sonic Bacon Double Cheeseburger with Mayo	1	1240	87	790	35	3.5	255	1690	44	8	2	67	3 carb, 8 med-fat protein, 9 fat

FAST FOOD

	Serving	Calories	Fat (g)	Cal. from Fat	Sat. Fat (g)	Trans Fat (g)	Chol. (mg)	Sod. (mg)	Carb. (g)	Sugar (g)	Fiber (g)	Prot. (g)	Servings/Exchanges
Super Sonic Double Cheeseburger with Ketchup	1	1130	76	680	32	3.5	235	1590	47	11	2	63	3 carb, 8 med-fat protein, 7 fat
Veggie Burger with Ketchup	1	460	14	130	4	0	10	1390	68	11	5	15	4 1/2 carb, 2 fat
Toaster Sandwiches & Wraps													
Bacon Cheeseburger Toaster Sandwich	1	850	50	450	19	2	130	1490	59	14	3	40	4 carb, 4 med-fat protein, 5 fat
BLT Toaster Sandwich	1	510	26	230	7	0	35	1050	53	8	2	16	3 1/2 carb, 1 med-fat protein, 3 1/2 fat
Chicken Club Toaster Sandwich	1	690	36	330	10	0	80	1540	58	8	2	30	4 carb, 3 med-fat protein, 3 fat
Chicken Wrap, Crispy	1	510	22	200	5	0	45	1260	57	4	3	22	4 carb, 1 med-fat protein, 3 fat
Chicken Wrap, Grilled	1	430	14	130	4	0	80	1720	42	4	2	31	3 carb, 3 lean protein, 1 fat
Country Fried Steak Toaster Sandwich	1	650	29	260	9	0	50	1440	80	8	3	15	5 carb, 6 fat

Chicken

Food	Amount												Exchanges/Choices
Asiago-Chicken Club Sandwich, Crispy	1	680	39	350	9	0	80	1120	53	7	4	31	3 1/2 carb, 3 med-fat protein, 4 fat
Asiago-Chicken Club Sandwich, Grilled	1	610	30	270	7	0	110	1570	44	8	3	40	3 carb, 4 med-fat protein, 1 fat
Asian Sweet Chili Boneless Wings	6 wings	550	21	190	4	0	70	2060	62	25	2	30	4 carb, 3 med-fat protein
Buffalo Boneless Wings	6 wings	540	32	290	6	0	80	2330	35	1	3	28	2 carb, 3 med-fat protein, 3 fat
Classic Chicken Sandwich, Crispy	1	580	29	260	4.5	0	60	900	57	7	5	28	4 carb, 2 med-fat protein, 3 fat
Classic Chicken Sandwich, Grilled	1	450	17	150	2	0	80	1240	44	7	3	32	3 carb, 3 med-fat protein
Honey BBQ Boneless Wings	6 wings	510	21	190	4	0	70	1500	50	16	2	28	3 carb, 3 med-fat protein, 1 fat
Jumbo Popcorn Chicken	1 medium order	380	22	190	4	0	45	1260	27	1	3	18	2 carb, 2 med-fat protein, 2 fat
Spicy Jumbo Popcorn Chicken	1 medium order	360	17	150	3	0	45	870	30	0	2	21	2 carb, 2 med-fat protein, 1 fat

FAST FOOD

	Serving	Calories	Fat (g)	Cal. from Fat	Sat. Fat (g)	Trans Fat (g)	Chol. (mg)	Sod. (mg)	Carb. (g)	Sugar (g)	Fiber (g)	Prot. (g)	Servings/Exchanges
Super Crunch Chicken Strip Dinner	1 (3-piece) order	970	46	410	8	1	55	2160	109	9	7	30	7 carb, 1 med-fat protein, 7 fat
Super Crunch Chicken Strips	3 pieces	330	16	140	3	0	55	670	25	0	2	22	1 1/2 carb, 2 med-fat protein, 1 fat
Hot Dogs													
All-American Dog	1	380	18	160	7	0	35	1170	40	15	1	11	2 1/2 carb, 1/2 med-fat protein, 3 fat
Cheesy Bacon Pretzel Dog	1	500	26	240	10	0	50	1410	46	7	2	15	3 carb, 1 med-fat protein, 4 fat
Chicago Dog	1	410	19	170	7	0	35	2330	48	17	2	13	3 carb, 1 med-fat protein, 2 fat
Chili Cheese Coney	1	420	26	240	11	0	55	1280	30	4	2	17	2 carb, 1 med-fat protein, 4 fat
Corn Dog	1	230	15	130	4	0	25	570	19	6	1	6	1 carb, 3 fat
Footlong 1/4 Pounder Coney	1	830	55	490	23	0	105	1970	54	9	3	31	3 1/2 carb, 3 med-fat protein, 7 fat

Item	Serving												Exchanges
New York Dog	1	340	19	170	7	0	35	1170	30	3	3	13	2 carb, 1 med-fat protein, 2 fat
Original Pretzel Dog	1	320	18	160	7	0	35	910	27	2	1	11	2 carb, 1 med-fat protein, 2 fat

Breakfast Items

Item	Serving												Exchanges
Bagel Breakfast Sandwich with Ham	1	550	16	150	6	0.5	315	1990	68	6	2	32	4 1/2 carb, 3 lean protein, 1 fat
Bagel Breakfast Sandwich with Sausage	1	680	32	290	12	1	340	1730	68	5	2	31	4 1/2 carb, 3 med-fat protein, 2 1/2 fat
Breakfast Burrito with Ham	1	460	22	190	10	0.5	320	1900	40	1	1	29	2 1/2 carb, 3 med-fat protein, 1 fat
Breakfast Burrito with Sausage	1	500	29	260	12	1	320	1480	39	0	1	24	2 1/2 carb, 2 med-fat protein, 3 fat
Breakfast Toaster with Ham	1	540	23	210	1	0.5	315	1770	53	8	2	29	3 1/2 carb, 3 med-fat protein, 1 fat
Breakfast Toaster with Sausage	1	670	39	350	13	1	340	1510	52	7	2	27	3 1/2 carb, 2 med-fat protein, 5 fat
Cinnasnacks without Frosting	3 pieces	340	15	140	5	0	10	210	44	17	4	7	3 carb, 1 med-fat protein, 1 fat

FAST FOOD

	Serving	Calories	Fat (g)	Cal. from Fat	Sat. Fat (g)	Trans Fat (g)	Chol. (mg)	Sod. (mg)	Carb. (g)	Sugar (g)	Fiber (g)	Prot. (g)	Servings/Exchanges
Cream Cheese Frosting	1 order	290	18	160	9	0	15	260	31	34	1	0	2 carb, 4 fat
French Toast Sticks without Syrup	4 pieces	500	31	280	5	0	15	490	49	9	2	7	3 carb, 6 fat
Super Sonic Breakfast Burrito	1	580	32	290	13	1	320	1920	49	1	2	25	3 carb, 2 med-fat protein, 4 fat
Syrup	1 order	90	0	0	0	0	0	0	22	15	0	0	1 1/2 carb
Ultimate Meat & Cheese Breakfast Burrito	1	800	56	510	18	1	355	2140	46	1	2	29	3 carb, 3 med-fat protein, 8 fat
Snacks & Sides													
Apple Slices	1 order	35	0	0	0	0	0	0	9	7	2	0	1/2 carb
Ched 'R' Peppers	6 pieces	710	48	43	12	1.5	55	2130	56	4	3	13	3 1/2 carb, 9 fat
Chili Cheese Natural Cut Fries	1 medium order	450	26	240	10	0	35	940	43	2	4	13	3 carb, 1 med-fat protein, 4 fat

	Serving											
Chili Cheese Tots	1 medium order	520	32	290	11	0.5	35	1540	47	2	5	12	3 carb, 6 fat
Handmade Onion Rings	1 medium order	580	29	260	5	0	0	570	74	19	4	8	5 carb, 5 fat
Mozzarella Sticks	6 pieces	540	27	240	11	1	50	1510	52	3	2	23	3 1/2 carb, 2 med-fat protein, 3 fat
Natural Cut Fries	1 medium order	290	13	120	2.5	0	0	300	38	0	3	3	2 1/2 carb, 2 fat
Tots	1 medium order	360	19	170	3.5	0	0	890	43	0	4	3	3 carb, 3 fat

Ultimate Drink Shop

	Serving											
Blue Coconut Slush	1 medium	260	0	0	0	0	0	45	69	0	69	0	4 1/2 carb
Blue Raspberry with Jolly Rancher Hard Candy Slush	1 medium	420	2.5	25	2.5	0	0	320	103	0	99	0	7 carb, 1/2 fat

FAST FOOD

	Serving	Calories	Fat (g)	Cal. from Fat	Sat. Fat (g)	Trans Fat (g)	Chol. (mg)	Sod. (mg)	Carb. (g)	Sugar (g)	Fiber (g)	Prot. (g)	Servings/Exchanges
Blue Raspberry with Rainbow Candy Slush	1 medium	500	0	0	0	0	0	50	131	128	0	0	8 1/2 carb
Cherry Limeade	1 medium	230	0	0	0	0	0	40	61	60	0	0	4 carb
Diet Cherry Limeade	1 medium	20	0	0	0	0	0	15	3	2	0	0	free
Green Apple Slush	1 medium	270	0	0	0	0	0	45	73	73	0	0	5 carb
Lemonberry Real Fruit Slush	1 medium	280	0	0	0	0	0	45	75	73	1	0	5 carb
Limeade	1 medium	170	0	0	0	0	0	40	47	46	0	0	3 carb
Frozen Zone													
Brownie & Cookie Dough Madness Master Blast	1 mini	620	31	280	20	0	80	350	80	67	1	7	5 carb, 5 fat
Chocolate Malt	1 mini	530	26	230	19	0	80	260	69	47	0	7	4 1/2 carb, 4 fat

Chocolate Shake	1 mini	570	26	230	19	0	80	270	78	45	0	6	5 carb, 4 fat
Fudge Brownie Molten Cake Sundae	1	800	34	310	18	0	65	610	117	73	4	8	8 carb, 5 fat
Hot Fudge Real Ice Cream Sundae	1	520	26	240	20	0	80	280	64	57	1	7	4 carb, 4 fat
Oreo Chocolate Master Malt	1 mini	770	33	300	22	0	90	470	107	64	1	9	7 carb, 5 fat
Oreo Chocolate Master Shake	1 mini	740	33	300	22	0	90	450	102	61	1	8	7 carb, 5 fat
Peanutty Swirl Master Blast with Snickers Bars	1 mini	710	46	420	23	0	75	370	67	59	1	12	4 1/2 carb, 8 fat
Snickers Bars & Caramel Waffle Cone Sundae	1	450	19	170	13	0	60	270	63	48	1	6	4 carb, 3 fat
Sonic Blast with Butterfinger	1 mini	520	27	240	18	0	65	240	63	51	0	7	4 carb, 5 fat
Sonic Blast with Oreo	1 mini	530	28	250	18	0	65	380	62	50	1	6	4 carb, 5 fat
Vanilla Malt	1 mini	490	28	250	20	0	90	260	54	51	0	7	3 1/2 carb, 5 fat
Vanilla Shake	1 mini	480	28	250	20	0	90	250	52	49	0	7	3 1/2 carb, 5 fat

FAST FOOD

STARBUCKS

Iced Coffee & Iced Tea

	Serving	Calories	Fat (g)	Cal. from Fat	Sat. Fat (g)	Trans Fat (g)	Chol. (mg)	Sod. (mg)	Carb. (g)	Sugar (g)	Fiber (g)	Prot. (g)	Servings/Exchanges
Iced Coffee, 2% Milk	1 tall	80	1	10	0.5	0	5	30	17	17	0	2	1 carb
Iced Espresso Classics, Caffè Latte, 2% Milk	1 tall	100	3.5	35	2	0	15	90	10	9	0	6	1 low-fat milk
Iced Espresso Classics, Caramel Macchiato	1 tall	170	5	45	2.5	0	20	105	25	23	0	7	1 reduced-fat milk, 1 carb
Iced Espresso Classics, Mocha, 2% Milk	1 tall	260	12	110	8	0	40	80	29	23	3	7	1 reduced-fat milk, 1 carb, 1 fat
Iced Espresso Classics, Vanilla Latte, 2% Milk	1 tall	140	3	30	1.5	0	15	75	23	22	0	6	1 low-fat milk, 1 carb
Iced Green Tea Latte	1 tall	160	4.5	40	2.5	0	15	105	22	21	1	8	1 low-fat milk, 1 carb
Iced Skinny Mocha, Nonfat Milk	1 tall	70	1	5	0.5	0	5	70	9	8	0	7	1 low-fat milk
Shaken Sweet Tea	1 tall	80	0	0	0	0	0	10	19	19	0	0	1 carb

Item	Serving											
Shaken Sweet Tea Lemonade	1 tall	110	0	0	0	0	0	29	29	0	0	2 carb
Teavana Shaken Iced Black Tea Lemonade	1 tall	120	0	0	0	0	0	32	32	0	0	2 carb
Teavana Shaken Iced Peach Green Tea	1 tall	60	0	0	0	0	0	15	15	0	0	1 carb
Espresso Beverages, 2% Milk												
Caffè Latte	1 tall	150	6	3.5	0	25	115	14	13	0	10	1 reduced-fat milk
Caffè Mocha	1 tall	290	13	8	0	40	120	34	28	3	11	1 reduced-fat milk, 1 1/2 carb, 1 fat
Cappuccino	1 tall	90	3.5	1.5	0	15	80	9	8	0	6	1 low-fat milk
Caramel Macchiato	1 tall	180	5	3	0	20	115	25	23	0	8	1 reduced-fat milk, 1 carb
Flat White (Whole Milk)	1 tall	170	9	5	0	25	115	14	13	0	9	1 whole milk
Skinny Mocha	1 tall	70	1	0.5	0	5	70	9	8	2	7	1 low-fat milk
Vanilla Latte	1 tall	200	5	2.5	0	20	125	28	27	0	9	1 reduced-fat milk, 1 carb
White Chocolate Mocha with Whipped Cream	1 tall	370	15	10	0	45	200	47	46	0	11	1 reduced-fat milk, 2 carb, 2 fat

FAST FOOD

Frappucino Blended Beverages

	Serving	Calories	Fat (g)	Cal. from Fat	Sat. Fat (g)	Trans Fat (g)	Chol. (mg)	Sod. (mg)	Carb. (g)	Sugar (g)	Fiber (g)	Prot. (g)	Servings/Exchanges
Caffè Vanilla Frappuccino with Whipped Cream	1 tall	300	11	90	6	0	35	160	50	48	0	3	3 carb, 2 fat
Caffè Vanilla Light Frappuccino	1 tall	130	0	0	0	0	0	150	30	29	0	3	2 carb
Caramel Frappuccino with Whipped Cream	1 tall	300	11	100	7	0	40	170	47	45	0	3	3 carb, 2 fat
Caramel Light Frappuccino	1 tall	100	0	0	0	0	0	150	22	22	0	3	1 1/2 carb
Chai Crème Frappuccino with Whipped Cream	1 tall	250	11	100	7	0	40	160	35	34	0	4	2 carb, 2 fat
Coffee Frappuccino	1 tall	180	2.5	25	1.5	0	10	160	36	36	0	3	2 1/2 carb
Coffee Light Frappuccino	1 tall	90	0	0	0	0	0	150	18	18	0	3	1 carb
Double Chocolaty Chip Crème Frappuccino with Whipped Cream	1 tall	310	14	130	9	0	40	200	42	38	2	5	3 carb, 2 fat

Item	Serving												Exchanges
Green Tea Crème Frappuccino with Whipped Cream	1 tall	320	12	100	7	0	40	180	50	48	1	5	3 carb, 2 fat
Java Chip Frappuccino with Whipped Cream	1 tall	340	13	120	9	0	35	190	51	47	2	4	3 1/2 carb, 2 fat
Java Chip Light Frappuccino	1 tall	150	3	25	2	0	0	170	29	26	2	4	2 carb
Mocha Frappuccino with Whipped Cream	1 tall	290	11	100	7	0	35	170	44	42	1	4	3 carb, 2 fat
Mocha Light Frappuccino	1 tall	110	0.5	5	0	0	0	150	23	21	1	3	1 1/2 carb
Strawberries & Crème Frappuccino with Whipped Cream	1 tall	270	11	100	7	0	40	150	40	39	0	3	2 1/2 carb, 2 fat
Teavana Oprah Cinnamon Chai Crème Frappuccino with Whipped Cream	1 tall	240	11	100	7	0	40	140	33	31	0	3	2 carb, 2 fat
Vanilla Bean Crème Frappuccino with Whipped Cream	1 tall	280	11	100	7	0	40	170	41	39	0	4	2 1/2 carb, 2 fat

FAST FOOD

	Serving	Calories	Fat (g)	Cal. from Fat	Sat. Fat (g)	Trans Fat (g)	Chol. (mg)	Sod. (mg)	Carb. (g)	Sugar (g)	Fiber (g)	Prot. (g)	Servings/Exchanges
Hot Tea Lattes, 2% Milk													
Classic Chai Tea Latte	1 tall	190	3.5	30	1.5	0	15	90	34	32	0	6	1 low-fat milk, 1 1/2 carb
Green Tea Latte	1 tall	190	5	50	3.5	0	20	125	25	24	1	10	1 reduced-fat milk, 1 carb
Teavana London Fog Tea Latte	1 tall	140	3	30	2	0	15	80	23	23	0	5	1 low-fat milk, 1 carb
Teavana Oprah Cinnamon Chai Tea Latte	1 tall	150	3	30	2	0	15	80	25	23	0	5	1 low-fat milk, 1 carb
Bakery Sweets													
Banana Nut Bread	1	420	22	190	3	0	65	320	52	30	2	6	3 1/2 carb, 4 fat
Birthday Cake Pop	1	170	9	80	5	0	10	110	23	18	0	1	1 1/2 carb, 1 1/2 fat
Blueberry Scone	1	420	17	150	10	0.5	60	510	61	20	2	5	4 carb, 3 fat
Chewy Chocolate Cookie	1	170	5	45	2.5	0	0	110	30	26	2	2	2 carb, 1 fat
Classic Coffee Cake	1	390	16	150	10	0	75	400	57	31	1	5	4 carb, 2 fat

Double Chocolate Chunk Brownie	1	380	23	200	7	0	70	170	41	28	2	4	2 1/2 carb, 4 fat
Gluten-Free Marshmallow Dream Bar	1	240	5	45	3	0	15	260	45	23	0	2	3 carb
Iced Lemon Pound Cake	1	470	20	180	9	0.5	100	310	68	42	1	6	4 1/2 carb, 3 fat
Oatmeal Cookie	1	290	12	100	7	0	45	190	40	20	3	5	2 1/2 carb, 2 fat
Old-Fashioned Glazed Doughnut	1	480	27	240	13	0	20	410	56	30	1	5	3 1/2 carb, 5 fat
Petite Vanilla Bean Scone	1	120	2.5	40	2	0	15	95	18	8	0	2	1 carb
Reduced-Fat Cinnamon Swirl Coffee Cake	1	370	9	80	5	0	20	280	67	41	2	5	4 1/2 carb, 1 fat
Salted Caramel Square with Pecans	1	380	22	190	12	0	40	280	45	28	1	3	3 carb, 4 fat

Bistro Boxes

Cheese & Fruit	1 box	470	28	250	10	0	50	470	38	17	6	14	2 1/2 carb, 1 med-fat protein, 4 fat
Protein Bistro Box	1 box	370	19	170	6	0	200	460	37	18	5	13	2 1/2 carb, 1 med-fat protein, 2 fat

FAST FOOD

	Serving	Calories	Fat (g)	Cal. from Fat	Sat. Fat (g)	Trans Fat (g)	Chol. (mg)	Sod. (mg)	Carb. (g)	Sugar (g)	Fiber (g)	Prot. (g)	Servings/Exchanges
Thai-Style Peanut Chicken Wrap	1 box	450	20	180	7	0	35	510	51	20	4	11	3 1/2 carb, 3 fat
Hot Breakfast													
Bacon & Gouda Breakfast Sandwich	1	350	18	160	7	0	160	820	30	0	0	15	2 carb, 1 med-fat protein, 2 fat
Classic Whole-Grain Oatmeal	1	160	2.5	25	0.5	0	0	0	28	0	4	5	2 carb
Double-Smoked Bacon, Cheddar & Egg Sandwich	1	490	27	240	13	0	215	910	40	7	1	17	2 1/2 carb, 1 med-fat protein, 4 fat
Egg & Cheddar Breakfast Sandwich	1	280	13	110	5	0	160	460	27	2	2	12	2 carb, 1 med-fat protein, 1 fat
Reduced-Fat Turkey Bacon Breakfast Sandwich	1	230	6	50	2.5	0	20	560	28	3	2	13	2 carb, 1 med-fat protein
Spinach & Feta Breakfast Wrap	1	290	10	90	3.5	0	20	830	33	4	6	19	2 carb, 2 med-fat protein

Sandwiches, Paninis, Salads & Foldovers

Ancho Chipotle Chicken	1	440	18	160	7	0	60	1020	46	3	3	20	3 carb, 2 med-fat protein, 1 fat
Chicken Artichoke on Ancient Grain Flatbread	1	510	27	240	8	0	70	1120	37	1	5	24	2 1/2 carb, 2 med-fat protein, 3 fat
Chicken BLT Salad Sandwich	1	470	25	220	4.5	0	60	890	35	3	3	21	2 carb, 2 med-fat protein, 3 fat
Ham & Cheese Savory Foldover	1	250	11	100	6	0	50	480	24	4	<1	13	1 1/2 carb, 1 med-fat protein, 1 fat
Ham & Swiss Panini	1	380	11	100	5	0	50	1080	46	1	2	19	3 carb, 1 med-fat protein, 1 fat
Hearty Veggie & Brown Rice Salad Bowl	1	430	22	200	3	0	0	640	50	8	8	10	3 carb, 4 fat
Italian-Style Ham & Spicy Salami	1	480	20	180	8	0	65	1100	49	3	3	22	3 carb, 2 med-fat protein, 1 fat
Old-Fashioned Grilled Cheese	1	580	29	260	13	0.5	65	1110	57	7	5	28	4 carb, 2 med-fat protein, 3 fat
Roasted Tomato & Mozzarella Panini	1	420	18	160	6	0	35	620	47	3	3	11	3 carb, 3 fat

FAST FOOD

	Serving	Calories	Fat (g)	Cal. from Fat	Sat. Fat (g)	Trans Fat (g)	Chol. (mg)	Sod. (mg)	Carb. (g)	Sugar (g)	Fiber (g)	Prot. (g)	Servings/Exchanges
Wheat Spinach Savory Foldover	1	250	15	140	8	0	50	380	23	4	3	4	1 1/2 carb, 3 fat
Zesty Chicken & Black Bean Salad Bowl	1	360	15	130	2.5	0	30	840	38	9	8	14	2 1/2 carb, 1 med-fat protein, 1 1/2 fat
SUBWAY													
6-Inch Low Fat Sandwiches													
Black Forest Ham	1	290	4.5	40	1	0	20	800	46	8	5	18	3 carb, 1 lean protein
Oven Roasted Chicken	1	320	5	40	1.5	0	40	610	47	8	5	23	3 carb, 2 lean protein
Roast Beef	1	320	5	40	1.5	0	40	660	45	7	5	24	3 carb, 2 lean protein
Sweet Onion Chicken Teriyaki	1	370	4.5	40	1	0	50	770	57	16	5	25	4 carb, 2 lean protein
Turkey Breast	1	280	3.5	30	1	0	20	670	46	7	5	18	3 carb, 1 lean protein
Veggie Delite	1	230	2.5	20	0.5	0	0	280	44	6	5	8	3 carb

6-Inch Sandwiches

Chicken & Bacon Ranch Melt	1	610	30	270	10	0.5	95	1290	48	8	5	38	3 carb, 4 med-fat protein, 1 fat
Cold Cut Combo	1	360	12	110	3.5	0	45	1030	46	7	5	17	3 carb, 1 med-fat protein, 1 fat
Italian BMT	1	410	16	150	6	0	45	1260	46	8	5	20	3 carb, 2 med-fat protein, 1 fat
Meatball Marinara	1	480	18	160	7	0.5	30	920	59	12	8	21	4 carb, 1 med-fat protein, 2 fat
Spicy Italian	1	480	24	220	9	0.5	50	1490	46	8	5	20	3 carb, 2 med-fat protein, 2 fat
Steak & Cheese	1	380	10	90	4.5	0	50	1030	48	8	5	26	3 carb, 2 med-fat protein
Tuna	1	480	25	210	4	0	35	600	44	6	5	20	3 carb, 2 med-fat protein, 2 fat
Turkey Italiano Melt	1	510	25	230	9	0.5	50	1490	48	9	5	24	3 carb, 2 med-fat protein, 2 fat

FAST FOOD

	Serving	Calories	Fat (g)	Cal. from Fat	Sat. Fat (g)	Trans Fat (g)	Chol. (mg)	Sod. (mg)	Carb. (g)	Sugar (g)	Fiber (g)	Prot. (g)	Servings/Exchanges
Flatizza													
Cheese	1	390	16	140	8	0	35	810	42	3	2	21	3 carb, 2 med-fat protein, 1 fat
Pepperoni	1	500	26	230	12	0	60	1340	43	4	2	26	3 carb, 2 med-fat protein, 3 fat
Spicy Italian	1	490	25	220	11	0	60	1290	43	4	2	25	3 carb, 2 med-fat protein, 2 fat
Veggie	1	410	17	150	8	0	35	850	44	4	3	21	3 carb, 2 med-fat protein, 1 fat
Low Fat Salads (No Dressing)													
Black Forest Ham	1	110	3	25	1	0	20	600	12	6	4	12	1 carb, 1 lean protein
Chicken Teriyaki with Spinach	1	220	3	30	1	0	70	610	23	14	4	27	1 1/2 carb, 3 lean protein
Oven Roasted Chicken	1	140	2.5	25	0.5	0	50	280	10	4	4	19	1/2 carb, 2 lean protein
Roast Beef	1	140	3.5	30	1	0	40	460	11	5	4	19	1 carb, 2 lean protein
Subway Club	1	140	3.5	30	1	0	40	590	12	5	4	18	1 carb, 2 lean protein

Sweet Onion Chicken Teriyaki	1	230	3	25	0.5	0	50	650	32	22	4	20	2 carb, 2 lean protein
Turkey	1	110	2	20	0.5	0	20	460	12	5	4	12	1 carb, 1 lean protein
Veggie Delite	1	60	1	10	0	0	0	75	10	4	4	3	2 vegetable
Salads (No Dressing)													
Big Hot Pastrami Melt	1	400	29	300	11	0	85	1250	12	4	4	23	1 carb, 3 med-fat protein, 3 fat
Chipotle Chicken with Guacamole	1	520	40	360	9	0	75	880	19	6	8	24	1 carb, 3 med-fat protein, 5 fat
Double Chicken Chopped	1	220	4.5	35	1.5	0	100	490	10	4	4	36	1/2 carb, 5 lean protein
Monterey Chicken Melt	1	190	7	60	3.5	0	65	360	10	4	4	22	1/2 carb, 3 lean protein
Turkey & Bacon Guacamole	1	330	20	180	4.5	0	30	1080	19	6	8	19	1 carb, 2 med-fat protein, 2 fat
Turkey Italiano	1	390	29	260	9	0.5	50	1450	16	8	4	18	1 carb, 2 med-fat protein, 4 fat
Salad Dressing													
Fat Free Italian	2 oz	35	0	0	0	0	0	720	7	4	0	1	1/2 carb
Ranch	2 oz	320	35	310	6	0.5	30	560	3	2	0	0	7 fat

FAST FOOD

Breakfast Sandwiches, 6-Inch Bread

	Serving	Calories	Fat (g)	Cal. from Fat	Sat. Fat (g)	Trans Fat (g)	Chol. (mg)	Sod. (mg)	Carb. (g)	Sugar (g)	Fiber (g)	Prot. (g)	Servings/Exchanges
Bacon, Egg & Cheese	1	440	17	160	6	0	240	1290	45	7	5	25	3 carb, 2 med-fat protein, 1 fat
Bacon, Egg (White) & Cheese	1	400	13	120	5	0	15	1330	45	5	4	25	3 carb, 2 med-fat protein
Black Forest Ham, Egg & Cheese	1	390	13	120	5	0	240	1120	45	7	5	24	3 carb, 2 med-fat protein
Egg & Cheese	1	360	12	110	4.5	0	230	860	44	6	5	19	3 carb, 1 med-fat protein, 1 fat
Egg (White) & Cheese	1	320	8	70	3	0	10	910	44	5	4	19	3 carb, 1 med-fat protein
Egg (White) & Cheese with Ham	1	350	9	80	3.5	0	25	1170	45	6	4	24	3 carb, 2 lean protein
Steak, Egg & Cheese	1	430	15	130	5	0	255	1190	47	7	5	28	3 carb, 3 med-fat protein
Steak, Egg (White) & Cheese	1	390	10	90	4	0	35	1240	47	6	4	28	3 carb, 3 lean protein

Soup

Beef Chili	1 bowl	350	24	220	10	0	80	730	17	7	4	15	1 carb, 2 med-fat protein, 3 fat
Black Bean	1 bowl	210	1	10	0	0	0	860	39	6	15	12	2 1/2 carb, 1 lean protein
Broccoli & Cheddar	1 bowl	170	9	70	5	0	25	630	18	4	1	5	1 carb, 2 fat
Creamy Chicken & Dumpling	1 bowl	150	4.5	40	2	0	35	740	20	3	3	8	1 carb, 1 med-fat protein
Creamy Wild & Brown Rice	1 bowl	190	11	90	6	0.5	40	820	16	3	1	7	1 carb, 1 med-fat protein, 1 fat
Homestyle Chicken Noodle	1 bowl	110	3	30	1.5	0	30	720	14	2	1	8	1 carb, 1 lean protein
Loaded Baked Potato	1 bowl	210	13	120	7	0	35	800	15	4	1	5	1 carb, 2 fat
Poblano Corn Chowder	1 bowl	150	7	60	4	0.5	20	560	18	7	2	5	1 carb, 1 fat
Thai Coconut	1 bowl	210	3	30	0	0	25	680	17	7	1	5	1 carb
Tomato Basil	1 bowl	140	7	60	4	0	25	750	15	8	2	5	1 carb, 1 fat

FAST FOOD

	Serving	Calories	Fat (g)	Cal. from Fat	Sat. Fat (g)	Trans Fat (g)	Chol. (mg)	Sod. (mg)	Carb. (g)	Sugar (g)	Fiber (g)	Prot. (g)	Servings/Exchanges
Cookies & Desserts													
Apple Slices	1 pkg (2.5 oz)	35	0	0	0	0	0	0	9	7	2	0	1/2 carb
Chocolate Chip	1 cookie	210	10	90	5	0	15	130	30	18	1	2	2 carb, 2 fat
Gingerbread	1 cookie	190	7	60	3	0	15	110	31	17	1	2	2 carb, 1 fat
M&M	1 cookie	210	10	90	5	0	15	100	30	18	1	2	2 carb, 2 fat
Oatmeal Raisin	1 cookie	200	8	70	3.5	0	15	130	30	16	1	3	2 carb, 2 fat
Peanut Butter	1 cookie	220	12	110	5	0	10	130	26	16	1	4	2 carb, 2 fat
Raspberry Cheesecake	1 cookie	200	9	80	4.5	0	15	120	29	16	0	2	2 carb, 1 fat
Sugar	1 cookie	230	12	110	6	0	15	130	28	14	1	4	2 carb, 2 fat
White Macadamia Nut	1 cookie	220	11	100	5	0	15	130	28	18	1	2	2 carb, 2 fat
TACO BELL													
Breakfast													
A.M. Grilled Taco, Egg & Cheese	1	170	9	80	3	0	90	330	15	<1	<1	7	1 carb, 1 med-fat protein, 1 fat

Item	Amount												Exchanges
A.M. Grilled Taco, Sausage	1	280	19	170	7	0	110	460	16	1	1	11	1 carb, 1 med-fat protein, 3 fat
Biscuit Taco, Egg & Cheese	1	310	17	160	7	0	100	610	29	7	<1	10	2 carb, 1 med-fat protein, 2 fat
Biscuit Taco, Sausage & Cheese	1	370	23	210	10	0	135	650	29	7	<1	11	2 carb, 1 med-fat protein, 3 fat
Breakfast Crunchwrap, California	1	630	38	340	11	0	125	1400	52	3	5	21	3 1/2 carb, 1 med-fat protein, 6 fat
Breakfast Crunchwrap, Country	1	660	41	360	13	0	135	1290	54	5	4	21	3 1/2 carb, 1 med-fat protein, 6 fat
Breakfast Crunchwrap, Sausage	1	710	47	430	14	0	135	1180	51	3	4	20	3 1/2 carb, 1 med-fat protein, 8 fat
Cheesy Burrito, Fiesta Potato	1	520	27	240	10	0	195	1060	49	3	3	20	3 carb, 2 med-fat protein, 3 fat
Cinnabon Delights (2 pack)	1	160	9	80	2	0	5	80	17	10	0	2	1 carb, 2 fat
Grande Scrambler, Sausage	1	690	39	350	11	0	200	1380	65	5	5	20	4 carb, 1 med-fat protein, 6 fat
Grilled Breakfast Burrito, Country	1	440	23	200	7	0	105	930	45	3	3	14	3 carb, 1 med-fat protein, 3 fat

FAST FOOD

	Serving	Calories	Fat (g)	Cal. from Fat	Sat. Fat (g)	Trans Fat (g)	Chol. (mg)	Sod. (mg)	Carb. (g)	Sugar (g)	Fiber (g)	Prot. (g)	Servings/Exchanges
Hashbrown (Side)	1	160	12	100	1	0	0	270	13	0	2	1	1 carb, 2 fat
Tacos, Gorditas, Chalupas													
Chalupa Supreme, Beef	1	360	21	190	5	0	30	580	31	4	4	13	2 carb, 1 med-fat protein, 3 fat
Cheesy Gordita Crunch	1	500	29	260	10	1	55	880	41	5	5	20	2 1/2 carb, 2 med-fat protein, 3 fat
Chicken Soft Taco	1	160	5	50	2.5	0	25	480	16	1	2	12	1 carb, 1 med-fat protein
Crunchy Taco	1	170	10	90	3.5	0	25	320	13	<1	3	8	1 carb, 1 med-fat protein, 1 fat
Crunchy Taco Supreme	1	190	11	100	4.5	0	30	340	15	2	3	8	1 carb, 1 med-fat protein, 1 fat
Double Decker	1	320	14	120	5	0	25	710	36	2	7	13	2 1/2 carb, 1 med-fat protein, 1 fat
Double Decker Supreme	1	340	15	140	6	0	30	730	38	3	7	14	2 1/2 carb, 1 med-fat protein, 1 1/2 fat

Gordita Supreme, Beef	1	290	12	110	4.5	0	30	580	31	5	3	13	2 carb, 1 med-fat protein, 1 fat
Grilled Steak Soft Taco	1	200	10	90	3.5	0	35	490	16	2	1	13	1 carb, 1 med-fat protein, 1 fat
Nacho Cheese Doritos Cheesy Gordita Crunch	1	500	29	260	10	1	55	930	41	5	5	20	2 1/2 carb, 2 med-fat protein, 3 fat
Nacho Cheese Doritos Locos	1	170	10	90	3.5	0	25	370	13	1	3	8	1 carb, 1 med-fat protein, 1 fat
Nacho Cheese Doritos Locos Supreme	1	190	11	100	4.5	0	30	390	15	2	3	8	1 carb, 1 med-fat protein, 1 fat
Soft Taco, Beef	1	190	9	80	4	0	25	500	17	1	3	9	1 carb, 1 med-fat protein, 1 fat
Soft Taco Supreme, Beef	1	210	10	90	5	0	30	520	20	2	3	10	1 carb, 1 med-fat protein, 1 fat
Burritos & Grillers													
7-Layer Burrito	1	430	16	140	6	0	15	1020	57	4	7	14	4 carb, 2 fat
Bean Burrito	1	370	11	100	4	0	5	1050	55	3	8	15	3 1/2 carb, 1 med-fat protein, 1 fat

FAST FOOD

	Serving	Calories	Fat (g)	Cal. from Fat	Sat. Fat (g)	Trans Fat (g)	Chol. (mg)	Sod. (mg)	Carb. (g)	Sugar (g)	Fiber (g)	Prot. (g)	Servings/Exchanges
Beefy 5-Layer Burrito	1	500	19	170	7	0	30	1290	64	5	8	19	4 carb, 1 med-fat protein, 2 fat
Beefy Nacho Loaded Griller	1	380	16	140	4	0	20	830	47	3	5	12	3 carb, 3 fat
Black Bean Burrito	1	380	11	100	4	0	10	1030	57	3	8	14	4 carb, 1 fat
Burrito Supreme, Beef	1	410	15	140	6	0	30	1140	51	4	7	17	3 1/2 carb, 1 med-fat protein, 2 fat
Cantina Power Burrito, Steak	1	470	21	190	8	0	70	1180	41	4	4	28	2 1/2 carb, 3 med-fat protein, 1 fat
Chipotle Chicken Loaded Griller	1	350	16	140	4	0	40	810	37	3	2	15	2 1/2 carb, 1 med-fat protein, 2 fat
Loaded Potato Griller	1	410	18	160	5	0	20	1030	50	4	3	12	3 carb, 3 fat
Quesarito, Chicken	1	620	30	270	10	0	60	1460	65	4	5	21	4 carb, 1 med-fat protein, 4 fat
Shredded Chicken Burrito	1	400	18	160	4.5	0	30	960	45	3	3	16	3 carb, 1 med-fat protein, 2 fat

Smothered Burrito, Beef	1	700	35	310	13	1	70	2260	68	4	9	28	4 1/2 carb, 2 med-fat protein, 4 fat
XXL Grilled Stuft Burrito, Beef	1	860	41	370	14	1	65	2200	91	6	12	32	6 carb, 2 med-fat protein, 5 fat
Other Specialties													
Cantina Power Bowl, Steak	1	500	21	190	7	0	70	1280	47	3	8	29	3 carb, 3 med-fat protein, 1 fat
Crunchwrap Supreme	1	540	21	190	6	0	25	1210	71	6	6	16	4 1/2 carb, 3 fat
Fiesta Taco Salad, Beef	1	770	40	360	10	1	55	1590	76	7	11	26	5 carb, 2 med-fat protein, 5 fat
Mexican Pizza	1	550	30	270	8	0.5	40	990	49	3	7	20	3 carb, 2 med-fat protein, 3 fat
Meximelt	1	250	14	120	7	0.5	40	730	19	2	3	14	1 carb, 2 med-fat protein, 1 fat
Nachos Bellgrande	1	760	38	340	6	0	25	1310	85	5	13	19	5 1/2 carb, 6 1/2 fat
Nachos Supreme	1	440	23	210	4.5	0	25	860	46	3	8	12	3 carb, 4 fat
Quesadilla, Cheese	1	460	26	230	11	0.5	50	980	37	3	4	19	2 1/2 carb, 2 med-fat protein, 4 fat

FAST FOOD

Dollar Cravings

	Serving	Calories	Fat (g)	Cal. from Fat	Sat. Fat (g)	Trans Fat (g)	Chol. (mg)	Sod. (mg)	Carb. (g)	Sugar (g)	Fiber (g)	Prot. (g)	Servings/Exchanges
Beefy Fritos Burrito	1	430	18	160	4.5	0	20	1030	55	3	4	13	3 1/2 carb, 3 fat
Caramel Apple Empanada	1	310	15	140	2.5	0	0	310	39	13	2	3	2 1/2 carb, 2 1/2 fat
Cheese Roll-Up	1	180	9	80	5	0	20	430	15	<1	2	9	1 carb, 1 med-fat protein, 1 fat
Cheesy Bean & Rice Burrito	1	420	17	160	3.5	0	<5	930	55	4	6	11	3 1/2 carb, 3 fat
Cinnamon Twists	1	170	6	50	0	0	0	210	27	12	<1	1	2 carb, 1 fat
Shredded Chicken Mini Quesadilla	1	180	8	70	2.5	0	25	540	15	1	2	12	1 carb, 1 med-fat protein
Spicy Potato Soft Taco	1	240	12	110	3	0	10	480	27	1	2	5	2 carb, 2 fat
Spicy Tostada	1	210	10	90	3	0	10	450	22	1	4	7	1 1/2 carb, 2 fat
Triple Layer Nachos	1	320	15	140	1.5	0	0	600	41	2	6	7	2 1/2 carb, 1 med-fat protein, 1 1/2 fat

TACO JOHN'S

Breakfast

Junior Breakfast Burrito, Sausage	1	240	12	110	4.5	0	170	630	22	2	1	10	1 1/2 carb, 1 med-fat protein, 1 fat
Meat & Potato Breakfast Burrito, Sausage	1	640	36	320	11	0	245	1720	57	2	4	21	4 carb, 1 med-fat protein, 5 fat
Potato Olés Scrambler, Sausage	1 regular	1190	79	710	24	0	375	3360	87	5	9	31	6 carb, 2 med-fat protein, 12 fat
Scrambler Breakfast Burrito, Sausage	1	650	34	300	11	0	245	1840	58	4	4	21	4 carb, 1 med-fat protein, 5 fat
Spicy Chorizo Breakfast Burrito	1	510	28	250	9	0	245	1540	44	3	2	20	3 carb, 2 med-fat protein, 3 fat

Tacos

Crispy Taco	1	170	10	90	4	0	25	290	11	1	2	9	1 carb, 1 med-fat protein, 1 fat
Fish Taco	1	280	14	130	4.5	0	35	1160	29	3	2	10	2 carb, 1 med-fat protein, 1 fat
Soft Shell Taco	1	220	10	90	4.5	0	25	580	23	2	2	11	1 1/2 carb, 1 med-fat protein, 1 fat

FAST FOOD

	Serving	Calories	Fat (g)	Cal. from Fat	Sat. Fat (g)	Trans Fat (g)	Chol. (mg)	Sod. (mg)	Carb. (g)	Sugar (g)	Fiber (g)	Prot. (g)	Servings/Exchanges
Soft Shell Taco, Chicken	1	190	6	50	3	0	30	680	21	2	2	14	1 1/2 carb, 1 lean protein, 1/2 fat
Stuffed Grilled Taco	1	540	27	240	10	1	40	1320	58	1	3	18	4 carb, 1 med-fat protein, 4 fat
Taco Bravo	1	330	13	120	5	0	25	750	38	2	6	14	2 1/2 carb, 1 med-fat protein, 1 fat
Taco Burger	1	280	12	110	4.5	0.5	30	570	29	4	2	14	2 carb, 1 med-fat protein, 1 fat
Burritos													
Bean Burrito	1	370	11	100	5	0	10	1090	53	1	7	14	3 1/2 carb, 1/2 med-fat protein, 1 fat
Beef & Bean Combo Burrito	1	410	16	150	7	1	30	1120	47	1	5	18	3 carb, 1 med-fat protein, 2 fat
Beefy Burrito	1	440	21	190	9	1	45	1150	42	1	3	21	3 carb, 2 med-fat protein, 2 fat
Chicken & Potato Burrito	1	480	21	190	7	0	35	1590	56	2	4	18	3 1/2 carb, 1 med-fat protein, 2 1/2 fat

Crunchy Chicken & Potato Burrito	1	580	27	240	8	0	25	1670	67	2	4	18	4 1/2 carb, 1 med-fat protein, 3 1/2 fat
Grilled Burrito, Beef	1	590	32	290	14	1	55	1680	53	1	4	24	3 1/2 carb, 2 med-fat protein, 4 fat
Grilled Burrito, Chicken	1	590	30	270	12	1	70	1960	50	1	3	29	3 carb, 3 med-fat protein, 2 fat
Meat & Potato Burrito	1	520	25	230	8	0.5	30	1490	57	2	5	15	4 carb, 4 fat
Super Burrito	1	450	20	180	9	1	35	1190	50	2	6	19	3 carb, 1 med-fat protein, 2 fat
Specialties													
Chicken Taco Salad (No Dressing)	1	500	27	250	11	0	60	950	39	6	5	25	2 1/2 carb, 2 med-fat protein, 3 fat
Crunchy Chicken	1 order	370	18	160	3	0	40	920	29	0	0	22	2 carb, 2 med-fat protein, 1 fat
Crunchy Chicken Taco Salad (No Dressing)	1	630	36	320	12	0	50	1070	53	6	5	26	3 1/2 carb, 1 med-fat protein, 5 1/2 fat
Mexi Rolls (No Nacho Cheese)	4 pieces	550	21	190	9	1	45	800	61	1	9	28	4 carb, 2 med-fat protein, 1 fat

FAST FOOD

	Serving	Calories	Fat (g)	Cal. from Fat	Sat. Fat (g)	Trans Fat (g)	Chol. (mg)	Sod. (mg)	Carb. (g)	Sugar (g)	Fiber (g)	Prot. (g)	Servings/Exchanges
Quesadilla	1	450	24	220	12	1	55	1400	40	0	1	19	2 1/2 carb, 2 med-fat protein, 2 fat
Quesadilla with Chicken	1	520	25	230	12	1	75	1690	45	2	2	28	3 carb, 3 med-fat protein, 1 fat
Super Nachos	1 regular	790	47	430	15	1	55	1650	72	2	7	22	5 carb, 1 med-fat protein, 7 fat
Super Potato Olés	1 regular	1090	67	600	21	1	55	3300	98	3	14	24	6 1/2 carb, 1 med-fat protein, 11 fat
Taco Salad	1	540	33	300	13	1	50	820	40	6	6	22	2 1/2 carb, 2 med-fat protein, 4 fat
TJ Baja Boneless Wings, Bold Buffalo	1 order	410	22	200	3.5	0	40	1880	30	0	0	22	2 carb, 2 med-fat protein, 2 fat
Snacks & Sides													
Chips & Nacho Cheese	1 order	380	23	200	5	0	15	940	39	0	1	6	2 1/2 carb, 4 fat
Chips & Queso	1 order	430	25	220	6	0	20	1130	43	1	2	9	3 carb, 4 fat
Nacho Cheese	3 oz	110	9	80	3.5	0	15	520	5	0	0	3	2 fat

Item	Serving												Exchanges/Choices
Potato Olés	1 small	480	27	250	6	0	0	1380	52	1	6	5	3 1/2 carb, 5 fat
Refried Beans	1 order	320	7	70	4	0	10	1060	46	1	15	18	3 carb, 1 med-fat protein
Salad Dressing, House	1.5 oz	70	7	60	1	0	0	280	2	2	1	0	1 fat
Side Salad	1	40	2.5	20	1.5	0	5	50	3	2	1	2	1 vegetable, 1/2 fat
Desserts													
Churro	1	200	9	80	2.5	0	20	170	29	10	4	3	2 carb, 1 fat
Mexican Donut Bites	1 order	290	12	100	3	0	5	220	47	21	4	4	3 carb, 2 fat
Oreo Churro	1	280	10	90	2	0	0	280	45	20	2	3	3 carb, 1 fat
WENDY'S													
Breakfast													
Artisan Egg Sandwich	1	360	19	170	8	0	250	760	29	4	1	20	2 carb, 2 med-fat protein, 1 fat
Fresh Baked Biscuit	1	570	37	330	18	0	265	1350	38	5	2	20	2 1/2 carb, 2 med-fat protein, 5 fat
Honey Butter Biscuit	1	510	25	220	11	0	55	1400	52	9	2	21	3 1/2 carb, 1 med-fat protein, 3 fat

FAST FOOD

	Serving	Calories	Fat (g)	Cal. from Fat	Sat. Fat (g)	Trans Fat (g)	Chol. (mg)	Sod. (mg)	Carb. (g)	Sugar (g)	Fiber (g)	Prot. (g)	Servings/Exchanges
Mornin Melt Panini	1	520	33	290	17	1	285	800	33	3	1	30	2 carb, 3 med-fat protein, 3 fat
Oatmeal Bar	1	290	10	90	4.5	0	20	230	47	23	5	4	3 carb, 1 fat
Sausage Biscuit	1	460	29	260	14	2	45	1070	37	4	2	12	2 1/2 carb, 1 med-fat protein, 2 1/2 fat
Sausage Egg Burrito	1	280	20	180	7	0	210	770	14	3	1	12	1 carb, 1 med-fat protein, 3 fat
Steel Cut Oatmeal	1	330	12	100	1	0	0	250	57	33	4	5	4 carb, 2 fat
Burgers													
Baconator	1	930	62	560	24	3	205	1810	33	8	1	58	2 carb, 7 med-fat protein, 5 fat
Dave's Double	1	790	51	460	20	3	175	1460	35	8	2	48	2 carb, 6 med-fat protein, 4 fat
Dave's Single	1	550	34	300	13	1.5	100	1180	35	8	2	28	2 carb, 3 med-fat protein, 3 fat

Dave's Triple	1	1070	72	650	30	4	260	1930	36	9	2	70	2 1/2 carb, 9 med-fat protein, 5 fat
Double Stack	1	390	21	190	9	1.5	90	1070	25	5	1	25	1 1/2 carb, 3 med-fat protein, 1 fat
Jr. Bacon Cheeseburger	1	380	22	200	8	1	65	850	26	5	1	19	2 carb, 2 med-fat protein, 2 fat
Jr. Cheeseburger	1	280	13	120	6	0.5	50	820	25	5	1	16	1 1/2 carb, 2 med-fat protein
Jr. Cheeseburger Deluxe	1	330	19	170	7	1	55	810	27	6	2	16	2 carb, 1 med-fat protein, 2 fat
Jr. Hamburger	1	240	10	90	3.5	1	40	620	25	5	1	14	1 1/2 carb, 1 med-fat protein, 1 fat
Son of Baconator	1	620	39	360	15	1.5	130	1590	33	7	1	33	2 carb, 4 med-fat protein, 3 fat

Chicken, Wraps & More

Asiago Ranch Chicken Club	1	650	33	300	9	0	110	1550	50	6	3	37	3 carb, 4 med-fat protein, 2 fat
Chicken Nuggets, 4 Piece	1 order	180	13	110	2.5	0	30	390	10	0	1	10	1/2 carb, 1 med-fat protein, 1 1/2 fat

FAST FOOD

	Serving	Calories	Fat (g)	Cal. from Fat	Sat. Fat (g)	Trans Fat (g)	Chol. (mg)	Sod. (mg)	Carb. (g)	Sugar (g)	Fiber (g)	Prot. (g)	Servings/Exchanges
Chicken Nuggets, 6 Piece	1 order	270	19	170	4	0	20	580	15	0	1	14	1 carb, 2 med-fat protein, 2 fat
Chicken Nuggets, 10 Piece	1 order	450	32	290	7	0	80	960	26	0	2	24	2 carb, 3 med-fat protein, 3 fat
Crispy Chicken BLT	1	440	24	220	7	0	55	950	37	5	1	20	2 1/2 carb, 2 med-fat protein, 2 fat
Crispy Chicken Sandwich	1	350	17	150	3	0	35	600	35	4	1	15	2 carb, 1 med-fat protein, 2 fat
Grilled Chicken Sandwich	1	350	9	80	1.5	0	100	880	35	9	2	33	2 carb, 4 lean protein
Grilled Chicken Wrap	1	270	10	90	3.5	0	60	730	24	3	2	20	1 1/2 carb, 2 med-fat protein
Homestyle Chicken Sandwich	1	500	21	190	4	0	75	1140	48	5	2	28	3 carb, 3 med-fat protein, 1 fat
Spicy Chicken Sandwich	1	490	21	190	4	0	75	1060	46	5	1	28	3 carb, 3 med-fat protein, 1 fat

Spicy Chicken Wrap	1	370	19	170	5	0	50	840	30	2	2	18	2 carb, 2 med-fat protein, 1 fat
Ultimate Chicken Grill	1	340	8	80	1.5	0	105	930	34	7	1	32	2 carb, 4 lean protein

Fresh Made Salads (with Dressing)

Apple Pecan Chicken Salad	1 full	590	27	240	9	0.5	125	1350	52	40	7	37	3 1/2 carb, 4 med-fat protein, 1 fat
Asian Cashew Chicken Salad	1 full	380	14	120	2	0	100	1070	32	18	6	36	2 carb, 4 lean protein, 1 fat
BBQ Ranch Chicken Salad	1 full	600	30	270	9	0	150	1560	44	27	5	42	3 carb, 5 med-fat protein
Power Mediterranean Chicken Salad	1 full	430	14	130	4	0	115	1220	38	18	8	39	2 1/2 carb, 4 lean protein, 1 fat
Spicy Chicken Caesar Salad	1 full	790	51	460	16	1	140	1640	42	6	6	42	3 carb, 5 med-fat protein, 5 fat

Fries & Sides

Bacon Cheese Baked Potato	1	480	17	150	8	0	40	780	66	6	7	17	4 1/2 carb, 2 1/2 fat
Broccoli Cheese Baked Potato	1	430	11	100	6	0	25	570	70	7	10	15	4 1/2 carb, 1 fat

FAST FOOD

	Serving	Calories	Fat (g)	Cal. from Fat	Sat. Fat (g)	Trans Fat (g)	Chol. (mg)	Sod. (mg)	Carb. (g)	Sugar (g)	Fiber (g)	Prot. (g)	Servings/Exchanges
Caesar Side Salad with Dressing	1	250	18	160	4.5	0	25	460	18	2	3	7	1 carb, 1 med-fat protein, 2 fat
Garden Salad with Ranch Dressing	1	210	13	120	2	0	10	380	18	4	2	4	1 carb, 2 fat
Natural Cut Fries, Kids/Value	1 order	230	10	90	2	0	0	230	30	0	3	3	2 carb, 2 fat
Natural Cut Fries, Large	1 order	530	24	220	4.5	0	0	520	70	0	6	7	4 1/2 carb, 4 fat
Natural Cut Fries, Medium	1 order	420	19	170	3.5	0	0	420	56	0	5	6	3 1/2 carb, 3 fat
Natural Cut Fries, Small	1 order	320	15	130	2.5	0	0	320	43	0	4	5	3 carb, 2 fat
Rich & Meaty Chili	1 small	170	5	45	3	0	35	780	16	6	4	15	1 carb, 2 lean protein
Rich & Meaty Chili	1 large	250	7	60	3	0.5	50	1170	23	9	5	23	1 1/2 carb, 3 lean protein
Sour Cream & Chive Baked Potato	1	310	2.5	20	1.5	0	10	35	63	4	7	8	4 carb

Frosty

Chocolate Frosty, Jr.	1	200	5	45	3	0	20	90	32	27	0	5	2 carb, 1 fat
Chocolate Frosty, Large	1	580	15	130	9	0.5	60	270	96	79	1	16	6 1/2 carb, 2 fat
Chocolate Frosty, Medium	1	460	12	110	8	0.5	50	210	76	63	0	13	5 carb, 1 fat
Chocolate Frosty, Small	1	340	9	80	6	0	35	160	56	46	0	9	3 1/2 carb, 1 fat

FROZEN DINNERS, ENTRÉES, CHICKEN, FISH

	Serving	Calories	Fat (g)	Cal. from Fat	Sat. Fat (g)	Trans Fat (g)	Chol. (mg)	Sod. (mg)	Carb. (g)	Sugar (g)	Fiber (g)	Prot. (g)	Servings/Exchanges
FROZEN DINNERS, ENTRÉES													
Aunt Jemima Entrées													
Eggs & Bacon	1 entrée	300	20	180	6	0	340	910	14	3	1	15	1 carb, 2 med-fat protein, 2 fat
Ham & Cheese Omelet	1 entrée	250	14	126	6	0	265	810	19	4	1	13	1 carb, 1 med-fat protein, 2 fat
Pancakes & Bacon	1 entrée	450	17	153	4.5	0	65	1100	61	15	3	14	4 carb, 3 fat
Pancakes & Sausage	1 entrée	490	23	207	6	0	90	1000	58	17	1	14	4 carb, 5 fat
Sausage & Egg Scramble	1 entrée	300	18	162	5	0	200	890	21	3	2	15	1 1/2 carb, 2 med-fat protein, 2 fat
Banquet Meals													
All-American Patty & Fries	1 entrée	280	16	140	5	0	35	970	23	3	3	12	1 1/2 carb, 1 med-fat protein, 2 fat
Beef Pot Pie	1 pie	380	23	210	9	0.5	30	710	36	4	3	8	2 1/2 carb, 5 fat
Boneless Pork Riblet	1 entrée	370	14	120	4.5	0	50	1100	45	13	6	15	3 carb, 1 med-fat protein, 2 fat

Food	Serving												Exchanges/Choices
Cheesy Macaroni & Beef	1 entrée	230	9	80	3.5	0	20	800	27	4	2	9	2 carb, 2 fat
Chicken Fingers with Mac & Cheese	1 entrée	310	12	110	2.5	0	25	730	33	4	4	16	2 carb, 2 med-fat protein, 1 fat
Chicken Fried Chicken	1 entrée	330	14	120	3	0	20	1100	40	5	4	11	2 1/2 carb, 1 med-fat protein, 2 fat
Chicken Nugget with Fries	1 entrée	260	10	90	1.5	0	15	460	32	1	4	11	2 carb, 1 med-fat protein, 1 fat
Chicken Parmesan	1 entrée	320	11	100	2	0	20	630	41	5	5	14	2 1/2 carb, 1 med-fat protein, 1 fat
Chicken Pot Pie	1 pie	350	19	170	7	0	55	930	33	2	3	12	2 carb, 1 med-fat protein, 3 fat
Chicken Strips	1 entrée	440	19	170	4	0	35	1050	45	4	8	23	3 carb, 2 med-fat protein, 2 fat
Country Fried Beef Patty	1 entrée	400	21	190	6	0.5	40	1030	43	4	5	10	3 carb, 4 fat
Fettuccine Alfredo	1 entrée	300	12	110	5	0	20	690	36	2	4	10	2 1/2 carb, 1 med-fat protein, 1 fat
Fish Sticks with Mac & Cheese	1 entrée	260	9	80	2	0	20	640	33	11	4	2	2 carb, 2 fat

FROZEN DINNERS, ENTRÉES, CHICKEN, FISH

	Serving	Calories	Fat (g)	Cal. from Fat	Sat. Fat (g)	Trans Fat (g)	Chol. (mg)	Sod. (mg)	Carb. (g)	Sugar (g)	Fiber (g)	Prot. (g)	Servings/Exchanges
Homestyle Patty Meal	1 entrée	340	17	160	6	0	85	1040	32	2	4	15	2 carb, 1 med-fat protein, 2 fat
Lasagna with Meat Sauce	1 entrée	250	9	80	3	0	15	510	31	6	4	11	2 carb, 1 med-fat protein, 1 fat
Macaroni & Cheese	1 entrée	240	9	80	3	0	10	930	32	5	3	8	2 carb, 2 fat
Meatloaf	1 entrée	330	11	100	3.5	0	50	1350	43	11	5	13	3 carb, 1 med-fat protein, 1 fat
Pepper Steak	1 entrée	320	13	120	4	0	45	1110	39	2	3	12	2 1/2 carb, 1 med-fat protein, 2 fat
Pizza Meal	1 entrée	310	11	100	3	0	10	980	39	8	4	12	2 1/2 carb, 1 med-fat protein, 1 fat
Rigatoni & Italian Sausage	1 entrée	300	12	110	4	0	30	650	35	6	4	13	2 carb, 1 med-fat protein, 1 fat
Salisbury Steak Deep Dish	1 pie	400	23	210	8	0	30	780	40	4	4	9	2 1/2 carb, 1 med-fat protein, 4 fat
Salisbury Steak with Mashed Potatoes	1 entrée	350	14	120	4.5	0	55	1340	44	11	4	12	3 carb, 1 med-fat protein, 2 fat

Spaghetti & Chicken Nuggets	1 entrée	230	7	60	1.5	0	10	540	32	5	4	10	2 carb, 1 med-fat protein
Swedish Meatballs	1 entrée	360	19	170	7	0	100	640	31	1	3	16	2 carb, 2 med-fat protein, 2 fat
Sweet & Sour Chicken	1 entrée	420	10	90	1.5	0	15	520	70	24	4	11	4 1/2 carb, 2 fat
Turkey	1 entrée	280	11	100	3	0	45	1460	29	4	5	17	2 carb, 2 med-fat protein
Turkey Pot Pie	1 pie	320	18	160	6	0	40	740	31	3	2	10	2 carb, 1 med-fat protein, 3 fat
Boston Market													
BBQ Pork & Biscuits	1 entrée	480	18	160	10	0	60	1360	56	23	2	22	3 1/2 carb, 2 med-fat protein, 2 fat
Beef Pot Roast	1 entrée	340	9	80	4	0	65	1440	41	5	5	22	2 1/2 carb, 2 med-fat protein
Beef Steak & Pasta	1 entrée	470	14	130	6	0	80	970	52	3	2	30	3 1/2 carb, 3 med-fat protein
Boneless Pork Rib Shaped Patty	1 entrée	640	35	320	13	0	80	1560	56	20	4	24	3 1/2 carb, 2 med-fat protein, 5 fat

FROZEN DINNERS, ENTRÉES, CHICKEN, FISH

	Serving	Calories	Fat (g)	Cal. from Fat	Sat. Fat (g)	Trans Fat (g)	Chol. (mg)	Sod. (mg)	Carb. (g)	Sugar (g)	Fiber (g)	Prot. (g)	Servings/Exchanges
Buffalo Style Chicken Strips	1 entrée	510	22	200	6	0	35	1340	53	3	2	23	3 1/2 carb, 2 med-fat protein, 2 fat
Chicken Breast with BBQ Sauce	1 entrée	370	6	50	1.5	0	55	1300	59	27	3	20	4 carb, 1 med-fat protein
Chicken, Broccoli & Cheese Casserole	1 entrée	460	14	130	6	0	70	1050	56	3	2	27	3 1/2 carb, 2 med-fat protein, 1 fat
Chicken Fettuccine Alfredo	1 entrée	400	14	120	7	0	75	900	43	5	3	26	3 carb, 2 med-fat protein, 1 fat
Chicken Fritters & Mashed Potatoes	1 entrée	410	16	140	4	0	45	1650	45	4	2	22	3 carb, 2 med-fat protein, 1 fat
Chicken Parmesan	1 entrée	500	13	110	3	0	40	900	70	10	4	23	4 1/2 carb, 1 med-fat protein, 2 fat
Chicken Pot Pie	1 pie	450	30	260	13	1	15	380	35	4	2	10	2 carb, 1 med-fat protein, 5 fat
Chicken Primavera	1 entrée	480	15	130	7	0	80	1150	55	9	5	30	3 1/2 carb, 3 med-fat protein

Country Fried Beef Steak	1 entrée	520	29	260	12	1	80	1220	45	5	2	19	3 carb, 2 med-fat protein, 4 fat
Fried Chicken & Biscuit	1 entrée	550	30	270	15	0	65	2010	49	4	1	19	3 carb, 1 med-fat protein, 5 fat
Meatloaf	1 entrée	430	23	210	9	0.5	70	770	40	5	3	19	2 1/2 carb, 2 med-fat protein, 3 fat
Oven Roasted Chicken	1 entrée	280	7	60	2	0	55	1250	32	6	5	23	2 carb, 2 lean protein
Salisbury Steak	1 entrée	530	32	290	13	1	85	1410	38	4	3	26	2 1/2 carb, 3 med-fat protein, 3 fat
Spaghetti & Meatballs	1 entrée	600	25	230	9	0	60	1030	63	10	6	31	4 carb, 3 med-fat protein, 2 fat
Swedish Meatballs	1 entrée	570	26	230	10	0	60	1210	55	8	4	27	3 1/2 carb, 2 med-fat protein, 3 fat
Sweet & Sour Chicken	1 entrée	580	16	140	2	0	70	1710	91	34	3	19	6 carb, 3 fat
Turkey Breast Medallions	1 entrée	240	5	45	2.5	0	55	1410	28	3	4	21	2 carb, 2 lean protein

Eating Right

Cashew Chicken	1	270	5	45	1.5	0	25	700	43	11	2	14	3 carb, 1 med-fat protein

FROZEN DINNERS, ENTRÉES, CHICKEN, FISH

	Serving	Calories	Fat (g)	Cal. from Fat	Sat. Fat (g)	Trans Fat (g)	Chol. (mg)	Sod. (mg)	Carb. (g)	Sugar (g)	Fiber (g)	Prot. (g)	Servings/Exchanges
Cheese Ravioli	1	240	5	45	2.5	0	45	550	38	10	3	11	2 1/2 carb, 1 med-fat protein
Chicken Poblano	1	310	8	70	3	0	40	490	37	3	2	22	2 1/2 carb, 2 med-fat protein
Chicken Teriyaki	1	240	3.5	32	0.5	0	20	530	40	15	2	11	2 1/2 carb, 1 med-fat protein
Five Grain Beef & Vegetables	1	290	5	45	1	0	25	500	43	6	4	13	3 carb, 1 med-fat protein
Lemongrass Chicken	1	230	7	60	3	0	40	500	26	5	3	16	2 carb, 1 med-fat protein
Macaroni & Cheese	1	330	8	72	4.5	0	25	770	46	4	2	18	3 carb, 1 med-fat protein, 1 fat
Roasted Turkey	1	320	9	81	2	0	55	790	40	11	3	21	2 1/2 carb, 2 med-fat protein
Spaghetti with Meat Sauce	1	330	9	80	3	0	15	800	47	7	4	14	3 carb, 1 med-fat protein, 1 fat

Turkey Lasagna	1	230	3	27	1.5	0	20	720	36	7	3	14	2 1/2 carb, 1 lean protein
Green Giant Create A Meal													
Stir-Fry Lo Mein	21 oz bag	510	4.5	30	0	0	0	2550	102	27	9	18	7 carb, 1 fat
Green Giant Complete Skillet Meal													
Cheesy Macaroni & Beef	1/4 cup	270	6	54	3	0	30	740	38	5	4	17	2 1/2 carb, 1 med-fat protein
Chicken Alfredo	1/4 cup	186	4	35	2	0	10	593	27	6	6	10	2 carb
Mexican Style Rice & Beef	1/4 cup	260	6	54	2	0	20	940	43	5	2	9	3 carb, 1 fat
Pasta Primavera	1/4 cup	270	40	4.5	2	0	25	700	42	6	4	17	3 carb, 1 med-fat protein, 7 fat
Healthy Choice Simply Café Steamers													
Beef and Broccoli	1 meal	270	6	60	2	0	40	580	34	6	3	20	2 carb, 2 lean protein
Chicken Fried Rice	1 meal	320	7	60	1.5	0	85	580	43	9	4	22	3 carb, 2 lean protein
Chicken Pasta Primavera	1 meal	220	2.5	25	0.5	0	40	390	29	8	5	20	2 carb, 2 lean protein

FROZEN DINNERS, ENTRÉES, CHICKEN, FISH

	Serving	Calories	Fat (g)	Cal. from Fat	Sat. Fat (g)	Trans Fat (g)	Chol. (mg)	Sod. (mg)	Carb. (g)	Sugar (g)	Fiber (g)	Prot. (g)	Servings/Exchanges
Chicken & Vegetable Stir Fry	1 meal	190	4	35	1	0	75	500	15	8	4	22	1 carb, 2 lean protein
Grilled Chicken & Broccoli Alfredo	1 meal	190	6	60	2.5	0	85	600	8	2	4	27	1/2 carb, 4 lean protein
Grilled Chicken Pesto & Vegetables	1 meal	200	6	60	2.5	0	85	600	11	3	5	27	1 carb, 3 lean protein
Lemon Herb Chicken	1 meal	260	5	45	2	0	40	550	33	3	5	20	2 carb, 2 lean protein
Meatball Marinara	1 meal	280	6	50	2	0	35	500	39	8	6	18	2 1/2 carb, 2 lean protein
Southwestern Style Chicken	1 meal	200	3	25	0.5	0	75	500	20	6	6	23	1 carb, 3 lean protein
Healthy Choice Café Steamers													
Balsamic Garlic Chicken	1 meal	250	5	45	1	0	30	600	34	7	6	18	2 carb, 2 lean protein
Barbecue Seasoned Steak with Red Potatoes	1 meal	260	3.5	30	1	0	35	470	39	18	6	17	2 1/2 carb, 1 lean protein

Beef Teriyaki	1 meal	270	5	45	1.5	0	25	600	39	14	5	16	2 1/2 carb, 1 med-fat protein
Chicken Fettuccini Alfredo	1 meal	280	2.5	70	2.5	0	45	580	31	2	6	21	2 carb, 2 lean protein
Chicken Linguini with Red Pepper Alfredo	1 meal	250	6	50	2	0	40	520	27	3	6	21	2 carb, 2 lean protein
Chicken Margherita with Balsamic	1 meal	280	7	60	1.5	0	35	530	36	9	4	19	2 1/2 carb, 2 lean protein
Chicken & Noodles	1 meal	270	8	70	2	0	60	590	29	3	4	19	2 carb, 2 med-fat protein
Chicken & Potatoes with BBQ Sauce	1 meal	250	3.5	30	0.5	0	35	1040	40	20	5	15	2 1/2 carb, 1 med-fat protein
Crustless Chicken Pot Pie	1 meal	280	8	70	2	0	65	600	34	3	7	19	2 carb, 2 med-fat protein
Four Cheese Ravioli & Chicken Marinara	1 meal	270	6	60	2.5	0	45	600	34	11	7	19	2 carb, 2 lean protein
General Tso's Spicy Chicken	1 meal	290	3.5	30	1	0	25	580	47	11	4	16	3 carb, 1 med-fat protein
Grilled Chicken Marinara with Parmesan	1 meal	270	6	60	2	0	25	580	31	7	6	21	2 carb, 2 lean protein

FROZEN DINNERS, ENTRÉES, CHICKEN, FISH

	Serving	Calories	Fat (g)	Cal. from Fat	Sat. Fat (g)	Trans Fat (g)	Chol. (mg)	Sod. (mg)	Carb. (g)	Sugar (g)	Fiber (g)	Prot. (g)	Servings/Exchanges
Grilled Chicken Marsala with Mushrooms	1 meal	250	7	60	1.5	0	30	550	30	6	6	18	2 carb, 2 lean protein
Grilled Chicken Pesto with Vegetables	1 meal	300	7	70	2	0	35	590	36	2	4	22	2 1/2 carb, 2 lean protein
Honey Balsamic Chicken	1 meal	210	4.5	40	1	0	25	500	29	10	7	14	2 carb, 1 med-fat protein
Honey Glazed Turkey & Potatoes	1 meal	220	2	15	0.5	0	20	500	37	9	8	14	2 1/2 carb, 1 lean protein
Spaghetti & Meatballs	1 meal	300	7	70	2.5	0	20	400	40	5	5	19	2 1/2 carb, 2 lean protein
Sweet Sesame Chicken	1 meal	280	7	70	1.5	0	60	520	31	23	5	21	2 carb, 2 lean protein
Sweet & Sour Chicken	1 meal	350	3.5	30	0.5	0	25	590	68	22	3	12	4 1/2 carb, 1 fat
Healthy Choice Whole Grain Café Steamers													
Grilled Basil Chicken	1 meal	240	5	45	1.5	0	30	550	30	3	5	17	2 carb, 2 lean protein
Kung Pao Chicken	1 meal	280	4.5	40	1	0	40	550	41	11	4	17	2 1/2 carb, 1 med-fat protein

Food	Serving											Exchanges
Pineapple Chicken	1 meal	310	5	45	1	0	30	510	49	21	5	16	3 carb, 1 med-fat protein
Sweet & Spicy Orange Zest Chicken	1 meal	320	5	45	1	0	40	500	49	16	6	18	3 carb, 1 med-fat protein
Healthy Choice Meals													
Beef Pot Roast	1 meal	260	7	60	2.5	0	45	570	32	14	4	18	2 carb, 1 med-fat protein
Beef Strips Portabella	1 meal	280	7	70	2.5	0	50	500	33	15	5	19	2 carb, 2 lean protein
Chicken Parmigiana	1 meal	330	10	90	2	0	30	560	43	13	6	17	3 carb, 1 med-fat protein, 1 fat
Classic Meatloaf	1 meal	280	5	50	2	0	30	550	42	13	6	15	3 carb, 1 med-fat protein
Country Fried Chicken	1 meal	340	8	70	2	0	25	600	52	16	5	15	3 1/2 carb, 1 med-fat protein, 1 fat
Country Herb Chicken	1 meal	280	5	50	2	0	45	470	39	15	5	18	2 1/2 carb, 2 lean protein
Four Cheese Tortellini	1 meal	300	6	60	3	0	20	560	45	9	9	15	3 carb, 1 med-fat protein

FROZEN DINNERS, ENTRÉES, CHICKEN, FISH

	Serving	Calories	Fat (g)	Cal. from Fat	Sat. Fat (g)	Trans Fat (g)	Chol. (mg)	Sod. (mg)	Carb. (g)	Sugar (g)	Fiber (g)	Prot. (g)	Servings/Exchanges
Golden Roast Turkey Breast	1 meal	260	4.5	45	1	0	30	500	35	16	8	18	2 carb, 2 lean protein
Herb Crusted Fish	1 meal	270	5	45	1.5	0	25	370	40	8	5	16	2 1/2 carb, 1 med-fat protein
Homestyle Salisbury Steak	1 meal	240	4.5	40	2	0	30	560	33	12	6	16	2 carb, 1 med-fat protein
Lemon Pepper Fish	1 meal	340	4	40	1	0	25	530	59	17	4	16	4 carb, 1 fat
Oven Roasted Chicken	1 meal	240	5	45	1.5	0	55	560	30	10	4	18	2 carb, 2 lean protein
Jimmy Dean													
Bacon, Egg, Cheese Biscuit	1	410	24	220	10	0	340	1230	19	0	2	28	1 carb, 3 med-fat protein, 2 fat
Eggs, Potato, Ham Breakfast Bowl	1	340	19	170	8	0	315	810	20	1	2	21	1 carb, 3 med-fat protein, 1 fat
Pancakes & Sausage on a Stick	1	230	12	110	3.5	0	25	480	22	9	1	6	1 1/2 carb, 2 fat
Sausage Biscuit	1	320	22	200	9	0	25	620	24	3	2	7	1 1/2 carb, 4 fat

Kashi

Amaranth Polenta Plantain Bowl	1	340	9	80	1	0	0	390	59	19	7	9	4 carb, 2 fat
Black Bean Mango	1	330	9	80	1	0	0	270	56	12	11	10	4 carb, 2 fat
Chimichurri Quinoa Bowl	1	260	8	70	1.5	0	0	350	42	5	10	10	3 carb, 2 fat
Sweet Potato Quinoa Bowl	1	300	8	80	1.5	0	0	440	50	9	7	9	3 carb, 2 fat

Lean Cuisine—American

Apple Cranberry Chicken	1 meal	280	4	30	1	0	30	470	48	23	5	14	3 carb, 1 med-fat protein
Baked Chicken	1 meal	250	6	50	2	0	30	600	34	5	2	14	2 carb, 1 med-fat protein
Cheddar Potatoes with Broccoli	1 meal	220	3	30	2	0	10	670	38	5	4	9	2 1/2 carb, 1 fat
Chicken with Almonds	1 meal	290	5	45	0	0	25	490	44	8	4	16	3 carb, 1 med-fat protein
Chicken Carbonara	1 meal	240	6	50	1	0	30	660	29	4	2	18	2 carb, 1 med-fat protein

FROZEN DINNERS, ENTRÉES, CHICKEN, FISH

	Serving	Calories	Fat (g)	Cal. from Fat	Sat. Fat (g)	Trans Fat (g)	Chol. (mg)	Sod. (mg)	Carb. (g)	Sugar (g)	Fiber (g)	Prot. (g)	Servings/Exchanges
Chicken Club Panini	1 meal	350	9	80	3	0	40	680	45	6	4	23	3 carb, 2 med-fat protein
Chicken Parmesan	1 meal	310	4	80	2	0	30	660	39	10	1	18	2 1/2 carb, 2 lean protein
Chicken Ranch Club Flatbread Melt	1 meal	370	9	80	3	0	30	530	52	9	4	21	3 1/2 carb, 2 med-fat protein
Chicken in Sweet BBQ Sauce	1 meal	280	8	70	3	0	40	710	20	14	3	20	1 carb, 2 med-fat protein
Glazed Chicken	1 meal	250	4	40	1	0	35	470	31	7	2	22	2 carb, 2 lean protein
Glazed Turkey Tenderloins	1 meal	270	5	45	1	0	25	530	41	19	3	14	2 1/2 carb, 1 med-fat protein
Macaroni & Cheese	1 meal	300	6	50	4	0	20	560	48	5	2	13	3 carb, 1 med-fat protein
Pepperoni Pizza	1 meal	390	9	80	3	0	25	580	58	6	3	20	4 carb, 1 med-fat protein, 1 fat
Roasted Chicken & Garden Vegetables	1 meal	220	4	35	1	0	25	620	31	6	5	16	2 carb, 1 med-fat protein

Roasted Turkey & Vegetables	1 meal	190	6	50	1	0	30	580	18	10	4	15	1 carb, 2 lean protein
Southwest-Style Chicken Panini	1 meal	320	8	70	3	0	30	500	43	6	6	20	3 carb, 2 med-fat protein
Supreme Pizza	1 meal	340	8	70	3	0	20	470	50	7	4	16	3 carb, 1 med-fat protein, 1 fat
Wood Fire–Style Margherita Pizza	1 meal	320	7	60	3	0	15	525	48	7	3	16	3 carb, 1 med-fat protein
Lean Cuisine—Asian													
Asian-Style Pot Stickers	1 meal	280	4	35	1	0	15	530	52	9	3	9	3 1/2 carb, 1 fat
Chicken with Peanut Sauce	1 meal	290	7	25	1	0	25	600	35	11	4	21	2 carb, 2 lean protein
Fajita-Style Chicken Spring Rolls	1 meal	220	8	70	1	0	22	470	22	3	2	15	1 1/2 carb, 2 med-fat protein
Garlic Chicken Spring Rolls	1 meal	210	7	60	1	0	20	430	25	4	2	11	1 1/2 carb, 1 med-fat protein
Ginger Garlic Stir Fry with Chicken	1 meal	290	3	30	1	0	30	630	48	17	5	17	3 carb, 1 lean protein

FROZEN DINNERS, ENTRÉES, CHICKEN, FISH

	Serving	Calories	Fat (g)	Cal. from Fat	Sat. Fat (g)	Trans Fat (g)	Chol. (mg)	Sod. (mg)	Carb. (g)	Sugar (g)	Fiber (g)	Prot. (g)	Servings/Exchanges
Orange Chicken	1 meal	310	8	70	1	0	20	690	46	13	2	14	3 carb, 1 med-fat protein, 1 fat
Sesame Chicken	1 meal	330	9	80	1	0	25	650	48	15	3	14	3 carb, 1 med-fat protein, 1 fat
Sesame Stir Fry with Chicken	1 meal	280	5	40	1	0	40	650	38	13	6	21	2 1/2 carb, 2 lean protein
Sweet & Sour Chicken	1 meal	300	2	25	0	0	30	550	54	20	1	16	3 1/2 carb, 1 lean protein
Sweet & Spicy Korean-Style Beef	1 meal	320	7	60	2	0	35	650	50	15	3	15	3 carb, 1 med-fat protein
Thai-Style Chicken Spring Rolls	1 meal	190	7	60	1	0	25	390	22	4	1	10	1 1/2 carb, 1 med-fat protein
Vegetable Eggroll	1 meal	300	4	35	2	0	0	550	59	13	3	7	4 carb, 1 fat
Lean Cuisine—Italian													
Alfredo Pasta with Chicken & Broccoli	1 meal	280	4	35	2	0	30	600	45	4	2	17	3 carb, 1 med-fat protein

Food	Serving												Exchanges
Angel Hair Pomondoro	1 meal	220	3	30	1	0	5	550	39	9	4	8	2 1/2 carb, 1 fat
Cheese Ravioli	1 meal	250	6	50	3	0	30	620	40	10	3	10	2 1/2 carb, 1 fat
Chicken Fettuccini	1 meal	280	5	45	2	0	30	600	43	3	3	15	3 carb, 1 med-fat protein
Classic Five Cheese Lasagna	1 meal	350	7	60	3	0	20	620	51	11	4	20	3 1/2 carb, 1 med-fat protein
Fettuccini Alfredo	1 meal	260	5	45	2	0	10	570	45	3	2	9	3 carb, 1 fat
Five Cheese Rigatoni	1 meal	360	8	70	4	0	15	560	56	7	4	15	3 1/2 carb, 1 med-fat protein, 1 fat
Four Cheese Cannelloni	1 meal	230	6	50	3	0	30	690	33	11	3	11	2 carb, 1 med-fat protein
French Bread Pepperoni Pizza	1 meal	310	7	60	2	0	15	700	46	4	3	15	3 carb, 1 med-fat protein
French Bread Supreme Pizza	1 meal	330	7	60	2	0	19	730	49	5	3	17	3 carb, 1 med-fat protein
Lasagna with Meat Sauce	1 meal	320	8	70	4	0	25	650	45	9	4	18	3 carb, 1 med-fat protein, 1 fat
Pasta Romano with Bacon	1 meal	260	5	45	1	0	10	600	42	9	3	12	3 carb, 1 fat

FROZEN DINNERS, ENTRÉES, CHICKEN, FISH

	Serving	Calories	Fat (g)	Cal. from Fat	Sat. Fat (g)	Trans Fat (g)	Chol. (mg)	Sod. (mg)	Carb. (g)	Sugar (g)	Fiber (g)	Prot. (g)	Servings/Exchanges
Spaghetti with Meat Sauce	1 meal	310	4	35	1	0	10	520	53	8	4	15	3 1/2 carb, 1 med-fat protein
Lean Cuisine—Mediterranean													
Butternut Squash Ravioli	1 meal	260	7	60	2	0	20	580	40	11	5	9	2 1/2 carb, 1 fat
Grilled Chicken Caesar	1 meal	230	6	50	2	0	30	550	25	2	3	18	1 1/2 carb, 2 lean protein
Lemon Chicken	1 meal	270	7	60	1	0	25	560	40	9	2	11	2 1/2 carb, 1 med-fat protein
Lemon Pepper Fish	1 meal	310	8	70	2	0	25	550	46	4	2	13	3 carb, 1 med-fat protein, 1 fat
Parmesan Crusted Fish	1 meal	290	7	60	1	0	25	570	42	8	3	15	3 carb, 1 med-fat protein
Salmon with Basil	1 meal	250	2	25	0	0	20	500	38	6	4	19	2 1/2 carb, 2 lean protein
Steak Portabella	1 meal	160	3	30	1	0	25	610	16	3	3	15	1 carb, 2 lean protein

Lean Cuisine—Mexican

Cheese & Fire-Roasted Chile Tamale	1 meal	330	9	80	3	0	10	580	55	10	5	8	3 1/2 carb, 2 fat
Chicken Enchilada Suiza	1 meal	280	4	35	2	0	20	520	51	7	3	10	3 1/2 carb, 1 fat
Ranchero Braised Beef	1 meal	250	6	30	2	0	30	570	33	22	2	15	2 carb, 1 med-fat protein
Spicy Beef & Bean Enchilada	1 meal	300	6	50	2	0	15	680	50	9	5	11	3 carb, 1 fat
Tortilla Crusted Fish	1 meal	300	9	30	2	0	30	490	41	6	2	14	2 1/2 carb, 1 med-fat protein, 1 fat

Marie Callender's Meals

Cheesy Chicken Breast & Rice	1	380	12	110	5	0	55	900	45	4	4	22	3 carb, 2 med-fat protein
Chicken Parmigiana	1	530	27	220	7	0	40	710	47	5	7	25	3 carb, 2 med-fat protein, 3 fat
Chunky Chicken & Noodles	1	440	18	160	6	0	65	1150	46	3	4	23	3 carb, 2 med-fat protein, 2 fat
Country Fried Beef Steak & Gravy	1	660	31	280	10	0.5	50	1220	75	5	7	20	5 carb, 1 med-fat protein, 5 fat

FROZEN DINNERS, ENTRÉES, CHICKEN, FISH

	Serving	Calories	Fat (g)	Cal. from Fat	Sat. Fat (g)	Trans Fat (g)	Chol. (mg)	Sod. (mg)	Carb. (g)	Sugar (g)	Fiber (g)	Prot. (g)	Servings/Exchanges
Country Fried Chicken & Gravy	1	560	27	240	8	0	50	1020	61	3	6	20	4 carb, 1 med-fat protein, 4 fat
Country Fried Pork Chop	1	460	19	170	5	0	40	1060	55	12	6	17	3 1/2 carb, 1 med-fat protein, 3 fat
Creamy Chicken & Shrimp Parmesan	1	420	14	130	6	0	75	1040	75	1	5	26	5 carb, 2 med-fat protein, 1 fat
Fettuccini Alfredo & Garlic Bread	1	610	31	280	13	0.5	45	1080	59	3	9	23	4 carb, 2 med-fat protein, 4 fat
Golden Battered Fish Fillet	1	410	11	100	3	0	35	1260	58	6	4	19	4 carb, 1 med-fat protein, 1 fat
Grilled Chicken Alfredo Bake	1	480	21	190	8	0.5	60	900	45	4	6	28	3 carb, 3 med-fat protein, 1 fat
Herb Roasted Chicken	1	470	17	160	5	0	135	680	46	3	5	32	3 carb, 3 med-fat protein
Meatloaf & Gravy	1	450	17	160	7	0	55	1400	43	2	8	31	3 carb, 3 med-fat protein

Roasted Turkey Breast & Stuffing	1	320	8	70	2	0	35	990	37	2	6	24	2 1/2 carb, 2 med-fat protein
Salisbury Steak	1	420	19	170	8	0.5	55	1100	39	2	5	23	2 1/2 carb, 2 med-fat protein, 2 fat
Spaghetti & Meatballs	1	420	13	120	4.5	0	35	770	52	4	8	23	3 1/2 carb, 2 med-fat protein, 1 fat
Steak & Roasted Potatoes	1	350	11	100	4	0	45	930	40	4	6	22	2 1/2 carb, 2 med-fat protein
Sweet & Sour Chicken	1	560	13	120	2	0	15	500	93	33	5	16	6 carb, 3 fat
Three Meat & Four Cheese Lasagna	1	280	11	100	5	0	30	860	30	6	4	14	2 carb, 1 med-fat protein, 1 fat
Michael Angelo's												
Chicken Alfredo	11 oz	410	12	110	7	0	70	690	47	1	2	28	3 carb, 3 lean protein
Eggplant Parmesan	11 oz	430	28	250	9	0	110	760	26	7	6	21	2 carb, 2 med-fat protein, 4 fat
Lasagna with Meat Sauce	11 oz	420	13	120	7	0	75	760	51	8	4	27	3 1/2 carb, 2 med-fat protein, 1 fat
Vegetable Lasagna	11 oz	390	15	130	7	0	50	760	44	10	5	23	3 carb, 2 med-fat protein, 1 fat

FROZEN DINNERS, ENTRÉES, CHICKEN, FISH

	Serving	Calories	Fat (g)	Cal. from Fat	Sat. Fat (g)	Trans Fat (g)	Chol. (mg)	Sod. (mg)	Carb. (g)	Sugar (g)	Fiber (g)	Prot. (g)	Servings/Exchanges
Michellina's Budget Gourmet													
Buffalo-Style Chicken Snackers	11 snacks	200	7	70	1.5	0	10	500	25	2	1	9	1 1/2 carb, 1 med-fat protein
Chicken Fried Rice	1	410	11	100	2.5	0	35	1140	65	2	2	12	4 carb, 2 fat
Fettuccine Alfredo	1	300	10	90	6	0	30	630	43	3	2	11	3 carb, 2 fat
Lasagna Alfredo with Broccoli	1	280	10	90	6	0	35	650	36	3	2	11	2 1/2 carb, 1 med-fat protein, 1 fat
Lasagna with Meat Sauce	1	240	7	60	2.5	0	15	680	34	5	3	10	2 carb, 1 med-fat protein
Macaroni & Cheese	1	310	12	110	4.5	0	20	660	40	2	2	12	2 1/2 carb, 2 fat
Spaghetti Marinara	1	230	3	25	0.5	0	0	440	45	5	3	8	3 carb, 1 fat
Spaghetti & Meatballs	1	290	8	70	2.5	0	15	720	42	7	3	13	3 carb, 1 med-fat protein, 1 fat
Sriracha Chicken & Pasta	1	290	3.5	30	0.5	0	10	780	53	7	2	13	3 1/2 carb, 1 fat
Stuffed Cheese Rigatoni	1	230	5	50	2.5	0	30	540	36	7	3	8	2 1/2 carb, 1 fat

Sweet & Sour Chicken	1	330	3	25	0.5	0	15	620	66	17	1	10	4 1/2 carb, 1 fat
Teriyaki Chicken	1	310	3	30	0.5	0	10	830	60	10	1	10	4 carb, 1 fat
Michelina's Lean Gourmet													
Beef & Peppers	1	280	5	45	1.5	0	10	780	48	4	2	10	3 carb, 1 fat
Beef Supreme	1	290	8	80	3	0	20	890	37	3	2	13	2 1/2 carb, 1 med-fat protein, 1 fat
Buffalo-Style Chicken Snackers	11 snacks	200	7	70	1.5	0	10	500	25	2	1	9	1 1/2 carb, 1 med-fat protein
Chicken Alfredo Florentine	1	260	7	60	3.5	0	35	730	36	3	1	13	2 1/2 carb, 1 med-fat protein
Creamy Rigatoni with Broccoli & Chicken	1	260	8	70	3.5	0	30	630	34	2	2	13	2 carb, 1 med-fat protein, 1 fat
Enchilada Bake	1	310	8	70	2.5	0.5	15	770	47	4	6	12	3 carb, 1 med-fat protein, 1 fat
Five Cheese Lasgna	1	280	5	45	2.5	0	10	560	42	6	4	13	3 carb, 1 med-fat protein
Penne Primavera	1	260	6	50	3.5	0	15	490	40	2	2	10	2 1/2 carb, 1 fat
Pepperoni Pizza Snackers	11 snacks	200	8	70	1.5	0	10	290	26	3	2	7	2 carb, 2 fat

FROZEN DINNERS, ENTRÉES, CHICKEN, FISH

	Serving	Calories	Fat (g)	Cal. from Fat	Sat. Fat (g)	Trans Fat (g)	Chol. (mg)	Sod. (mg)	Carb. (g)	Sugar (g)	Fiber (g)	Prot. (g)	Servings/Exchanges
Salisbury Steak	1	180	3	60	3	0	20	690	21	2	2	8	1 1/2 carb, 1 lean protein
Sante Fe Style Rice & Beans	1	300	8	70	3	0	20	630	49	2	3	11	3 carb, 2 fat
Sesame Chicken	1	260	3.5	30	0.5	0	15	590	46	12	2	12	3 carb, 1 med-fat protein
Southwestern-Style Mac 'n' Cheese	1	250	3	50	3	0	25	550	35	3	2	14	2 carb, 1 med-fat protein
Spaghetti & Meat Sauce	1	330	8	70	2.5	0	15	620	50	6	3	13	3 carb, 1 med-fat protein, 1 fat
Swedish Meatballs	1	310	8	70	3.5	0	25	650	43	5	2	14	3 carb, 1 med-fat protein, 1 fat
Teriyaki Chicken	1	330	6	50	1	0	15	840	59	11	1	11	4 carb, 1 fat
Michellina's Authentico													
Chicken Fried Rice	1	410	11	100	2.5	0	35	1140	65	2	2	12	4 carb, 1 med-fat protein, 1 fat

Fettucine Alfredo	1	300	10	90	6	0	30	630	43	3	2	11	3 carb, 2 fat
Five-Cheese Ziti	1	270	7	60	2.5	0	10	670	42	4	3	10	3 carb, 1 fat
Four Cheese Lasagna	1	270	6	60	3	0	15	520	42	4	3	11	3 carb, 1 fat
Macaroni & Cheese Bake	1	310	12	110	4.5	0	20	660	40	2	2	10	2 1/2 carb, 1 med-fat protein, 1 fat
Orange Chicken	1	280	2.5	20	0	0	10	580	55	9	1	9	3 1/2 carb, 1 fat
Pasta & Chicken	1	290	10	90	4	0	30	830	39	4	2	12	2 1/2 carb, 1 med-fat protein, 1 fat
Penne with Chicken	1	290	9	80	4	0	30	560	40	2	2	13	2 1/2 carb, 1 med-fat protein, 1 fat
Spaghetti with Meat Sauce	1	270	6	50	1.5	0	10	760	44	6	3	10	3 carb, 1 fat
Sriracha Chicken & Pasta	1	290	3.5	30	0.5	0	10	780	53	7	2	13	3 1/2 carb, 1 fat
Sweet & Sour Chicken	1	330	3	25	0.5	0	15	620	66	17	1	10	4 1/2 carb, 1 fat
Vegetable & Rice Stir Fry	1	460	20	180	4	0	10	850	62	2	2	8	4 carb, 4 fat
Wheels & Cheese	1	320	12	100	4.5	0	25	650	44	2	2	11	3 carb, 2 fat

FROZEN DINNERS, ENTRÉES, CHICKEN, FISH

	Serving	Calories	Fat (g)	Cal. from Fat	Sat. Fat (g)	Trans Fat (g)	Chol. (mg)	Sod. (mg)	Carb. (g)	Sugar (g)	Fiber (g)	Prot. (g)	Servings/Exchanges
Red Baron													
Biscuit Style Bacon Scramblers	1	440	21	190	11	0	100	890	47	10	1	17	3 carb, 1 med-fat protein, 3 fat
Biscuit Style Sausage Scramblers	1	430	20	180	9	0	60	740	47	11	2	16	3 carb, 1 med-fat protein, 3 fat
Stouffer's													
Baked Chicken Breast	1	240	8	70	3	0	75	760	17	1	1	24	1 carb, 3 lean protein
Beef Pot Roast	1	320	8	70	3	0	30	1570	41	9	8	20	2 1/2 carb, 2 med-fat protein
Beef Stroganoff	1	380	17	150	5	0	70	990	34	4	2	22	2 carb, 2 med-fat protein, 1 fat
Chicken in BBQ Sauce	1	430	19	170	6	0	70	1120	42	17	3	23	3 carb, 2 med-fat protein, 2 fat
Chicken Fettuccini Alfredo	1	840	38	340	13	0	75	1050	94	3	5	31	6 carb, 2 med-fat protein, 6 fat

Escalloped Chicken & Noodles	1	450	22	200	4	0	65	940	43	7	5	19	3 carb, 1 med-fat protein, 3 fat
Fish Filet with Macaroni & Cheese	1	400	19	170	5	0	55	800	35	2	1	22	2 carb, 2 med-fat protein, 2 fat
Fried Chicken Breast	1	340	16	140	4.5	0	60	810	28	1	1	20	2 carb, 2 med-fat protein, 1 fat
Grandma's Chicken & Vegetable Rice Bake	1	330	14	130	5	0	45	740	34	4	1	17	2 carb, 2 med-fat protein, 1 fat
Green Pepper Steak	1	240	4	35	1.5	0	30	910	32	5	3	18	2 carb, 2 lean protein
Lasagna with Meat Sauce	1	350	10	90	4	0	30	960	49	11	5	17	3 carb, 1 med-fat protein, 1 fat
Macaroni & Beef	1	410	16	140	7	0	40	990	45	12	4	22	3 carb, 2 med-fat protein, 1 fat
Macaroni & Cheese with Broccoli	1	480	20	180	8	0	35	1000	52	8	5	22	3 1/2 carb, 2 med-fat protein, 2 fat
Meatloaf	1	530	26	230	12	0	95	1280	40	7	4	33	2 1/2 carb, 4 med-fat protein, 1 fat
Monterey Chicken	1	530	21	190	6	0	80	1300	54	19	5	31	3 1/2 carb, 3 med-fat protein, 1 fat

FROZEN DINNERS, ENTRÉES, CHICKEN, FISH

	Serving	Calories	Fat (g)	Cal. from Fat	Sat. Fat (g)	Trans Fat (g)	Chol. (mg)	Sod. (mg)	Carb. (g)	Sugar (g)	Fiber (g)	Prot. (g)	Servings/Exchanges
Rigatoni Pasta in Pesto Sauce	1	400	15	140	5	0	40	770	44	2	3	22	3 carb, 2 med-fat protein, 1 fat
Roast Turkey Breast	1	440	16	140	6	0	25	1320	47	4	4	26	3 carb, 2 med-fat protein, 1 fat
Salisbury Steak	1	630	34	310	34	14	0	1540	41	6	3	39	2 1/2 carb, 4 med-fat protein, 3 fat
Sausage & Egg Scramble	1	360	20	180	9	0	200	780	21	4	3	26	1 1/2 carb, 3 med-fat protein, 1 fat
Smoked Turkey Club Panini	1	380	15	140	6	0	55	870	37	3	4	24	2 1/2 carb, 2 med-fat protein, 1 fat
Spaghetti with Meatballs	1	360	12	110	3.5	0	35	850	45	9	6	19	3 carb, 1 med-fat protein, 1 fat
Spinach Soufflé	1	150	10	90	2	0	110	390	9	4	1	6	1/2 carb, 1 med-fat protein, 1 fat
Stuffed Green Pepper	1	210	9	80	3	0	15	990	23	9	3	10	1 1/2 carb, 1 med-fat protein, 1 fat

Three Cheese and Ham Panini	1	420	18	160	8	0	60	940	42	5	4	22	3 carb, 2 med-fat protein, 2 fat
Tuna Noodle Casserole	1	450	20	180	6	0	70	990	45	3	3	22	3 carb, 2 med-fat protein, 2 fat
White Meat Chicken Pot Pie	1	590	34	310	13	0	50	930	54	10	1	19	3 1/2 carb, 1 med-fat protein, 6 fat

Stouffer's Easy Express Skillets

Garlic Chicken	1	330	5	45	0	0	40	870	48	6	5	23	3 carb, 2 lean protein
Grilled Chicken & Vegetables	1	370	9	80	0	0	45	740	46	6	4	25	3 carb, 2 med-fat protein
Savory Chicken & Rice	1	300	6	50	1.5	0	45	880	44	3	3	21	3 carb, 2 lean protein
Teriyaki Chicken	1	310	3	25	0	0	30	740	54	10	0	17	3 1/2 carb, 1 lean protein

Swanson Hungry-Man

Beer Battered Chicken	1	760	34	307	8	0	105	1640	74	20	6	32	5 carb, 2 med-fat protein, 5 fat
Boneless Fried Chicken	1	820	39	351	12	0	75	1130	86	22	5	32	5 1/2 carb, 2 med-fat protein, 6 fat

FROZEN DINNERS, ENTRÉES, CHICKEN, FISH

	Serving	Calories	Fat (g)	Cal. from Fat	Sat. Fat (g)	Trans Fat (g)	Chol. (mg)	Sod. (mg)	Carb. (g)	Sugar (g)	Fiber (g)	Prot. (g)	Servings/Exchanges
Country Fried Chicken	1	580	26	233	6	0	55	1860	56	14	5	20	3 1/2 carb, 1 med-fat protein, 4 fat
Grilled Bourbon Steak Strips	1	480	12	108	3	0	40	980	72	39	4	20	5 carb, 1 med-fat protein, 1 fat
Grilled Southwest Style Chicken	1	630	19	172	5	0	60	1650	85	11	3	29	5 1/2 carb, 2 med-fat protein, 2 fat
Meatloaf	1	680	36	323	12	0	90	1650	66	25	5	26	4 1/2 carb, 2 med-fat protein, 5 fat
Mexican Style Fiesta	1	593	21	191	9.5	0	26	1557	86	13	10	18	5 1/2 carb, 4 fat
Roasted Carved Turkey	1	680	35	315	8	0	85	2240	57	5	3	32	4 carb, 3 med-fat protein, 4 fat
Salisbury Steak	1	600	35	315	12	0	80	1390	50	19	5	24	3 carb, 2 med-fat protein, 5 fat
Weight Watchers Smart Ones													
Angel Hair Marinara	1	180	2	20	1.5	0	0	660	34	6	6	7	2 carb

Asian-Style Beef and Broccoli	1	160	4.5	40	1.5	0	30	640	16	7	4	14	1 carb, 1 med-fat protein
Bacon Macaroni & Cheese	1	290	8	70	3.5	0	25	720	42	4	5	14	3 carb, 1 med-fat protein, 1 fat
Brick Oven–Style Pizza Pepperoni	1	430	13	120	5	0	30	780	57	7	5	21	4 carb, 1 med-fat protein, 2 fat
Chicken Carbonara	1	290	6	50	2.5	0	40	570	39	3	5	22	2 1/2 carb, 2 lean protein
Chicken Enchiladas Suiza	1	290	6	60	2.5	0	25	780	46	6	3	12	3 carb, 1 med-fat protein
Chicken Fajitas	1	260	5	45	1.5	0	30	550	39	4	4	16	2 1/2 carb, 1 med-fat protein
Chicken Fettucini	1	300	4	35	1.5	0	25	670	45	2	4	20	3 carb, 2 lean protein
Chicken Oriental	1	250	2.5	20	1	0	15	670	44	3	2	12	3 carb, 1 fat
Chicken Parmesan	1	280	5	50	1.5	0	35	580	37	4	5	21	2 1/2 carb, 2 lean protein
Chicken Sante Fe	1	160	3	30	0.5	0	45	800	13	4	3	19	1 carb, 2 lean protein
Chicken Strips & Sweet Potato Fries	1	270	12	110	2.5	0	30	620	28	5	3	11	2 carb, 1 med-fat protein, 1 fat

FROZEN DINNERS, ENTRÉES, CHICKEN, FISH

	Serving	Calories	Fat (g)	Cal. from Fat	Sat. Fat (g)	Trans Fat (g)	Chol. (mg)	Sod. (mg)	Carb. (g)	Sugar (g)	Fiber (g)	Prot. (g)	Servings/Exchanges
Creamy Basil Chicken with Broccoli	1	180	4.5	40	2	0	45	520	18	6	4	18	1 carb, 2 lean protein
Homestyle Turkey Breast with Stuffing	1	280	6	50	1.5	0	25	690	36	5	4	22	2 1/2 carb, 2 lean protein
Orange Sesame Chicken	1	250	6	50	1	0	15	480	39	10	4	11	2 1/2 carb, 1 med-fat protein
Pulled Pork & Black Beans	1	230	4	35	1.5	0	40	480	30	12	7	19	2 carb, 2 lean protein
Slow-Roasted Turkey Breast	1	210	3.5	30	1.5	0	40	690	22	0	2	22	1 1/2 carb, 2 lean protein
Thai Style Chicken & Rice Noodles	1	270	4.5	40	1	0	30	540	42	12	3	15	3 carb, 1 med-fat protein
Three Cheese Ziti Marinara with Meatballs	1	320	10	90	4.5	0	25	690	43	3	6	14	3 carb, 1 med-fat protein, 1 fat
Tomato Basil Chicken with Spinach	1	160	4.5	40	1.5	0	50	600	13	4	3	18	1 carb, 2 lean protein

FROZEN CHICKEN

Banquet

Food	Serving												Exchanges
Chicken Breast Patty	1	170	9	80	1.5	0	15	300	13	1	2	8	1 carb, 1 med-fat protein, 1 fat
Chicken Breast Tenders	5 pieces	210	11	100	2	0	20	390	17	1	2	10	1 carb, 1 med-fat protein, 1 fat
Chicken, Buffalo Boneless Wings	2 pieces	210	12	110	2	0	30	610	14	2	1	12	1 carb, 1 med-fat protein, 1 fat
Chicken, Crispy Fried	1 piece	220	12	110	3	0.5	60	600	11	0	<1	15	1 carb, 2 med-fat protein
Chicken, Drumstick	3 oz	240	15	140	3.5	0.5	70	410	9	0	<1	17	1/2 carb, 2 med-fat protein, 1 fat
Chicken, Hot & Spicy Wings	3 oz	240	15	140	3.5	1	65	690	8	0	<1	17	1/2 carb, 2 med-fat protein, 1 fat
Chicken Nuggets	6 pieces	220	12	100	2	0	15	360	17	1	2	11	1 carb, 1 med-fat protein, 1 fat
Chicken, Popcorn	10 pieces	230	10	90	1.5	0	15	380	25	1	2	9	1 1/2 carb, 1 med-fat protein, 1 fat

FROZEN DINNERS, ENTRÉES, CHICKEN, FISH

	Serving	Calories	Fat (g)	Cal. from Fat	Sat. Fat (g)	Trans Fat (g)	Chol. (mg)	Sod. (mg)	Carb. (g)	Sugar (g)	Fiber (g)	Prot. (g)	Servings/Exchanges
Chicken Wings, Honey BBQ	2 pieces	230	13	120	2.5	0	30	590	17	4	1	11	1 carb, 1 med-fat protein, 2 fat
Foster Farms													
Breast Nuggets	4 pieces	220	14	130	4	0	30	320	13	0	0	10	1 carb, 1 med-fat protein, 2 fat
Buffalo Style Strips	3 oz	190	8	70	2	0	30	680	15	<1	0	14	1 carb, 2 med-fat protein
Crispy Strips	3 oz	170	8	60	1.5	0	35	400	11	0	0	17	1 carb, 2 med-fat protein
Honey BBQ Wings	3 wings	190	11	100	3.5	0	85	350	7	4	0	16	1/2 carb, 2 med-fat protein
Hot 'n Spicy Wings	3 wings	190	14	130	4	0	65	360	1	1	0	15	2 med-fat protein, 1 fat
Tyson													
Batter Dipped Chicken Breast Tenders	4 pieces	190	12	100	2.5	0	20	420	12	0	3	9	1 carb, 1 med-fat protein, 1 fat

Breaded Chicken Breast Fillets	1 piece	250	11	100	2	0	40	510	22	1	1	17	1 carb, 2 med-fat protein
Buffalo Style Chicken Strips	3 oz	190	9	80	1.5	0	35	1040	17	0	1	12	1 carb, 1 med-fat protein, 1 fat
Chicken Breast Nuggets	5 pieces	220	13	110	3.5	0	30	470	15	1	1	12	1 carb, 1 med-fat protein, 2 fat
Chicken Breast Patties	1 patty	200	13	120	3	0	35	400	13	0	0	9	1 carb, 1 med-fat protein, 1 fat
Chicken Breast Tenderloins	4 oz	100	0.5	5	0	0	45	190	0	0	0	22	3 lean protein
Crispy Chicken Strips	3 oz	190	9	80	1.5	0	30	480	12	0	1	15	1 carb, 2 med-fat protein
Drumstick	4 oz	150	2.5	80	2.5	0	90	210	0	0	0	17	2 lean protein
Fun Shaped Chicken Nuggets	4 pieces	180	11	90	2.5	0	30	480	10	0	1	10	1/2 carb, 1 med-fat protein, 1 fat
Honey BBQ Wings	3 oz	200	8	80	1.5	0	20	580	20	5	1	11	1 carb, 1 med-fat protein, 1 fat

FROZEN DINNERS, ENTRÉES, CHICKEN, FISH

	Serving	Calories	Fat (g)	Cal. from Fat	Sat. Fat (g)	Trans Fat (g)	Chol. (mg)	Sod. (mg)	Carb. (g)	Sugar (g)	Fiber (g)	Prot. (g)	Servings/Exchanges
FROZEN FISH													
Fisher Boy													
Crunchiest Fish Sticks	4 pieces	250	11	100	2	0	15	750	26	2	2	10	2 carb, 1 med-fat protein, 1 fat
Fish Fillets	2 portions	230	9	80	1.5	0	35	740	26	2	1	11	2 carb, 1 med-fat protein, 1 fat
Fish Sticks	6 sticks	210	9	80	1.5	0	10	540	24	2	2	9	1 1/2 carb, 1 med-fat protein, 1 fat
Shrimp Poppers	3/4 cup	230	12	110	2	0	35	860	25	1	2	8	1 1/2 carb, 1 med-fat protein, 1 fat
Gorton's													
Classic Crispy Battered Fillets	1 portion	150	10	90	2.5	0	10	320	10	1	2	5	1/2 carb, 1 med-fat protein, 1 fat
Classic Crunchy Golden Fish Fillets	2 fillets	240	12	108	2.5	0	30	500	23	3	0	9	1 1/2 carb, 1 med-fat protein, 1 fat

Crunchy Fish Portions	2 fillets	250	13	117	3	0	30	470	23	3	1	10	1 1/2 carb, 1 med-fat protein, 2 fat
Crunchy Golden Popcorn Shrimp	22 shrimp	260	13	117	4	0	60	680	26	3	0	10	2 carb, 1 med-fat protein, 2 fat
Garlic Herb Butter Grilled Fillets	2 fillets	260	15	135	4	0	25	580	21	4	1	9	1 1/2 carb, 1 med-fat protein, 2 fat
Grilled Shrimp Classic	8 shrimp	110	1.5	13	0	0	50	920	5	1	0	18	3 lean protein
Lemon Pepper Grilled Fillets	1 fillet	90	3	27	0.5	0	70	310	0	0	0	15	2 lean protein
Original Batter Fish Tenders	2 fillets	230	14	126	3.5	0	25	550	20	2	1	7	1 carb, 1 med-fat protein, 2 fat
Salmon Classic Grilled Fillets	1 fillet	90	2	18	0	0	35	350	3	1	0	15	2 lean protein

Mrs. Paul's

Beer Battered Fish Fillets	1 fillet	210	10	90	3	0	25	680	21	4	1	10	1 1/2 carb, 1 med-fat protein, 1 fat
Crunchy Fish Fillets	1 fillet	280	14	100	3.5	0	40	510	25	1	1	13	1 1/2 carb, 1 med-fat protein, 2 fat

FROZEN DINNERS, ENTRÉES, CHICKEN, FISH

	Serving	Calories	Fat (g)	Cal. from Fat	Sat. Fat (g)	Trans Fat (g)	Chol. (mg)	Sod. (mg)	Carb. (g)	Sugar (g)	Fiber (g)	Prot. (g)	Servings/Exchanges
Crunchy Fish Sticks	6 sticks	220	10	90	2.5	0	35	420	20	0	1	10	1 carb, 1 med-fat protein, 1 fat
Lightly Breaded Flounder Fillets	1 fillet	160	7	60	2	0	25	200	12	1	0	8	1 carb, 1 med-fat protein
Van de Kamp's													
Beer Battered Fish Fillets	2 fillets	210	10	90	3	0	25	680	21	4	1	10	1 1/2 carb, 1 med-fat protein, 1 fat
Breaded Popcorn Fish	8 pieces	270	13	100	3	0	40	510	25	1	1	14	1 1/2 carb, 1 med-fat protein, 2 fat
Crunchy Breaded Fish Fillets	1 fillet	90	4	0	4	0	10	170	13	1	1	4	1 carb, 1 fat
Garlic Herb Cod	1 fillet	260	10	90	1.5	0	34	580	26	<1	1	18	2 carb, 2 med-fat protein
Lemon Pepper Cod	1 fillet	280	10	90	1	0	45	650	26	2	1	20	2 carb, 2 med-fat protein

FROZEN PIZZA & SNACKS

FROZEN PIZZA

California Pizza Kitchen

	Serving	Calories	Fat (g)	Cal. from Fat	Sat. Fat (g)	Trans Fat (g)	Chol. (mg)	Sod. (mg)	Carb. (g)	Sugar (g)	Fiber (g)	Prot. (g)	Servings/Exchanges
Crispy Thin Crust, BBQ Chicken	1/2 pizza	300	11	100	5	0	40	640	35	8	1	16	2 carb, 1 med-fat protein, 1 fat
Crispy Thin Crust, Margherita	1/3 pizza	320	16	150	7	0	30	480	31	4	2	12	2 carb, 1 med-fat protein, 2 fat
Crispy Thin Crust, Sicilian	1/3 pizza	360	18	170	7	0	45	870	32	4	2	17	2 carb, 2 med-fat protein, 2 fat
Crispy Thin Crust, White Pizza	1/3 pizza	320	17	150	7	0	30	420	30	2	2	13	2 carb, 1 med-fat protein, 2 fat
Hand-Tossed Style Crust, BBQ Chicken with Bacon	1/3 pizza	360	9	80	4	0	30	720	50	7	2	17	3 carb, 1 med-fat protein, 1 fat
Hand-Tossed Style Crust, The Works	1/3 pizza	350	11	100	4.5	0	25	710	48	5	3	14	3 carb, 1 med-fat protein, 1 fat

FROZEN PIZZA & SNACKS

DiGiorno

	Serving	Calories	Fat (g)	Cal. from Fat	Sat. Fat (g)	Trans Fat (g)	Chol. (mg)	Sod. (mg)	Carb. (g)	Sugar (g)	Fiber (g)	Prot. (g)	Servings/Exchanges
Cheese Stuffed Crust, Pepperoni	1/5 pizza	380	16	150	8	0	40	790	41	5	2	18	2 1/2 carb, 2 med-fat protein, 1 fat
Cheese Stuffed Crust, Supreme	1/6 pizza	350	16	150	7	0	40	780	35	5	2	17	2 carb, 2 med-fat protein, 1 fat
Cheese Stuffed Crust, Three Meat	1/6 pizza	300	12	120	5	0	30	590	31	5	2	10	2 carb, 1 med-fat protein, 1 fat
Garlic Bread Pizza, Pepperoni	1/6 pizza	360	14	130	6	0	25	660	41	6	1	16	2 1/2 carb, 1 med-fat protein, 2 fat
Garlic Bread Pizza, Supreme	1/8 pizza	280	12	110	5	0	20	540	32	4	1	13	2 carb, 1 med-fat protein, 1 fat
Rising Crust, Four Cheese	1/6 pizza	290	10	90	5	0	25	670	36	5	1	14	2 1/2 carb, 1 med-fat protein, 1 fat
Rising Crust, Hawaiian	1/6 pizza	270	8	70	4	0	20	670	38	6	1	13	2 1/2 carb, 1 med-fat protein, 1 fat
Rising Crust, Pepperoni	1/6 pizza	300	11	100	5	0	25	730	36	5	1	14	2 1/2 carb, 1 med-fat protein, 1 fat

	Serving											Exchanges
Rising Crust, Supreme	1/6 pizza	330	13	120	5	0	30	840	37	5	2	15	2 1/2 carb, 1 med-fat protein, 2 fat
Thin Crispy Crust, Margherita	1/4 pizza	300	11	100	6	0	35	690	32	3	2	16	2 carb, 1 med-fat protein, 1 fat
Thin Crispy Crust, Supreme	1/4 pizza	310	14	130	6	0	30	750	32	4	2	13	2 carb, 1 med-fat protein, 2 fat

Freschetta

	Serving											Exchanges
Brick Oven, 5 Italian Cheese	1/4 pizza	380	18	160	7	0	30	930	40	9	3	15	2 1/2 carb, 1 med-fat protein, 3 fat
Brick Oven, Pepperoni	1/5 pizza	340	17	150	6	0	30	930	33	9	2	14	2 carb, 1 med-fat protein, 2 fat
Brick Oven, Roasted Portabella Mushrooms & Spinach	1/5 pizza	270	10	90	3.5	0	15	610	34	10	2	11	2 carb, 1 med-fat protein, 1 fat
Brick Oven, Supreme	1/5 pizza	310	14	130	5	0	25	780	34	9	2	12	2 carb, 1 med-fat protein, 2 fat
Naturally Rising Crust, Canadian Style Bacon & Pineapple	1/6 pizza	290	9	80	4.5	0	15	760	40	7	2	13	2 1/2 carb, 1 med-fat protein, 1 fat
Naturally Rising Crust, Supreme	1/6 pizza	350	15	130	6	0	30	910	41	6	2	15	2 1/2 carb, 1 med-fat protein, 2 fat

FROZEN PIZZA & SNACKS

	Serving	Calories	Fat (g)	Cal. from Fat	Sat. Fat (g)	Trans Fat (g)	Chol. (mg)	Sod. (mg)	Carb. (g)	Sugar (g)	Fiber (g)	Prot. (g)	Servings/Exchanges
Totino's													
Cheese	1/2 pizza	320	15	140	4	0	0	560	35	4	2	10	2 carb, 1 med-fat protein, 2 fat
Combination	1/2 pizza	360	19	170	5	0	15	720	36	4	2	12	2 1/2 carb, 1 med-fat protein, 3 fat
Hamburger	1/2 pizza	350	18	160	5	0	5	690	36	4	2	12	2 1/2 carb, 1 med-fat protein, 3 fat
Pepperoni	1/2 pizza	360	19	170	5	0	10	720	35	4	2	12	2 carb, 1 med-fat protein, 3 fat
Sausage	1/2 pizza	360	18	160	5	0	15	700	36	4	2	12	2 1/2 carb, 1 med-fat protein, 3 fat
Supreme	1/2 pizza	360	18	160	5	0	15	710	36	4	2	12	2 1/2 carb, 1 med-fat protein, 3 fat
Red Baron													
Classic 4-Cheese	1/4 pizza	390	17	150	9	0.5	35	780	42	8	2	16	2 1/2 carb, 1 med-fat protein, 2 fat

Classic 4-Meat	1/4 pizza	380	17	150	8	0	35	860	42	8	2	16	2 1/2 carb, 1 med-fat protein, 2 fat
Classic Hamburger	1/4 pizza	370	16	140	8	0	30	840	42	8	2	16	2 1/2 carb, 1 med-fat protein, 2 fat
Classic Mexican Style Supreme	1/4 pizza	370	16	140	8	0	30	660	44	7	2	13	3 carb, 1 med-fat protein, 2 fat
Classic Pepperoni	1/4 pizza	380	18	160	8	0	35	830	41	8	2	15	2 1/2 carb, 1 med-fat protein, 2 fat
Classic Supreme	1/5 pizza	320	15	130	7	0	30	690	34	7	2	12	2 carb, 1 med-fat protein, 2 fat
Deep Dish Singles, Cheese	1 pizza	400	16	150	9	0	25	820	48	16	2	15	3 carb, 1 med-fat protein, 2 fat
Deep Dish Singles, Pepperoni	1 pizza	420	19	170	10	0	35	990	48	15	2	17	3 carb, 1 med-fat protein, 3 fat
Deep Dish Singles, Supreme	1 pizza	410	18	170	9	0	30	900	48	15	2	14	3 carb, 1 med-fat protein, 3 fat
French Bread 5 Cheese & Garlic	1 pizza	420	22	200	8	0	30	660	41	1	2	14	2 1/2 carb, 1 med-fat protein, 3 fat
French Bread Pepperoni	1 pizza	380	15	140	6	0	40	890	42	4	2	15	3 carb, 1 med-fat protein, 2 fat

FROZEN PIZZA & SNACKS

	Serving	Calories	Fat (g)	Cal. from Fat	Sat. Fat (g)	Trans Fat (g)	Chol. (mg)	Sod. (mg)	Carb. (g)	Sugar (g)	Fiber (g)	Prot. (g)	Servings/Exchanges
Thin & Crispy 5-Cheese	1/3 pizza	360	16	150	9	0	30	840	40	9	2	13	2 1/2 carb, 1 med-fat protein, 2 fat
Thin & Crispy Pepperoni	1/3 pizza	390	19	170	9	0	45	1010	41	9	2	14	2 1/2 carb, 1 med-fat protein, 3 fat
Thin & Crispy Supreme	1/4 pizza	300	15	130	7	0	30	790	31	8	2	11	2 carb, 1 med-fat protein, 2 fat
Tombstone													
Original 4 Meat	1/5 pizza	280	13	120	5	0	30	620	27	3	1	14	2 carb, 1 med-fat protein, 2 fat
Original 5 Cheese	1/4 pizza	350	16	140	7	0	30	570	34	4	2	17	2 carb, 2 med-fat protein, 1 fat
Original Pepperoni	1/4 pizza	360	18	160	7	0	35	770	35	4	2	16	2 carb, 1 med-fat protein, 3 fat
Original Pepperoni & Sausage	1/4 pizza	330	15	140	6	0	35	690	34	4	2	16	2 carb, 1 med-fat protein, 2 fat

Original Supreme	1/5 pizza	270	12	110	5	0	30	570	27	3	1	13	2 carb, 1 med-fat protein, 1 fat

Tony's

Original Cheese	1/4 pizza	330	13	120	7	0	30	600	41	7	2	12	2 1/2 carb, 1 mec-fat protein, 2 fat
Original Meat Trio	1/4 pizza	360	16	140	7	0	35	750	41	7	2	13	2 1/2 carb, 1 med-fat protein, 2 fat
Original Pepperoni	1/4 pizza	330	14	130	7	0	30	650	40	7	2	12	2 1/2 carb, 1 med-fat protein, 2 fat
Original Sausage & Pepperoni	1/4 pizza	350	15	140	7	0	30	700	41	7	2	12	2 1/2 carb, 1 med-fat protein, 2 fat
Original Supreme	1/4 pizza	350	15	140	7	0	30	700	41	7	2	12	2 1/2 carb, 1 med-fat protein, 2 fat

FROZEN SNACKS

Bagel Bites

Supreme	4 bites	190	5	45	2	0	10	330	30	3	2	6	2 carb, 1 fat
Three Cheese	4 bites	200	5	45	2.5	0	10	350	32	3	2	7	2 carb, 1 fat

FROZEN PIZZA & SNACKS

	Serving	Calories	Fat (g)	Cal. from Fat	Sat. Fat (g)	Trans Fat (g)	Chol. (mg)	Sod. (mg)	Carb. (g)	Sugar (g)	Fiber (g)	Prot. (g)	Servings/Exchanges
Delimex													
Beef Taquitos	3 pieces	230	7	65	1.5	0	5	230	37	0	3	6	2 1/2 carb, 1 fat
Chicken Taquitos	5 pieces	370	17	155	3	0	20	480	43	1	4	12	3 carb, 1 med-fat protein, 2 fat
Hot Pockets													
BBQ Beef	1	320	13	110	6	1	20	690	44	9	1	9	3 carb, 3 fat
Ham & Cheese	1	310	15	130	8	0	20	490	35	3	1	9	2 carb, 3 fat
Meatballs & Mozarella	1	310	13	120	5	0	15	480	38	3	2	10	2 1/2 carb, 3 fat
Pizzeria Four Cheese Pizza	1	320	13	120	6	0	20	740	39	4	1	11	2 1/2 carb, 1 med-fat protein, 2 fat
Pizzeria Pepperoni	1	320	15	140	6	0	25	700	35	3	1	11	2 carb, 1 med-fat protein, 2 fat
Lean Pockets													
Chicken, Broccoli & Cheddar	1	250	7	60	4	0	20	380	39	6	2	10	2 1/2 carb, 1 fat

	Amount	Cal.	Fat (g)	Cal. from Fat	Sat. Fat (g)	Trans Fat (g)	Chol. (mg)	Sod. (mg)	Carb. (g)	Fiber (g)	Sugars (g)	Pro. (g)	Exchanges/Choices
Chicken, Jalapeño & Cheese	1	260	8	70	4	0	50	580	11	2	1	12	1 carb, 1 med-fat protein, 1 fat
Four Cheese Pizza	1	260	6	50	3	0	20	460	42	4	1	12	3 carb, 1 med-fat protein
Ham & Cheddar	1	270	8	70	4	0	25	540	38	5	2	12	2 1/2 carb, 1 med-fat protein, 2 fat
Meatballs & Mozzarella	1	280	9	80	4	0	25	490	41	5	1	10	2 1/2 carb, 2 fat
Pepperoni Pizza	1	270	7	60	4	0	25	480	41	5	1	12	2 1/2 carb, 1 med-fat protein
Philly Steak & Cheese	1	270	8	70	4	0	25	510	41	4	1	9	2 1/2 carb, 2 fat
Ling Ling Potstickers													
Chicken & Vegetable Dumplings	5 pieces	260	7	63	1.5	0	0	35	600	39	4	2	12	2 1/2 carb, 1 med-fat protein
Pork & Vegetable Dumplings	5 pieces	280	8	72	2.5	0	0	25	640	38	4	2	12	2 1/2 carb, 1 med-fat protein, 2 fat
Jose Ole Mexi-Minis													
Beef & Cheese Mini Tacos	4 pieces	220	11	100	4	0	20	430	23	<1	3	8	1 1/2 carb, 1 med-fat protein, 1 fat
Beef Taquitos	3 pieces	230	12	110	3	0	15	320	26	<1	2	6	2 carb, 2 fat

FROZEN PIZZA & SNACKS

	Serving	Calories	Fat (g)	Cal. from Fat	Sat. Fat (g)	Trans Fat (g)	Chol. (mg)	Sod. (mg)	Carb. (g)	Sugar (g)	Fiber (g)	Prot. (g)	Servings/Exchanges
Chicken Taquitos	3 pieces	200	8	70	1.5	0	10	400	26	<1	3	7	2 carb, 2 fat
Michelina's													
Pepperoni Pizza Snack Rolls	1 package	330	16	140	4	0.5	15	690	37	3	2	10	2 1/2 carb, 3 fat
Rockin' Taco Snack Rolls	1 package	320	16	150	5	0	20	790	31	1	2	10	2 carb, 3 fat
Poppers													
Cream Cheese Jalapeños	3 pieces	230	15	135	6	0	25	430	19	3	1	4	1 carb, 3 fat
Totino's													
Pizza Rolls Cheese	6 rolls	190	6	54	1.5	0	5	480	26	4	1	8	2 carb, 1 fat
Pizza Rolls Supreme	6 rolls	200	8	72	2.5	0	5	330	25	3	1	7	1 1/2 carb, 2 fat
Pizza Rolls Taco	6 rolls	200	8	72	3	0	15	470	24	3	1	7	1 1/2 carb, 2 fat

FRUIT, JUICE, FRUIT DRINKS

	Serving	Calories	Fat (g)	Cal. from Fat	Sat. Fat (g)	Trans Fat (g)	Chol. (mg)	Sod. (mg)	Carb. (g)	Sugar (g)	Fiber (g)	Prot. (g)	Servings/Exchanges
FRUIT													
Apple, Unpeeled	1 small	77	0	0	0	0	0	1	14	15	3	0	1 fruit
Apple, Unpeeled	1 large	116	0	0	0	0	0	0	32	23	6	0	2 fruit
Apples, Dried	4 rings	60	0	0	0	0	0	23	17	16	2	0	1 fruit
Applesauce, Sweetened	1/2 cup	84	0	0	0	0	0	35	51	18	2	<1	1 fruit, 2 1/2 carb
Applesauce, Unsweetened	1/2 cup	53	0	0	0	0	0	3	14	12	2	<1	1 fruit
Apricots, Canned, Extra Light Syrup	1/2 cup	60	0	0	0	0	0	10	16	15	1	0	1 fruit
Apricots, Canned, Heavy Syrup	1/2 cup	107	0	0	0	0	0	5	28	26	2	<1	1 fruit, 1 carb
Apricots, Canned, Juice Pack	1/2 cup	59	0	0	0	0	0	5	15	13	2	<1	1 fruit
Apricots, Canned, Light Syrup	1/2 cup	80	0	0	0	0	0	5	21	19	2	<1	1 fruit, 1/2 carb

FRUIT, JUICE, FRUIT DRINKS

	Serving	Calories	Fat (g)	Cal. from Fat	Sat. Fat (g)	Trans Fat (g)	Chol. (mg)	Sod. (mg)	Carb. (g)	Sugar (g)	Fiber (g)	Prot. (g)	Servings/Exchanges
Apricots, Canned, Water Pack	1/2 cup	33	0	0	0	0	0	4	8	6	2	<1	1/2 fruit
Apricots, Dried	8 halves	64	0	0	0	0	0	3	18	15	2	0	1 fruit
Banana	6-inch	90	0	0	0	0	0	1	19	6	2	<1	1 fruit
Blackberries, Canned, Heavy Syrup	1/2 cup	118	0	0	0	0	0	4	29	25	4	2	1 fruit, 1 carb
Blackberries, Fresh	3/4 cup	56	0	0	0	0	0	0	14	5	6	<1	1 fruit
Blackberries, Frozen, Unsweetened	1 cup	97	0	0	0	0	0	2	24	16	8	2	1 1/2 fruit
Blueberries, Canned, Heavy Syrup	1/2 cup	113	0	0	0	0	0	8	28	26	4	<1	1 fruit, 1 carb
Blueberries, Dried	1/2 cup	130	1	1	0	0	0	10	32	30	1	1	2 fruit
Blueberries, Fresh	1 cup	84	0	0	0	0	0	1	22	15	4	<1	1 1/2 fruit
Blueberries, Frozen, Sweetened	1 cup	186	0	0	0	0	0	2	50	45	5	<1	1 fruit, 2 carb

Blueberries, Frozen, Unsweetened	1 cup	79	0	0	0	0	2	19	13	4	<1	1 fruit
Boysenberries, Canned, Heavy Syrup	1/2 cup	118	0	0	0	0	4	30	25	4	2	1 fruit, 1 carb
Boysenberries, Frozen, Unsweetened	1 cup	66	0	0	0	0	1	16	9	7	1	1 fruit
Cantaloupe, Fresh	1 cup	60	0	0	0	0	14	13	14	1	1	1 fruit
Cherries, Dried	1 oz	98	0	0	0	0	0	16	13	1	0	1 fruit
Cherries, Sour, Canned, Extra Heavy Syrup	1/2 cup	149	0	0	0	0	9	38	0	1	1	1 fruit, 1 1/2 carb
Cherries, Sour, Canned, Heavy Syrup	1/2 cup	117	0	0	0	0	9	30	28	1	1	1 fruit, 1 carb
Cherries, Sour, Canned, Light Syrup	1/2 cup	95	0	0	0	0	9	25	9	1	1	1 fruit, 1/2 carb
Cherries, Sour, Canned, Water Pack	1/2 cup	44	0	0	0	0	9	11	10	1	2	1 fruit
Cherries, Sour, Frozen, Unsweetened	1 cup	71	0	0	0	0	2	17	14	25	1	1 fruit
Cherries, Sweet, Canned, Extra Heavy Syrup	1/2 cup	133	0	0	0	0	4	34	0	2	<1	1 fruit, 1 carb

FRUIT, JUICE, FRUIT DRINKS

	Serving	Calories	Fat (g)	Cal. from Fat	Sat. Fat (g)	Trans Fat (g)	Chol. (mg)	Sod. (mg)	Carb. (g)	Sugar (g)	Fiber (g)	Prot. (g)	Servings/Exchanges
Cherries, Sweet, Canned, Heavy Syrup	1/2 cup	105	0	0	0	0	0	4	27	25	2	<1	1 fruit, 1 carb
Cherries, Sweet, Canned, Juice Pack	1/2 cup	68	0	0	0	0	0	4	18	16	2	<1	1 fruit
Cherries, Sweet, Canned, Light Syrup	1/2 cup	85	0	0	0	0	0	4	22	20	2	<1	1 fruit, 1/2 carb
Cherries, Sweet, Canned, Water Pack	1/2 cup	57	0	0	0	0	0	1	15	13	2	1	1 fruit
Cherries, Sweet, Fresh	12 cherries	60	0	0	0	0	0	0	14	12	2	1	1 fruit
Cherries, Sweet, Frozen, Unsweetened	1 cup	231	0	0	0	0	0	3	17	14	5	3	1 fruit
Cranberries	1 cup	47	<1	0	<1	0	0	<1	12	4	4	<1	1 fruit
Cranberries, Dried	1 oz	86	0	0	0	0	0	0	13	18	<1	0	1 fruit
Cranberry Sauce, Canned, Sweetened	1/2 cup	209	0	0	0	0	0	40	54	53	1	<1	1 fruit, 2 1/2 carb

Food	Serving	Calories										Exchange
Currants, Red/White, Fresh	1 cup	63	0	0	0	0	1	15	8	5	2	1 fruit
Figs, Canned, Extra Heavy Syrup	1/2 cup	140	0	0	0	0	2	37	0	0	<1	1 fruit, 1 1/2 carb
Figs, Canned, Heavy Syrup	1/2 cup	114	0	0	0	0	2	30	27	3	<1	1 fruit, 1 carb
Figs, Canned, Light Syrup	1/2 cup	87	0	0	0	0	2	23	21	2	<1	1 fruit, 1/2 carb
Figs, Canned, Water Pack	1/2 cup	66	0	0	0	0	1	18	15	3	<1	1 fruit
Figs, Dried	1 cup	371	0	0	0	0	3	18	71	3	<1	1 fruit
Figs, Fresh	2 medium	94	0	0	0	0	1	19	16	3	<1	1 fruit
Fruit Cocktail, Canned, Extra Heavy Syrup	1/2 cup	114	0	0	0	0	10	25	21	1	<1	1 fruit, 1 carb
Fruit Cocktail, Canned, Extra Light Syrup	1/2 cup	55	0	0	0	0	15	18	16	1	0	1 fruit
Fruit Cocktail, Canned, Heavy Syrup	1/2 cup	91	0	0	0	0	15	24	22	1	<1	1 fruit, 1/2 carb
Fruit Cocktail, Canned, Juice Pack	1/2 cup	104	0	0	0	0	5	14	13	1	<1	1 fruit

FRUIT, JUICE, FRUIT DRINKS

	Serving	Calories	Fat (g)	Cal. from Fat	Sat. Fat (g)	Trans Fat (g)	Chol. (mg)	Sod. (mg)	Carb. (g)	Sugar (g)	Fiber (g)	Prot. (g)	Servings/Exchanges
Fruit Cocktail, Canned, Light Syrup	1/2 cup	69	0	0	0	0	0	8	18	17	1	<1	1 fruit
Fruit Cocktail, Canned, Waterpack	1/2 cup	38	0	0	0	0	0	5	10	9	1	<1	1/2 fruit
Fruit Salad, Canned, Extra Heavy Syrup	1/2 cup	114	0	0	0	0	0	7	30	25	1	<1	1 fruit, 1 carb
Fruit Salad, Canned, Heavy Syrup	1/2 cup	93	0	0	0	0	0	8	25	20	1	<1	1 fruit, 1/2 carb
Fruit Salad, Canned, Juice Pack	1/2 cup	55	0	0	0	0	0	5	16	14	2	1	1 fruit
Fruit Salad, Canned, Light Syrup	1/2 cup	73	0	0	0	0	0	8	19	10	1	<1	1 fruit
Fruit Salad, Canned, Water Pack	1/2 cup	37	0	0	0	0	0	4	10	6	1	<1	1/2 fruit
Grapefruit, Fresh	1/2	52	0	0	0	0	0	0	13	8	2	1	1 fruit

Food	Serving										
Grapefruit Sections, Canned, Juice Pack	1/2 cup	46	0	0	0	0	9	12	11	<1	<1	1 fruit
Grapefruit Sections, Canned, Light Syrup	1/2 cup	76	0	0	0	0	3	20	19	<1	<1	1 fruit
Grapefruit Sections, Canned, Waterpack	1/2 cup	44	0	0	0	0	3	11	11	<1	<1	1 fruit
Grapes, Canned, Heavy Syrup	1/2 cup	98	0	0	0	0	7	25	25	<1	<1	1 fruit, 1/2 carb
Grapes, Canned, Water Pack	1/2 cup	49	0	0	0	0	8	13	12	<1	<1	1 fruit
Grapes, Fresh, Seedless	1 cup	104	0	0	0	0	2	27	23	<1	<1	1 fruit
Guava, Fresh	1	46	0	0	0	0	3	11	5	5	1	1 fruit
Honeydew Melon, Fresh	1 cup	61	0	0	0	0	31	16	14	1	<1	1 fruit
Kiwi, Fresh	1 large	56	0	0	0	0	3	13	7	3	1	1 fruit
Kumquats, Fresh	2	26	0	0	0	0	4	6	4	2	1	1/2 fruit
Mixed Fruit, Canned, Heavy Syrup	1/2 cup	92	0	0	0	0	5	24	22	2	<1	1 fruit, 1/2 carb
Nectarine, Fresh	1 medium	62	0	0	0	0	0	15	11	2	1	1 fruit

FRUIT, JUICE, FRUIT DRINKS

	Serving	Calories	Fat (g)	Cal. from Fat	Sat. Fat (g)	Trans Fat (g)	Chol. (mg)	Sod. (mg)	Carb. (g)	Sugar (g)	Fiber (g)	Prot. (g)	Servings/Exchanges
Orange, Fresh	1 medium	62	0	0	0	0	0	0	18	12	3	1	1 fruit
Oranges, Mandarin, Canned, Juice Pack	1 cup	72	0	1	0	0	0	9	18	16	2	1	1 fruit
Papaya, Fresh	1 cup	55	0	0	0	0	0	4	16	8	3	<1	1 fruit
Peach, Fresh	1 medium	58	0	0	0	0	0	0	14	13	2	1	1 fruit
Peaches, Canned, Heavy Syrup	1/2 cup	86	0	0	0	0	0	6	22	20	2	1	1 fruit, 1/2 carb
Peaches, Canned, Light Syrup	1/2 cup	68	0	0	0	0	0	7	18	16	1	<1	1 fruit
Peaches, Canned, Water Pack	1/2 cup	30	0	0	0	0	0	7	7	6	1	1	1/2 fruit
Peaches, Frozen, Sweetened	1 cup	235	0	0	0	0	0	15	60	55	4	2	2 fruit, 2 carb
Pear, Fresh	1 medium	101	0	0	0	0	0	1	27	17	6	1	2 fruit

Pears, Canned, Heavy Syrup	1/2 cup	98	0	0	0	0	7	25	20	2	<1	1 fruit, 1/2 carb
Pears, Canned, Juice Pack	1/2 cup	62	0	0	0	0	5	16	12	2	<1	1 fruit
Pears, Canned, Light Syrup	1/2 cup	71	0	0	0	0	6	19	15	2	<1	1 fruit
Pears, Canned, Water Pack	1/2 cup	35	0	0	0	0	3	10	7	2	0	1/2 fruit
Pineapple, Canned, Heavy Syrup	1/2 cup	99	0	0	0	0	1	25	21	1	1	1 fruit, 1/2 carb
Pineapple, Canned, Juice Pack	1/2 cup	54	0	0	0	0	1	14	13	1	<1	1 fruit
Pineapple, Canned, Light Juice Pack	1/2 cup	66	0	0	0	0	2	17	16	1	<1	1 fruit
Pineapple, Canned, Water Pack	1/2 cup	40	0	0	0	0	1	10	9	1	<1	1/2 fruit
Pineapple, Fresh	1 cup	82	0	0	0	0	2	22	16	2	0	1 1/2 fruit
Pineapple, Frozen, Sweetened	1 cup	211	0	0	0	0	5	54	52	3	<1	1 fruit, 2 1/2 carb

FRUIT, JUICE, FRUIT DRINKS

	Serving	Calories	Fat (g)	Cal. from Fat	Sat. Fat (g)	Trans Fat (g)	Chol. (mg)	Sod. (mg)	Carb. (g)	Sugar (g)	Fiber (g)	Prot. (g)	Servings/Exchanges
Plum, Fresh	2	61	0	0	0	0	0	0	15	14	2	<1	1 fruit
Plums, Canned, Heavy Syrup	1/2 cup	115	1	0	0	0	0	25	30	29	1	<1	1 fruit, 1 carb
Plums, Canned, Juice Pack	1/2 cup	126	0	0	0	0	0	2	19	18	1	<1	1 fruit
Plums, Canned, Light Syrup	1/2 cup	84	0	0	0	0	0	25	21	20	1	<1	1 fruit, 1/2 carb
Plums, Canned, Water Pack	1/2 cup	51	0	0	0	0	0	1	15	14	1	<1	1 fruit
Plums, Dried	2	68	0	0	0	0	0	1	16	12	2	<1	1 fruit
Pomegranate, Fresh	1/2 cup	72	1	0	0	0	0	3	16	12	4	1	1 fruit
Raisins, Seedless	small box (1.5 oz)	129	0	0	0	0	0	5	34	25	2	1	3 fruit
Raspberries, Canned, Heavy Syrup	1/2 cup	117	0	0	0	0	0	4	30	25	4	1	1 fruit, 1 carb

Food	Amount												Exchanges
Raspberries, Fresh	1 cup	64	0	0	0	0	0	1	15	5	8	1	1 fruit
Raspberries, Frozen, Sweetened	1 cup	258	0	3	0	0	0	3	65	54	11	2	1 fruit, 2 1/2 carb
Rhubarb, Frozen, Unsweetened	1 cup	35	0	0	0	0	0	3	7	3	3	<1	1/2 fruit
Star Fruit (Carambola), Fresh	1 cup	41	0	0	0	0	0	3	9	5	4	1	1/2 fruit
Strawberries, Canned, Heavy Syrup	1/2 cup	117	0	0	0	0	0	5	30	27	2	1	1 fruit, 1 carb
Strawberries, Fresh	1 cup	46	0	0	0	0	0	1	11	7	3	1	1 fruit
Strawberries, Frozen, Unsweetened	1 cup	38	0	0	0	0	0	2	10	5	3	<1	1/2 fruit
Tangerine, Fresh	1 medium	47	0	0	0	0	0	2	12	9	2	1	1 fruit
Tangerines, Juice Pack	1/2 cup	36	0	0	0	0	0	5	9	8	1	<1	1/2 fruit
Tangerines, Light Syrup	1/2 cup	77	0	0	0	0	0	7	20	20	1	<1	1 fruit
Watermelon, Fresh	1 cup	46	0	0	0	0	0	2	12	9	<1	1	1 fruit

FRUIT, JUICE, FRUIT DRINKS

	Serving	Calories	Fat (g)	Cal. from Fat	Sat. Fat (g)	Trans Fat (g)	Chol. (mg)	Sod. (mg)	Carb. (g)	Sugar (g)	Fiber (g)	Prot. (g)	Servings/Exchanges
FRUIT JUICES													
Apple Juice/Cider, Canned/Bottled	1/2 cup	58	0	0	0	0	0	4	15	14	0	0	1 fruit
Apricot Nectar, Canned	1/2 cup	70	0	0	0	0	0	4	18	17	0	0	1 fruit
Cranberry Juice Cocktail, Bottled	1/2 cup	68	0	0	0	0	0	2	17	15	0	0	1 fruit
Cranberry Juice Cocktail, Reduced-Calorie	1 cup	45	0	0	0	0	0	7	11	11	0	0	1 fruit
Fruit Juice Blends, 100% Juice	1/2 cup	60	0	0	0	0	0	12	15	13	0	0	1 fruit
Grapefruit Juice, Canned	1/2 cup	48	0	0	0	0	0	1	11	12	0	<1	1 fruit
Orange Juice, Canned	1/2 cup	58	0	0	0	0	0	5	13	11	0	<1	1 fruit
Orange Juice, Fresh	1/2 cup	56	0	0	0	0	0	1	13	10	0	<1	1 fruit
Orange Juice, Frozen, Reconstituted	1/2 cup	56	0	0	0	0	0	1	13	13	<1	<1	1 fruit
Pineapple Juice, Canned	1/2 cup	66	0	0	0	0	0	2	16	14	<1	<1	1 fruit

Prune Juice, Bottled	1/2 cup	91	0	0	0	0	0	5	22	21	<1	1	1 1/2 fruit

FRUIT DRINKS, JUICES

Capri-Sun (Single Serving Pouch)

100% Juice, Apple Juice	1 pouch	80	0	0	0	0	0	25	20	20	0	0	1 1/2 fruit
Juice Drink, Strawberry Kiwi	1 pouch	50	0	0	0	0	0	15	19	13	0	0	1 carb
Lemonade	1 pouch	50	0	0	0	0	0	25	14	13	0	0	1 carb
Roarin Waters, Fruit Flavored Water, Fruit Punch	1 pouch	30	0	0	0	0	0	15	8	8	0	0	1/2 carb

Dole

100% Juice Paradise Blend	8 oz	120	0	0	0	0	0	60	28	25	0	<1	2 fruit
Orange Peach Mango Fruit Juice Blend	8 oz	120	0	0	0	0	0	10	29	27	0	<1	2 fruit
Orange Strawberry Banana Fruit Juice Blend	8 oz	120	0	0	0	0	0	10	29	27	0	1	2 fruit

FRUIT, JUICE, FRUIT DRINKS

	Serving	Calories	Fat (g)	Cal. from Fat	Sat. Fat (g)	Trans Fat (g)	Chol. (mg)	Sod. (mg)	Carb. (g)	Sugar (g)	Fiber (g)	Prot. (g)	Servings/Exchanges
Pina Colada Fruit Juice Blend	8 oz	120	0	0	0	0	0	10	29	24	0	0	2 fruit
Pineapple Juice	8 oz	150	0	0	0	0	0	0	36	31	0	0	2 1/2 fruit
Pineapple Peach Mango Juice	8 oz	120	0	0	0	0	0	10	29	27	0	<1	2 fruit
Strawberry Kiwi	8 oz	120	0	0	0	0	0	25	31	NA	0	0	2 fruit
Donald Duck													
Orange Juice No Pulp Plus Calcium	8 oz	110	0	0	0	0	0	20	27	24	0	2	2 fruit
Florida's Natural													
Orange Juice with Calcium & Vitamin D	8 oz	110	0	0	0	0	0	0	26	22	0	2	2 fruit
Original Orange Juice	8 oz	110	0	0	0	0	0	0	26	22	0	2	2 fruit
Ruby Red Grapefruit Juice	8 oz	90	0	0	0	0	0	0	22	20	0	1	1 1/2 fruit

Hansen's Natural

Food	Serving											
Smoothie, Assorted Flavors, Single Serving	11.5 oz	180	0	0	0	0	20	45	45	0	0	3 carb

Hawaiian Punch

Fruit Punch, Assorted Flavors	8 oz	70	0	0	0	0	105	17	17	0	0	1 carb

Hollywood

Carrot Juice, Single Serving	11-oz can	120	0	0	0	0	250	27	14	1	2	2 fruit

Kool-Aid (Single Serving)

Bursts Soft Drink, Assorted Flavors	6.8 oz	35	0	0	0	0	30	9	9	0	0	1/2 carb
Jammers Juice Drink, Cherry	5.9 oz	90	0	0	0	0	15	24	24	0	0	1 1/2 carb
Jammers Juice Drink, Tropical	6.7 oz	70	0	0	0	0	15	19	19	0	0	1 carb

Langers

Apple Cider	8 oz	120	0	0	0	0	0	28	26	0	0	2 carb
Apple Juice	8 oz	120	0	0	0	0	15	27	26	0	0	2 fruit

FRUIT, JUICE, FRUIT DRINKS

	Serving	Calories	Fat (g)	Cal. from Fat	Sat. Fat (g)	Trans Fat (g)	Chol. (mg)	Sod. (mg)	Carb. (g)	Sugar (g)	Fiber (g)	Prot. (g)	Servings/Exchanges
Cranberry Juice Cocktail	8 oz	140	0	0	0	0	0	15	35	32	0	0	2 carb
Cranberry Raspberry	8 oz	120	0	0	0	0	0	10	30	30	0	0	2 carb
Diet Low Carb Apple Juice Cocktail	8 oz	30	0	0	0	0	0	10	7	6	0	0	1/2 carb
Diet Low Carb Cranberry Juice Cocktail	8 oz	30	0	0	0	0	0	10	8	8	0	0	1/2 carb
Diet Low Carb Ruby Red Grapefruit Juice Cocktail	8 oz	30	0	0	0	0	0	10	8	8	0	0	1/2 carb
Ruby Red Grapefruit Juice Cocktail	8 oz	130	0	0	0	0	0	10	33	32	0	0	2 carb
Juicy Juice 100% Juice													
Apple Juice	8 oz	110	0	0	0	0	0	20	28	26	0	0	2 fruit
Kern's													
Kern's Aguas Frescas Limeade Juice Drink	8 oz	120	0	0	0	0	0	5	31	NA	0	0	2 carb

Kern's Apricot Nectar, Single Serving	8 oz	95	0	0	0	0	5	24	21	0	1 1/2 carb
Kern's Guava Nectar	8 oz	160	0	0	0	0	10	39	38	0	2 1/2 carb
Kern's Peach Nectar, Single Serving	11.5-oz can	190	0	0	0	0	20	46	45	0	3 carb
Kern's Pear Nectar	8 oz	220	0	0	0	0	20	54	35	0	3 1/2 carb
Kern's Strawberry Banana Nectar	8 oz	153	0	0	0	0	7	36	32	0	2 1/2 carb
Martinelli's										
Apple Juice	10 oz	180	0	0	0	0	0	43	39	0	3 fruit
Apple Pomegranate Juice	8 oz	150	0	0	0	0	10	38	32	0	2 1/2 fruit
Minute Maid										
Apple Juice, Single Serving	10 oz	140	0	0	0	0	25	35	32	0	2 fruit
Apple Strawberry Juice	15.2 oz	210	0	0	0	0	35	56	53	0	3 1/2 carb
Berry Punch	8 oz	90	0	0	0	0	15	25	25	0	1 1/2 carb
Cherry Limeade	8 oz	120	0	0	0	0	15	34	33	0	2 carb

FRUIT, JUICE, FRUIT DRINKS

	Serving	Calories	Fat (g)	Cal. from Fat	Sat. Fat (g)	Trans Fat (g)	Chol. (mg)	Sod. (mg)	Carb. (g)	Sugar (g)	Fiber (g)	Prot. (g)	Servings/Exchanges
Country Style Orange Juice	8 oz	110	0	0	0	0	0	0	27	24	0	0	2 fruit
Fruit Punch	10 oz	140	0	0	0	0	0	25	36	32	0	0	2 1/2 carb
Heart Wise Orange Juice	8 oz	110	0	0	0	0	0	20	27	24	0	2	2 fruit
Home Squeezed Orange Juice/Calcium & Vitamin D	8 oz	110	0	0	0	0	0	15	27	24	0	2	2 fruit
Kids+ Orange Juice	8 oz	110	0	0	0	0	0	15	27	24	0	2	2 fruit
Lemonade	8 oz	150	0	0	0	0	0	50	42	40	0	0	3 carb
Light Orange Juice Beverage	8 oz	50	0	0	0	0	0	10	12	10	0	0	1 carb
Light Raspberry Passion	8 oz	15	0	0	0	0	0	15	4	2	0	0	free
Limeade	8 oz	90	0	0	0	0	0	0	26	23	C	0	2 carb
Mixed Berry Juice, Single Serving	15.2 oz	130	0	0	0	0	0	45	34	31	0	0	2 carb
Orange Juice, Multi-Vitamin	8 oz	120	0	0	0	0	0	0	27	24	0	0	2 fruit

Original Orange Juice	8 oz	110	0	0	0	0	15	27	24	0	2	2 fruit
Original Orange Juice with Calcium	8 oz	120	0	0	0	0	0	27	24	0	0	2 fruit
Pink Lemonade, Single Serving	12 oz	150	0	0	0	0	50	42	40	0	0	3 carb
Mott's												
Plus Light Apple Juice	8 oz	50	0	0	0	0	30	12	12	0	0	1 carb
Naked Single Serving												
Berry Blast	15.2 oz	250	0	0	0	0	20	55	49	0	2	3 1/2 carb
Mighty Mango	15.2 oz	290	0	0	0	0	20	68	57	0	2	4 1/2 carb
Protein Zone	15.2 oz	420	4	40	2	55	270	65	53	0	30	4 carb, 4 lean protein
Strawberry Banana	15.2 oz	250	0	0	0	0	10	59	44	0	2	4 carb
Superfood Green Machine	15.2 oz	270	0	0	0	0	25	63	53	0	4	4 carb
Ocean Spray												
Cran-Apple Juice Drink	8 oz	110	0	0	0	0	45	31	31	0	0	2 carb
Cranberry Juice Cocktail	8 oz	110	0	0	0	0	5	28	28	0	0	2 carb

FRUIT, JUICE, FRUIT DRINKS

	Serving	Calories	Fat (g)	Cal. from Fat	Sat. Fat (g)	Trans Fat (g)	Chol. (mg)	Sod. (mg)	Carb. (g)	Sugar (g)	Fiber (g)	Prot. (g)	Servings/Exchanges
Cranergy Juice Drink	8 oz	35	0	0	0	0	0	50	9	9	0	0	1/2 carb
Cran-Grape Juice Drink	8 oz	110	0	0	0	0	0	40	28	28	0	0	2 carb
Cran-Pomegranate	8 oz	110	0	0	0	0	0	30	28	28	0	0	2 carb
Cran-Raspberry Juice Drink	8 oz	110	0	0	0	0	0	40	28	28	0	0	2 carb
Diet Cranberry	8 oz	5	0	0	0	0	0	20	2	<1	0	0	free
Light Cran-Grape Juice Drink	8 oz	50	0	0	0	0	0	35	13	13	0	0	1 carb
No Sugar Added 100% Cranberry Juice Blend	8 oz	110	0	0	0	0	0	15	28	28	0	0	2 carb
Old Orchard													
Apple Cranberry 100% Juice Blend	8 oz	120	0	0	0	0	0	25	29	27	0	0	2 fruit
Berry Blend 100% Juice Blend	8 oz	120	0	0	0	0	0	25	29	27	0	0	2 fruit

Healthy Balance Grape Juice Cocktail	8 oz	15	0	0	0	0	5	6	6	0	0	1/2 carb
Healthy Balance Ruby Red Grapefruit Cocktail	8 oz	25	0	0	0	0	5	5	5	0	0	1/2 carb
Peach Mango 100% Juice Blend	8 oz	120	0	0	0	0	25	29	27	0	0	2 fruit
SunnyD												
Fruit Punch	6.75 oz	50	0	0	0	0	110	13	12	0	0	1 carb
Tangy Original	16 oz	110	0	0	0	0	310	28	27	0	0	2 carb
Sunsweet												
Prune Juice	8 oz	180	0	0	0	0	30	43	NA	3	2	3 fruit
Prune Juice with Pulp	8 oz	180	0	0	0	0	30	43	NA	3	2	3 fruit
Tree Top												
Apple Juice	8 oz	120	0	0	0	0	25	29	NA	0	0	1 1/2 fruit
Apple Orange Banana Fiber Rich	8 oz	160	0	0	0	0	30	38	NA	6	<1	2 fruit
Tropicana												
Antioxidant Advantage	8 oz	110	0	0	0	0	0	26	26	0	2	2 fruit

FRUIT, JUICE, FRUIT DRINKS

	Serving	Calories	Fat (g)	Cal. from Fat	Sat. Fat (g)	Trans Fat (g)	Chol. (mg)	Sod. (mg)	Carb. (g)	Sugar (g)	Fiber (g)	Prot. (g)	Servings/Exchanges
Healthy Heart Orange Juice	8 oz	120	0.5	5	0	0	0	15	26	22	0	2	2 fruit
Low Acid Orange Juice	8 oz	110	0	0	0	0	0	0	26	22	0	2	2 fruit
Orange Juice with Calcium and Vitamin D	8 oz	110	0	0	0	0	0	0	26	22	0	2	2 fruit
Orange Strawberry Banana Juice Blend	8 oz	130	0	0	0	0	0	0	30	26	0	2	2 fruit
Orange Tangerine Juice	8 oz	110	0	0	0	0	0	0	25	22	0	2	1 1/2 fruit
Original Orange Juice	8 oz	110	0	0	0	0	0	0	26	22	0	2	2 fruit
Ruby Red Grapefruit Juice	8 oz	90	0	0	0	0	0	0	22	17	0	1	1 1/2 fruit
V8 V-Fusion													
Acai Mixed Berry	8 oz	100	0	0	0	0	0	75	25	23	0	0	1 1/2 carb
Peach Mango	8 oz	80	0	0	0	0	0	70	29	26	0	0	2 carb
Pomegranate Blueberry	8 oz	100	0	0	0	0	0	65	25	22	0	0	1 1/2 carb

Welch's

	Serving	Cal												Exchanges
100% Grape Juice	8 oz	140	0	0	0	0	0	0	15	36	36	0	1	2 1/2 fruit
100% White Grape Juice	8 oz	140	0	0	0	0	0	0	15	38	36	0	1	2 1/2 fruit
Grape Cranberry Juice Cocktail	8 oz	150	0	0	0	0	0	0	20	37	36	0	0	2 1/2 carb
Guava Pineapple Juice Cocktail	8 oz	140	0	0	0	0	0	0	20	34	33	0	0	2 carb
Light Grape Juice Cocktail	8 oz	45	0	0	0	0	0	0	75	12	11	0	0	1 carb
Mango Twist Juice Cocktail	8 oz	50	0	0	0	0	0	0	50	12	11	0	0	1 carb
Mountain Berry Juice Cocktail	8 oz	140	0	0	0	0	0	0	5	34	33	0	0	2 carb
Orange Pineapple Apple Juice Drink	8 oz	120	0	0	0	0	0	0	20	32	31	0	0	2 carb
Passion Fruit Juice Cocktail	8 oz	150	0	0	0	0	0	0	60	38	37	0	0	2 1/2 carb
Strawberry Breeze Fruit Juice Cocktail	8 oz	130	0	0	0	0	0	0	5	33	32	0	0	2 carb

GLUTEN-FREE FOODS

	Serving	Calories	Fat (g)	Cal. from Fat	Sat. Fat (g)	Trans Fat (g)	Chol. (mg)	Sod. (mg)	Carb. (g)	Sugar (g)	Fiber (g)	Prot. (g)	Servings/Exchanges
Ancient Quinoa Harvest													
Shells, Elbows, Rotelle Pasta	2 oz	205	1	7	0	0	0	4	46	<1	4	4	3 carb
Bakery On Main													
Extreme Fruit & Nut Granola	1/3 cup	140	7	60	1	0	0	15	18	2	2	2	1 carb, 1 fat
Nutty Maple Cranberry Granola	1/3 cup	140	6	60	0.5	0	0	15	20	8	2	2	1 carb, 1 fat
Rainforest Granola	1/3 cup	150	7	70	1	0	0	15	19	6	2	2	1 carb, 1 fat
Betty Crocker (Gluten Free)													
Chocolate Chip Cookie Mix	2 cookies	110	2	60	1	0	0	125	23	13	1	1	1 1/2 carb
Yellow Cake Mix	1/10 cake	150	0	90	0	0	0	230	37	17	0	1	2 1/2 carb

DeBoles

Food	Serving	Cal.	Fat (g)	Cal. from Fat	Sat. Fat (g)	Chol. (mg)	Sodium (mg)	Carb (g)	Fiber (g)	Sugar (g)	Protein (g)	Exchanges
Rice Angel Hair Pasta	1/4 pkg	210	0.5	5	0	0	15	46	0	<1	4	3 carb
Rice Angel Hair Pasta Plus Golden Flax	1/4 pkg	210	1.5	15	0	0	10	44	0	1	4	3 carb
Rice Fettucini	1/4 pkg	210	0.5	5	0	0	15	46	0	1	4	3 carb
Rice Lasagna	1/4 pkg	260	0.5	5	0	0	15	56	0	<1	5	3 1/2 carb
Rice Spaghetti Style Pasta	1/4 pkg	210	0.5	5	0	0	15	46	0	<1	4	3 carb
Rice Spirals	1/4 pkg	210	0.5	5	0	0	15	46	0	<1	4	3 carb
Wheat Free Corn Spaghetti Style Pasta	1/4 pkg	200	2	20	0	0	15	43	0	5	4	3 carb

Ener-G Foods

Food	Serving	Cal.	Fat (g)	Cal. from Fat	Sat. Fat (g)	Chol. (mg)	Sodium (mg)	Carb (g)	Fiber (g)	Sugar (g)	Protein (g)	Exchanges
Cinnamon Crackers	7 crackers	100	4	35	0	0	75	19	7	1	0	1 carb, 1 fat
Corn Loaf	1 slice	40	2	15	0	0	50	7	1	3	0	1/2 carb
Doughnut Holes (Plain)	1	90	3.5	30	1.5	25	210	14	10	3	4	1 carb, 1 fat
Light White Rice Flax Loaf	1 slice	50	2	20	0	0	60	7	1	1	1	1/2 carb

GLUTEN-FREE FOODS

	Serving	Calories	Fat (g)	Cal. from Fat	Sat. Fat (g)	Trans Fat (g)	Chol. (mg)	Sod. (mg)	Carb. (g)	Sugar (g)	Fiber (g)	Prot. (g)	Servings/Exchanges
Original Pretzels	40 crackers	140	4	35	2	0	0	360	24	0	2	1	1 1/2 carb, 1 fat
Plain Croutons	1/2 cup	135	6	50	0.5	0	0	165	20	2	3	1	1 carb, 1 fat
Seattle Brown Hamburger Buns	1 bun	190	6	50	0.5	0	0	270	32	4	3	2	2 carb, 1 fat
Seattle Brown Hot Dog Buns	1 bun	190	6	50	0.5	0	0	270	32	4	3	2	2 carb, 1 fat
Seattle Crackers	8 crackers	110	6	50	0	0	0	240	10	3	1	1	1/2 carb, 1 fat
Sesame Pretzels	19 crackers	150	8	70	3	0	0	390	19	0	0	1	1 carb, 2 fat
Tapioca Hamburger Buns	1 bun	120	3	30	0	0	0	150	21	3	4	1	1 1/2 carb, 1 fat
Tapioca Hot Dog Buns	1 bun	120	3	30	0	0	0	150	21	3	4	1	1 1/2 carb, 1 fat
Tapioca Loaf (Thin Sliced)	1 slice	80	3	30	0	0	0	95	11	1	2	1	1 carb, 1 fat

Enjoy Life Foods

Chewy Chocolate Chip Cookies	2	120	5	45	1	0	0	100	19	10	1	1	1 carb, 1 fat
Plentils Garlic & Parmesan	1 bag	100	5	45	0	0	0	320	13	0	2	1	1 carb, 1 fat
Plentils Sea Salt Lentil Chips	1 bag	110	5	50	0	0	0	220	12	0	1	2	1 carb, 1 fat
Seed & Fruit Beach Bash	1/4 cup	130	7	60	1	0	0	45	14	9	2	3	1 carb, 1 fat
Seed & Fruit Mountain Meadow	1/4 cup	140	8	70	1.5	0	0	25	13	9	2	4	1 carb, 2 fat
Soft Baked Gingerbread Spice Cookies	2	120	4	35	0	0	0	95	20	9	1	1	1 carb, 1 fat
Soft & Chewy Caramel Apple Snack Bar	1	110	3	25	0	0	0	100	20	7	1	1	1 carb, 1 fat
Soft & Chewy Mixed Berry Bar	1	110	2.5	25	0	0	0	80	21	8	1	1	1 1/2 carb, 1 fat

General Mills Gluten Free

Corn Chex	1 cup	120	0.5	5	0	0	0	220	26	3	2	2	2 carb

GLUTEN-FREE FOODS

	Serving	Calories	Fat (g)	Cal. from Fat	Sat. Fat (g)	Trans Fat (g)	Chol. (mg)	Sod. (mg)	Carb. (g)	Sugar (g)	Fiber (g)	Prot. (g)	Servings/Exchanges
Rice Chex	1 cup	100	0.5	5	0	0	0	220	23	2	1	2	1 1/2 carb
Gillian's Foods													
Caramelized Onion Gluten-Free Rolls	1 roll	130	4	35	0.5	0	0	160	20	1	1	3	1 carb, 1 fat
Cinnamon Raisin Rolls	1/2 roll	150	3.5	30	0	0	0	130	24	7	1	7	1 1/2 carb, 1 fat
Foods By George													
Blueberry Muffins	1	220	8	70	1	0	25	450	33	11	1	3	2 carb, 2 fat
Brownies	1/9 tray	180	9	80	1	0	40	45	24	16	1	2	1 1/2 carb, 2 fat
Corn Muffins	1	240	9	80	1	0	30	480	36	8	1	4	2 1/2 carb, 2 fat
English Muffins	1	210	3.5	30	0	0	0	270	39	3	1	4	2 1/2 carb, 1 fat
Pecan Tarts	1	470	28	250	7	0	95	160	51	26	3	6	3 1/2 carb, 6 fat
French Meadow Bakery													
Chocolate Chip Cookie	1	190	10	90	4.5	0	15	150	25	14	1	1	1 1/2 carb, 2 fat
Cinnamon Raisin Bread	1 slice	150	5	45	3	0	0	270	22	NA	2	2	1 1/2 carb, 1 fat

Food	Serving												Exchanges
Fudge Brownie	1	170	8	72	1	0	30	120	24	17	1	1	1 1/2 carb, 2 fat
Italian Rolls	1	340	9	81	1	0	40	470	63	7	8	3	4 carb, 2 fat
Multigrain Bread	1 slice	150	4.5	41	2	0	0	230	23	3	3	4	1 1/2 carb, 1 fat
Sandwich Bread	1 slice	120	4	36	2.5	0	0	310	20	0	1	2	1 carb, 1 fat
Tortilla	1	120	1	9	0	0	0	290	24	1	1	1	1 1/2 carb
Glutino													
Apple Breakfast Bar	1	140	2	20	0	0	0	45	29	14	3	2	2 carb
Blueberry Breakfast Bar	1	140	2	20	0	0	0	45	29	14	3	2	2 carb
Cheddar Crackers	8	130	4	40	2	0	5	280	22	1	1	1	1 1/2 carb, 1 fat
Parmesan Garlic Bagel Chips	7 chips	110	4	40	0	0	0	190	17	3	0	1	1 carb, 1 fat
Plain Bagel	1/2 bagel	200	6	50	1	0	5	330	36	5	1	3	2 1/2 carb, 1 fat
Pretzels Sticks	33	120	3	30	1.5	0	0	490	24	1	3	0	1 1/2 carb, 1 fat
Heartland's Finest													
All Natural Macaroni & Cheese	3 oz	340	7	63	4.5	0	20	800	53	7	6	14	3 1/2 carb, 1 med-fat protein

GLUTEN-FREE FOODS

	Serving	Calories	Fat (g)	Cal. from Fat	Sat. Fat (g)	Trans Fat (g)	Chol. (mg)	Sod. (mg)	Carb. (g)	Sugar (g)	Fiber (g)	Prot. (g)	Servings/Exchanges
Elbow Macaroni Pasta	2 oz	210	1.5	14	0.5	0	0	0	41	1	5	7	2 1/2 carb
Lasagna Pasta	2 oz	210	1.5	14	0.5	0	0	0	41	1	5	7	2 1/2 carb
Linguini Pasta	2 oz	210	1.5	14	0.5	0	0	0	41	1	5	7	2 1/2 carb
Original CerOs Cereal	1/2 cup	240	6	50	1	0	0	130	40	13	4	6	2 1/2 carb, 1 fat
Spaghetti Pasta	2 oz	210	1.5	14	0.5	0	0	0	41	1	5	7	2 1/2 carb
Hodgson Mill Brown Rice Pasta													
Elbows, Penne, Spaghetti, Angel Hair, Linguine	2 oz	190	1	10	0	0	0	0	41	1	3	8	2 1/2 carb
Kay's Naturals Better Balance													
Apple Cinnamon Cereal	1.2 oz	120	1.5	10	0	0	0	150	19	3	4	12	1 carb
Chili Nacho Cheese Protein Chips	1.2 oz	120	2.5	30	0	0	0	240	15	1	4	12	1 carb, 1 fat
Crispy Parmesan Protein Chips	5 oz	110	3.5	30	0	0	0	230	14	0	3	10	1 carb, 1 med-fat protein

Golden Butter Twists Pretzels	1 oz	110	5	30	1.5	0	0	220	12	1	2	10	1 carb, 1 med-fat protein
Honey Almond Cereal	1.2 oz	120	1.5	10	0	0	0	150	19	2	4	12	1 carb
White Cheddar Cheese Kruncheeze	1.2 oz	130	4	35	0.5	0	0	240	14	1	2	12	1 carb, 1 fat
Kinnikinnick Foods													
Blueberry Muffin	1	140	7	65	1	0	20	160	23	12	1	1	1 1/2 carb, 1 fat
Chocolate Chip Muffin	1	170	8	80	2	0	20	160	26	15	1	1	2 carb, 2 fat
Chocolate Dipped Donuts	1	210	7	55	3	0	15	220	36	17	1	2	2 1/2 carb, 1 fat
Chocolate Vanilla Sandwich Cookies	3	150	6	35	3	0	0	95	23	11	1	1	1 1/2 carb, 1 fat
Cinnamon Sugar Donuts	1	180	7	40	3	0	15	220	29	11	1	2	2 carb, 1 fat
English Muffins	1	210	3.5	30	<1	0	0	350	43	6	4	3	3 carb, 1 fat
Ginger Snap Cookies	4	140	4	30	2	0	5	170	25	8	2	1	1 1/2 carb, 1 fat
Hamburger Bun	1	150	5	65	1	0	0	210	26	1	5	2	2 carb, 1 fat
Hot Dog Bun	1	180	5	70	1	0	0	250	30	1	6	3	2 carb, 1 fat
White Sandwich Bread	2 slices	140	4	40	1	0	0	200	24	1	2	5	1 1/2 carb, 1 fat

GLUTEN-FREE FOODS

	Serving	Calories	Fat (g)	Cal. from Fat	Sat. Fat (g)	Trans Fat (g)	Chol. (mg)	Sod. (mg)	Carb. (g)	Sugar (g)	Fiber (g)	Prot. (g)	Servings/Exchanges
Whole Grain Sandwich Bread	2 slices	160	5	30	1	0.5	0	220	25	2	5	3	1 1/2 carb, 1 fat
Lundberg Organic Brown Rice Pasta													
Rotini, Penne, Spaghetti	2 oz	190	3	30	0.5	0	0	0	41	1	4	4	2 1/2 carb, 1 fat
Mary's Gone Crackers													
Black Pepper Crackers	13	140	5	45	0.5	0	0	180	21	0	3	3	1 1/2 carb, 1 fat
Hot 'n Spicy Jalapeño Crackers	15	140	5	45	0.5	0	0	180	21	0	3	3	1 1/2 carb, 1 fat
Lightly Salted Crackers	15	140	6	50	2	0	0	230	20	3	2	2	1 carb, 1 fat
Original Crackers	13	140	5	45	0.5	0	0	190	21	0	3	3	1 1/2 carb, 1 fat
Mi-Del													
Arrowroot Cookies	10	130	4	35	1	0	10	85	23	9	2	2	1 1/2 carb, 1 fat
Chocolate Chip Cookies	5	130	4.5	40	1.5	0	0	130	21	11	1	2	1 1/2 carb, 1 fat
Ginger Snaps	5	140	6	50	0	0	0	85	21	12	1	2	1 1/2 carb, 1 fat
Mini Pecan Cookies	5	120	4.5	40	1	0	5	130	18	9	1	2	1 carb, 1 fat

Royal Vanilla Sandwich Cookies	2	140	6	60	1.5	0	5		19	11	0	1	1 carb, 1 fat
Nature's Path												
Crunchy Maple Sunrise	2/3 cup	110	1	10	0	0	0	130	25	7	3	2	1 1/2 carb
Crunchy Vanilla Sunrise	2/3 cup	110	1	10	0	0	0	135	25	6	3	2	1 1/2 carb
EnviroKidz Panda Puffs	3/4 cup	130	3.5	30	1	0	0	125	23	7	2	2	1 1/2 carb, 1 fat
Whole O's Cereal	2/3 cup	120	1.5	10	0	0	0	115	25	4	3	2	1 1/2 carb
Pamela's Products												
Butter Shortbread Cookies	1	110	7	60	4	0	13	70	13	3	0	0	1 carb, 1 fat
Chunky Chocolate Chip Cookies	1	120	6	60	1	0	10	80	14	7	0.5	1	1 carb, 1 fat
Lemon Shortbread Cookies	1	120	6	60	4	0	15	50	15	5	0	0.5	1 carb, 1 fat
Peanut Butter Cookies	1	100	5	45	1	0	15	120	11	7	0.5	3	1 carb, 1 fat
Schär												
Chocolate Dipped Cookies	3	150	6	60	3.5	0	0	60	21	7	1	2	1 1/2 carb, 1 fat

GLUTEN-FREE FOODS

	Serving	Calories	Fat (g)	Cal. from Fat	Sat. Fat (g)	Trans Fat (g)	Chol. (mg)	Sod. (mg)	Carb. (g)	Sugar (g)	Fiber (g)	Prot. (g)	Servings/Exchanges
Crispbread	4 slices	110	0	0	0	0	0	160	24	2	<1	2	1 1/2 carb
Italian Breadsticks	5	110	1.5	20	1	0	0	220	23	<1	0	1	1 1/2 carb
Ladyfingers	3	120	2	20	1	0	45	50	23	10	1	2	1 1/2 carb
Multigrain Bread	2 slices	180	2	20	0	0	0	210	38	4	5	3	2 1/2 carb
Shortbread Cookies	4	130	4	40	2.5	0	10	45	22	6	0	2	1 1/2 carb, 1 fat
Table Crackers	5 crackers	140	3	30	2	0	0	240	24	2	<1	2	1 1/2 carb, 1 fat
Vanilla Wafers	4	160	8	80	6	0	0	20	20	11	0	2	1 carb, 2 fat
White Bread	2 slices	170	1.5	15	0	0	0	210	38	4	4	2	2 1/2 carb
Tinkyada Brown Rice Pasta													
Fettucini, Lasagna, Penne, Spaghetti, Shells, Spirals	2 oz	200	2	15	0	0	0	25	43	0	2	4	3 carb
Trader Joe's													
Brown Rice Tortillas	1 tortilla	130	2.5	25	0	0	0	160	24	0	2	2	1 1/2 carb, 1 fat

Organic Brown Rice Penne Pasta	1 cup	200	0	10	1.5	0	0	0	43	0	2	4	3 carb

Whole Foods Gluten Free Bakehouse

Banana Bread	1 slice	150	5	0	0	0	45	250	24	3	0	0	1 1/2 carb, 1 fat
Blueberry Muffin	1	330	13	110	1	0	60	380	53	26	1	4	3 1/2 carb, 3 fat
Chocolate Chip Cookies	1	160	8	80	4.5	0	30	95	22	9	0	2	1 1/2 carb, 2 fat
Cornbread	1 slice	160	7	60	1	0	45	320	21	5	2	3	1 1/2 carb, 1 fat
Cream Biscuits	1	220	13	120	8	0	50	400	24	1	<1	2	1 1/2 carb, 3 fat
Honey Oat Bread	1 slice	140	3.5	35	0	0	35	200	24	4	1	2	1 1/2 carb, 1 fat
Lemon Poppy Seed Muffin	1	390	2	18	0	0	120	300	48	26	1	5	3 carb
Morning Glory Muffin	1	310	18	160	1.5	0	70	310	36	13	1	4	2 1/2 carb, 4 fat
Prairie Bread	1 slice	150	4.5	41	0.5	0	40	230	23	3	<1	4	1 1/2 carb, 1 fat
Sandwich Bread	1 slice	170	6	54	6	0	0	450	28	2	1	1	2 carb, 1 fat

ICE CREAM, FROZEN YOGURT, NOVELTIES, PUDDING, GELATIN

	Serving	Calories	Fat (g)	Cal. from Fat	Sat. Fat (g)	Trans Fat (g)	Chol. (mg)	Sod. (mg)	Carb. (g)	Sugar (g)	Fiber (g)	Prot. (g)	Servings/Exchanges
Frozen Yogurt, Fat-Free	1/2 cup	82	0	0	0	0	0	43	18	14	0	3	1 carb
Frozen Yogurt, Regular	1/2 cup	114	4	30	2.5	0	1	63	17	17	0	3	1 carb, 1 fat
Fruit Juice Bar, Frozen, 100% Juice	1 (3-oz) bar	67	<1	0	0	0	0	3	16	13	1	1	1 carb
Gelatin, Dessert	1/2 cup	83	0	0	0	0	0	101	19	18	0	2	1 carb
Ice Cream	1/2 cup	137	7	90	5	0	29	53	16	14	0	2	1 carb, 1 fat
Ice Cream, Fat-Free	1/2 cup	95	0	0	0	0	0	67	21	9	1	6	1 1/2 carb
Ice Cream, Light	1/2 cup	107	3	28	2	0	18	48	17	14	0	3	1 carb, 1 fat
Ice Cream, No Sugar Added	1/2 cup	97	4	38	3	0	12	46	15	4	0	3	1 carb, 1 fat
Ice Pops	1	34	0	1	0	0	0	3	8	6	0	0	1/2 carb
Pudding, Chocolate	1 oz	40	1	0	0	0	1	43	7	5	0	0	1/2 carb
Pudding, Fat-Free	4 oz	100	0	0	0	0	0	180	23	17	1	2	1 1/2 carb
Pudding, Tapioca	1/2 cup	143	4	38	1	0	1	159	24	16	0	2	1 1/2 carb, 1 fat
Pudding, Vanilla	1 cup	90	1	9	0.5	0	1	160	21	15	0	0	1 1/2 carb, 1 fat

Sherbet, Orange	1/2 cup	107	1	1	0	0	1	34	22	18	1	1	1 1/2 carb
Sorbet	1/2 cup	65	0.5	5	0	0	0	70	28	20	2	2	2 carb
Sugar/Rolled Ice Cream Cone	1	40	0	0	0	0	0	32	8	3	<1	<1	1/2 carb
Topping, Butterscotch	2 Tbsp	120	1	8	0	0	2	28	31	12	0	1	2 carb
Topping, Hot Fudge	2 Tbsp	130	5	41	2	0	0	50	22	18	1	2	1 1/2 carb, 1 fat
Topping, Marshmallow Cream	2 Tbsp	91	0	1	0	0	0	23	22	13	0	0	1 1/2 carb
Topping, Whipped	2 Tbsp	63	4	33	3	0	1	20	7	7	0	1	1/2 carb, 1 fat
Topping, Whipped, Light	2 Tbsp	20	1	5	5	0	0	0	2	0	1	0	free

ICE CREAM/FROZEN YOGURT

Ben & Jerry's

Frozen Yogurt, Cherry Garcia	1/2 cup	170	3	25	2	0	20	55	32	24	1	5	2 carb, 1 fat
Frozen Yogurt, Chocolate Fudge Brownie	1/2 cup	180	2.5	25	1	0	15	85	35	27	2	5	2 carb, 1 fat
Frozen Yogurt, Half Baked	1/2 cup	180	3	25	1.5	0	20	75	35	25	1	5	2 carb, 1 fat

ICE CREAM, FROZEN YOGURT, NOVELTIES, PUDDING, GELATIN

	Serving	Calories	Fat (g)	Cal. from Fat	Sat. Fat (g)	Trans Fat (g)	Chol. (mg)	Sod. (mg)	Carb. (g)	Sugar (g)	Fiber (g)	Prot. (g)	Servings/Exchanges
Ice Cream, Cake Batter	1/2 cup	270	16	140	10	0	65	65	27	23	1	5	2 carb, 3 fat
Ice Cream, Cherry Garcia	1/2 cup	260	15	140	9	0.5	70	40	27	23	1	4	2 carb, 3 fat
Ice Cream, Chocolate Chip Cookie Dough	1/2 cup	280	15	140	9	0.5	75	50	32	25	0	4	2 carb, 3 fat
Ice Cream, Chocolate Fudge Brownie	1/2 cup	200	11	100	6	0	0	45	23	16	2	3	1 1/2 carb, 2 fat
Ice Cream, Chubby Hubby	1/2 cup	340	21	190	11	0	65	160	33	26	2	7	2 carb, 4 fat
Ice Cream, Chunky Monkey	1/2 cup	260	14	130	8	0	0	15	31	26	1	2	2 carb, 3 fat
Ice Cream, Coffee Caramel Fudge	1/2 cup	240	12	110	9	0	0	40	31	23	1	2	1 1/2 carb, 2 fat
Ice Cream, Mint Chocolate Cookie	1/2 cup	280	17	150	10	0.5	80	120	28	23	0	5	2 carb, 3 fat
Ice Cream, Original Vanilla	1/2 cup	250	16	140	10	0.5	90	50	21	20	0	4	1 1/2 carb, 3 fat

Ice Cream, P.B. & Cookies	1/2 cup	290	17	150	8	0	0	160	31	22	2	4	2 carb, 3 fat
Ice Cream, Peanut Butter Cup	1/2 cup	370	26	230	14	0.5	70	140	29	25	1	7	2 carb, 5 fat
Ice Cream, Red Velvet	1/2 cup	260	14	130	9	0	70	110	29	23	0	4	2 carb, 3 fat
Ice Cream, Vanilla Caramel Fudge	1/2 cup	290	16	140	10	0.5	80	115	33	32	0	4	2 carb, 3 fat
Sorbet, Berry Berry Extraordinary	1/2 cup	80	0	0	0	0	0	10	20	16	1	0	1 carb
Sorbet, Lemonade	1/2 cup	80	0	0	0	0	0	10	20	16	1	0	1 carb
Sorbet, Mango Mango Sorbet	1/2 cup	80	0	0	0	0	0	10	20	14	1	0	1 carb
Breyers													
Carb Smart, Chocolate	1/2 cup	110	6	50	3.5	0	15	80	13	4	4	2	1 carb, 1 fat
Carb Smart, Vanilla	1/2 cup	120	6	50	3.5	0	15	50	14	4	4	2	1 carb, 1 fat
Ice Cream, Chocolate	1/2 cup	140	7	60	4.5	0	20	50	17	16	1	2	1 carb, 1 fat
Ice Cream, Chocolate Chip Cookie Dough	1/2 cup	150	5	45	3	0	10	45	25	16	0	2	1 1/2 carb, 1 fat

ICE CREAM, FROZEN YOGURT, NOVELTIES, PUDDING, GELATIN

	Serving	Calories	Fat (g)	Cal. from Fat	Sat. Fat (g)	Trans Fat (g)	Chol. (mg)	Sod. (mg)	Carb. (g)	Sugar (g)	Fiber (g)	Prot. (g)	Servings/Exchanges
Ice Cream, Chocolate Peanut Butter	1/2 cup	180	11	100	4.5	0	15	135	19	14	2	4	1 1/2 carb, 2 fat
Ice Cream, Cookies and Cream	1/2 cup	140	4.5	40	2.5	0	10	80	23	15	0	2	1 1/2 carb, 1 fat
Ice Cream, Mint Chocolate Chip	1/2 cup	150	8	70	6	0	15	40	18	17	1	2	1 carb, 2 fat
Ice Cream, Natural Vanilla	1/2 cup	130	7	60	4	0	20	35	14	14	0	3	1 carb, 1 fat
Ice Cream, Rocky Road	1/2 cup	140	5	45	3	0	10	40	22	16	1	2	1 1/2 carb, 1 fat
Ice Cream, Strawberry	1/2 cup	110	5	45	3	0	15	30	14	14	0	2	1 carb, 1 fat
Ice Cream, Vanilla Fudge Twirl	1/2 cup	120	3	25	2	0	10	40	21	14	0	2	1 1/2 carb, 1 fat
Häagen-Dazs													
Frozen Yogurt, Coffee	1/2 cup	180	2.5	25	1	0	45	45	31	21	0	8	2 carb, 1 fat
Frozen Yogurt, Dulce de Leche	1/2 cup	270	16	145	10	0.5	75	75	27	27	0	5	2 carb, 3 fat

Frozen Yogurt, Vanilla	1/2 cup	170	2.5	25	1	0	45	45	29	21	0	9	2 carb, 1 fat
Frozen Yogurt, Vanilla Raspberry Swirl	1/2 cup	140	1	10	0.5	0	25	25	31	25	0	5	1 1/2 carb
Ice Cream, Chocolate	1/2 cup	260	17	155	10	0.5	90	45	22	19	0	5	1 1/2 carb, 3 fat
Ice Cream, Chocolate Chocolate Chip	1/2 cup	300	18	160	11	0.5	75	90	30	23	0	4	2 carb, 4 fat
Ice Cream, Mint Chip	1/2 cup	250	16	145	10	0	70	70	23	20	0	4	1 1/2 carb, 3 fat
Ice Cream, Rocky Road	1/2 cup	290	17	155	8	0	70	60	29	22	1	5	2 carb, 3 fat
Kraft													
Cool Whip Free Whipped Topping	2 Tbsp	20	0	0	0	0	0	5	3	1	0	0	free
Cool Whip Lite Whipped Topping	2 Tbsp	20	1	10	1	0	0	0	2	1	0	0	free
Cool Whip, Sugar Free	2 Tbsp	20	1	10	1	0	0	0	3	2	0	0	free
Cool Whip Topping, Regular	2 Tbsp	25	1.5	15	1.5	0	0	0	2	2	0	0	free
Dream Whip Whipped Topping Mix	2 Tbsp	10	0.5	0.5	0.5	0	0	0	2	1	0	0	free

ICE CREAM, FROZEN YOGURT, NOVELTIES, PUDDING, GELATIN

	Serving	Calories	Fat (g)	Cal. from Fat	Sat. Fat (g)	Trans Fat (g)	Chol. (mg)	Sod. (mg)	Carb. (g)	Sugar (g)	Fiber (g)	Prot. (g)	Servings/Exchanges
Marshmallow Creme	2 Tbsp	45	0	0	0	0	0	10	11	8	0	0	1/2 carb
Marshmallows, Jet Puffed	4	100	0	0	0	0	0	24	24	20	0	3	1 1/2 carb
Marshmallows, Miniature	2/3 cup	100	0	0	0	0	0	25	25	18	0	0.5	1 1/2 carb
Smuckers													
Topping, Butterscotch	2 Tbsp	100	0	0	0	0	0	110	25	20	0	1	1 1/2 carb
Topping, Hot Fudge	2 Tbsp	130	4.5	40	1.5	0	0	50	22	18	<1	2	1 1/2 carb, 1 fat
Topping, Magic Shell Chocolate Fudge	2 Tbsp	210	15	140	7	0	0	25	18	16	1	1	1 carb, 3 fat
Topping, Strawberry	2 Tbsp	100	0	0	0	0	0	15	26	21	0	0	2 carb
Topping, Sugar Free Caramel	2 Tbsp	90	0	0	0	0	0	65	24	13	0	0	1 1/2 carb
Topping, Sugar Free Hot Fudge	2 Tbsp	90	0.5	5	0	0	0	40	23	17	1	1	1 1/2 carb

FROZEN NOVELTIES

Blue Bunny

Item	Serving	Cal.	Fat (g)	Cal. from Fat	Sat. Fat (g)	Trans Fat (g)	Chol. (mg)	Sodium (mg)	Carb. (g)	Sugar (g)	Fiber (g)	Prot. (g)	Exchanges
Banana Pops	1 bar	35	0	0	0	0	0	5	9	7	0	0	1/2 carb
Big Star Bars	1	130	8	72	7	0	5	40	13	11	0	2	1 carb, 2 fat
Caramel Lovers Ice Cream Cone	1	310	16	140	9	0	15	110	38	24	2	6	2 1/2 carb, 3 fat
Chips Galore! Ice Cream Sandwich	1	310	14	130	8	0	30	220	43	27	1	4	3 carb, 3 fat
Chocolate Raspberry Ice Cream Bar	1	260	16	140	11	0	20	45	26	20	1	3	2 carb, 3 fat
Cookies 'N Cream Ice Cream Sandwich	1	240	10	90	5	0	20	210	37	18	1	4	2 1/2 carb, 2 fat
Hot Fudge Bars	1	360	24	220	13	0	30	100	33	25	2	7	2 carb, 5 fat
Jolly Rancher Bomb Pop	1	80	0	0	0	0	0	15	20	15	0	0	1 carb
Krunch Bars	1	110	7	60	6	0	5	30	11	8	1	2	1 carb, 2 fat
Malt Cups	1 cup	330	11	99	7	0	45	160	52	42	0	6	3 1/2 carb, 2 fat
Neapolitan Sandwich	1	160	5	45	3	0	15	115	27	15	<1	3	2 carb, 1 fat

ICE CREAM, FROZEN YOGURT, NOVELTIES, PUDDING, GELATIN

	Serving	Calories	Fat (g)	Cal. from Fat	Sat. Fat (g)	Trans Fat (g)	Chol. (mg)	Sod. (mg)	Carb. (g)	Sugar (g)	Fiber (g)	Prot. (g)	Servings/Exchanges
Orange Dream Bar	1	80	1.5	14	1	0	5	35	16	14	0	1	1 carb
Original Bomb Pop	1	40	0	0	0	0	0	5	10	8	0	0	1/2 carb
Root Beer Float Bar	1	80	2	18	1.5	0	10	25	14	11	0	<1	1 carb
Simply Vanilla Ice Cream Sandwich	1	160	5	45	3	0	15	110	27	15	<1	3	2 carb, 1 fat
Slush Pops	1	58	1	0	0	0	0	10	12	6	4	4	1/2 carb
Sour Power Bomb Pop	1	50	0	0	0	0	0	5	12	10	0	0	1/2 carb
Star Bars	1	130	8	72	7	0	5	40	13	11	0	2	1 carb, 2 fat
Sugar Free Bomb Pop	1	15	0	0	0	0	0	10	6	3	0	0	1/2 carb
Sweet Freedom No Sugar Added Bunny Tracks Ice Cream	1/2 cup	140	7	60	3.5	0	10	60	22	10	4	3	1 1/2 carb, 1 fat
Sweet Freedom No Sugar Added Butter Pecan Ice Cream	1/2 cup	110	4.5	40	2	0	10	60	19	9	5	3	1 carb, 2 fat

Sweet Freedom No Sugar Added Chocolate Ice Cream	1/2 cup	100	3	30	2	0	10	50	19	9	5	3	1 carb, 1 fat
Sweet Freedom No Sugar Added Vanilla Krunch Bar	1	110	7	60	6	0	5	30	11	8	1	2	1 carb, 1 fat
The Champ! Chocolate Lovers	1	270	13	110	9	0	15	130	36	22	2	4	2 1/2 carb, 3 fat
Turtle Bars	1	350	23	210	13	0	30	95	33	28	1	5	2 carb, 5 fat
Twin Pops	1	70	0	0	0	0	0	10	18	13	0	0	1 carb
Breyers													
All Natural Fruit Bars (All Varieties)	1	50	0	0	0	0	0	0	12	8	0	0	1 carb
Carb Smart Fudge Bars	1	70	3	25	3	2	10	35	11	8	1	2	1 carb, 1 fat
Carb Smart Vanilla Ice Cream Bars	1	150	11	100	8	0	5	60	13	10	0	2	1 carb, 2 fat
Double Churn Creamy Vanilla Ice Cream Bars	1	170	9	81	5	0	5	55	21	15	3	4	1 1/2 carb, 2 fat

ICE CREAM, FROZEN YOGURT, NOVELTIES, PUDDING, GELATIN

	Serving	Calories	Fat (g)	Cal. from Fat	Sat. Fat (g)	Trans Fat (g)	Chol. (mg)	Sod. (mg)	Carb. (g)	Sugar (g)	Fiber (g)	Prot. (g)	Servings/Exchanges
Oreo Ice Cream Sandwich	1	140	5	45	2.5	0	10	70	22	15	0	2	1 1/2 carb, 1 fat
Smooth & Dreamy 1/2 Fat Creamy Chocolate	1	100	3	25	2	0	10	40	16	11	1	2	1 carb, 1 fat
Dole													
Fruit Juice Bars (All Varieties)	1	70	0	0	0	0	0	10	18	17	0	0	1 carb
Dove													
Dove Bars, Dark Chocolate with Vanilla	1	250	16	150	10	0	25	30	25	20	2	3	1 1/2 carb, 3 fat
Dove Bars, Milk Chocolate with Almonds	1	250	17	150	9	0	25	100	21	18	1	4	1 1/2 carb, 3 fat
Dove Bars, Milk Chocolate with Vanilla	1	250	16	140	10	0	30	45	24	21	1	3	1 1/2 carb, 3 fat
Outshine													
Fruit Bars, Mango	1	70	0	0	0	0	0	0	17	16	0	0	1 carb

Food													
Fruit Bars, Strawberry	1	60	0	0	0	0	0	15	14	1	0		1 carb
Whole Fruit, Creamy Coconut	1	120	3	25	2.5	0	5	40	20	18	1	4	1 carb, 1 fat
Good Humor													
Chocolate Chip Cookie Sandwich	1	280	12	108	6	0	15	230	41	22	1	3	2 1/2 carb, 2 fat
Chocolate Éclair Bars	1	220	10	90	5	0	10	55	30	4	1	2	2 carb, 2 fat
Strawberry Shortcake Bars	1	230	12	108	5	0	10	55	31	17	1	2	2 carb, 2 fat
Sundae Cones	1	260	15	135	9	0	15	80	29	18	1	4	2 carb, 3 fat
Toasted Almond Bars	1	240	12	108	3.5	0	10	40	30	23	1	2	2 carb, 2 fat
Vanilla Ice Cream Sandwiches	1	160	5	45	3	0	10	90	26	13	0	2	2 carb, 1 fat
Häagen-Daz													
Chocolate & Dark Chocolate Ice Cream Bars	1	300	21	189	13	0	70	40	24	21	1	4	1 1/2 carb, 4 fat
Vanilla & Almonds Ice Cream Bars	1	320	12	108	12	0	75	55	22	20	1	5	1 1/2 carb, 2 fat

ICE CREAM, FROZEN YOGURT, NOVELTIES, PUDDING, GELATIN

	Serving	Calories	Fat (g)	Cal. from Fat	Sat. Fat (g)	Trans Fat (g)	Chol. (mg)	Sod. (mg)	Carb. (g)	Sugar (g)	Fiber (g)	Prot. (g)	Servings/Exchanges
Vanilla & Dark Chocolate Ice Cream Bar	1	280	20	180	13	0	55	30	21	20	<1	4	1 1/2 carb, 4 fat
Vanilla & Milk Chocolate Ice Cream Bars	1	300	22	198	13	0	65	40	21	19	1	5	1 1/2 carb, 4 fat
Healthy Choice													
Caramel Swirl Sandwiches	1	140	3	27	1	0	5	120	27	17	1	2	2 carb, 1 fat
Fudge Bars	1	80	1.5	14	2	0	5	65	13	4	4	3	1 carb
Ice Cream Sandwiches	1	130	3	27	1	0	5	150	24	14	1	2	1 1/2 carb, 1 fat
Mocha Swirl Bars	1	90	1	9	0.5	0	4	35	17	11	1	3	1 carb
Sorbet & Cream Bars	1	90	1	9	0.5	0	5	35	17	12	0	1	1 carb
Klondike													
Caramel Pretzel Bars	1	270	15	135	13	0	10	140	32	22	1	3	2 carb, 3 fat
Choco Taco	1	290	15	135	11	0	5	125	38	25	1	4	2 1/2 carb, 3 fat
Dark Chocolate Bars	1	250	17	153	12	0	20	50	22	17	1	3	1 1/2 carb, 3 fat

Double Chocolate Bar	1	240	14	126	11	0	10	75	27	24	1	3	2 carb, 3 fat
Heath Bars	1	230	15	135	11	0	10	80	25	20	1	2	1 1/2 carb, 3 fat
Krunch Bars	1	250	14	126	11	0	10	70	24	23	1	3	1 1/2 carb, 3 fat
Neapolitan Bars	1	250	17	153	13	0	20	50	22	18	1	3	1 1/2 carb, 3 fat
Oreo Cookie Sandwich	1	200	7	63	2	0	5	250	34	17	2	3	2 carb, 1 fat
Original Vanilla Bars	1	250	14	126	11	0	10	70	29	23	1	3	2 carb, 3 fat
Reese's Bars	1	270	18	162	11	0	15	90	24	20	1	3	1 1/2 carb, 3 fat
Slim-a-Bear 100 Calorie English Toffee Bar	1	100	6	50	4.5	0	5	30	12	8	2	1	1 carb, 1 fat
Slim-a-Bear 100 Calorie Fudge Bar	1	100	2.5	23	1.5	0	5	65	19	12	4	3	1 carb, 1 fat
Slim-a-Bear 100 Calorie Vanilla Sandwich	1	100	2	18	1	0	5	90	20	3	2	3	1 carb
Slim-a-Bear No Sugar Added Krunch Bar	1	170	10	90	8	0	5	85	22	7	4	4	1 1/2 carb, 2 fat
Slim-a-Bear No Sugar Added Vanilla Bars	1	170	9	90	8	0	5	65	21	13	4	4	1 1/2 carb, 2 fat
Triple Chocolate Bars	1	250	16	144	11	0	15	60	24	20	1	3	1 1/2 carb, 3 fat

ICE CREAM, FROZEN YOGURT, NOVELTIES, PUDDING, GELATIN

	Serving	Calories	Fat (g)	Cal. from Fat	Sat. Fat (g)	Trans Fat (g)	Chol. (mg)	Sod. (mg)	Carb. (g)	Sugar (g)	Fiber (g)	Prot. (g)	Servings/Exchanges
Whitehouse Cherry Bar	1	250	17	153	13	0	20	55	24	20	1	2	1 1/2 carb, 3 fat
Luigi's													
Italian Ice (All Varieties)	6-oz cup	120	0	0	0	0	0	10	30	23	1	0	2 carb
Italian Ice No Sugar Added	6-oz cup	60	0	0	0	0	0	10	20	1	0	0	1 carb
Nestlé/Carnation													
Drumstick Classic, Vanilla	1	290	15	140	8	0	10	90	34	22	2	4	2 carb, 3 fat
Drumstick Simply Dipped, Peppermint	1	260	12	110	9	0	10	100	36	25	1	2	2 1/2 carb, 2 fat
Drumstick Simply Dipped, Vanilla	1	260	12	110	9	0	10	100	37	25	1	2	2 1/2 carb, 2 fat
Drumstick, Vanilla Caramel	1	300	15	140	8	0	10	100	38	25	2	4	2 1/2 carb, 3 fat
Lil' Drums Cones, Vanilla and Fudge Sauce	1	110	4	35	2.5	0	5	45	18	11	0	1	1 carb, 1 fat

Popsicle

	Serving	Cal	Fat (g)	% Fat Cal	Sat Fat (g)	Chol (mg)	Sod (mg)	Carb (g)	Sugar (g)	Fiber (g)	Prot (g)	Choices/Exchanges
All Natural Ice Pops	1	50	0	0	0	0	5	12	9	0	0	1 carb
Big Stick Cherry Pineapple Swirl Ice Pop	1	80	0	0	0	0	0	19	18	0	0	1 carb
Cotton Candy Swirl Bar	1	45	0	0	0	0	5	12	8	0	0	1 carb
Creamsicle 100 Calorie Pops	1	100	2	18	0.5	5	30	20	12	0	1	1 carb
Firecracker Ice Pops	1	35	0	0	0	0	0	9	7	0	0	1/2 carb
Firecracker Super Heroes	1	40	0	0	0	0	0	9	9	0	0	1/2 carb
Fudgsicle Triple Chocolate Bars	1	70	0	0	0	0	50	14	10	1	3	1 carb
Lemon Lime Shots	1	25	1.5	13	1	1	35	3	3	0	0	free
Lick-A-Color Ice Pops	1	50	0	0	0	0	0	13	12	0	0	1 carb
Low Fat Creamsicle Bars	1	100	2	18	0.5	5	30	20	12	0	1	1 carb
No Sugar Added Creamsicle Pops	1	45	4	0	0.5	5	25	10	2	2	1	1/2 carb, 1 fat
Orange Burst Pop-Ups	1	80	1	9	0	0	15	19	15	0	1	1 carb

ICE CREAM, FROZEN YOGURT, NOVELTIES, PUDDING, GELATIN

	Serving	Calories	Fat (g)	Cal. from Fat	Sat. Fat (g)	Trans Fat (g)	Chol. (mg)	Sod. (mg)	Carb. (g)	Sugar (g)	Fiber (g)	Prot. (g)	Servings/Exchanges
Rainbow Ice Pops	1	40	0	0	0	0	0	0	10	7	0	0	1/2 carb
Rootbeer, Banana & Lemon Lime Ice Pops	1	45	0	0	0	0	0	0	11	8	0	0	1 carb
Scribblers	1	60	0	0	0	0	0	5	15	10	0	0	1 carb
Slow Melt Swirl Winds	1	40	0	0	0	0	0	0	10	7	0	0	1/2 carb
Snow Cone	1	30	0	0	0	0	0	5	7	5	0	0	1/2 carb
Spider Man Bar	1	100	1.5	14	0	0	0	20	25	13	0	0	1 1/2 carb
SpongeBob SquarePants Pop Ups	1	90	0	0	0	0	0	20	17	13	0	1	1 carb
Sugar Free Fudgsicle	1	40	1	7	0.5	0	2	48	10	5	2	2	1/2 carb
Sugar Free Ice Pops (All Varieties)	1	15	0	0	0	0	0	0	4	0	0	0	free
Snickers													
Snickers Ice Cream Bars	1	180	11	99	6	0	15	60	18	15	1	3	1 carb, 2 fat

Skinny Cow/Silhouette

Chocolate Fudge Cone	1	160	3	25	2	0	5	75	30	16	3	4	2 carb, 1 fat
Fudge Bars	1	110	1	10	0.5	0	5	40	22	17	3	4	1 1/2 carb
Ice Cream Sandwich, Vanilla	1 sandwich	150	2.5	25	1	0	5	120	29	15	2	4	2 carb, 1 fat
No Sugar Added Vanilla Ice Cream Sandwich	1 sandwich	140	2	20	1	0	0	125	29	4	4	4	2 carb

Weight Watchers

Smart Ones Chocolate Chip Cookie Dough Sandwich	1	140	3	30	1	0	5	60	26	16	0	2	2 carb, 1 fat
Smart Ones Mocha Fudge Sundae	1	160	4	36	2	0	5	85	27	15	1	3	2 carb, 1 fat
Smart Ones Peanut Butter-Cup Sundae	1	130	3	27	1.5	0	0	55	23	13	1	2	1 1/2 carb, 1 fat

ICE CREAM, FROZEN YOGURT, NOVELTIES, PUDDING, GELATIN

	Serving	Calories	Fat (g)	Cal. from Fat	Sat. Fat (g)	Trans Fat (g)	Chol. (mg)	Sod. (mg)	Carb. (g)	Sugar (g)	Fiber (g)	Prot. (g)	Servings/Exchanges
PUDDING & GELATIN													
Hunt's Gelatin													
Gel Snacks	3.5 oz	100	0	0	0	0	0	35	24	20	0	0	1 1/2 carb
Gel Snacks, Sugar Free	3.5 oz	5	0	0	0	0	0	30	1	0	0	0	free
Hunt's Snack Pack Pudding Cups													
Banana Cream Pie	3.5 oz	110	3.5	31	2	0	0	140	19	14	0	1	1 carb, 1 fat
Butterscotch	3.5 oz	110	2.5	30	1	0	0	140	21	14	0	1	1 1/2 carb, 1 fat
Caramel Cream	3.5 oz	120	3	25	1.5	0	0	160	21	17	0	1	1 1/2 carb, 1 fat
Chocolate	3.5 oz	110	2.5	20	1	0	0	115	20	13	2	1	1 carb, 1 fat
Fat Free Chocolate	3.5 oz	90	0	0	0	0	0	140	20	15	1	1	1 carb
Fat Free Tapioca	3.5 oz	80	0	0	0	0	0	140	19	11	0	1	1 carb
Fat Free Vanilla	3.5 oz	80	0	0	0	0	0	140	18	14	0	1	1 carb
Lemon Meringue	3.5 oz	120	2.5	23	0.5	0	0	65	25	20	0	0	1 1/2 carb, 1 fat

No Sugar Added Chocolate	3.5 oz	60	3	27	1	0	0	110	7	1	0	1	1/2 carb, 1 fat
No Sugar Added Vanilla	3.5 oz	60	3	25	1.5	0	0	105	5	0	2	0	1 fat
Tapioca	3.5 oz	120	2	36	2	0	0	140	21	16	0	2	1 1/2 carb
Vanilla	3.5 oz	110	2.5	20	1	0	0	125	20	13	1	1	1 carb, 1 fat

Jell-O Gelatin

Gelatin Dessert, Dry Mix (All Varieties)	1/2 cup	84	0	0	0	0	0	101	19	18	0	2	1 carb
Gelatin Snacks (All Flavors)	3.5 oz	70	0	0	0	0	0	40	17	16	0	1	1 carb
Gel Cups, X-treme Watermelon & Green Apple	3.5 oz	60	0	0	0	0	0	35	16	15	0	0	1 carb
Sugar-Free Snacks (All Flavors)	3.5 oz	0	0	0	0	0	0	1	0	0	0	1	free

Jell-O Pudding Snacks

Cheesecake	3.5 oz	130	2	18	1.5	0	5	125	25	22	0	2	1 1/2 carb, 4 fat
Chocolate	4 oz	90	1	9	1	0	0	130	23	17	1	1	1 1/2 carb

ICE CREAM, FROZEN YOGURT, NOVELTIES, PUDDING, GELATIN

	Serving	Calories	Fat (g)	Cal. from Fat	Sat. Fat (g)	Trans Fat (g)	Chol. (mg)	Sod. (mg)	Carb. (g)	Sugar (g)	Fiber (g)	Prot. (g)	Servings/Exchanges
Chocolate Fudge	4 oz	100	0	0	0	0	0	380	25	17	1	0	1 1/2 carb
Chocolate Vanilla Swirls	4 oz	110	1.5	15	1.5	0	0	190	24	19	0	2	1 1/2 carb
Fat Free Chocolate	4 oz	35	0	0	0	0	0	310	8	0	1	1	1/2 carb
Fat Free Chocolate Vanilla Swirls	4 oz	90	0	0	0	0	0	135	20	13	1	2	1 carb
Fat Free Tapioca	4 oz	100	0	0	0	0	0	200	23	17	0	1	1 1/2 carb
Oreo	4 oz	120	1.5	15	1.5	0	0	190	25	19	1	2	1 1/2 carb
Sugar Free Chocolate Vanilla Swirls	3.8 oz	60	1.5	13.5	1	0	0	170	6	0	1	1	1/2 carb
Sugar Free Creamy Caramel	3.8 oz	60	1	9	1	0	0	200	7	0	0	1	1/2 carb
Sugar Free Double Chocolate	3.8 oz	60	1.5	10	1	0	0	170	7	0	1	2	1/2 carb
Sugar Free Vanilla	3.8 oz	60	1	10	1	0	0	170	12	0	0	1	1 carb
Tapioca	4 oz	110	1.5	10	1.5	0	0	200	25	19	0	1	1 1/2 carb

Vanilla	4 oz	90	0	0	0	0	0	35	23	19	0	0	1 1/2 carb
Jell-O Pudding Snacks Crème Savers													
Strawberry & Crème Swirled	4 oz	130	3	27	2	0	10	85	25	19	0	2	1 1/2 carb, 1 fat
Sundae Toppers Chocolate with Chocolate Topping	3.8 oz	110	1.5	13	1	0	0	170	23	18	1	2	1 1/2 carb
Sundae Toppers Vanilla with Caramel	3.8 oz	106	1	10	1	0	0	160	23	18	0	1	1 1/2 carb
Jell-O Smoothie Snacks													
Mixed Berry	4 oz	100	2.5	23	1.5	0	10	40	18	15	0	1	1 carb, 1 fat
Strawberry Banana	4 oz	100	2.5	25	1.5	0	10	40	18	15	0	1	1 carb, 1 fat
Jell-O Pudding Sticks													
X-treme Chocolate	2.3 oz	80	2	20	1	0	0	100	16	12	1	1	1 carb
Kozy Shack													
Cinnamon Raisin Rice Pudding	1/2 cup	140	2.5	25	1.5	0	15	140	26	17	0	4	2 carb, 1 fat
Crème Caramel Flan	1/2 cup	160	4	35	2.5	0	50	100	28	28	0	5	2 carb, 1 fat

ICE CREAM, FROZEN YOGURT, NOVELTIES, PUDDING, GELATIN

	Serving	Calories	Fat (g)	Cal. from Fat	Sat. Fat (g)	Trans Fat (g)	Chol. (mg)	Sod. (mg)	Carb. (g)	Sugar (g)	Fiber (g)	Prot. (g)	Servings/Exchanges
No Sugar Added Chocolate	1/2 cup	90	2.5	25	1.5	0	10	160	13	5	3	4	1 carb, 1 fat
No Sugar Added Rice Pudding	1/2 cup	90	1.5	15	1	0	15	140	14	5	2	4	1 carb
No Sugar Added Tapioca	1/2 cup	90	1.5	10	1	0	5	135	14	5	3	3	1 carb
Old Fashioned Tapioca	1/2 cup	130	2	20	1.5	0	10	150	25	19	0	4	1 1/2 carb
Original Rice Pudding	1/2 cup	130	2.5	20	1.5	0	15	140	24	15	0	4	1 1/2 carb, 1 fat
Real Chocolate	1/2 cup	140	2.5	20	1.5	0	10	160	27	22	1	4	2 carb, 1 fat
Kraft Handi-Snacks Pudding Cups													
Banana Split	3.5 oz	100	1	10	1	0	0	170	21	16	0	1	1 1/2 carb
Butterscotch	3.5 oz	100	1	10	0.5	0	0	160	7	16	0	1	1/2 carb
Chocolate	3.5 oz	100	1	10	1	0	0	150	22	17	1	1	1 1/2 carb
Chocolate Chip Cookie	3.5 oz	120	4	35	1	0	0	160	22	16	0	2	1 1/2 carb, 1 fat
Chocolate Vanilla	3.5 oz	100	1	10	1	0	0	150	23	17	1	1	1 1/2 carb
Fat Free Chocolate	3.5 oz	100	1	10	0.5	0	0	150	23	17	0	2	1 1/2 carb

Vanilla	3.5 oz	100	1	10	1	0	0	150	23	17	1	1	1 1/2 carb
Swiss Miss Pudding Cups													
Banana Cream	1	130	3.5	32	3	0	0	170	23	17	0	2	1 1/2 carb, 1 fat
Chocolate Vanilla	1	140	3.5	32	3	0	0	160	27	20	0	2	2 carb, 1 fat
Classic Butterscotch	1	130	3.5	32	3	0	0	180	22	17	0	2	1 1/2 carb, 1 fat
Creamy Milk Chocolate	1	160	4	36	3	0	0	170	28	22	1	3	2 carb, 1 fat
Creamy Vanilla	1	160	5	45	3	0	0	160	28	21	3	1	2 carb, 1 fat
Lemon Meringue	1	140	3	30	3.5	0	0	600	28	21	0	0	2 carb, 1 fat
Low Fat Creamy Chocolate	1	160	4	36	3	0	0	180	28	22	1	3	2 carb, 1 fat
Old Fashioned Tapioca	1	140	3.5	32	0.5	0	0	180	24	18	0	2	1 1/2 carb, 1 fat
Triple Chocolate Dream	1	150	4	36	4	0	0	180	26	21	0	3	2 carb, 1 fat

MEAT, POULTRY, FISH, SEAFOOD (FRESH, COOKED)

	Serving	Calories	Fat (g)	Cal. from Fat	Sat. Fat (g)	Trans Fat (g)	Chol. (mg)	Sod. (mg)	Carb. (g)	Sugar (g)	Fiber (g)	Prot. (g)	Servings/Exchanges
BEEF (TRIMMED)													
Brisket													
Brisket, Flat Cut	3 oz	181	7	63	3	0	34	46	0	0	0	28	4 lean protein
Brisket, Whole	3 oz	247	17	153	6	0	79	55	0	0	0	23	3 med-fat protein
Chuck													
Arm Pot Roast	3 oz	238	14	126	6	0	85	53	0	0	0	25	3 med-fat protein
Blade Roast	3 oz	284	21	189	8	0	88	55	0	0	0	23	3 high-fat protein
Clod Roast	3 oz	176	9	81	3	0	59	60	0	0	0	22	3 lean protein
Flank	3 oz	160	7	63	3	0	38	48	0	0	0	24	3 lean protein
Mock Tender Steak	3 oz	136	5	45	2	0	54	60	0	0	0	22	3 lean protein
Top Blade Steak	3 oz	184	10	90	3	0	52	57	0	0	0	22	3 lean protein
Ground Beef													
75% Lean Ground Beef	3 oz	236	16	144	6	0	76	66	0	0	0	22	3 med-fat protein
80% Lean Ground Beef	3 oz	230	15	135	6	0	77	64	0	0	0	22	3 med-fat protein
85% Lean Ground Beef	3 oz	213	13	117	5	0	77	61	0	0	0	22	3 med-fat protein

90% Lean Ground Beef	3 oz	184	10	90	4	0	72	58	0	0	22	3 lean protein
95% Lean Ground Beef	3 oz	145	6	54	3	0	65	55	0	0	22	3 lean protein
Plate												
Inside Skirt Steak	3 oz	187	10	90	4	0	51	64	0	0	22	3 lean protein
Round												
Bottom Round	3 oz	159	7	63	2	0	73	31	0	0	23	3 lean protein
Eye of Round	3 oz	145	5	45	2	0	59	53	0	0	24	3 lean protein
Tip Round	3 oz	162	7	63	2	0	69	54	0	0	24	3 lean protein
Top Round	3 oz	178	5	45	2	0	77	38	0	0	30	4 lean protein
Ribs												
Rib Eye	3 oz	210	13	117	5	0	94	48	0	0	23	3 med-fat protein
Short Ribs	3 oz	400	36	324	15	0	80	45	0	0	18	3 high-fat protein
Shank												
Shank Crosscuts, Trimmed to 1/4-inch	3 oz	224	12	108	5	0	68	52	0	0	26	3 med-fat protein
Short Loin												
Porterhouse Steak	3 oz	235	16	144	6	0	57	55	0	0	20	3 med-fat protein

MEAT, POULTRY, FISH, SEAFOOD (FRESH, COOKED)

	Serving	Calories	Fat (g)	Cal. from Fat	Sat. Fat (g)	Trans Fat (g)	Chol. (mg)	Sod. (mg)	Carb. (g)	Sugar (g)	Fiber (g)	Prot. (g)	Servings/Exchanges
T-Bone Steak	3 oz	210	14	126	5	0	51	57	0	0	0	21	3 med-fat protein
Tenderloin	3 oz	200	11	99	4	0	72	53	0	0	0	23	3 med-fat protein
Top Loin	3 oz	180	9	81	3	0	65	57	0	0	0	24	3 lean protein
Sirloin													
Bottom Sirloin Tri-Tip Roast	3 oz	177	9	81	3	0	71	45	0	0	0	22	3 lean protein
Top Sirloin	3 oz	183	8	72	3	0	76	55	0	0	0	25	3 lean protein
Variety Cuts													
Liver	3 oz	162	4	36	1	0	337	67	0	0	0	25	3 lean protein
Tongue	3 oz	236	19	171	7	0	112	55	0	0	0	16	2 high-fat protein
BUFFALO	3 oz	120	2	18	<2	0	69	48	0	0	0	24	3 lean protein
LAMB													
Ground, Broiled	3 oz	240	17	153	7	0	81	69	0	0	0	21	3 med-fat protein
Leg, Sirloin, Roast, Lean	3 oz	174	8	70	3	0	78	60	0	0	0	24	3 lean protein

Loin, Roast/Chop, Cooked	3 oz	183	8	72	3	0	81	72	0	0	26	4 lean protein
Rib, Roasted	3 oz	198	11	99	3	0	75	69	0	0	22	3 med-fat protein
PORK												
Ground Pork	3 oz	252	18	162	7	0	80	62	0	0	22	3 high-fat protein
Leg (Ham)	3 oz	232	15	135	5	0	80	51	0	0	23	3 med-fat protein
Loin												
Back Ribs	3 oz	315	25	225	9	0	100	86	0	0	21	3 high-fat protein
Blade Chops	3 oz	272	21	189	8	0	73	60	0	0	19	3 high-fat protein
Center Loin Chops	3 oz	210	12	108	5	0	73	50	0	0	24	3 med-fat protein
Center Rib Roast	3 oz	214	13	117	5	0	69	41	0	0	23	3 med-fat protein
Country-Style Ribs	3 oz	279	22	198	8	0	78	44	0	0	20	3 high-fat protein
Sirloin Roast	3 oz	222	14	126	5	0	74	51	0	0	23	3 med-fat protein
Tenderloin	3 oz	147	5	45	2	0	67	47	0	0	24	3 lean protein
Top Loin Roast	3 oz	192	10	90	4	0	66	37	0	0	24	3 lean protein
Whole Loin	3 oz	211	12	108	5	0	70	50	0	0	23	3 med-fat protein

MEAT, POULTRY, FISH, SEAFOOD (FRESH, COOKED)

	Serving	Calories	Fat (g)	Cal. from Fat	Sat. Fat (g)	Trans Fat (g)	Chol. (mg)	Sod. (mg)	Carb. (g)	Sugar (g)	Fiber (g)	Prot. (g)	Servings/Exchanges
Shoulder													
Arm Picnic	3 oz	269	20	180	7	0	80	60	0	0	0	20	3 high-fat protein
Blade Boston Roast	3 oz	229	16	144	6	0	73	57	0	0	0	20	3 med-fat protein
Whole Shoulder	3 oz	248	18	162	7	0	77	58	0	0	0	20	3 med-fat protein
RABBIT	3 oz	174	6	54	2	0	72	30	0	0	0	27	3 lean protein
VEAL													
Breast	3 oz	226	14	126	6	0	96	55	0	0	0	23	3 med-fat protein
Ground Veal	3 oz	146	6	54	3	0	88	71	0	0	0	21	3 lean protein
Leg (Top Round)	3 oz	136	4	36	2	0	88	58	0	0	0	24	3 lean protein
Loin	3 oz	184	10	90	4	0	88	79	0	0	0	21	3 lean protein
Rib	3 oz	194	12	108	5	0	94	78	0	0	0	20	3 med-fat protein
Shank	3 oz	162	5	45	2	0	105	79	0	0	0	27	4 lean protein
Shoulder	3 oz	156	7	63	3	0	96	82	0	0	0	22	3 lean protein
Sirloin	3 oz	172	9	81	4	0	87	71	0	0	0	21	3 lean protein

VENISON	3 oz	135	2	18	2	0	96	45	0	0	27	3 lean protein
POULTRY												
Chicken Back, No Skin, Roasted	3 oz	203	11	99	3	0	76	82	0	0	24	3 med-fat protein
Chicken Breast, No Skin, Roasted	3 oz	141	3	27	1	0	72	63	0	0	26	3 lean protein
Chicken Capon	3 oz	195	10	90	3	0	73	42	0	0	25	3 lean protein
Chicken, Dark Meat, No Skin, Roasted	3 oz	174	8	76	2	0	78	78	0	0	23	3 lean protein
Chicken, Dark Meat with Skin, Roasted	3 oz	216	14	126	3.6	0	78	75	0	0	22	3 med-fat protein
Chicken Drumstick, No Skin, Roasted	3 oz	146	5	45	1	0	79	81	0	0	24	3 lean protein
Chicken Leg, No Skin, Roasted	3 oz	162	7	63	2	0	80	77	0	0	23	3 lean protein
Chicken, Light Meat with Skin, Roasted	3 oz	189	9	81	3	0	72	63	0	0	25	3 lean protein
Chicken Neck, No Skin, Simmered	3 oz	152	7	63	2	0	67	54	0	0	21	3 lean protein

MEAT, POULTRY, FISH, SEAFOOD (FRESH, COOKED)

	Serving	Calories	Fat (g)	Cal. from Fat	Sat. Fat (g)	Trans Fat (g)	Chol. (mg)	Sod. (mg)	Carb. (g)	Sugar (g)	Fiber (g)	Prot. (g)	Servings/Exchanges
Chicken Thigh, No Skin, Roasted	3 oz	178	9	81	3	0	81	75	0	0	0	22	3 lean protein
Chicken Wing, No Skin, Roasted	3 oz	173	7	63	2	0	72	78	0	0	0	26	4 lean protein
Chicken, with Skin, Roasted	3 oz	204	11	99	3	0	75	69	0	0	0	23	3 med-fat protein
Cornish Game Hen, Whole Bird, No Skin, Cooked	3 oz	114	3	27	1	0	90	54	0	0	0	20	3 lean protein
Duck, Domestic, No Skin, Roasted	3 oz	171	10	86	3	0	75	54	0	0	0	20	3 lean protein
Goose, No Skin, Roasted	3 oz	201	11	97	3	0	81	66	0	0	0	25	3 med-fat protein
Ostrich, Cooked	3 oz	120	2	18	0	0	81	66	0	0	0	23	3 lean protein
Pheasant, No Skin, Roasted	3 oz	114	3	27	0	0	57	30	0	0	0	20	3 lean protein

	Serving	Cal	Fat	Cal Fat	Sat	Trans	Chol	Sod	Carb	Fiber	Prot	Exchanges
Turkey Back, No Skin, Roasted	3 oz	144	5	45	2	0	81	62	0	0	24	3 lean protein
Turkey Breast, Roasted	3 oz	114	1	9	0	0	69	45	0	0	26	3 lean protein
Turkey, Dark Meat, No Skin, Cooked	3 oz	159	6	54	3	0	72	66	0	0	24	3 lean protein
Turkey, Ground, Cooked	3 oz	201	11	99	3	0	87	90	0	0	23	3 med-fat protein
Turkey Leg, No Skin, Roasted	3 oz	135	3	27	1	0	101	69	0	0	25	3 lean protein
Turkey Neck, No Skin, Roasted	3 oz	153	6	54	2	0	104	48	0	0	23	3 lean protein
Turkey Wing, No Skin, Roasted	3 oz	139	3	27	1	0	87	66	0	0	26	4 lean protein
FISH/SEAFOOD												
Bluefish, Baked	3 oz	130	5	35	1	0	65	65	0	0	22	3 lean protein
Catfish, Baked	3 oz	129	7	63	2	0	54	68	0	0	16	2 lean protein
Caviar, Black/Red, Granular	2 Tbsp	81	6	54	1	0	188	480	1	0	8	1 med-fat protein
Clams, Fresh, Steamed	1 oz	42	<1	5	<1	0	19	32	1	0	7	1 lean protein

MEAT, POULTRY, FISH, SEAFOOD (FRESH, COOKED)

	Serving	Calories	Fat (g)	Cal. from Fat	Sat. Fat (g)	Trans Fat (g)	Chol. (mg)	Sod. (mg)	Carb. (g)	Sugar (g)	Fiber (g)	Prot. (g)	Servings/Exchanges
Cod, Baked	3 oz	89	1	9	0	0	47	66	0	0	0	19	3 lean protein
Crab	3 oz	114	6	54	2	0	81	453	2	0	0	15	3 lean protein
Escargot/Snails	1 oz	51	<1	5	<1	0	28	34	1	0	0	9	1 lean protein
Flounder/Sole, Baked	3 oz	99	1	14	0	0	58	89	0	0	0	21	3 lean protein
Haddock, Baked	3 oz	95	1	7	0	0	63	74	0	0	0	21	3 lean protein
Halibut, Baked	3 oz	119	2	22	0	0	35	59	0	0	0	23	3 lean protein
Herring, Atlantic, Baked	3 oz	173	10	89	2	0	65	98	0	0	0	20	3 lean protein
Imitation Shellfish, from Surimi	1 oz	29	<1	0	<1	0	6	238	3	0	0	3	1 lean protein
Lobster, Fresh, Steamed	1 oz	28	<1	0	<1	0	20	108	<1	0	0	6	1 lean protein
Mackerel, Atlantic/Pacific, Baked	3 oz	223	15	120	4	0	64	71	0	0	0	20	3 med-fat protein
Mackerel, King, Baked	3 oz	114	2	20	0	0	58	173	0	0	0	22	3 lean protein
Ocean Perch, Baked	3 oz	102	2	16	0	0	46	82	0	0	0	20	3 lean protein
Octopus, Cooked	1 oz	46	<1	0	<1	0	27	130	1	0	0	9	1 lean protein

Food	Serving										Exchange
Orange Roughy, Baked	3 oz	76	1	7	0	22	69	0	0	16	2 lean protein
Oyster, Medium	6	58	2	18	<1	44	177	3	0	6	1 lean protein
Pollock, Baked	3 oz	100	1	9	0	77	94	0	0	21	3 lean protein
Rainbow Trout, Baked	3 oz	144	6	55	2	58	36	0	0	21	3 lean protein
Rockfish, Baked	3 oz	103	2	15	0	37	65	0	0	20	3 lean protein
Sablefish, Baked	3 oz	212	17	152	3	54	61	0	0	15	2 high-fat protein
Salmon, Atlantic/Coho, Baked	3 oz	175	10	94	2	54	52	0	0	19	3 lean protein
Salmon, Chum/Pink, Baked	3 oz	130	4	32	0	81	54	0	0	22	3 lean protein
Salmon, Sockeye, Baked	3 oz	184	9	84	2	75	55	0	0	23	3 lean protein
Scallops, Fresh, Steamed	1 oz	32	<1	0	<1	15	78	0	0	7	1 lean protein
Sea Bass, Baked	3 oz	105	2	20	0	45	74	0	0	20	3 lean protein
Shark, Baked	3 oz	140	5	22	1	50	85	0	0	22	3 lean protein
Shrimp, Fresh, Cooked in Water	1 oz	28	<1	0	<1	56	64	0	0	6	1 lean protein
Swordfish, Baked	3 oz	130	4	39	1	43	98	0	0	22	3 lean protein

MEAT, POULTRY, FISH, SEAFOOD (FRESH, COOKED)

	Serving	Calories	Fat (g)	Cal. from Fat	Sat. Fat (g)	Trans Fat (g)	Chol. (mg)	Sod. (mg)	Carb. (g)	Sugar (g)	Fiber (g)	Prot. (g)	Servings/Exchanges
Tilefish, Baked	3 oz	125	4	36	1	0	54	50	0	0	0	20	3 lean protein
Trout, Baked	3 oz	162	6	54	2	0	63	57	0	0	0	24	3 lean protein
Tuna, Yellowfin, Baked	3 oz	118	1	9	0	0	49	40	0	0	0	25	3 lean protein
Whiting, Baked	3 oz	98	1	13	0	0	71	112	0	0	0	20	3 lean protein

MILK, YOGURT, NON-DAIRY MILK

	Serving	Calories	Fat (g)	Cal. from Fat	Sat. Fat (g)	Trans Fat (g)	Chol. (mg)	Sod. (mg)	Carb. (g)	Sugar (g)	Fiber (g)	Prot. (g)	Servings/Exchanges
Buttermilk, Fat-Free	1 cup	98	2	19	1	0	10	257	12	12	0	8	1 low-fat milk
Buttermilk, Low-Fat 1%	1 cup	98	2	20	1	0	10	257	12	12	0	8	1 low-fat milk
Eggnog, Whole	1/2 cup	171	10	84	6	0	75	69	17	10	0	5	1 whole milk
Kefir, 2%	1 cup	110	2	18	1.5	0	10	125	12	12	0	11	1 low-fat milk
Milk, 1%, Low-Fat	1 cup	102	2	21	2	0	12	107	13	13	0	8	1 low-fat milk
Milk, 2%, Low-Fat, Acidophilus	1 cup	122	5	43	3	0	20	100	11	12	0	8	1 reduced-fat milk
Milk, 2%, Reduced-Fat	1 cup	122	5	43	3	0	20	100	12	12	0	8	1 reduced-fat milk
Milk, 2%, Reduced-Fat, Lactaid	1 cup	130	5	45	3	0	20	125	13	12	0	8	1 reduced-fat milk
Milk, Evaporated Fat Free	1 cup	100	<1	2	0	0	5	147	15	14.5	0	10	1 fat-free milk
Milk, Evaporated Whole	1/2 cup	169	10	86	6	0	37	134	13	13	0	9	1 whole milk
Milk, Fat-Free, Acidophilus	1 cup	102	2	21	2	0	12	106	12	13	0	8	1 low-fat milk

MILK, YOGURT, NON-DAIRY MILK

	Serving	Calories	Fat (g)	Cal. from Fat	Sat. Fat (g)	Trans Fat (g)	Chol. (mg)	Sod. (mg)	Carb. (g)	Sugar (g)	Fiber (g)	Prot. (g)	Servings/Exchanges
Milk, Fat-Free, Chocolate	1 cup	140	1	6	0	0	5	98	27	25	1	9	1 fat-free milk, 1 carb
Milk, Fat Free, Lactaid	1 cup	80	0	0	0	0	0	125	13	12	0	8	1 fat-free milk
Milk, Fat-Free, Nonfat, Skim	1 cup	83	0	2	0	0	5	103	12	12	0	8	1 fat-free milk
Milk, Goat, Whole	1 cup	168	10	89	7	0	27	122	11	11	0	9	1 whole milk
Milk, Whole	1 cup	208	8	74	5	0	30	150	26	24	2	8	1 whole milk
Milk, Whole, Chocolate	1 cup	208	8	74	5	0	30	150	26	24	2	8	1 whole milk, 1 carb
Rice Drink, Fat-Free or 1%, Plain	1 cup	86	0	4	0	0	5	128	12	12	0	8	1 carb
Rice Drink, Low-Fat, Flavored	1 cup	120	2.5	23	0	0	0	100	24	11	0	1	1 1/2 carb, 1 fat
Soy Milk, Light	1 cup	70	2	18	2	0	0	119	8	6	1	6	1/2 carb
Soy Milk, Regular, Plain	1 cup	100	4	36	1	0	0	119	8	6	1	7	1/2 carb, 1 fat
Yogurt with Fruit, Low-Fat	1 cup	250	3	23	2	0	10	142	47	47	0	11	1 low-fat milk, 2 carb

Food	Amount	Cal	Fat (g)	Fat Cal	Sat Fat (g)	Trans Fat (g)	Chol (mg)	Sodium (mg)	Carb (g)	Sugars (g)	Fiber (g)	Protein (g)	Choices/Exchanges
Yogurt & Juice Blend	1 cup	150	0	0	0	0	0	55	34	32	0	3	1 fat-free milk, 1 1/2 carb
Yogurt, Low-Fat, Plain	1 cup	154	4	33	2	0	15	171	17	17	0	13	1 low-fat milk
Yogurt, Nonfat, Plain	6 oz	96	0	0	0	0	0	75	6	6	0	18	1/2 fat-free milk
Yogurt, Whole-Milk, Plain	1 cup	149	8	70	5	0	32	113	11	11	0	9	1 whole milk
YOGURT													
Breyers													
99% Fat Free, Peaches 'N Cream	4 oz	240	2	20	1	0	20	105	20	38	0	7	1 low-fat milk, 1/2 carb
Crème Savers, Orange & Crème	6 oz	170	1.5	14	1	0	10	180	33	27	0	6	1 low-fat milk, 1 1/2 carb
Fat Free, Strawberry	6 oz	90	0	0	0	0	0	40	20	13	3	3	1 fat-free milk, 1/2 carb
Fruit on the Bottom, Peach Orange Mango	6 oz	160	1.5	10	1	0	10	85	32	28	0	6	1 low-fat milk, 1 1/2 carb
Fruit on the Bottom, Strawberry Banana	6 oz	240	2	18	1	0	20	105	48	39	0	7	1 low-fat milk, 2 1/2 carb
Inspirations, Chocolate Chip	4 oz	140	3.5	32	3	0	5	65	22	19	0	4	1 reduced-fat milk, 1/2 carb
Inspirations, Strawberry	4 oz	110	1	9	0.5	0	5	55	22	19	0	4	1 low-fat milk, 1/2 carb

MILK, YOGURT, NON-DAIRY MILK

	Serving	Calories	Fat (g)	Cal. from Fat	Sat. Fat (g)	Trans Fat (g)	Chol. (mg)	Sod. (mg)	Carb. (g)	Sugar (g)	Fiber (g)	Prot. (g)	Servings/Exchanges
Light, Mixed Berry	6 oz	80	0	0	0	0	5	85	12	11	0	6	1 fat-free milk
Smooth & Creamy, Strawberry	8 oz	232	2	18	1	0	20	125	45	39	1	9	1 low-fat milk, 2 carb
Brown Cow													
Cream Top Greek, Blueberry	6 oz	190	6	50	3.5	0	20	75	29	28	<1	5	1 reduced-fat milk, 1 carb
Cream Top Greek, Maple	6 oz	170	7	60	4	0	25	85	23	23	0	5	1 reduced-fat milk, 1 carb
Cream Top Smooth & Creamy, Pom-Berry	6 oz	160	7	60	4	0	25	85	20	20	0	6	1 reduced-fat milk, 1/2 carb
Cream Top Smooth & Creamy, Vanilla	6 oz	160	7	60	4	0	25	85	20	19	0	6	1 reduced-fat milk, 1/2 carb
Lowfat Fruit on the Bottom, Cherry-Vanilla	6 oz	180	6	50	3.5	0	20	20	28	27	0	5	1 reduced-fat milk, 1 carb
Lowfat Fruit on the Bottom, Strawberry	6 oz	190	6	50	3.5	0	20	75	29	28	<1	5	1 reduced-fat milk, 1 carb

Lowfat Smooth & Creamy, Apricot Mango	6 oz	170	6	50	3.5	0	20	80	25	24	0	5	1 reduced-fat milk, 1 carb
Lowfat Smooth & Creamy, Peach	6 oz	180	6	50	3.5	0	20	75	28	27	<1	5	1 fat-free milk, 1 carb
Nonfat Fruit on the Bottom, Strawberry	6 oz	130	0	0	0	0	0	65	18	17	0	13	1 fat-free milk, 1/2 carb
Nonfat Greek Fruit on the Bottom, Blueberry	5.3 oz	100	0	0	0	0	0	45	13	13	0	10	1 fat-free milk
Chobani Greek													
Apple Cinnamon Mighty Oats	5.3 oz	170	2	20	1	0	10	60	27	16	3	10	1 low-fat milk, 1 carb
Flip, Sriracha Mango	5.3 oz	190	6	2	0	0	15	190	23	14	<1	12	1 reduced-fat milk, 1 carb
Flip, Tropical Escape	5.3 oz	230	9	80	0	0	10	85	25	18	3	12	1 whole milk, 1 carb
Nonfat, Plain	6 oz	100	0	0	0	0	0	80	7	18	0	20	1 fat-free milk
Nonfat, Strawberry	5.3 oz	120	0	0	0	0	5	60	19	15	<1	12	1 fat-free milk, 1/2 carb
Raisin Brown Sugar Mighty Oats	5.3 oz	160	1	20	1	0	10	45	26	16	3	10	1 low-fat milk, 1 carb

MILK, YOGURT, NON-DAIRY MILK

	Serving	Calories	Fat (g)	Cal. from Fat	Sat. Fat (g)	Trans Fat (g)	Chol. (mg)	Sod. (mg)	Carb. (g)	Sugar (g)	Fiber (g)	Prot. (g)	Servings/Exchanges
Dannon Yogurt													
Activia													
Fiber, Strawberry & Cereal	4 oz	110	2	15	1	0	5	60	20	16	3	4	1 low-fat milk, 1/2 carb
Light, Strawberry	4 oz	60	0	0	0	0	<5	75	10	7	0	4	1 fat-free milk
Peach	4 oz	100	1.5	0	1	0	5	60	19	16	0	4	1 low-fat milk, 1/2 carb
Prune	4 oz	100	1.5	15	1	0	5	55	18	15	0	4	1 low-fat milk, 1/2 carb
Strawberry	4 oz	100	1.5	20	1	0	5	70	18	16	0	4	1 low-fat milk, 1/2 carb
All Natural													
Coffee	8 oz	160	2.5	23	1.5	0	10	105	26	25	0	8	1 low-fat milk, 1 carb
Lowfat, Plain	8 oz	100	2.5	25	1.5	0	10	110	12	12	0	8	1 low-fat milk
Nonfat, Plain	8 oz	100	0	0	0	0	0	150	15	15	0	11	1 fat-free milk
Vanilla	8 oz	100	2.5	23	1.5	0	10	110	12	23	0	9	1 low-fat milk

DanActive													
Strawberry	1	90	1.5	14	1	0	5	45	17	17	0	3	1 low-fat milk
Fruit on the Bottom													
Cherry	6 oz	140	1.5	14	1	0	5	85	26	24	0	6	1 low-fat milk, 1 carb
Strawberry	6 oz	150	1.5	14	1	0	10	105	25	25	0	6	1 low-fat milk, 1 carb
Light & Fit													
Carb & Sugar Controlled, Vanilla Cream	1	45	1.5	15	1	0	10	25	3	2	0	5	1/2 low-fat milk
Greek, Pineapple	1	80	0	0	0	0	10	45	8	7	0	12	1/2 fat-free milk
Greek, Strawberry	1	80	0	0	0	0	10	55	8	6	0	12	1/2 fat-free milk
Nonfat, Strawberry	1	80	0	0	0	0	<5	80	14	9	0	5	1 fat-free milk
Passion Fruit	1	80	0	0	0	0	10	45	9	7	0	12	1/2 fat-free milk
Fage													
Total 0%, Nonfat Greek	1	100	0	0	0	0	10	65	7	7	0	18	1 fat-free milk
Total 0%, Nonfat Raspberry	1	120	0	0	0	0	5	45	18	16	0	13	1 fat-free milk
Total 2%, Lowfat Greek	1	150	4	35	3	0	20	65	8	15	0	20	1 reduced-fat milk

MILK, YOGURT, NON-DAIRY MILK

	Serving	Calories	Fat (g)	Cal. from Fat	Sat. Fat (g)	Trans Fat (g)	Chol. (mg)	Sod. (mg)	Carb. (g)	Sugar (g)	Fiber (g)	Prot. (g)	Servings/Exchanges
Total 2%, Lowfat Strawberry	1	140	2.5	25	1.5	0	10	40	17	16	0	12	1 low-fat milk
Total Classic, Cherry	1	170	6	50	4.5	0	20	45	17	16	0	11	1 reduced-fat milk
Total Classic, Strawberry	1	170	6	50	4.5	0	20	45	17	16	0	11	1 reduced-fat milk
Oikos Greek													
Fat Free, Strawberry	1	120	0	0	0	0	5	50	19	18	0	12	1 fat-free milk, 1/2 carb
Fat Free, Strawberry Banana	1	130	0	0	0	0	10	45	20	19	<1	12	1 fat-free milk, 1/2 carb
Traditional, Café Latte	1	160	4.5	40	3	0	15	50	20	19	2	11	1 reduced-fat milk, 1/2 carb
Traditional, Strawberry	1	160	4.5	40	3	0	15	55	19	18	0	11	1 reduced-fat milk, 1/2 carb
Siggi's													
2% Skyr, Coconut	5.3 oz	170	8	70	5	0	10	55	11	9	1	13	1 whole milk
2% Skyr, Plain	5.3 oz	110	3	25	2	0	10	65	6	4	0	14	1 low-fat milk

Probiotic Drinkable Yogurt, Blueberry	3.9 oz	60	0	0	0	0	50	11	9	0	4	1 fat-free milk
Probiotic Drinkable Yogurt, Plain	3.9 oz	40	0	0	0	0	50	7	5	0	4	1 fat-free milk
Skyr, Blueberry	5.3 oz	110	0	0	0	0	55	13	11	0	14	1 fat-free milk
Skyr, Plain	5.3 oz	80	0	0	0	0	60	5	4	0	15	1 fat-free milk
Skyr, Strawberry	5.3 oz	120	0	0	0	10	50	14	11	0	16	1 fat-free milk
Silk (Blended Cultured Soymilk)												
Fruity & Creamy, Black Cherry	5.3 oz	140	3.5	30	0.5	0	85	21	17	2	6	1 1/2 carb, 1 fat
Fruity & Creamy, Strawberry	5.3 oz	130	3.5	30	0	0	85	19	14	2	6	1 carb, 1 fat
Fruity & Creamy, Vanilla	5.3 oz	140	3.5	30	0.5	0	90	20	16	2	6	1 carb, 1 fat
Stonyfield Organic												
Drinkable Lowfat Greek Yogurt, Honey Vanilla	1	160	2	15	1	5	135	27	26	0	9	1 low-fat milk, 1 carb
Honey Fig	1	110	0	0	0	0	65	14	14	0	14	1 fat-free milk

MILK, YOGURT, NON-DAIRY MILK

	Serving	Calories	Fat (g)	Cal. from Fat	Sat. Fat (g)	Trans Fat (g)	Chol. (mg)	Sod. (mg)	Carb. (g)	Sugar (g)	Fiber (g)	Prot. (g)	Servings/Exchanges
Strawberry	1	200	2.5	22.5	1.5	0	15	130	36	35	0	9	1 low-fat milk, 1 1/2 carb
Trader Joe's													
French Village Nonfat Fruit on the Bottom, Black Cherry	6 oz	130	0	0	0	0	0	100	26	24	0	6	1 fat-free milk, 1 carb
French Village Nonfat Fruit on the Bottom, Mixed Berry	6 oz	130	0	0	0	0	0	95	26	24	0	6	1 fat-free milk, 1 carb
Greek, Strawberry Vanilla	8 oz	310	19	170	10	0	60	160	29	23	0	8	1 whole milk, 1 carb
Greek Nonfat, Mango	5.3 oz	120	0	0	0	0	5	50	18	16	0	12	1 fat-free milk
Greek Nonfat, Strawberry	5.3 oz	120	0	0	0	0	5	40	17	14	3	12	1 fat-free milk
Low Fat Apricot Mango with Granola	4.6 oz	140	2.5	22.5	1	0	10	80	27	18	3	5	1 low-fat milk, 1 carb
Low Fat Vanilla with Almonds	4.6 oz	160	7	60	2	0	10	70	20	17	3	6	1 reduced-fat milk, 1/2 carb

Food	Serving												Exchanges/Choices
Mocha European Style Low Fat, Chocolate	5.3 oz	130	2	18	0	0	10	90	20	16	0	8	1 low-fat milk, 1/2 carb
Organic Greek Nonfat, Plain	1 cup	130	0	0	0	0	5	95	9	9	0	23	1 fat-free milk
Organic Greek Nonfat, Vanilla	5.3 oz	130	0	0	0	0	5	45	20	17	0	12	1 fat-free milk, 1/2 carb
Organic Low Fat, Blueberry	6 oz	140	2.5	25	1.5	0	15	75	24	20	0	7	1 low-fat milk, 1/2 carb
Organic Low Fat, Strawberry	6 oz	120	1.5	10	1	0	15	120	21	20	0	6	1 low-fat milk, 1/2 carb
Strawberry	8 oz	310	19	170	10	0	60	160	320	23	0	8	1 whole milk, 1 carb
Yoplait Yogurt													
Delights, All Flavors	4 oz	100	1.5	13	1	0	5	90	18	13	0	5	1 low-fat milk, 1/2 carb
Fiber One Nonfat Yogurt	4 oz	80	0	0	0	0	3	65	19	11	4	5	1 fat-free milk, 1/2 carb
GoGurt, Fruit Flavors	1 tube	60	0.5	5	0	0	<5	30	12	9	0	2	1 carb
Light, Fruit Flavors	6 oz	90	0	0	0	0	<5	80	16	10	0	5	1 fat-free milk
Original, Fruit Flavors	6 oz	150	2	15	1	0	10	95	25	18	0	5	1 low-fat milk, 1 carb

MILK, YOGURT, NON-DAIRY MILK

	Serving	Calories	Fat (g)	Cal. from Fat	Sat. Fat (g)	Trans Fat (g)	Chol. (mg)	Sod. (mg)	Carb. (g)	Sugar (g)	Fiber (g)	Prot. (g)	Servings/Exchanges
Thick & Creamy, Fruit Flavors	6 oz	180	2.5	1.5	2	0	15	110	31	28	0	7	1 low-fat milk, 1 carb
Trix Yogurt, Fruit Flavors	4 oz	100	0.5	5	0.5	0	<5	50	20	13	0	3	1 fat-free milk, 1/2 carb
Whips! (Whipped Yogurt), Fruit Flavors	4 oz	140	2.5	20	1.5	0	10	75	25	21	0	5	1 low-fat milk, 1 carb
Yoplait Kids, Strawberry	4 oz	70	1	20	0.5	0	5	75	12	8	0	3	1 low-fat milk
Yoplus	4 oz	110	1.5	13	1	0	10	70	21	16	3	4	1 low-fat milk, 1/2 carb
Yoplus Light	4 oz	70	0	0	0	0	6	65	15	10	3	4	1 fat-free milk
ALMOND MILK													
Almond Dream (Shelf Stable)													
Original	1 cup	70	3	25	0	0	0	135	12	7	5	1	1 carb, 1 fat
Unsweetened	1 cup	50	3.5	30	0	0	0	135	3	<1	<1	1	1 fat
Unsweetened Vanilla	1 cup	50	3.5	30	0	0	0	170	3	<1	<1	1	1 fat
Vanilla	1 cup	80	2.5	25	0	0	0	125	13	11	<1	1	1 carb, 1 fat

Blue Diamond Almond Breeze (Shelf Stable)

Chocolate	1 cup	130	3	20	0	0	190	24	22	1	2	1 1/2 carb, 1 fat
Original	1 cup	60	2.5	25	0	0	130	8	7	1	1	1/2 carb, 1 fat
Unsweetened, Chocolate	1 cup	40	3.5	30	0	0	160	2	0	1	2	1 fat
Unsweetened, Original	1 cup	30	2.5	20	0	0	150	1	0	1	1	1 fat
Unsweetened, Vanilla	1 cup	30	2.5	20	0	0	150	1	0	1	1	1 fat
Vanilla	1 cup	100	3	25	0	0	180	17	16	1	1	1 carb, 1 fat

Blue Diamond Almond Breeze (Refrigerated)

Chocolate	1 cup	120	3	25	0	0	150	22	20	1	1	1 1/2 carb, 1 fat
Original	1 cup	60	2.5	25	0	0	150	8	7	1	1	1/2 carb, 1 fat
Original Reduced Sugar	1 cup	40	2.5	20	0	0	150	4	3	1	1	1 fat
Unsweetened, Original	1 cup	30	2.5	20	0	0	180	1	0	1	1	1 fat
Unsweetened, Vanilla	1 cup	30	2.5	25	0	0	180	1	0	1	1	1 fat
Vanilla	1 cup	80	2.5	25	0	0	150	14	13	13	1	1 carb, 1 fat
Vanilla Reduced Sugar	1 cup	60	2.5	25	0	0	150	9	8	1	1	1/2 carb, 1 fat

MILK, YOGURT, NON-DAIRY MILK

	Serving	Calories	Fat (g)	Cal. from Fat	Sat. Fat (g)	Trans Fat (g)	Chol. (mg)	Sod. (mg)	Carb. (g)	Sugar (g)	Fiber (g)	Prot. (g)	Servings/Exchanges
Pacific Organic (Shelf Stable)													
Chocolate	1 cup	100	3	25	0	0	0	150	19	17	1	1	1 carb, 1 fat
Original	1 cup	60	3	30	0	0	0	150	8	7	0	1	1/2 carb, 1 fat
Unsweetened, Original	1 cup	35	2.5	25	0	0	0	190	2	0	0	1	1 fat
Unsweetened, Vanilla	1 cup	35	2.5	25	0	0	0	190	3	0	0	1	1 fat
Vanilla	1 cup	70	3	30	0	0	0	150	11	10	0	1	1 carb, 1 fat
Silk (Refrigerated)													
Dark Chocolate	1 cup	100	2.5	20	0	0	0	240	19	17	1	1	1 carb, 1 fat
Light Original	1 cup	40	2	20	0	0	0	160	5	5	0	<1	1 fat
Light Vanilla	1 cup	60	2	15	0	0	0	160	11	11	0	<1	1 carb
Original	1 cup	60	2.5	25	0	0	0	160	8	7	<1	1	1/2 carb, 1 fat
Unsweetened, Original	1 cup	30	2.5	25	0	0	0	160	<1	0	<1	1	1 fat
Unsweetened, Vanilla	1 cup	30	2.5	25	0	0	0	160	<1	0	<0	1	1 fat
Vanilla	1 cup	90	2.5	25	0	0	0	160	16	16	<1	1	1 carb, 1 fat

Vanilla Protein + Fiber	1 cup	100	2.5	25	0	0	150	13	12	5	5	1 carb, 1 fat

CASHEW MILK

Cashew Dream

Original Cashew Drink	1 cup	50	2.5	25	0.5	0	120	7	5	0	<1	1/2 carb, 1 fat
Unsweetened Cashew Drink	1 cup	40	3	0.5	25	0	120	3	0	0	<1	1 fat

Silk

Enriched Unsweetened	1 cup	60	5	45	0	0	150	1	<1	0	0	1 fat
Original	1 cup	60	2.5	20	0	0	170	9	7	0	<1	1/2 carb, 1 fat
Unsweetened	1 cup	25	2	15	0	0	160	1	0	0	<1	free

COCONUT MILK

Coconut Dream (Shelf Stable)

Enriched Original	1 cup	80	5	45	0	0	140	7	7	0	0	1/2 carb, 1 fat
Enriched Vanilla	1 cup	90	5	45	0	0	140	9	8	0	0	1/2 carb, 1 fat

Silk

Original	1 cup	80	5	45	0	0	45	7	6	0	<1	1/2 carb, 1 fat
Unsweetened	1 cup	45	4.5	40	0	0	40	<1	0	0	0	1 fat

MILK, YOGURT, NON-DAIRY MILK

	Serving	Calories	Fat (g)	Cal. from Fat	Sat. Fat (g)	Trans Fat (g)	Chol. (mg)	Sod. (mg)	Carb. (g)	Sugar (g)	Fiber (g)	Prot. (g)	Servings/Exchanges
Vanilla	1 cup	90	5	45	5	0	0	45	9	9	0	<1	1/2 carb, 1 fat
GRAIN MILK													
Pacific (Shelf Stable)													
Organic Oat, Low Fat, Vanilla	1 cup	130	2.5	20	0	0	0	110	24	20	2	4	1 1/2 carb, 1 fat
HAZELNUT MILK													
Pacific (Shelf Stable)													
Chocolate	1 cup	120	5	45	0.5	0	0	140	19	15	1	2	1 carb, 1 fat
Original	1 cup	110	3.5	30	0	0	0	120	19	14	1	2	1 carb, 1 fat
HEMP MILK													
Pacific All Natural (Shelf Stable)													
Chocolate	1 cup	190	5	45	1	0	0	150	35	23	2	3	2 carb, 1 fat
Original	1 cup	140	5	45	0.5	0	0	130	20	14	1	3	1 carb, 1 fat
Unsweetened, Original	1 cup	70	5	45	0.5	0	0	140	1	0	2	3	1 fat

Unsweetened, Vanilla	1 cup	70	5	45	0.5	0	0	140	1	0	2	3	1 fat
Vanilla	1 cup	160	5	45	0.5	0	0	135	24	16	1	3	1 1/2 carb, 1 fat

RICE MILK

Pacific (Shelf Stable)

Low Fat, Plain	1 cup	130	2	20	0	0	0	60	27	14	0	1	2 carb

Rice Dream (Refrigerated)

Enriched, Original	1 cup	130	2	20	0	0	0	60	27	14	0	1	2 carb
Enriched, Vanilla	1 cup	130	2	20	0	0	0	60	27	14	0	1	2 carb

Rice Dream (Shelf Stable)

Classic, Carob	1 cup	150	2.5	23	0	0	0	80	30	26	0	1	2 carb, 1 fat
Enriched, Original	1 cup	100	2	18	0	0	0	90	20	15	0	0	1 carb
Enriched, Vanilla	1 cup	120	2	18	0	0	0	100	26	18	0	0	2 carb
Heartwise, Original	1 cup	130	2	18	0	0	0	80	30	9	3	1	2 carb
Heartwise, Vanilla	1 cup	140	2	18	0	0	0	80	30	10	3	1	2 carb
Horchata	1 cup	140	2.5	23	1.5	0	5	35	27	23	0	3	2 carb, 1 fat
Original	1 cup	120	2	18	0	0	1	25	25	0	0	0	1 1/2 carb
Vanilla	1 cup	130	2	18	0	0	0	60	27	14	0	1	2 carb

MILK, YOGURT, NON-DAIRY MILK

	Serving	Calories	Fat (g)	Cal. from Fat	Sat. Fat (g)	Trans Fat (g)	Chol. (mg)	Sod. (mg)	Carb. (g)	Sugar (g)	Fiber (g)	Prot. (g)	Servings/Exchanges
WestSoy (Shelf Stable)													
Rice Beverage, Plain	1 cup	110	2.5	25	0	0	0	105	20	13	0	1	1 carb, 1 fat
Rice Beverage, Vanilla	1 cup	110	2.5	22	0	0	0	110	20	13	0	1	1 carb, 1 fat
SOY MILK													
Pacific (Shelf Stable)													
Organic Soy, Unsweetened, Original	1 cup	100	0.5	40	0.5	0	0	30	5	1	4	9	1/2 carb
Select Soy, Low Fat, Plain	1 cup	70	2.5	20	0	0	0	115	9	6	1	5	1/2 carb, 1 fat
Select Soy, Low Fat, Vanilla	1 cup	80	2.5	20	0	0	0	115	11	9	1	5	1 carb, 1 fat
Ultra Soy, Plain	1 cup	140	5	45	0.5	0	0	150	12	8	1	10	1 carb, 1 fat
Ultra Soy, Vanilla	1 cup	140	5	45	0.5	0	0	150	14	10	1	10	1 carb, 1 fat
Silk (Refrigerated)													
Chocolate	1 cup	120	3	25	0.5	0	0	80	21	17	2	5	1 1/2 carb, 1 fat

Light, Chocolate	1 cup	90	1.5	15	0	0	85	16	14	1	3	1 carb
Light, Original	1 cup	60	1.5	15	0	0	135	5	3	1	6	1/2 carb
Light, Vanilla	1 cup	70	2	15	0	0	90	7	5	1	6	1/2 carb
Plain Original	1 cup	110	4.5	40	0.5	0	95	9	6	2	8	1/2 carb, 1 fat
Unsweetened	1 cup	80	4	35	0.5	0	75	4	1	2	7	1 fat
Vanilla	1 cup	100	3.5	30	0.5	0	90	12	9	1	6	1/2 carb, 1 fat
Very Vanilla	1 cup	130	3.5	30	0.5	0	110	18	15	1	6	1 carb, 1 fat
Silk (Shelf Stable)												
Plain Original	1 cup	100	4	35	0.5	0	120	8	6	1	7	1/2 carb, 1 fat
Unsweetened	1 cup	30	2.5	25	0	0	170	1	0	1	1	1 fat
Vanilla	1 cup	100	3.5	30	0.5	0	100	10	7	1	6	1/2 carb, 1 fat
Soy Dream (Refrigerated)												
Classic Original	1 cup	130	4	36	0.5	0	150	16	9	2	7	1 carb, 1 fat
Enriched, Vanilla	1 cup	100	4	35	0.5	0	135	8	6	2	7	1 carb, 1 fat
Soy Dream (Shelf Stable)												
Classic Vanilla	1 cup	140	4	36	0.5	0	135	18	10	2	7	1 carb, 1 fat

MILK, YOGURT, NON-DAIRY MILK

	Serving	Calories	Fat (g)	Cal. from Fat	Sat. Fat (g)	Trans Fat (g)	Chol. (mg)	Sod. (mg)	Carb. (g)	Sugar (g)	Fiber (g)	Prot. (g)	Servings/Exchanges
Enriched, Chocolate	1 cup	150	4	36	0.5	0	0	125	21	15	3	7	1 1/2 carb, 1 fat
Enriched, Original	1 cup	100	4	36	0.5	0	0	135	8	4	2	7	1/2 carb, 1 fat
Enriched, Vanilla	1 cup	120	4	36	0.5	0	0	135	14	10	2	7	1 carb, 1 fat
WestSoy (Shelf Stable)													
Lite, Plain	1 cup	60	2	18	0	0	0	80	6	6	1	4	1/2 carb
Low Fat, Plain	1 cup	90	2	18	0	0	0	80	15	5	2	4	1 carb
Low Fat, Vanilla	1 cup	120	1.5	13	0	0	0	90	21	10	2	4	1 1/2 carb
Non Fat, Plain	1 cup	70	1.5	10	0	0	0	105	10	9	1	6	1/2 carb
Non Fat, Vanilla	1 cup	80	1.5	10	0	0	0	105	12	10	1	6	1 carb
Organic Plus, Plain	1 cup	70	3.5	30	0.5	0	0	125	7	6	1	7	1/2 carb, 1 fat
Organic Plus, Vanilla	1 cup	110	4.5	41	0.5	0	0	125	11	10	1	8	1/2 carb, 1 fat
Organic, Unsweetened, Original	1 cup	90	4.5	41	0.5	0	0	30	5	1	4	9	1 fat
Organic, Unsweetened, Vanilla	1 cup	100	4.5	41	0.5	0	0	30	5	1	4	9	1 fat

NUTS, SEEDS, NUT/SEED PRODUCTS

	Serving	Calories	Fat (g)	Cal. from Fat	Sat. Fat (g)	Trans Fat (g)	Chol. (mg)	Sod. (mg)	Carb. (g)	Sugar (g)	Fiber (g)	Prot. (g)	Servings/Exchanges
Almond Butter, Plain	1 Tbsp	101	9	79	1	0	0	2	3	0	1	2	2 fat
Almond Butter, Salted	1 Tbsp	101	9	80	<1	0	0	72	3	1	1	2	2 fat
Almonds, Dried, Whole	1 oz	169	15	125	1	0	0	0	5	1	3	6	3 fat
Almonds, Dry-Roasted	1 oz	169	15	125	1	0	0	96	5	1	3	6	3 fat
Almonds, Dry-Roasted, Whole, Unsalted	1 oz	169	15	135	1	0	0	0	5	1	3	6	3 fat
Almonds, Oil-Roasted	1 oz	171	16	130	1	0	0	96	5	1	3	6	3 fat
Almonds, Toasted	1 oz	169	15	135	1	0	0	0	6	1	3	6	1/2 carb, 3 fat
Beechnuts, Dried	1 oz	163	14	127	2	0	0	11	10	0	0	2	1 carb, 1 fat
Brazilnuts, Dried	1 oz	185	19	157	4	0	0	1	4	1	2	4	4 fat
Cashew Butter, Plain	1 Tbsp	94	8	71	2	0	0	3	4	0	<1	3	2 fat
Cashews, Dry-Roasted	1 oz	161	13	109	3	0	0	179	9	1	1	4	1/2 carb, 3 fat
Cashews, Oil-Roasted	1 oz	164	13	113	2	0	0	87	9	1	1	5	1/2 carb, 3 fat
Chinese Chestnuts, Dried	1 oz	103	1	4	0	0	0	1	22	0	0	2	1 1/2 carb

NUTS, SEEDS, NUT/SEED PRODUCTS

	Serving	Calories	Fat (g)	Cal. from Fat	Sat. Fat (g)	Trans Fat (g)	Chol. (mg)	Sod. (mg)	Carb. (g)	Sugar (g)	Fiber (g)	Prot. (g)	Servings/Exchanges
Chinese Chestnuts, Roasted	1 oz	68	<1	3	0	0	0	1	15	0	0	1	1 carb
Coconut, Dried, Shredded, Sweetened	1 oz	140	10	86	9	0	0	73	13	12	1	1	1 carb, 2 fat
Coconut, Fresh	1 cup	283	27	224	24	0	0	16	12	5	7	3	1 carb, 5 fat
Coconut Milk, Raw	1 Tbsp	35	4	30	0	0	0	2	1	1	0	0	1 fat
Coconut, Toasted	1 oz	166	13	110	12	0	0	9	7	2	4	2	1/2 carb, 3 fat
English Walnut Halves, Dried	1 oz	185	18	154	2	0	0	0	1	1	2	4	4 fat
European Chestnuts, Roasted	1 oz	69	1	5	0	0	0	1	15	2	1	1	1 carb
Filberts/Hazelnuts, Dried, Whole	0.5 oz	87	8	76	0	0	0	0	3	<1	1	2	2 fat
Filberts/Hazelnuts, Dry-Roasted, Salted	1 oz	181	17	146	1	0	0	146	0	1	3	4	3 fat
Flaxseed, Whole	1 Tbsp	55	4	36	0	0	0	3	3	0	3	2	1 fat

Ginkgo Nuts	1 oz	51	0	4	0	0	2	11	0	0	1	1 carb
Hickory Nuts, Dried	1 oz	186	18	165	2	0	2	5	1	2	4	4 fat
Japanese Chestnuts, Dried	1 oz	101	0	3	0	0	10	23	1	<1	1	1 1/2 carb
Japanese Chestnuts, Roasted	1 oz	56	0	2	0	0	5	13	1	0	1	1 carb
Macadamia Nuts	1 oz	203	21	179	3	0	1	4	1	2	2	4 fat
Macadamia Nuts, Oil-Roasted	1 oz	202	21	180	3	0	75	4	1	2	2	4 fat
Mixed Nuts, Dry-Roasted	1 oz	166	14	121	2	0	187	7	1	3	5	1/2 carb, 3 fat
Mixed Nuts, Oil-Roasted	1 oz	172	16	132	3	0	86	6	1	2	4	1/2 carb, 3 fat
Mixed Nuts, Oil-Roasted, No Peanuts	1 oz	172	16	132	3	0	3	6	1	2	4	1/2 carb, 3 fat
Mixed Nuts, Oil-Roasted, Unsalted	1 oz	173	16	132	2	0	117	6	1	3	5	1/2 carb, 3 fat
Peanut Butter, Chunky or Smooth	2 Tbsp	190	16	138	3	0	117	6	4	2	8	1/2 carb, 3 fat
Peanut Butter, Natural, Salted	2 Tbsp	188	16	135	3	0	5	6	3	2	8	1/2 carb, 3 fat

NUTS, SEEDS, NUT/SEED PRODUCTS

	Serving	Calories	Fat (g)	Cal. from Fat	Sat. Fat (g)	Trans Fat (g)	Chol. (mg)	Sod. (mg)	Carb. (g)	Sugar (g)	Fiber (g)	Prot. (g)	Servings/Exchanges
Peanut Butter, Natural, Unsalted	1 oz	175	13	118	3	0	0	0	6	2	2	8	1/2 carb, 3 fat
Peanuts, Dry-Roasted, Unsalted	1 oz	166	14	127	2	0	0	2	6	1	2	7	1/2 carb, 3 fat
Peanuts, Oil-Roasted	1 oz	168	15	123	2	0	0	90	4	1	3	8	3 fat
Peanuts, Spanish, Raw	1 oz	160	14	116	2	0	0	6	4	1	3	7	3 fat
Pecans, Dried Halves	1 oz	162	14	127	2	0	0	6	4	1	2	7	3 fat
Pecans, Dry-Roasted	1 oz	199	21	174	2	0	0	0	4	1	3	3	4 fat
Pecans, Oil-Roasted	1 oz	200	21	176	2	0	0	0	4	1	3	3	4 fat
Pine Nuts (Pignoli), Dried	1 oz	61	6	56	0	0	0	0	1	0	0	1	1 fat
Pistachio Nuts, Dry-Roasted	1 oz	161	13	109	2	0	0	3	8	2	3	6	1/2 carb, 3 fat
Pumpkin Seeds, Roasted	1 oz	163	14	46	2	0	0	73	4	0	2	8	3 fat
Sesame Seeds, Dried, Whole	1 Tbsp	52	4	37	1	0	0	1	2	0	1	2	1 fat

Soy Nut Butter	2 Tbsp	190	14	120	2.5	0	0	100	10	3	3	7	1/2 carb, 3 fat
Soy Nuts, Dry-Roasted, No Salt	0.75 oz	96	5	45	<1	0	0	0	7	1	2	8	1/2 carb, 1 fat
Sunflower Seeds, Dried	1 oz	165	14	125	1.5	0	0	1	7	3	1	5	1/2 carb, 3 fat
Sunflower Seeds, Dry-Roasted	1 oz	163	14	117	1	0	0	1	7	3	1	5	1/2 carb, 3 fat
Sunflower Seeds, Oil-Roasted	1 oz	166	14	120	2	0	0	1	6	3	1	6	1/2 carb, 3 fat
Tahini/Sesame Butter	1 Tbsp	89	8	68	1	0	0	17	3	0	1	3	2 fat

PEANUT BUTTER, REDUCED-FAT PEANUT BUTTER, & FLAVORED PEANUT BUTTER

Better'n Peanut Butter

Low Sodium	2 Tbsp	100	2	22	0	0	0	95	13	2	2	4	1 carb, 1 lean protein
Regular Creamy	2 Tbsp	100	2	18	0	0	0	190	13	2	2	4	1 carb, 1 lean protein

Fifty50

Creamy Peanut Butter, No Added Sugar	2 Tbsp	190	16	144	2	0	0	0	7	1	3	7	1 high-fat protein, 1 fat

Jif

Creamy	2 Tbsp	190	16	130	3	0		135	8	3	2	7	1 high-fat protein, 1 fat

NUTS, SEEDS, NUT/SEED PRODUCTS

	Serving	Calories	Fat (g)	Cal. from Fat	Sat. Fat (g)	Trans Fat (g)	Chol. (mg)	Sod. (mg)	Carb. (g)	Sugar (g)	Fiber (g)	Prot. (g)	Servings/Exchanges
Creamy Peanut Butter & Honey	2 Tbsp	180	14	120	2.5	0	0	120	10	5	2	7	1/2 carb, 1 high-fat protein, 1 fat
Creamy Peanut Butter with Omega-3 DHA & EPA	2 Tbsp	190	16	140	3	0	0	135	8	3	2	7	1 high-fat protein, 1 fat
Creamy Peanut Butter TO GO	1.5-oz cup	250	22	180	3.5	0	0	180	11	4	3	9	1 carb, 1 high-fat protein, 2 fat
Crunchy Peanut Butter	2 Tbsp	190	16	130	2.5	0	0	105	8	3	2	7	1 high-fat protein, 1 fat
Extra Crunchy	2 Tbsp	190	16	130	3	0	0	130	8	3	2	7	1 high-fat protein, 1 fat
Natural Creamy Peanut Butter Spread 90% Peanuts	2 Tbsp	190	16	130	3	0	0	80	8	3	2	7	1 high-fat protein, 1 fat
Natural Creamy Peanut Butter Spread & Honey 80% Peanuts	2 Tbsp	190	15	130	2.5	0	0	85	10	6	2	7	1/2 carb, 1 high-fat protein, 1 fat

Food	Serving											
Peanut Butter & Chocolate Flavored Spread TO GO	1.5-oz cup	250	18	160	3.5	0	0	95	18	14	2	5	1 carb, 1 high-fat protein, 2 fat
Peanut Powder, Chocolate	3 Tbsp	70	2	15	0	0	0	0	4	1	2	8	1 lean protein
Peanut Powder, Regular	3 Tbsp	70	2	15	0	0	0	0	4	1	2	8	1 lean protein
Reduced-Fat, Creamy Peanut Butter 60% Peanuts	2 Tbsp	190	12	100	2	0	0	200	15	4	2	7	1 carb, 1 high-fat protein
Reduced-Fat, Crunchy Peanut Butter 60% Peanuts	2 Tbsp	190	12	100	2	0	0	180	15	4	2	7	1 carb, 1 high-fat protein
Simply Jif, Creamy	2 Tbsp	180	16	130	2.5	0	0	65	7	2	2	7	1 high-fat protein, 1 fat
Whipped Creamy Peanut Butter Spread	2 Tbsp	140	12	100	2	0	0	95	6	2	2	5	1 high-fat protein
Whipped Peanut Butter & Chocolate Flavored Spread	2 Tbsp	150	11	100	2	0	0	55	11	8	1	3	1 carb, 1 high-fat protein

NUTS, SEEDS, NUT/SEED PRODUCTS

	Serving	Calories	Fat (g)	Cal. from Fat	Sat. Fat (g)	Trans Fat (g)	Chol. (mg)	Sod. (mg)	Carb. (g)	Sugar (g)	Fiber (g)	Prot. (g)	Servings/Exchanges
Whipped Peanut Butter & Salty Caramel Flavored Spread	2 Tbsp	140	12	100	2	0	0	90	6	3	2	5	1 carb, 1 high-fat protein
Laura Scudder's													
No-Stir Smooth Peanut Butter	2 Tbsp	210	17	140	3	0	0	160	6	1	2	7	1 high-fat protein, 1 fat
Nutty Peanut Butter	2 Tbsp	200	16	140	2.5	0	0	90	6	1	2	8	1 high-fat protein, 1 fat
Smooth Peanut Butter	2 Tbsp	200	16	140	2.5	0	0	105	6	1	2	8	1 high-fat protein, 1 fat
Smooth Reduced Fat Peanut Butter	2 Tbsp	190	12	110	2	0	0	115	12	2	2	8	1 carb, 1 high-fat protein
Smooth Unsalted Peanut Butter	2 Tbsp	210	16	140	2.5	0	0	0	6	1	2	8	1 high-fat protein, 1 fat
MaraNatha													
Natural No Stir Creamy Peanut Butter	2 Tbsp	190	16	140	2.5	0	0	70	8	3	2	7	1 high-fat protein, 1 fat

Food	Serving											Exchanges
Organic Creamy Peanut Butter No Salt Added	2 Tbsp	190	16	140	2	0	0	7	1	3	8	1 high-fat protein, 1 fat
Organic Crunchy Peanut Butter with Salt	2 Tbsp	190	16	140	2	0	0	7	1	3	8	1 high-fat protein, 1 fat
Organic No Stir Creamy Peanut Butter	2 Tbsp	190	16	140	2.5	0	0	8	3	2	7	1 high-fat prote.n, 1 fat
PB2												
Powdered Chocolate Peanut Butter	2 Tbsp	45	1	10	0	0	0	6	3	1	4	1 lean protein
Powdered Peanut Butter	2 Tbsp	45	1.5	13	0	0	0	5	1	2	5	1 lean protein
Peter Pan												
Chunky Reduced Fat	2 Tbsp	200	13	120	2.5	0	0	14	4	2	8	1 carb, 1 high-fat protein, 1 fat
Creamy	2 Tbsp	210	17	150	3	0	0	6	3	2	8	1 high-fat protein, 1 fat
Creamy Honey Roast	2 Tbsp	210	14	150	3	0	0	6	3	2	8	1 high-fat protein, 1 fat
Creamy Plus	2 Tbsp	210	17	150	3	0	0	7	3	2	8	1 high-fat protein, 1 fat
Creamy Spread, Reduced Fat	2 Tbsp	200	13	120	2	0	0	14	2	2	8	1 carb, 1 high-fat protein, 1 fat

NUTS, SEEDS, NUT/SEED PRODUCTS

	Serving	Calories	Fat (g)	Cal. from Fat	Sat. Fat (g)	Trans Fat (g)	Chol. (mg)	Sod. (mg)	Carb. (g)	Sugar (g)	Fiber (g)	Prot. (g)	Servings/Exchanges
Creamy Whipped	2 Tbsp	150	12	110	2.5	0	0	105	5	2	2	6	1 high-fat protein
Crunchy	2 Tbsp	200	16	140	3	0	0	110	6	3	2	8	1 high-fat protein, 1 fat
Skippy													
Creamy	2 Tbsp	190	16	140	3	0	0	150	7	3	2	7	1 high-fat protein, 1 fat
Natural Creamy	2 Tbsp	190	16	150	3.5	0	0	150	6	3	2	7	1 high-fat protein, 1 fat
Reduced-Fat Creamy	2 Tbsp	180	12	110	2	0	0	170	14	4	2	7	1 carb, 1 high-fat protein
Reduced-Fat Super Chunk	2 Tbsp	180	12	110	2	0	0	160	14	4	2	7	1 carb, 1 high-fat protein
Roasted Honey Nut Super Chunk	2 Tbsp	200	16	140	3	0	0	125	6	3	2	7	1 high-fat protein, 1 fat
Super Chunk	2 Tbsp	190	16	140	3	0	0	125	6	3	2	7	1 high-fat protein, 1 fat
Trader Joe's													
Creamy Salted Peanut Butter	2 Tbsp	190	16	140	2	0	0	140	7	1	2	7	1 high-fat protein, 1 fat

Food	Serving											Exchanges/Choices
Creamy Unsalted Peanut Butter	2 Tbsp	190	16	150	2.5	0	0	0	7	1	3	7	1 high-fat protein, 1 fat
Crunchy Salted Peanut Butter with Flax & Chia Seeds	2 Tbsp	170	14	130	2	0	0	10	7	1	3	7	1 high-fat protein, 1 fat
Organic Creamy No Salt Peanut Butter	2 Tbsp	200	14	140	2	0	0	0	7	2	3	8	1 high-fat protein, 1 fat

Smart Balance

Food	Serving											Exchanges/Choices
Chunky	2 Tbsp	190	15	135	13	0	0	0	8	3	2	7	1 high-fat protein, 1 fat

ALMOND, CASHEW, HAZELNUT, AND OTHER NUT BUTTERS

Jif

Food	Serving											Exchanges/Choices
Chocolate Cheesecake Flavored Hazelnut Spread	2 Tbsp	210	13	120	3.5	0	0	25	22	22	1	1	1 1/2 carb, 3 fat
Chocolate Flavored Hazelnut Spread	2 Tbsp	230	14	120	3	0	<5	25	23	22	1	2	1 1/2 carb, 3 fat
Cookies & Cream Hazelnut Spread	2 Tbsp	210	13	120	3.5	0	0	30	22	21	1	1	1 1/2 carb, 3 fat
Creamy Almond Butter	2 Tbsp	190	16	150	2	0	0	0	8	3	3	7	1 high-fat protein, 1 fat

NUTS, SEEDS, NUT/SEED PRODUCTS

	Serving	Calories	Fat (g)	Cal. from Fat	Sat. Fat (g)	Trans Fat (g)	Chol. (mg)	Sod. (mg)	Carb. (g)	Sugar (g)	Fiber (g)	Prot. (g)	Servings/Exchanges
Creamy Cashew Butter	2 Tbsp	200	18	150	3.5	0	0	105	10	3	1	4	1 high-fat protein, 2 fat
Crunchy Almond Butter	2 Tbsp	190	16	150	2	0	0	95	7	3	3	7	1 high-fat protein, 1 fat
Crunchy Cashew Butter	2 Tbsp	200	17	150	3.5	0	0	90	10	3	1	4	1 high-fat protein, 1 fat
Mocha Cappuccino Flavored Hazelnut Spread	2 Tbsp	230	14	130	3	0	<5	35	22	22	1	2	1 1/2 carb, 3 fat
Salted Caramel Flavored Hazelnut Spread	2 Tbsp	230	14	130	3	0	<5	70	23	23	1	2	1 1/2 carb, 3 fat
Justin's													
Chocolate Hazelnut Butter	2 Tbsp	180	14	120	2.5	0	0	65	12	8	3	4	1 carb, 1 high-fat protein, 1 fat
Maple Almond Butter	2 Tbsp	190	13	120	0	0	65	9	3	3	6	4	1 high-fat protein, 1 fat
MaraNatha													
Caramel Almond Spread	2 Tbsp	190	14	120	4	0	0	40	13	11	1	4	1 carb, 1 high-fat protein, 1 fat

Dark Chocolate Almond Spread	2 Tbsp	180	14	130	3	0	0	15	12	9	2	4	1 carb, 1 high-fat protein, 1 fat
Natural Cashew Butter	2 Tbsp	190	15	140	3	0	0	0	10	2	2	5	1 high-fat protein, 1 fat
Natural Creamy No Salt Almond Butter	2 Tbsp	190	16	150	1.5	0	0	0	6	2	4	7	1 high-fat protein, 1 fat
Natural Creamy Raw Almond Butter	2 Tbsp	195	16	150	1	0	0	0	6	2	4	7	1 high-fat protein, 1 fat
Natural No Stir Creamy Coconut Almond Butter	2 Tbsp	190	17	150	4	0	0	55	7	3	4	6	1 high-fat protein, 1 fat
No Stir Creamy Almond Butter	2 Tbsp	190	17	150	2.5	0	0	65	7	3	3	6	1 high-fat protein, 1 fat
Nutella													
Hazelnut Spread	2 Tbsp	200	12	110	4	0	0	15	21	21	1	2	1 1/2 carb, 2 fat
Trader Joe's													
Creamy Raw No Salt Almond Butter	2 Tbsp	190	16	140	1	0	0	0	7	1	4	7	1 high-fat protein, 1 fat
Creamy Salted Almond Butter	2 Tbsp	190	17	150	1.5	0	0	100	7	2	3	7	1 high-fat protein, 1 fat

NUTS, SEEDS, NUT/SEED PRODUCTS

	Serving	Calories	Fat (g)	Cal. from Fat	Sat. Fat (g)	Trans Fat (g)	Chol. (mg)	Sod. (mg)	Carb. (g)	Sugar (g)	Fiber (g)	Prot. (g)	Servings/Exchanges
Creamy Salted Cashew Butter	2 Tbsp	190	16	150	3	0	0	100	9	1	1	4	1 high-fat protein, 1 fat
SOY & SUNFLOWER SEED BUTTER													
MaraNatha													
All Natural Sunflower Seed Butter	2 Tbsp	180	12	110	1.5	0	0	65	8	1	4	9	1 high-fat protein, 1 fat
SunButter Organic													
Creamy Sunflower Spread	2 Tbsp	200	16	140	2	0	0	120	7	3	4	7	1 high-fat protein, 1 fat
Crunch Sunflower Spread	2 Tbsp	200	16	140	2	0	0	120	7	3	4	7	1 high-fat protein, 1 fat
Natural No Added Sugar Sunflower Spread	2 Tbsp	210	18	160	2	0	0	100	4	1	2	8	1 high-fat protein, 2 fat
No-Stir Creamy Sunflower Spread	2 Tbsp	200	16	140	2.5	0	0	120	7	3	4	7	1 high-fat protein, 1 fat

On The Go Sunflower Spread	2 Tbsp	200	16	140	2	0	0	120	7	3	4	7	1 high-fat protein, 1 fat
Trader Joe's													
Sunflower Seed Butter	2 Tbsp	200	16	140	2	0	0	120	7	3	4	7	1 high-fat protein, 1 fat
Wowbutter													
Toasted Soy Spread	2 Tbsp	200	15	135	3	0	0	100	8	4	4	7	1 high-fat protein, 1 fat

PASTA, PASTA MIXES & PASTA SAUCE

	Serving	Calories	Fat (g)	Cal. from Fat	Sat. Fat (g)	Trans Fat (g)	Chol. (mg)	Sod. (mg)	Carb. (g)	Sugar (g)	Fiber (g)	Prot. (g)	Servings/Exchanges
Lasagna, Cooked	1 noodle	86	<1	5	<1	0	0	128	17	<1	1	3	1 carb
Linguine, Cooked	1 cup	220	1	12	<1	0	0	326	43	1	3	8	3 carb
Macaroni, Cooked	1 cup	221	1	11	0	0	0	1	43	1	3	8	3 carb
Macaroni, Vegetable, Cooked	1 cup	116	<1	1	<1	0	0	90	24	1	4	4	1 1/2 carb
Macaroni, Whole-Wheat, Cooked	1 cup	174	1	6	0	0	0	4	37	1	6	7	2 1/2 carb
Noodles, Egg, Cooked	1 cup	221	3	28	1	0	46	8	40	1	2	7	2 1/2 carb, 1 fat
Noodles, Chow Mein	1 cup	237	14	116	2	0	0	198	26	0	2	4	2 carb, 3 fat
Noodles, Ramen, Cooked	1 cup	156	2	18	<1	0	38	1349	29	1.3	3	6	2 carb
Noodles, Rice, Cooked	1/2 cup	80	<1	0	<1	0	0	5	20	NA	<1	<1	1 carb
Noodles, Spinach Egg, Cooked	1 cup	211	3	21	1	0	53	19	39	1	4	8	2 1/2 carb, 1 fat
Pasta, Homemade without Egg, Cooked	2 oz	74	1	8	0	0	23	47	13	1	0	3	1 carb

Pasta/Noodles, Egg, Homemade, Cooked	2 oz	53	<1	8	<1	0	26	36	9	<1	2	1/2 carb
Pasta/Noodles, Fresh, Cooked	2 oz	88	<1	2	0	0	0	37	9	0	2	1/2 carb
Pasta/Noodles, Spinach, Fresh, Cooked	2 oz	74	1	5	0	0	19	3	14	1	3	1 carb
Pasta/Spirals, Cooked	1/2 cup	86	<1	0	<1	0	4	<1	18	1	6	1 carb
Pasta/Wagon Wheels, Cooked	3/4 cup	210	1	9	0	0	0	<1	41	2	7	2 1/2 carb
Rotini, Cooked	1/2 cup	110	<1	6	<1	0	0	163	22	<1	4	1 1/2 carb
Shells, Jumbo, Cooked	1 shell	36	<1	2	<1	0	0	53	7	<1	1	1/2 carb
Shells, Small, Cooked	1/2 cup	91	<1	10	<1	0	0	<1	17	<1	3	1 carb
Shells, Whole-Wheat, Cooked	1/2 cup	87	<1	0	<1	0	0	2	19	<1	4	1 carb
Spaghetti, Cooked	1/2 cup	110	1	0	11	0	0	91	21	2	4	1 1/2 carb
Spaghetti, Whole-Wheat, Cooked	1/2 cup	87	<1	0	<1	0	0	2	19	2	4	1 carb
Vermicelli, Cooked	1/2 cup	110	1	6	<1	0	0	163	22	1	4	1 1/2 carb

PASTA, PASTA MIXES & PASTA SAUCE

	Serving	Calories	Fat (g)	Cal. from Fat	Sat. Fat (g)	Trans Fat (g)	Chol. (mg)	Sod. (mg)	Carb. (g)	Sugar (g)	Fiber (g)	Prot. (g)	Servings/Exchanges
PASTA MIXES													
Kraft													
Macaroni & Cheese	1 cup	259	3	23	1	0	10	561	48	7	1	11	3 carb, 1 fat
Macaroni & Cheese, Deluxe Original	1 cup	310	10	90	2.5	0	15	890	45	3	1	12	3 carb, 2 fat
Macaroni & Cheese, Easy Mac, Original	1 pouch	230	4	36	2.5	0	5	550	42	5	1	7	3 carb, 1 fat
Macaroni & Cheese, Thick'n Creamy	1 cup	250	18	140	2	1	5	570	50	8	2	9	3 carb, 4 fat
Macaroni & Cheese, Three Cheese Blend	1 cup	380	2.5	140	1	0	5	580	48	8	3	9	3 carb, 1 fat
Velveeta Shells & Cheese, Original	1 cup	360	12	110	4	0	20	870	49	4	2	13	3 carb, 1 med-fat protein, 1 fat
Knorr													
Pasta Sides, Alfredo	1 cup	240	3.5	30	2	0	10	660	42	3	2	9	3 carb, 1 fat
Pasta Sides, Chicken	1 cup	220	2	20	0.5	0	5	700	42	2	2	8	3 carb

Pasta Sides, Parmesan	1 cup	230	4	35	2	0	10	530	39	1	2	9	2 1/2 carb, 1 fat
ASIAN PASTA													
Dynasty													
Maifun Rice Sticks	2 oz	200	0.5	5	0	0	0	130	48	0	1	0	3 carb
Saifun Bean Threads	1 cup	190	0	0	0	0	0	0	50	0	1	0	3 carb
Eden													
40% Buckwheat Soba	2 oz	190	1	9	0	0	0	490	37	2	3	8	2 1/2 carb
100% Buckwheat Soba	2 oz	207	1	9	0	0	0	5	45	2	3	6	3 carb
Bifun (Rice) Pasta	2 oz	200	5	0.5	0	0	0	5	44	0	0	5	3 carb
Brown Rice Udon	2 oz	190	1	9	0	0	0	510	38	2	2	8	2 1/2 carb
Kamut Soba, Organic	1/2 cup	200	1	9	0	0	0	60	38	1	3	7	2 1/2 carb
Kamut Udon, Organic	1/2 cup	200	1.5	13	0	0	0	120	37	0	3	10	2 1/2 carb
Kuzu Noodles	2 oz	200	0	0	0	0	0	0	48	0	2	0	3 carb
Lotus Root Soba	2 oz	190	1	9	0	0	0	470	37	2	4	9	2 1/2 carb
Mugwort Soba	2 oz	190	0.5	5	0	0	0	550	37	2	2	8	2 1/2 carb
Mung Bean Pasta	2 oz	190	0	0	0	0	0	5	47	0	0	0	3 carb

PASTA, PASTA MIXES & PASTA SAUCE

	Serving	Calories	Fat (g)	Cal. from Fat	Sat. Fat (g)	Trans Fat (g)	Chol. (mg)	Sod. (mg)	Carb. (g)	Sugar (g)	Fiber (g)	Prot. (g)	Servings/Exchanges
Soba, Organic	2 oz	200	1.5	15	0	0	0	120	39	3	2	8	2 1/2 carb
Spelt Soba, Organic	2 oz	200	1.5	15	0	0	0	120	37	0	2	9	2 1/2 carb
Udon	2 oz	200	1	10	0	0	0	120	39	<1	2	8	2 1/2 carb
La Choy													
Chow Mein Noodles	1/2 cup	130	6	50	2	0	0	260	18	0	2	3	1 carb, 1 fat
Rice Noodles	1/2 cup	130	4	35	0.5	0	0	380	21	2	1	2	1 1/2 carb, 1 fat
Wel-Pac													
Chinese Noodles	2 oz	200	0	0	0	0	0	400	42	2	1	7	3 carb
Chow Mein Stir-Fry Noodles	2 oz	200	1	5	0	0	0	125	42	0	0	7	3 carb
Japanese Udon Noodles	2 oz	190	0.5	5	0	0	0	950	40	0	1	5	2 1/2 carb
Thai Kitchen													
Stir-Fry Rice Noodles	2 oz	180	5	0.5	0	0	0	0	40	0	1	3	2 1/2 carb
Thin Rice Noodles	2 oz	196	0	0	0	0	0	0	46	0	2	3	3 carb

PASTA, PASTA MIXES & PASTA SAUCE 575

DRY PASTA

Al Dente

Carba–Nada	1 1/2 cups	140	1	9	0	0	15	20	24	0	6	12	1 1/2 carb
Garlic Parsley Fettucini	2 oz	220	2	18	0.5	0	33	15	41	6	2	8	2 1/2 carb

American Beauty

Angel Hair	2 oz	210	1	9	0	0	0	0	42	2	2	7	3 carb
Ditalini	2 oz	210	1	10	0	0	0	0	42	2	2	7	3 carb
Elbow Macaroni	2 oz	210	1	9	0	0	0	0	42	2	2	7	3 carb
Extra Wide Egg Noodles	2 oz	210	2.5	23	1	0	70	15	40	2	2	8	2 1/2 carb, 1 fat
Fettuccine	2 oz	210	1	10	0	0	0	0	42	2	2	7	3 carb
Fideo Cortado (Fino)	2 oz	210	1	9	0	0	0	0	42	2	2	7	3 carb
Jumbo Shells	2 oz	210	1	10	0	0	0	0	42	2	2	7	3 carb
Large Elbows	2 oz	210	1	10	0	0	0	0	42	2	2	7	3 carb
Large Shells	2 oz	210	1	10	0	0	0	0	42	2	2	7	3 carb
Manicotti	2 oz	210	1	10	0	0	0	0	42	2	2	7	3 carb

PASTA, PASTA MIXES & PASTA SAUCE

	Serving	Calories	Fat (g)	Cal. from Fat	Sat. Fat (g)	Trans Fat (g)	Chol. (mg)	Sod. (mg)	Carb. (g)	Sugar (g)	Fiber (g)	Prot. (g)	Servings/Exchanges
Oven Ready Lasagna	2 oz	210	1	10	0	0	0	0	42	2	2	7	3 carb
Penne Rigate	2 oz	210	1	10	0	0	0	0	42	2	2	7	3 carb
Rainbow Twirls	2 oz	210	1	10	0	0	0	30	42	2	2	7	3 carb
Rotini	2 oz	210	1	10	0	0	0	0	42	2	2	7	3 carb
Sea Shells	2 oz	210	1	10	0	0	0	0	42	2	2	7	3 carb
Small Shells	2 oz	210	1	10	0	0	0	0	42	2	2	7	3 carb
Spaghetti	2 oz	210	1	10	0	0	0	0	42	2	2	7	3 carb
Thin Spaghetti	2 oz	210	1	10	0	0	0	0	42	2	2	7	3 carb
Vermicelli	2 oz	210	1	10	0	0	0	0	42	2	2	7	3 carb
Wide Egg Noodles	2 oz	210	2.5	23	1	0	70	15	40	2	2	8	2 1/2 carb, 1 fat
Barilla													
Angel Hair	2 oz	200	1	10	0	0	0	0	42	1	2	7	3 carb
Elbows	2 oz	200	1	10	0	0	0	0	42	2	2	7	3 carb
Farfalle	2 oz	200	1	10	0	0	0	0	42	2	2	7	3 carb

Fetuccine	2 oz	200	1	10	0	0	0	42	2	2	7	3 carb
Lasagna	2 pieces	180	1	10	0	0	0	38	1	2	6	2 1/2 carb
Lasagna, No Boil	3 pieces	190	2	20	0.5	50	20	36	1	2	7	2 1/2 carb
Linguine	2 oz	200	1	10	0	0	0	42	2	2	7	3 carb
Medium Shells	2 oz	200	1	10	0	0	0	42	2	2	7	3 carb
Mini Penne	2 oz	200	1	10	0	0	0	42	2	2	7	3 carb
Mostaccioli	2 oz	200	1	10	0	0	0	42	2	2	7	3 carb
Penne	2 oz	200	1	10	0	0	0	42	2	2	7	3 carb
Rigatoni	2 oz	200	1	10	0	0	0	42	2	2	7	3 carb
Rotini	2 oz	200	1	10	0	0	0	42	2	2	7	3 carb
Spaghetti	2 oz	200	1	10	0	0	0	42	2	2	7	3 carb
Spaghetti Rigati	2 oz	200	1	10	0	0	0	42	2	2	7	3 carb
Thin Spaghetti	2 oz	200	1	10	0	0	0	42	1	2	7	3 carb
Tortellini Ricotta & Spinach	3/4 cup	230	8	70	2.5	60	340	32	2	5	8	2 carb, 2 fat
Tortellini Three Cheese	2/3 cup	230	8	70	2.5	40	475	33	2	3	8	3 carb, 2 fat

PASTA, PASTA MIXES & PASTA SAUCE

	Serving	Calories	Fat (g)	Cal. from Fat	Sat. Fat (g)	Trans Fat (g)	Chol. (mg)	Sod. (mg)	Carb. (g)	Sugar (g)	Fiber (g)	Prot. (g)	Servings/Exchanges
Tri-Color Rotini	2 oz	200	1	9	0	0	0	15	42	1	2	7	3 carb
Barilla Plus													
Angel Hair	2 oz	210	2	18	0	0	0	25	38	2	4	10	2 1/2 carb
Elbows	2 oz	210	1	10	0	0	0	25	38	2	4	10	2 1/2 carb
Penne	2 oz	210	2	18	0	0	0	25	38	2	4	10	2 1/2 carb
Spaghetti	2 oz	190	1	20	0	0	0	25	38	2	4	10	2 1/2 carb
Thin Spaghetti	2 oz	210	1	10	0	0	0	25	38	2	4	10	2 1/2 carb
Buitoni (Refrigerated)													
Chicken & Prosciutto Tortellini	1 cup	330	9	80	3	0	40	610	46	3	2	15	3 carb, 2 fat
Four Cheese Ravioli	1 1/4 cups	330	12	110	4	0	55	630	42	2	3	14	3 carb, 2 fat
Linguine	1 1/4 cups	240	2	25	1	0	50	20	46	1	2	10	3 carb
Mixed Cheese Tortellini	1 cup	320	8	70	3	0	40	500	47	3	3	14	3 carb, 2 fat

Spinach & Cheese Tortellini	1 cup	320	7	60	3.5	0	50	540	49	3	3	15	3 carb, 1 fat
Colavita												
Angel Hair	2 oz	210	1	10	0	0	0	0	44	2	2	7	3 carb
Angel Hair Nests	2 nests	210	1	10	0	0	0	0	44	2	2	7	3 carb
Bow Ties	3/4 cup	210	1	10	0	0	0	0	44	2	2	7	3 carb
Fettuccine Nests	2 nests	210	1	10	0	0	0	0	44	2	2	7	3 carb
Linguine	2 oz	210	1	10	0	0	0	0	44	2	2	7	3 carb
Long Fusilli	2 oz	210	1	10	0	0	0	0	44	2	2	7	3 carb
Creamette												
Angel Hair	2 oz	210	1	10	0	0	0	0	42	2	2	7	3 carb
Elbow Macaroni	2 oz	210	1	10	0	0	0	0	42	2	2	7	3 carb
Extra Wide Egg Noodles	2 oz	210	2.5	25	0.5	0	65	5	38	2	2	8	2 1/2 carb, 1 fat
Lasagna	2 oz	210	1	10	0	0	0	0	42	2	2	7	3 carb
Spaghetti	2 oz	210	1	10	0	0	0	0	42	2	2	7	3 carb
Thin Spaghetti	2 oz	210	1	10	0	0	0	0	42	2	2	7	3 carb

PASTA, PASTA MIXES & PASTA SAUCE

	Serving	Calories	Fat (g)	Cal. from Fat	Sat. Fat (g)	Trans Fat (g)	Chol. (mg)	Sod. (mg)	Carb. (g)	Sugar (g)	Fiber (g)	Prot. (g)	Servings/Exchanges
DaVinci													
100% Whole Wheat Elbows	1/2 cup	210	1.5	14	0	0	0	0	41	2	5	7	2 1/2 carb
100% Whole Wheat Penne	2/3 cup	190	1.5	14	0	0	0	0	40	2	5	7	2 1/2 carb
Angel Hair	2 oz	170	1	9	0	0	0	0	42	5	2	6	3 carb
Bowties	1 cup	210	1	9	0	0	0	0	43	3	2	6	3 carb
Cut Ziti	3/4 cup	210	1	9	0	0	0	0	41	2	2	7	2 1/2 carb
Fettuccine	2 oz	210	1	9	0	0	0	0	43	3	2	6	3 carb
Fusilli Springs	3/4 cup	210	1	10	0	0	0	0	43	3	2	6	3 carb
Penne Rigate	3/4 cup	210	1	10	0	0	0	0	43	3	2	7	3 carb
Potato Gnocchi	3/4 cup	210	1	9	0	0	0	440	46	0	3	5	3 carb
Rotini	1 cup	210	1	9	0	0	0	0	43	3	2	6	3 carb
Spaghetti	2 oz	210	1	9	0	0	0	0	43	3	2	6	3 carb

DeBoles

Organic Whole Wheat Spaghetti Style Pasta	2 oz	210	1.5	13	0	0	0	10	42	2	5	7	3 carb
Rice Spirals	2 oz	210	0.5	5	0	0	0	15	46	0	<1	4	3 carb
Rice Style Spaghetti Pasta	2 oz	210	0.5	5	0	0	0	15	46	0	<1	4	3 carb
Tomato & Basil Angel Hair Pasta	2 oz	210	1	9	0	0	0	0	41	2	2	7	2 1/2 carb

De Cecco

Farfalle	1 cup	200	1	10	0	0	0	0	41	2	2	7	2 1/2 carb
Fusilli	3/4 cup	200	1	10	0	0	0	0	41	2	2	7	2 1/2 carb
Linguine	2 oz	200	1	10	0	0	0	0	41	2	2	7	2 1/2 carb
Penne Rigate	1/2 cup	200	1	10	0	0	0	0	41	2	2	7	2 1/2 carb
Spaghetti	2 oz	200	1	10	0	0	0	0	41	2	2	7	2 1/2 carb
Zita Cut	2/3 cup	200	1	10	0	0	0	0	41	2	2	7	2 1/2 carb

Dreamfields

Elbows	2 oz	190	1	9	0	0	0	10	41	1	5	7	2 1/2 carb
Lasagna	2 oz	190	1	9	0	0	0	10	41	1	5	7	2 1/2 carb

PASTA, PASTA MIXES & PASTA SAUCE

	Serving	Calories	Fat (g)	Cal. from Fat	Sat. Fat (g)	Trans Fat (g)	Chol. (mg)	Sod. (mg)	Carb. (g)	Sugar (g)	Fiber (g)	Prot. (g)	Servings/Exchanges
Linguine	2 oz	190	1	10	0	0	0	10	41	1	2	7	2 1/2 carb
Penne Rigate	2 oz	190	1	10	0	0	0	10	41	1	4	7	2 1/2 carb
Spaghetti	2 oz	190	1	10	0	0	0	10	41	1	5	7	2 1/2 carb
Fiber Wise													
High Fiber Elbows	2 oz	170	1	9	0	0	0	25	41	0	12	8	2 1/2 carb
High Fiber Penne	2 oz	170	1	9	0	0	0	25	41	0	12	8	2 1/2 carb
High Fiber Spaghetti	2 oz	170	1	9	0	0	0	25	41	0	12	8	2 1/2 carb
Hodgson Mill													
100% Whole Grain Fettuccine	2 oz	189	1	9	0	0	0	10	33	0	6	9	2 carb
100% Whole Grain Spaghetti	2 oz	210	1	9	0	0	0	0	41	1	6	9	2 1/2 carb
100% Whole Grain Spirals	2 oz	190	1	9	0	0	0	10	34	1	6	9	2 carb

Organic Whole Wheat Fettuccine with Milled Flax Seed	2 oz	200	2	18	0	0	0	10	40	0	6	9	2 1/2 carb
Organic Whole Wheat Penne with Milled Flax Seed	2 oz	215	2	20	0	0	0	0	40	0	6	9	2 1/2 carb
Organic Whole Wheat Spaghetti with Milled Flax Seed	2 oz	200	2	20	0	0	0	10	40	0	6	9	2 1/2 carb
Organic Whole Wheat Spirals with Milled Flax Seed	2 oz	200	2	20	0	0	0	10	40	0	6	9	2 1/2 carb
Veggie Rotini	2 oz	200	1	5	0	0	0	15	41	0	1	8	2 1/2 carb
No Yolks (Cholesterol Free)													
Dumplings	2 oz	210	0.5	5	0	0	0	30	41	3	3	8	2 1/2 carb
Extra Broad Noodles	2 oz	210	0.5	5	0	0	0	30	41	3	3	8	2 1/2 carb
Rao's Specialty Foods													
Fusilli	1/2 cup	197	1	0	0	0	0	0	41	2	2	6	2 1/2 carb
Penne Rigate	1/2 cup	190	1	9	0	0	0	0	39	1	3	7	2 1/2 carb

PASTA, PASTA MIXES & PASTA SAUCE

	Serving	Calories	Fat (g)	Cal. from Fat	Sat. Fat (g)	Trans Fat (g)	Chol. (mg)	Sod. (mg)	Carb. (g)	Sugar (g)	Fiber (g)	Prot. (g)	Servings/Exchanges
Ronzoni													
Healthy Harvest Multi-Grain Thin Spaghetti	2 oz	180	2	14	1.5	0	0	0	39	2	5	9	2 1/2 carb
Healthy Harvest Whole Wheat Fusilli	2 oz	180	2	20	0	0	0	0	40	0	5	8	2 1/2 carb
PASTA SAUCE													
Barilla													
Bacon and Cheese	1/2 cup	70	1.5	15	0	0	0	480	12	8	1	2	1 carb
Creamy Alfredo	1/2 cup	70	6	50	1.5	0	15	370	4	1	0	1	1 fat
Marinara	1/2 cup	70	1	5	0	0	0	400	15	9	3	2	1 carb
Meat Sauce	1/2 cup	70	1	10	0	0	0	550	12	9	3	2	1 carb
Three Cheese	1/2 cup	70	1	10	0	0	0	400	12	8	2	2	1 carb
Tomato & Basil	1/2 cup	70	1	10	0	0	0	410	14	9	3	2	1 carb
Traditional Pesto	1/2 cup	220	21	190	2.5	0	5	600	4	0	1	3	4 fat

Bertolli

Alfredo	1/4 cup	110	10	90	5	0	40	410	2	<1	0	2	2 fat
Arrabbiata	1/2 cup	60	1.5	15	0	0	0	450	11	4	2	1	1 carb
Italian Vodka	1/2 cup	150	9	80	4.5	0	25	700	11	8	2	3	1 carb, 2 fat
Marinara	1/2 cup	80	2	20	0	0	0	500	14	12	1	3	1 carb
Mushroom Alfredo	1/4 cup	80	7	60	3	0	30	380	2	<1	0	2	1 fat
Olive Oil & Garlic	1/2 cup	70	2	20	0	0	0	460	13	12	3	3	1 carb
Portobello Mushroom	1/2 cup	80	2.5	25	0	0	0	450	12	11	1	2	1 carb, 1 fat
Reduced Fat Alfredo	1/4 cup	50	4	35	2	0	15	320	1	<1	0	1	1 fat
Riserva Asiago Cheese & Artichoke	1/2 cup	110	6	50	2	0	<5	460	10	6	2	3	1 carb, 1 fat

Buitoni (Refrigerated)

Alfredo Sauce	1/4 cup	140	12	110	7	0	30	350	4	2	0	4	2 fat
Light Alfredo Sauce	1/4 cup	90	6	50	4	0	20	350	4	1	0	4	1 fat
Marinara	1/2 cup	70	3	25	0	0	0	560	10	6	2	1	1/2 carb, 1 fat
Pesto with Basil	1/4 cup	270	26	230	5	0	15	380	4	4	2	6	5 fat

PASTA, PASTA MIXES & PASTA SAUCE

	Serving	Calories	Fat (g)	Cal. from Fat	Sat. Fat (g)	Trans Fat (g)	Chol. (mg)	Sod. (mg)	Carb. (g)	Sugar (g)	Fiber (g)	Prot. (g)	Servings/Exchanges
Reduced Fat Pesto with Basil	1/4 cup	230	17	150	3	0	10	500	8	6	2	7	1/2 carb, 3 fat
Classico													
Creamy Alfredo	1/4 cup	60	4.5	40	2.5	0	35	370	3	1	0	2	1 fat
Four Cheese	1/2 cup	60	1	10	0	0	0	490	10	6	2	2	1/2 carb
Spicy Red Pepper	1/2 cup	50	1.5	15	0	0	0	310	8	4	2	2	1/2 carb
Tomato & Basil	1/2 cup	60	2	15	0	0	0	430	9	6	2	2	1/2 carb
Traditional Basil Pesto	1/4 cup	240	24	220	4.5	0	<5	590	5	0	<1	3	5 fat
Vodka Sauce	1/2 cup	90	4.5	40	1.5	0	10	440	9	6	2	2	1/2 carb, 1 fat
Dell'Amore													
Original	1/2 cup	80	4	35	0	0	0	250	10	6	2	2	1/2 carb, 1 fat
Sweet Basil & Garlic	1/2 cup	80	4.5	40	0.5	0	0	220	8	5	2	2	1/2 carb, 1 fat
Newman's Own													
Alfredo Sauce	1/4 cup	90	8	70	4.5	0	40	410	3	1	0	1	2 fat

Five Cheese	1/2 cup	80	2	20	1	0	5	460	11	6	3	4	1 carb
Italian Sausage & Peppers	1/2 cup	90	3.5	30	1	0	5	550	11	7	2	4	1 carb, 1 fat
Marinara Sauce	1/2 cup	70	1	10	0	0	0	460	12	7	3	3	1 carb
Sockarooni	1/2 cup	70	1	10	0	0	0	460	12	7	3	3	1 carb
Vodka Sauce	1/2 cup	120	5	45	1.5	0	5	440	13	8	2	5	1 carb, 1 fat
Prego													
Artisan Three Cheese	1/4 cup	70	6	50	3	0	25	310	3	1	1	0	1 fat
Creamy Vodka	1/2 cup	140	7	60	3	0	15	480	15	10	3	3	1 carb, 1 fat
Fresh Mushroom & Garlic	1/2 cup	70	1.5	15	0	0	0	480	13	11	3	2	1 carb
Heart Smart Mushroom Italian	1/2 cup	70	1.5	15	0	0	0	360	13	9	2	2	1 carb
Homestyle Alfredo	1/4 cup	80	7	60	3.5	0	25	390	3	1	0	1	1 fat
Light Homestyle Alfredo	1/4 cup	50	3.5	30	2	0	20	340	3	1	0	1	1 fat
Light Smart Traditional	1/2 cup	45	0	0	0	0	0	410	11	7	3	1	1 carb
Marinara	1/2 cup	80	3	30	0.5	0	0	480	10	7	3	2	1/2 carb, 1 fat

PASTA, PASTA MIXES & PASTA SAUCE

	Serving	Calories	Fat (g)	Cal. from Fat	Sat. Fat (g)	Trans Fat (g)	Chol. (mg)	Sod. (mg)	Carb. (g)	Sugar (g)	Fiber (g)	Prot. (g)	Servings/Exchanges
Mini Meatball	1/2 cup	100	3	30	1	0	10	480	13	10	3	4	1 carb, 1 fat
Pesto Marinara	1/2 cup	90	3.5	30	1	0	5	480	12	8	3	3	1 carb, 1 fat
Traditional Italian	1/2 cup	70	1.5	15	0	0	0	480	13	10	3	2	1 carb
Ragu													
Chunky Sundried Tomato & Sweet Basil	1/2 cup	90	2.5	25	0	0	0	460	15	10	2	2	1 carb, 1 fat
Classic Cheesy Alfredo	1/4 cup	90	8	70	2.5	0	20	330	2	<1	0	1	2 fat
Light Parmesan Alfredo	1/4 cup	60	4	35	2.5	0	20	320	2	0	0	2	1 fat
Old World Style Meat	1/2 cup	80	2.5	25	0.5	0	0	480	10	6	2	2	1/2 carb, 1 fat
Old World Style Mushroom	1/2 cup	70	2	20	0	0	0	460	11	7	2	2	1 carb
Old World Style Traditional	1/2 cup	80	2	20	0	0	0	480	13	8	2	2	1 carb, 1 fat
Six Cheese	1/2 cup	90	2.5	25	1	0	<5	480	14	9	2	3	1 carb, 1 fat

Super Chunky Mushroom	1/2 cup	90	2	20	0	0	0	470	16	11	2	2	1 carb
Rao's Specialty Foods													
Arrabiata Sauce	1/2 cup	80	7	60	1	0	0	340	4	3	1	1	1 fat
Four Cheese	1/2 cup	70	6	50	1	0	5	460	4	4	1	2	1 fat
Marinara	1/2 cup	80	7	60	1	0	0	340	4	3	1	1	1 fat
Puttanesca	1/2 cup	80	6	50	1	0	0	250	4	3	1	2	1 fat
Roasted Eggplant	1/2 cup	70	5	45	0.5	0	0	400	4	3	1	1	1 fat
Tomato & Basil	1/2 cup	70	5	45	0.5	0	0	340	4	3	1	1	1 fat
The Silver Palate													
Fra Diavolo Arribiata Hot & Spicy	1/2 cup	70	3.5	30	0.5	0	0	360	8	5	2	2	1/2 carb, 1 fat
Low Sodium Marinara	1/2 cup	70	3.5	30	0	0	0	115	7	5	2	2	1/2 carb, 1 fat
San Marzano Marinara	1/2 cup	50	3.5	30	0	0	0	360	6	3	1	1	1/2 carb, 1 fat
San Marzano Vodka Elegante Pasta Sauce	1/2 cup	160	11	100	3.5	0	15	400	9	6	1	5	1/2 carb, 2 fat

PASTA, PASTA MIXES & PASTA SAUCE

	Serving	Calories	Fat (g)	Cal. from Fat	Sat. Fat (g)	Trans Fat (g)	Chol. (mg)	Sod. (mg)	Carb. (g)	Sugar (g)	Fiber (g)	Prot. (g)	Servings/Exchanges
Trader Joe's													
Alfredo	1/4 cup	80	7	60	4.5	0	35	280	3	1	0	2	1 fat
Arrabiata Sauce	1/2 cup	70	3.5	30	0.5	0	0	400	8	5	1	1	1/2 carb, 1 fat
Bolognese Sauce	1/2 cup	80	4.5	40	1	0	5	480	8	5	2	3	1/2 carb, 1 fat
Creamy Tomato Basil	1/2 cup	120	8	70	3.5	0	15	460	9	5	1	3	1/2 carb, 2 fat
Organic Marinara, No Added Salt	1/2 cup	60	0	0	0	0	0	35	12	6	2	2	1 carb
Puttanesca Sauce	1/2 cup	120	9	80	1.5	0	<5	350	8	2	2	2	1/2 carb, 2 fat
Rustico Pasta Sauce	1/2 cup	45	1.5	15	0	0	0	480	6	3	2	1	1/2 carb
Three Cheese	1/2 cup	80	5	45	1.5	0	5	500	6	3	1	4	1/2 carb, 1 fat
Tomato Basil Marinara	1/2 cup	90	5	45	1	0	0	580	11	6	3	2	1 carb, 1 fat
Traditional Marinara	1/2 cup	30	0.5	5	0	0	0	580	6	3	1	1	1/2 carb
Vodka Sauce	1/2 cup	90	4	35	1	0	<5	600	12	8	2	3	1 carb, 1 fat

PROCESSED MEAT, BREAKFAST MEAT, LUNCH MEAT, HOT DOGS, CANNED MEAT, SEAFOOD & CHICKEN

	Serving	Calories	Fat (g)	Cal. from Fat	Sat. Fat (g)	Trans Fat (g)	Chol. (mg)	Sod. (mg)	Carb. (g)	Sugar (g)	Fiber (g)	Prot. (g)	Servings/Exchanges
BREAKFAST MEATS													
Applegate Farms Sausage													
Chicken & Apple Sausage	1 link	160	7	63	2	0	70	500	7	0	1	16	2 lean protein
Fire Roasted Red Pepper Sausage	1 link	120	6	60	1.5	0	65	500	2	0	1	14	2 lean protein
Pork Andouille	1 link	200	15	140	5	0	50	510	2	1	1	12	2 high-fat protein
Pork Bratwurst Sausage	1 link	170	12	110	4	0	45	660	2	1	0	12	2 med-fat protein
Pork Kielbasa	1 link	190	14	130	5	0	50	600	2	1	0	12	2 med-fat protein, 1 fat
Spinach & Feta Sausage	1 link	120	7	63	2.5	0	60	470	2	1	0	13	2 lean protein
Sweet Italian Sausage	1 link	150	8	72	2	0	75	500	1	0	1	17	2 lean protein
Applegate Farms Bacon													
Natural Canadian Bacon	2 slices	90	4	35	1.5	0	35	500	1	1	0	12	2 lean protein
Natural Dry Cured Bacon	2 slices	60	5	45	2	0	10	290	0	1	0	4	1 med-fat protein

PROCESSED MEAT, BREAKFAST MEAT, LUNCH MEAT, HOT DOGS, CANNED MEAT, SEAFOOD & CHICKEN

	Serving	Calories	Fat (g)	Cal. from Fat	Sat. Fat (g)	Trans Fat (g)	Chol. (mg)	Sod. (mg)	Carb. (g)	Sugar (g)	Fiber (g)	Prot. (g)	Servings/Exchanges
Natural Sunday Bacon	2 slices	60	5	45	2	0	10	290	0	0	0	4	1 med-fat protein
Natural Turkey Bacon	2 slices	35	1.5	15	0	0	25	200	0	0	0	6	1 lean protein
Organic Sunday Bacon	2 slices	60	5	45	2	0	10	290	0	0	0	4	1 med-fat protein
Organic Turkey Bacon	1 slice	35	1	9	0	0	25	200	0	0	0	6	1 lean protein
Banquet Brown 'N Serve													
Beef Fully Cooked Sausage Links	3	200	19	162	8	1	35	440	2	1	0	7	1 high-fat protein, 2 fat
Original Fully Cooked Sausage Links	3	200	18	160	6	0	33	456	2	1	0	8	1 high-fat protein, 2 fat
Turkey Fully Cooked Sausage Links	3	110	7	60	2	0	40	390	2	1	0	9	1 med-fat protein
Bob Evans													
Brown Sugar and Honey Links	3 links	200	11	99	0	0	25	290	4	4	0	9	1 high-fat protein
Canadian Bacon	4 slices	60	1.5	13	0.5	0	20	700	2	2	0	11	2 lean protein
Country Pepper Bacon	2 slices	100	8	72	3	0	20	510	0	0	0	6	1 high-fat protein

Express Fully Cooked Bacon	3 slices	80	6	54	0	0	15	280	1	0	5	1 med-fat protein
Express Fully Cooked Lite Sausage Links	2	80	5	45	0	0	15	220	0	0	8	1 med-fat protein
Express Fully Cooked Original Links	2	130	10	90	0	0	25	290	0	0	7	1 high-fat protein
Hickory Smoked Bacon	2 slices	80	7	63	2.5	0	15	270	0	0	5	1 med-fat protein
Original Sausage Links	1 link	110	9	81	3.5	0	20	250	0	0	7	1 high-fat protein
Original Sausage Patties	2 links	160	13	117	0	0	30	380	0	0	11	2 med-fat protein, 1 fat
Celebrity												
Healthy Canadian Style Bacon	3 slices	60	1	15	0.5	0	30	350	1	0	10	1 lean protein
Farmer John												
Premium Bacon	2	90	4	10	4	0	20	480	0	<1	12	2 lean protein
Premium Pork Links	2	140	12	108	4	0	30	400	1	0	6	1 high-fat protein, 1 fat
Farmland												
Hickory Smoked Bacon	2 slices	80	7	63	3	0	15	260	0	0	4	1 med-fat protein
Original Pork Sausage Links	2 links	170	15	135	6	0	30	260	1	0	6	1 high-fat protein, 1 fat

PROCESSED MEAT, BREAKFAST MEAT, LUNCH MEAT, HOT DOGS, CANNED MEAT, SEAFOOD & CHICKEN

	Serving	Calories	Fat (g)	Cal. from Fat	Sat. Fat (g)	Trans Fat (g)	Chol. (mg)	Sod. (mg)	Carb. (g)	Sugar (g)	Fiber (g)	Prot. (g)	Servings/Exchanges
Pork & Bacon Sausage Links	3 links	230	21	189	8	0	50	640	1	1	0	10	1 high-fat protein, 2 fat
Thick Sliced Bacon	1 slice	70	6	54	2.5	0	10	230	0	0	0	3	1 med-fat protein
Hormel													
Little Sizzlers Pork Sausage	3	200	19	170	7	0	40	580	0	2	0	8	1 high-fat protein, 2 fat
Jennie-O													
Breakfast Bacon	1 slice	20	4	4	0.5	0	10	120	0	0	0	3	1 fat
Breakfast Lover's Turkey Sausage	2 oz	130	10	100	3	0	45	310	0	0	0	8	1 high-fat protein
Breakfast Sausage Rolls	2 oz	110	6	60	1.5	0	60	570	0	0	0	14	2 lean protein
Extra Lean Turkey Bacon	1 slice	30	2.5	20	0.5	0	10	130	0	0	0	2	1 fat
Fully Cooked Turkey Breakfast Sausage Links	2.1 oz	110	7	63	2	0	50	430	0	0	0	11	2 lean protein

Fully Cooked Turkey Sausage Patties	1.2 oz	65	4	36	1	0	30	250	0	0	0	6	1 med-fat protein
Maple Turkey Breakfast Sausage Links	2 links	65	4	36	1	0	35	310	0	0	0	8	1 med-fat protein
Turkey Breakfast Sausage Links	2 oz	90	5	45	1.5	0	45	370	0	0	0	9	1 med-fat protein
Jimmy Dean (Uncooked)													
All Natural Regular Pork Sausage	2 oz	180	15	135	5	0	40	430	1	1	0	9	1 high-fat protein, 1 fat
Lower Sodium Premium Bacon	1 slice	50	4	36	1.5	0	10	105	0	0	0	4	1 med-fat protein
Maple Link Sausage	3 links	280	26	130	9	0	50	710	5	3	0	9	1 high-fat protein, 3 fat
Maple Sausage Patties	2 patties	125	11	99	4	0	23	255	1.5	1.5	0	4	1 high-fat protein, 1 fat
Original Sausage Links	3 links	260	24	216	8	0	50	710	2	0	0	8	1 high-fat protein, 3 fat
Original Sausage Patties	2 patties	230	22	198	8	0	45	500	0	0	0	9	1 high-fat protein, 2 fat
Premium Pork Bold Country Sausage	2 oz	190	17	153	6	0	40	340	2	1	1	8	1 high-fat protein, 1 fat
Premium Pork Maple Sausage	2 oz	180	16	144	5	0	40	450	1	1	1	8	1 high-fat protein, 1 fat

PROCESSED MEAT, BREAKFAST MEAT, LUNCH MEAT, HOT DOGS, CANNED MEAT, SEAFOOD & CHICKEN

	Serving	Calories	Fat (g)	Cal. from Fat	Sat. Fat (g)	Trans Fat (g)	Chol. (mg)	Sod. (mg)	Carb. (g)	Sugar (g)	Fiber (g)	Prot. (g)	Servings/Exchanges
Premium Pork Regular Sausage	2 oz	180	15	135	5	0	45	390	1	0	0	10	1 high-fat protein, 1 fat
Thick Sliced Premium Bacon	1 slice	70	6	54	2.5	0	15	220	0	0	0	4	1 med-fat protein
Jimmy Dean (Fully Cooked)													
Maple Bacon Links	3 links	260	24	216	8	0	50	870	2	0	0	8	1 high-fat protein, 3 fat
Maple Sausage Patties	1 patty	125	11	99	4	0	23	255	1.5	1.5	0	4	1 high-fat protein, 1 fat
Original Sausage Links	3 links	260	24	216	8	0	50	710	2	0	0	9	1 high-fat protein, 3 fat
Original Sausage Patties	2 patties	240	23	207	8	0	50	610	1	0	0	9	1 high-fat protein, 3 fat
Turkey Sausage Patties	2 patties	100	7	63	2	0	70	420	1	1	0	11	2 lean protein
Jimmy Dean (Heat 'n Serve)													
Sausage Links	3 links	250	24	216	8	0	45	200	2	1	0	7	1 high-fat protein, 3 fat
Sausage Patties	1 patty	100	8.5	77	3	0	20	280	1	0.5	0	4	1 high-fat protein

Jones Dairy Farm

Product	Serving	Calories	Fat (g)	Cal. from Fat	Sat. Fat (g)	Trans Fat (g)	Chol. (mg)	Sodium (mg)	Carb (g)	Fiber (g)	Protein (g)	Exchanges
Little Pork Sausages	2 links	170	16	144	5	0	40	320	0	0	7	1 high-fat protein, 1 fat
Light Pork Sausage & Rice Links	2	110	7	63	2.5	0	30	440	3	0	8	1 med-fat protein
Pork Sausage Patties	1	130	12	111	5	0	23	215	1	0	4	1 high-fat protein, 1 fat

Land O'Frost

Product	Serving	Calories	Fat (g)	Cal. from Fat	Sat. Fat (g)	Trans Fat (g)	Chol. (mg)	Sodium (mg)	Carb (g)	Fiber (g)	Protein (g)	Exchanges
Canadian Bacon	5 slices	60	1.5	14	0.5	0	30	630	1	0	9	1 lean protein

Oscar Mayer

Product	Serving	Calories	Fat (g)	Cal. from Fat	Sat. Fat (g)	Trans Fat (g)	Chol. (mg)	Sodium (mg)	Carb (g)	Fiber (g)	Protein (g)	Exchanges
Bacon	2 slices	60	3.5	31	1.5	0	15	210	0	0	6	1 med-fat protein
Bacon, Center Cut	2 slices	80	5	45	2	0	20	330	0	0	8	1 med-fat protein
Bacon, Smoked Uncured	2 slices	80	6	54	2.5	0	20	270	0	0	6	1 med-fat protein
Lower Sodium Bacon	2 slices	100	8	70	3	0	20	240	0	0	6	1 med-fat protein
Ready-to-Serve Bacon	1 slice	70	5	45	2	0	15	220	15	0	5	1 med-fat protein

Trader Joe's

Product	Serving	Calories	Fat (g)	Cal. from Fat	Sat. Fat (g)	Trans Fat (g)	Chol. (mg)	Sodium (mg)	Carb (g)	Fiber (g)	Protein (g)	Exchanges
Uncured Apple Smoked Bacon	1 slice	90	7	70	2.5	0	15	240	0	0	5	1 med-fat protein
Uncured Turkey Bacon	1 slice	30	1.5	15	0	0	25	180	0	0	6	1 lean protein

PROCESSED MEAT, BREAKFAST MEAT, LUNCH MEAT, HOT DOGS, CANNED MEAT, SEAFOOD & CHICKEN

	Serving	Calories	Fat (g)	Cal. from Fat	Sat. Fat (g)	Trans Fat (g)	Chol. (mg)	Sod. (mg)	Carb. (g)	Sugar (g)	Fiber (g)	Prot. (g)	Servings/Exchanges
LUNCH MEAT & HOT DOGS													
Applegate Farms													
Honey & Maple Turkey Breast	2 oz	60	1	5	0	0	25	450	0	2	0	11	2 lean protein
Roasted Turkey Breast	2 oz	50	0	0	0	0	25	360	0	0	0	10	1 lean protein
Slow Cooked Ham	2 oz	60	1.5	13	0.5	0	35	480	0	0	0	11	2 lean protein
Uncured Black Forest Ham	2 oz	50	1.5	14	0.5	0	35	480	0	0	0	10	1 lean protein
Uncured Turkey Bologna	2 oz	90	6	50	1.5	0	50	400	0	0	0	8	1 med-fat protein
Applegate Farms Organic													
Herb Turkey Breast	2 oz	50	0.5	5	0	0	30	420	0	0	0	11	2 lean protein
Roasted Chicken Breast	2 oz	60	1.5	13	0.5	0	30	360	0	1	0	10	1 lean protein
Roasted Turkey Breast	2 oz	50	0	0	0	0	25	360	0	0	0	10	1 lean protein
Uncured Ham	2 oz	70	1.5	14	0.5	0	35	530	0	0	0	10	1 lean protein

Healthy Ones 97% Fat Free

Deli Thin-Sliced

Black Forest Ham	6 slices	70	1.5	15	0.5	0	25	340	3	3	2	10	1 lean protein
Honey Ham	6 slices	70	1.5	15	0.5	0	25	340	3	3	3	10	1 lean protein
Oven Roasted Turkey Breast	6 slices	60	1.5	15	0.5	0	25	320	0	<1	2	10	1 lean protein

Ball Park Franks

Beef Franks	1	190	16	144	7	1	35	550	4	2	0	7	1 high-fat protein, 1 fat
Bun Size Franks	1	180	15	135	6	0	30	510	4	1	0	6	1 high-fat protein, 1 fat

Bar-S

Beef Bologna	1 oz	110	9	80	3.5	0	20	350	2	1	2	4	1 high-fat protein
Bologna	1 slice	180	15	135	5	0	60	620	0	1	0	5	1 high-fat protein, 1 fat
Chicken Bologna	1 oz	80	7	63	2	0	35	360	3	0	0	3	1 med-fat protein
Cooked Ham	1.3 oz	40	1	9	0	0	20	420	0	1	0	5	1 lean protein
Cotto Salami	1 oz	90	8	72	2.5	0	40	350	2	1	0	3	1 high-fat protein
Deli Thin Cut Ham	2 oz	70	2	30	1	0	30	720	4	0	0	9	1 lean protein

PROCESSED MEAT, BREAKFAST MEAT, LUNCH MEAT, HOT DOGS, CANNED MEAT, SEAFOOD & CHICKEN

	Serving	Calories	Fat (g)	Cal. from Fat	Sat. Fat (g)	Trans Fat (g)	Chol. (mg)	Sod. (mg)	Carb. (g)	Sugar (g)	Fiber (g)	Prot. (g)	Servings/Exchanges
Deli Thin Cut Turkey Breast	2 oz	60	1	9	0	0	25	580	0	0	0	9	1 lean protein
Extra Lean Cooked Ham	1 oz	60	2	18	1	0	30	660	2	0	0	9	1 lean protein
Extra Lean Honey Cured Ham	1 oz	45	1.5	13	1.5	0.5	15	450	3	2	0	5	1 lean protein
Oven Roasted Turkey	1 oz	35	0.5	4	0	0	15	350	0	1	0	5	1 lean protein
Thick Sliced Bologna	2 oz	150	12	108	3.5	0	35	630	0	1	0	8	1 high-fat protein, 1 fat
Turkey Bologna	1 oz	70	5	45	1.5	0	25	380	0	0	0	4	1 med-fat protein
Butterball													
All Natural													
Oven Roasted Turkey Breast	1 oz	35	0.5	5	0	0	15	210	0	1	0	5	1 lean protein
Deep Fried Lunchmeat													
Extra Thin Sliced Original Turkey Lunchmeat	2 slices	35	2.5	20	0	0	15	180	0	0	0	3	1 lean protein

Thick Sliced Original Turkey Lunchmeat	2 slices	60	1	10	0	0	30	520	0	0	0	10	1 lean protein
Deli Premium													
Honey Roasted & Smoked Turkey Breast	4 slices	30	1	9	0	0	15	390	1	0	0	6	1 lean protein
Oven Roasted Chicken Breast	2 oz	60	1	9	0	0	30	450	1	0	0	10	1 lean protein
Oven Roasted Turkey Breast	2 oz	60	1	9	0	0	30	450	1	0	0	10	1 lean protein
Extra Thin Sliced													
Oven Roasted Turkey	2 oz	50	1	10	0	0	20	450	0	0	0	9	1 lean protein
Thin Sliced													
Honey Roasted Turkey Breast	2 oz	60	1	10	0	0	25	400	3	2	0	10	1 lean protein
Oven Roasted Chicken Breast	2 oz	60	1.5	14	0	0	25	450	1	0	0	10	1 lean protein
Oven Roasted Turkey Breast	2 oz	50	1	10	0	0	25	400	2	1	0	10	1 lean protein

PROCESSED MEAT, BREAKFAST MEAT, LUNCH MEAT, HOT DOGS, CANNED MEAT, SEAFOOD & CHICKEN

	Serving	Calories	Fat (g)	Cal. from Fat	Sat. Fat (g)	Trans Fat (g)	Chol. (mg)	Sod. (mg)	Carb. (g)	Sugar (g)	Fiber (g)	Prot. (g)	Servings/Exchanges
Smoked Turkey Breast	2 oz	30	1	9	0	0	15	390	1	0	0	6	1 lean protein
Carl Buddig													
Beef	2 oz	100	7	60	3	0	45	600	1	1	0	9	1 med-fat protein
Chicken	2 oz	90	5	45	1.5	0	30	530	2	1	0	10	1 med-fat protein
Corned Beef	2 oz	100	7	60	3	0	45	300	0	1	0	9	1 med-fat protein
Ham	2 oz	90	5	45	2	0	35	760	0	1	0	10	1 med-fat protein
Honey Ham	2 oz	90	5	45	2	0	35	590	2	2	0	10	1 med-fat protein
Honey Turkey	2 oz	90	5	45	2	0	30	600	0	2	0	9	1 med-fat protein
Pastrami	2 oz	100	7	60	3	0	45	600	0	1	0	9	1 med-fat protein
Turkey	2 oz	90	5	45	2	0	30	600	0	1	0	10	1 med-fat protein
Deli Cuts													
Oven Roasted Turkey Breast	4 slices	80	5	45	1.5	0	25	420	2	1	0	7	1 med-fat protein
Smoked Honey Ham	4 slices	70	2.5	25	1	0	25	420	3	3	0	9	1 lean protein

Celebrity

Black Forest Smoked Ham, 99% Fat Free	1 oz	25	0	0	0	0	15	180	0.5	0.5	0	5	1 lean protein
Ham, 99% Fat Free	1 oz	20	0	0	0	0	15	180	0	0	0	5	1 lean protein

Columbus

Honey Cured Turkey Breast	1 oz	25	0	0	0	0	15	180	0.5	0.5	0	5	1 lean protein
Italian Style Salami	2 oz	60	0.5	5	0	0	20	400	2	1	0	12	2 lean protein
Pastrami	2 oz	80	2.5	23	1	0	35	390	0	1	0	12	2 lean protein
Peppered Salami	1 oz	90	7	63	2.5	0	25	430	1	0	0	6	1 med-fat protein
Reduced Sodium Turkey Breast	2 oz	60	0.5	5	0	0	20	220	1	0	0	13	2 lean protein
Roasted Turkey Breast	2 oz	60	0.5	5	0	0	20	400	1	1	0	12	2 lean protein
Seasoned Roast Beef	2 oz	80	3	27	1	0	40	190	1	0	0	13	2 lean protein

Farmer John Sliced Deli Meats

Bologna	2 oz	160	14	130	4.5	0.5	25	520	0	1	0	6	1 high-fat protein, 1 fat
Cotto Salami	2 oz	150	12	108	4.5	0	45	600	0	0	0	8	1 high-fat protein, 1 fat

PROCESSED MEAT, BREAKFAST MEAT, LUNCH MEAT, HOT DOGS, CANNED MEAT, SEAFOOD & CHICKEN

	Serving	Calories	Fat (g)	Cal. from Fat	Sat. Fat (g)	Trans Fat (g)	Chol. (mg)	Sod. (mg)	Carb. (g)	Sugar (g)	Fiber (g)	Prot. (g)	Servings/Exchanges
Ham Roll	2 oz	60	2	18	1	0	20	420	0	0	0	10	1 lean protein
Head Cheese	1 slice	110	9	81	3	0	30	370	0	0	0	9	1 high-fat protein
Mission Loaf	2 oz	80	4.5	41	1.5	0	25	380	0	0	0	9	1 med-fat protein
Oven Roasted Turkey Breast	1 oz	25	0	0	0	0	10	270	1	1	0	5	1 lean protein
Foster Farms Premium Thin Sliced													
Mesquite Smoked Turkey Breast	2 oz	60	1.5	14	0	0	10	520	2	0	0	9	1 lean protein
Oven Roasted Turkey	2 oz	50	1	10	0.5	0	20	430	2	<1	0	9	1 lean protein
Hebrew National													
Beef Bologna	1 oz	80	8	70	3.5	0	15	240	0	0	0	3	1 high-fat protein
Beef Salami	2 oz	150	13	120	6	0	35	420	0	0	0	8	1 high-fat protein, 1 fat
Lean Beef Salami	2 oz	90	5	45	2	0	30	510	1	0	1	9	1 med-fat protein
Hebrew National Franks													
97% Fat Free Beef Franks	1	45	1	10	0	0	15	490	2	0	0	6	1 lean protein

Beef Franks	1	150	13	5	0.5	25	450	2	0	0	6	1 high-fat protein, 1 fat
Jumbo Beef Franks	1	260	23	9	1	45	770	3	0	0	10	1 high-fat protein, 3 fat

Hillshire Farm

Deli Select

Brown Sugar Baked Ham	2 oz	60	1.5	0.5	0	30	620	3	3	0	10	1 lean protein
Honey Ham	2 oz	70	1.5	0.5	0	30	690	3	2	0	9	1 lean protein
Honey Roasted Turkey Breast	2 oz	60	0.5	0	0	25	480	3	2	0	9	1 lean protein
Oven Roasted Chicken Breast	2 oz	50	0.5	0	0	25	487	2	0	0	9	1 lean protein
Oven Roasted Turkey Breast	2 oz	50	0.5	0	0	20	620	2	1	0	9	1 lean protein
Pastrami	2 oz	60	1.5	0.5	0	25	620	0	0	0	10	1 lean protein
Roast Beef	2 oz	70	3	1	0	30	550	0	1	0	11	2 lean protein
Smoked Chicken Breast	2 oz	60	1	0.5	0	30	730	0	0	0	9	1 lean protein
Smoked Ham	2 oz	60	1.5	0.5	0	30	670	0	1	0	9	1 lean protein
Smoked Turkey Breast	2 oz	60	0.5	0	0	25	690	0	2	0	10	1 lean protein

PROCESSED MEAT, BREAKFAST MEAT, LUNCH MEAT, HOT DOGS, CANNED MEAT, SEAFOOD & CHICKEN

	Serving	Calories	Fat (g)	Cal. from Fat	Sat. Fat (g)	Trans Fat (g)	Chol. (mg)	Sod. (mg)	Carb. (g)	Sugar (g)	Fiber (g)	Prot. (g)	Servings/Exchanges
Hearty Slices													
Honey Ham	1 oz	35	1	9	0	0	15	310	2	2	0	5	1 lean protein
Honey Roasted Turkey	1 oz	35	0.5	5	0	0	15	340	2	1	0	5	1 lean protein
Ultra Thin Sliced													
Hard Salami	1 oz	110	10	90	4	0	30	500	0	0	0	6	1 high-fat protein
Honey Ham	2 oz	80	1.5	15	0.5	0	30	450	0	4	0	10	1 lean protein
Oven Roasted Turkey Breast	2 oz	70	0.5	5	0	0	25	410	5	3	0	10	1 lean protein
Roast Beef	2 oz	70	3	25	1	0	30	550	0	1	0	11	1 med-fat protein
Smoked Ham	2 oz	80	1.5	15	1	0	30	450	3	2	1	10	1 lean protein
Hormel Natural Choice													
Deli Roast Beef	2 oz	60	2	25	1	0	25	520	0	0	0	11	2 lean protein
Honey Deli Ham, 97% Fat Free	2 oz	60	1	9	0.5	0	30	520	0	1	0	12	1 lean protein

Land O'Frost

DeliShaved

Chicken	2 oz	90	6	50	1.5	0	40	720	0	0	0	9	1 med-fat protein
Honey Ham	2 oz	90	6	50	2	0	30	570	3	3	0	8	1 med-fat protein
Oven Roasted Turkey	2 oz	80	5	45	1	0	25	550	1	0	0	8	1 med-fat protein
Smoked Turkey	2 oz	90	6	45	1.5	0	25	510	3	2	0	8	1 med-fat protein

Premium

Chicken Breast	2 oz	80	5	45	1	0	30	650	2	0	0	7	1 med-fat protein
Honey Ham	1.8 oz	67	2	20	1	0	28	650	2	0	0	10	1 lean protein

Select

Honey Smoked White Turkey	3 oz	80	3.5	30	1	0	25	670	4	2	0	8	1 med-fat protein
Oven Roasted Turkey Breast	1.9 oz	80	5	45	1	0	25	550	5	0	0	8	1 med-fat protein
Smoked Ham	3 oz	90	5	50	2	0	30	660	1	0	0	8	1 med-fat protein

Taste Escapes

Black Peppered Ham	2 oz	60	1.5	15	0.5	0	30	590	1	1	0	9	1 lean protein

PROCESSED MEAT, BREAKFAST MEAT, LUNCH MEAT, HOT DOGS, CANNED MEAT, SEAFOOD & CHICKEN

	Serving	Calories	Fat (g)	Cal. from Fat	Sat. Fat (g)	Trans Fat (g)	Chol. (mg)	Sod. (mg)	Carb. (g)	Sugar (g)	Fiber (g)	Prot. (g)	Servings/Exchanges
Hickory Smoked Maple Ham	2 oz	70	2	15	0.5	0	25	590	0	1	0	8	1 lean protein
Peppered Beef	2 oz	60	2	20	0.5	0	25	590	0	1	0	8	1 lean protein
Oscar Mayer													
Lunchmeat													
Baked Ham	2.25 oz	80	2.5	20	1	0	12	610	0	1	0	12	2 lean protein
Beef Bologna	1 oz	90	8	70	3.5	0	7	240	0	0	0	3	1 high-fat protein
Beef Cotto Salami	1 oz	60	4.5	40	2	0	7	230	0	0	0	4	1 med-fat protein
Beef Summer Sausage	1 oz	80	7	80	3.5	0	7	400	0	0	0	4	1 high-fat protein
Boiled Ham	2.25 oz	70	2	20	0.5	0	12	590	0	0	0	12	2 lean protein
Bologna	1 oz	90	8	70	3	0	30	240	0	0	0	3	1 high-fat protein
Chopped Ham	1 oz	50	3	30	1	0	5	240	0	1	0	3	1 lean protein
Cotto Salami	1 oz	70	6	50	2	0	8	230	0	0	0	4	1 med-fat protein
Hard Salami	1 oz	100	8	70	3	0	8	510	0	0	0	7	1 high-fat protein

	Serving	Calories	Fat (g)	Cal. from Fat	Sat. Fat (g)	Trans Fat (g)	Cholesterol (mg)	Sodium (mg)	Carb (g)	Fiber/Sugar (g)	(g)	Protein (g)	Exchanges/Choices
Honey Ham	2 oz	60	1.5	15	0.5	0	10	510	0	2	0	9	1 lean protein
Liver Cheese	1.5 oz	120	10	90	3.5	0	70	420	0	0	0	6	1 high-fat protein
Oven Roasted White Turkey	2 oz	50	1	10	0	0	7	540	1	1	0	9	1 lean protein
Pickle & Pimiento Loaf	1 oz	80	6	50	2	0	7	340	0	2	0	3	1 med-fat protein
Turkey Cotto Salami	1 oz	40	3	25	1	0	7	230	0	0	0	4	1 lean protein
Turkey Ham	1 oz	35	1.5	10	0	0	5	310	0	0	0	4	1 lean protein
Turkey White Smoked	2 oz	50	1	5	0	0	8	510	0	1	0	9	1 lean protein
Deli Fresh Meats													
Brown Sugar Ham, Shaved	1.8 oz	50	1.5	13	0	0	25	740	3	3	0	9	1 lean protein
Chicken Breast Rotisserie Style, Shaved	1.8 oz	50	1.5	14	0	0	25	500	0	0	0	9	1 lean protein
Honey Ham, Shaved	1.8 oz	50	1	10	0.5	0	25	560	0	0	0	9	1 lean protein
Roast Beef Slow Roasted, Shaved	1.8 oz	60	2.5	20	1	0	30	520	0	0	0	10	1 med-fat protein
Smoked Ham, Shaved	1.8 oz	45	1	10	0	0	25	640	0	2	0	9	1 lean protein

PROCESSED MEAT, BREAKFAST MEAT, LUNCH MEAT, HOT DOGS, CANNED MEAT, SEAFOOD & CHICKEN

	Serving	Calories	Fat (g)	Cal. from Fat	Sat. Fat (g)	Trans Fat (g)	Chol. (mg)	Sod. (mg)	Carb. (g)	Sugar (g)	Fiber (g)	Prot. (g)	Servings/Exchanges
Smoked Turkey Breast, Shaved	2.25 oz	60	0.5	5	0	0	25	760	0	0	0	13	2 lean protein
Oscar Mayer Hot Dogs													
Beef Franks, Jumbo	1	160	6	130	0	0	30	420	1	<1	0	6	1 med-fat protein
Beef Franks, Regular	1	130	12	110	5	0	8	330	0	1	0	4	1 high-fat protein, 1 fat
Jumbo Meat Weiners	1	110	9	80	2.5	0	17	510	1	0	0	6	1 high-fat protein
Turkey Franks	1	90	7	70	2	0	12	320	1	1	0	5	1 high-fat protein
Trader Joe's													
Black Forest Ham	2 oz	70	1	10	0	0	35	730	0	1	2	12	2 lean protein
Oven Roasted Turkey Breast	2 oz	60	0	0	0	0	25	630	0	1	2	11	2 lean protein
Pastrami	2 oz	80	2	15	0.5	0	25	270	0	0	<1	13	2 lean protein
Roast Beef	2 oz	80	2	20	0.5	0	85	330	0	0	0	13	2 lean protein
Smoked Turkey Breast	2 oz	60	0	0	0	0	25	460	1	11	1	11	2 lean protein

CANNED MEAT

Beef

Food	Serving											
Liver Pâté, Canned	2 Tbsp	26	2	15	1	0	51	50	0	0	2	free
Pickled Beef Tripe	1 oz	27	0	1	0	0	45	19	1	0	3	1 lean protein

Pork

Food	Serving											
Ham, Canned	1 oz	67	5	48	2	0	14	382	0	0	6	1 med-fat protein
Sausage, Vienna, Canned	1 oz	64	5	49	2	0	24	271	0	0	3	1 med-fat protein

CANNED FISH/SEAFOOD

Food	Serving											
Anchovies in Oil, Canned, Drained	1 oz	59	3	24	1	0	24	1036	0	0	8	1 lean protein
Clams, Canned, Drained Solids	1 oz	41	1	5	0	0	19	31	1	0	7	1 lean protein
Clams, Smoked, Canned in Oil, Small	1 oz	50	3	30	1	0	11	120	1	0	4	1 med-fat protein
Crab, Canned, Drained Solids	3 oz	84	1	9	0	0	76	283	0	0	17	2 lean protein
Salmon, Canned in Water	1 oz	38	1	12	0	0	23	112	0	0	6	1 lean protein

PROCESSED MEAT, BREAKFAST MEAT, LUNCH MEAT, HOT DOGS, CANNED MEAT, SEAFOOD & CHICKEN

	Serving	Calories	Fat (g)	Cal. from Fat	Sat. Fat (g)	Trans Fat (g)	Chol. (mg)	Sod. (mg)	Carb. (g)	Sugar (g)	Fiber (g)	Prot. (g)	Servings/Exchanges
Sardines, Oil-Packed, Drained	1 oz	58	3	29	0	0	40	141	0	0	0	7	1 lean protein
Shrimp, Canned, Drained Solids	3 oz	85	1	11	0	0	214	661	0	0	0	7	1 lean protein
Squid, Pickled	1 oz	26	<1	3	0	0	63	240	1	0	0	4	1 lean protein
Tuna, Canned in Oil, Drained	1 oz	55	2	21	0	0	5	99	0	0	0	9	1 lean protein
Tuna, Canned, Water-Packed, Solids Only	1 oz	36	0	8	0	0	12	106	0	0	0	7	1 lean protein
Bumble Bee													
Blueback Salmon	2.2 oz	110	7	60	1.5	0	40	270	0	0	0	13	2 lean protein
Chunk Light Tuna in Oil	2 oz	72	3	25	0.5	0	25	180	0	0	0	13	2 lean protein
Chunk Light Tuna in Water	2 oz	50	0.5	5	0	0	3	180	0	0	0	13	2 lean protein

Chunk White Albacore Tuna, Very Low Sodium, in Water	2 oz	60	1	10	0	0	25	35	0	0	15	2 lean protein
Fancy Whole Baby Clams	2 oz	50	1	10	0.5	0	40	270	2	0	9	1 lean protein
Jumbo Shrimp	2 oz	40	0	0	0	1	115	430	0	0	10	1 lean protein
Keta Salmon	2.2 oz	90	4	35	1	0	40	270	0	0	13	2 lean protein
Medium Shrimp	2 oz	40	0	0	0	1	115	430	0	0	10	1 lean protein
Medium Red Salmon (Alaska Coho)	2.2 oz	90	5	45	1	0	40	270	0	0	12	2 lean protein
Minced Clams	2 oz	25	0	0	0	0	10	320	2	0	4	1 lean protein
Pink Crabmeat	2 oz	35	0.5	5	0	0	50	300	0	0	7	1 lean protein
Pink Salmon	2.2 oz	90	5	45	1	0	40	270	0	0	12	2 lean protein
Premium Light Tuna in Water, Pouch	2 oz	60	0.5	5	0	0	30	180	0	0	13	2 lean protein
Prime Fillet Albacore Steak Entrées, Mesquite Grilled	4 oz	150	1.5	10	0	0	40	370	0	0	35	5 lean protein
Prime Fillet Atlantic Salmon	2 oz	80	3	30	1.5	0	10	170	0	6	12	2 lean protein

PROCESSED MEAT, BREAKFAST MEAT, LUNCH MEAT, HOT DOGS, CANNED MEAT, SEAFOOD & CHICKEN

	Serving	Calories	Fat (g)	Cal. from Fat	Sat. Fat (g)	Trans Fat (g)	Chol. (mg)	Sod. (mg)	Carb. (g)	Sugar (g)	Fiber (g)	Prot. (g)	Servings/Exchanges
Prime Fillet Salmon Steaks, Teriyake	4 oz	160	3	25	0.5	0	45	690	8	6	0	24	3 lean protein
Prime Fillet Solid Light Tuna, Tonno in Olive Oil	2 oz	110	5	50	1	0	30	220	0	0	0	15	2 lean protein
Prime Fillet Solid White Albacore Tuna in Water	2 oz	70	1	10	0	0	25	180	0	0	0	16	2 lean protein
Red Salmon (Sockeye)	2.2 oz	110	7	60	1.5	0	40	270	0	0	0	13	2 lean protein
Sardines in Oil	2.7-oz can	130	9	80	2	0	35	340	0	0	0	13	2 med-fat protein
Sardines in Water	2.7-oz can	120	7	70	2	0	35	340	0	0	0	13	2 lean protein
Sensations Easy Peel Bowls, Lemon & Cracked Pepper	3 oz	110	4	35	1	0	25	300	2	0	0	16	2 lean protein
Sensations Easy Peel Bowls, Spicy Thai Chili	3 oz	110	3	30	0.5	0	25	350	2	0	0	18	2 lean protein

Item													
Skinless Boneless Pink Salmon	2 oz	70	1.5	10	0	0	30	240	0	0	0	12	2 lean protein
Small Shrimp	2 oz	40	0	0	0	0	115	430	0	1	0	10	1 lean protein
Smoked Clams	2 oz	130	8	80	2	0	40	460	1	0	0	11	2 med-fat protein
Smoked Oysters	2 oz	120	7	60	1.5	0	35	210	6	0	0	10	1 med-fat protein
Smoked Salmon Fillets in Oil	3 oz	150	9	80	2	0	55	400	0	0	0	16	2 med-fat protein
Solid White Albacore Tuna in Oil	2 oz	80	3	25	0.5	0	25	180	0	0	0	14	2 lean protein
Solid White Albacore Tuna in Water	2 oz	60	1	10	0	0	25	180	0	0	0	13	2 lean protein
White Crabmeat	2 oz	40	1	10	0	0	50	300	0	0	0	8	1 lean protein
Whole Oysters	2 oz	70	3	30	0.5	0	45	140	3	0	0	7	1 lean protein
Chicken of the Sea													
Chunk Light Tuna in Oil	2 oz	100	6	50	1	0	25	250	0	0	0	10	1 med-fat protein
Chunk Light Tuna in Water	2 oz	50	0.5	50	0	0	25	250	0	0	0	11	2 lean protein

PROCESSED MEAT, BREAKFAST MEAT, LUNCH MEAT, HOT DOGS, CANNED MEAT, SEAFOOD & CHICKEN

	Serving	Calories	Fat (g)	Cal. from Fat	Sat. Fat (g)	Trans Fat (g)	Chol. (mg)	Sod. (mg)	Carb. (g)	Sugar (g)	Fiber (g)	Prot. (g)	Servings/Exchanges
Chunk Light Tuna in Water, Low Sodium	2 oz	50	0.5	50	0	0	25	90	0	0	0	11	2 lean protein
Chunk Light Tuna, 50% Less Sodium	2 oz	50	0.5	5	0	0	25	125	0	0	0	11	2 lean protein
Chunk White Albacore Tuna	2 oz	50	1	10	0	0	25	250	0	0	0	11	2 lean protein
Chunk White Albacore, Low Sodium	3 oz	80	1	10	0	0	35	50	0	0	0	18	3 lean protein
Fancy Crabmeat	2 oz	40	0	0	0	0	50	400	2	0	0	7	1 lean protein
Genova Skinless Boneless Red Salmon in Water	2 oz	60	2	20	1	0	20	280	0	0	0	10	1 lean protein
Genova Solid White Albacore Tuna in Olive Oil	2 oz	110	6	50	1	0	25	250	0	0	0	13	2 lean protein
Genova Tonno Tuna in Olive Oil	2 oz	120	8	70	2	0	25	250	0	0	0	13	2 med-fat protein
Medium or Small Shrimp	2 oz	45	0.5	5	0	0	145	400	1	0	0	10	1 lean protein

Food	Serving										
Minced Clams	1/4 cup	30	0	0	0	12	370	2	0	0	5	1 lean protein
Pink Crabmeat	2 oz	30	0	0	0	50	400	0	0	0	7	1 lean protein
Sardines in Water	3.75-oz can	100	4	40	2	45	430	2	0	0	13	2 lean protein
Skinless & Boneless Pink Salmon	2 oz	60	2	20	0.5	20	280	0	0	0	10	1 lean protein
Smoked Oysters in Oil	3.75 oz	170	8	70	2	45	280	8	0	0	10	1 high-fat protein
Smoked Oysters in Water	3.75 oz	120	3	30	1	55	400	10	0	0	12	2 lean protein
Smoked Sardines in Oil	3.75-oz can	190	14	130	6	45	430	2	0	0	12	2 med-fat protein, 1 fat
Solid White Albacore Tuna in Oil	2 oz	90	4	40	0	25	180	0	0	0	13	2 lean protein
Solid White Albacore Tuna in Water	2 oz	80	4	40	0	25	180	0	0	0	11	2 lean protein
Traditional Pink Salmon	1/4 cup	90	5	45	1	40	270	0	0	0	12	2 lean protein
Very Low Sodium Chunk White Albacore Tuna	2 oz	50	0.5	5	0	25	35	0	0	0	12	2 lean protein
Whole Baby Clams	1/4 cup	30	0	0	0	10	290	1	0	0	6	1 lean protein
Whole Oysters	2 oz	80	3	30	1	35	220	6	0	0	7	1 lean protein

PROCESSED MEAT, BREAKFAST MEAT, LUNCH MEAT, HOT DOGS, CANNED MEAT, SEAFOOD & CHICKEN

	Serving	Calories	Fat (g)	Cal. from Fat	Sat. Fat (g)	Trans Fat (g)	Chol. (mg)	Sod. (mg)	Carb. (g)	Sugar (g)	Fiber (g)	Prot. (g)	Servings/Exchanges
Starkist													
Chunk Light Tuna in Water	2 oz	50	1	0	0	0	25	180	0	0	0	10	1 lean protein
Hickory Smoked Tuna Creations	2 oz	80	2.5	0	0	0	30	0	0	0	0	14	2 lean protein
Low Sodium Albacore	2 oz	80	0.5	0	0	0	20	70	0	0	0	12	2 lean protein
Low Sodium Chunk Light Tuna	2 oz	50	0.5	0	0	0	20	70	0	0	0	12	2 lean protein
Solid White Albacore Tuna in Water	2 oz	70	2	0	0.5	0	25	200	0	0	0	13	2 lean protein
CANNED CHICKEN													
Swanson													
Premium White Chunk Chicken Breast in Water	2 oz	50	1	10	0	0	25	260	1	0	0	9	1 lean protein

Tyson

Premium Chunk Chicken Breast Pouch (97% Fat Free)	2 oz	70	1	15	0	45	210	0	0	14	2 lean protein
Premium White & Dark Chunk Chicken	2 oz	60	2	20	0	30	200	0	0	10	1 lean protein

RICE & RICE MIXES

	Serving	Calories	Fat (g)	Cal. from Fat	Sat. Fat (g)	Trans Fat (g)	Chol. (mg)	Sod. (mg)	Carb. (g)	Sugar (g)	Fiber (g)	Prot. (g)	Servings/Exchanges
Brown Rice, Long-Grain, Cooked	1/2 cup	108	<1	0	<1	0	0	5	22	<1	2	3	1 1/2 carb
Brown Rice, Medium-Grain, Cooked	1/2 cup	109	<1	0	<1	0	0	1	23	<1	2	2	1 1/2 carb
White Rice, Glutinous, Cooked	1/2 cup	85	<1	0	0	0	0	5	19	<1	<1	2	1 carb
White Rice, Long-Grain, Cooked	1/2 cup	103	<1	0	<1	0	0	1	22	<1	<1	2	1 1/2 carb
White Rice, Long-Grain, Instant, Cooked	1/2 cup	97	<1	0	<1	0	0	4	21	<1	<1	2	1 1/2 carb
White Rice, Long-Grain, Parboiled, Cooked	1/2 cup	97	<1	0	<1	0	0	2	21	<1	<1	2	1 1/2 carb
White Rice, Medium-Grain, Cooked	1/2 cup	121	<1	0	<1	0	0	0	27	<1	<1	2	2 carb
White Rice, Short-Grain, Cooked	1/2 cup	121	<1	0	<1	0	0	0	27	<1	<1	2	2 carb
Wild Rice, Cooked	1/2 cup	83	<1	0	<1	0	0	3	18	<1	2	3	1 carb

Knorr Lipton Rice Sides

Cheddar Broccoli	1 cup	240	1.5	15	0.5	0	<5	580	48	2	1	6	3 carb
Chicken	1 cup	240	2.5	25	0.5	0	<5	660	47	<1	1	6	2 carb, 1 fat
Herb & Butter	1 cup	230	1	10	0	0	0	780	48	2	1	6	3 carb
Rice Medley	1 cup	240	2	20	0	0	5	730	47	2	2	7	3 carb
Rice Pilaf	1 cup	220	1	10	0	0	0	630	47	0	1	5	3 carb

Mahatma

Authentic Spanish Rice	2/3 cup	180	0	0	0	0	0	650	42	0	1	4	3 carb
Basmati Rice	3/4 cup	150	1	10	0	0	0	0	32	0	0	3	2 carb
Brown	3/4 cup	150	1	10	0	0	0	0	32	0	1	3	2 carb
Classic Pilaf	2/3 cup	190	0.5	5	0	0	0	790	43	1	1	5	3 carb
Extra Long Grain	3/4 cup	150	0	0	0	0	0	0	35	0	0	3	3 carb
Jasmine Rice	3/4 cup	160	0	0	0	0	0	0	36	0	0	3	2 1/2 carb

Minute Rice

Basmati Rice	1 cup	160	0	0	0	0	0	0	35	0	0	4	2 carb
Multi-Grain Medley	1 cup	160	1.5	10	0	0	0	15	33	0	2	4	2 carb

RICE & RICE MIXES

	Serving	Calories	Fat (g)	Cal. from Fat	Sat. Fat (g)	Trans Fat (g)	Chol. (mg)	Sod. (mg)	Carb. (g)	Sugar (g)	Fiber (g)	Prot. (g)	Servings/Exchanges
Premium Rice	1 cup	170	0	0	0	0	0	5	41	0	0	5	3 carb
Ready to Serve Bowl, Fried Rice	1 cup	210	2.5	25	0	0	0	620	42	2	4	3	3 carb, 1 fat
Ready to Serve Bowl, Jasmine	1 cup	240	3.5	35	0.5	0	0	160	46	1	4	4	3 carb, 1 fat
Ready to Serve Bowl, White	1 cup	190	1.5	10	0	0	0	170	42	0	2	4	3 carb
Thai Jasmine Rice	1 cup	160	0	5	0	0	0	5	36	0	0	3	2 1/2 carb
White Rice	1 cup	170	0	0	0	0	0	0	39	0	2	4	2 1/2 carb
Whole Grain Brown Rice	2/3 cup	180	1.5	10	0	0	0	0	39	0	2	4	2 1/2 carb
Near East													
Long Grain & Wild Rice													
Brown Rice Pilaf	1 cup	210	4	35	2.5	0	10	630	41	1	3	5	3 carb, 1 fat
Garlic & Herb	1 cup	220	3.5	30	0.5	0	0	500	44	0	1	4	3 carb, 1 fat
Original	1 cup	220	4	35	2	0	10	810	43	0	1	4	3 carb, 1 fat

Original Long Grain & Wild Rice	1 cup	220	4	35	2	0	10	750	43	0	1	5	3 carb, 1 fat
Roasted Chicken & Garlic	1 cup	210	3	25	1.5	0	5	540	43	1	1	5	3 carb, 1 fat
Roasted Vegetable & Chicken Long Grain & Wild Rice	1 cup	220	4	35	2	0	10	690	43	1	2	5	3 carb, 1 fat
Spanish Rice	1 cup	310	8	70	5	0	20	990	55	1	2	5	3 1/2 carb, 2 fat
Sundried Tomato & Basil	1 cup	290	7	60	1	0	0	900	54	2	2	6	3 1/2 carb, 1 fat
Toasted Almond	1 cup	230	6	50	2	0	10	610	40	1	2	5	2 1/2 carb, 1 fat
Wild Mushrooms & Herb	1 cup	220	3.5	30	2	0	10	510	43	0	1	5	3 carb, 1 fat
Rice-A-Roni													
Beef	1 cup	310	9	80	2	1.5	0	1020	51	2	2	7	3 1/2 carb, 2 fat
Chicken	1 cup	300	9	80	2	1.5	0	1060	50	2	3	7	3 carb, 2 fat
Chicken & Broccoli	1 cup	220	5	45	1	1	0	920	40	2	2	6	2 1/2 carb, 1 fat
Chicken & Mushroom	1 cup	350	13	120	3	2	5	1290	51	3	2	8	3 1/2 carb, 3 fat
Country Cheddar	1 cup	370	16	140	5	2	10	990	50	6	2	8	3 carb, 3 fat

RICE & RICE MIXES

	Serving	Calories	Fat (g)	Cal. from Fat	Sat. Fat (g)	Trans Fat (g)	Chol. (mg)	Sod. (mg)	Carb. (g)	Sugar (g)	Fiber (g)	Prot. (g)	Servings/Exchanges
Creamy Four Cheese	1 cup	270	12	110	3.5	1.5	5	740	37	3	1	6	2 1/2 carb, 2 fat
Fried Rice	1 cup	310	10	90	2	1.5	0	1350	50	4	2	7	3 carb, 2 fat
Long Grain & Wild Rice, Original	1 cup	240	6	50	1	1	0	840	43	2	1	5	3 carb, 1 fat
Lower Sodium Beef	1 cup	270	5	45	1	0	0	650	50	3	2	7	3 carb, 1 fat
Lower Sodium Chicken	1 cup	270	5	45	1	0.5	0	670	51	1	2	7	3 1/2 carb, 1 fat
Mexican Style	1 cup	250	8	70	1.5	1	0	720	40	3	2	6	2 1/2 carb, 2 fat
Rice Pilaf	1 cup	310	9	80	1.5	1.5	0	1060	52	1	2	7	3 1/2 carb, 2 fat
Spanish Rice	1 cup	260	8	70	1.5	1	0	1250	44	6	3	6	3 carb, 2 fat
Uncle Ben's													
Country Inn Rice													
Broccoli Rice Au Gratin	1 cup	200	2	20	1	0	5	680	41	3	1	5	3 carb
Chicken Broccoli	1 cup	200	1	10	0	0	0	790	42	0	1	4	3 carb
Chicken Flavored	1 cup	200	1	10	0	0	0	810	42	1	1	5	2 1/2 carb

Chicken & Vegetable	1 cup	200	1	10	0	0	0	650	43	1	1	4	2 1/2 carb
Chicken & Wild Rice	1 cup	200	1	10	0	0	0	740	43	1	1	4	3 carb
Rice Pilaf	1 cup	200	1	10	0	0	0	570	43	0	1	4	3 carb
Long-Grain White Rice													
Boil-In-Bag	1 cup	170	0.5	5	0	0	0	0	38	0	1	4	3 1/2 carb
Instant Rice	1 cup	150	0	0	0	0	0	0	33	0	1	3	2 carb
Original Converted Rice	1 cup	170	0	0	0	0	0	0	37	0	0	4	2 1/2 carb
Long Grain & Wild Rice													
5 Grain Medley, Quinoa Pilaf	1 cup	200	1.5	15	0	0	0	670	41	1	3	6	2 1/2 carb
Basmati Medley, Savory Herb	1 cup	200	0.5	5	0	0	0	620	43	1	1	5	2 1/2 carb
Brown Rice & Quinoa, Roasted Red Pepper	1 cup	200	2	15	0	0	0	510	40	2	3	6	2 1/2 carb
Fast Cook Recipe	1 cup	200	0.5	5	0	0	0	660	43	3	1	6	2 1/2 carb
Original Recipe	1 cup	200	0.5	5	0	0	0	650	42	1	1	6	3 carb
Roasted Garlic & Herb	1 cup	200	2	15	0	0	0	570	40	0	3	7	2 1/2 carb

RICE & RICE MIXES

	Serving	Calories	Fat (g)	Cal. from Fat	Sat. Fat (g)	Trans Fat (g)	Chol. (mg)	Sod. (mg)	Carb. (g)	Sugar (g)	Fiber (g)	Prot. (g)	Servings/Exchanges
Ready Rice													
Long Grain & Wild	1 cup	200	0.5	5	0	0	0	650	42	1	1	6	3 carb
Original Long Grain	1 cup	200	2.5	25	0	0	0	10	40	0	1	4	2 1/2 carb, 1 fat
Rice Pilaf	1 cup	210	2.5	20	0	0	0	450	41	2	4	6	2 1/2 carb, 1 fat
Roasted Chicken	1 cup	210	3	30	0	0	0	700	42	1	2	4	3 carb, 1 fat
Spanish Style	1 cup	200	2.5	20	0	0	0	620	40	3	2	4	2 1/2 carb, 1 fat
Teriyaki	1 cup	220	3	25	0	0	5	870	42	2	3	6	3 carb, 1 fat
Whole Grain Brown	1 cup	190	3	30	0	0	0	15	39	0	3	5	2 1/2 carb, 1 fat
Whole Grain Brown Rice													
Boil-In-Bag Whole Grain Brown Rice	1 cup	170	1.5	15	0	0	0	0	36	0	2	4	2 1/2 carb
Instant Brown Rice	1 cup	170	1.5	15	0	0	0	0	36	0	1	4	2 1/2 carb
Natural Whole Grain Brown Rice	1 cup	180	1.5	15	0	0	0	0	36	0	2	4	2 1/2 carb

Ready Whole Grain Medley

Brown & Wild	1 cup	210	2.5	25	0	0	0	690	41	1	3	5	3 carb, 1 fat
Santa Fe	1 cup	220	3	25	0	0	0	700	42	1	5	7	3 carb, 1 fat
Vegetable Harvest	1 cup	220	3	25	0	0	0	780	44	2	5	5	3 carb, 1 fat

SALAD DRESSING

	Serving	Calories	Fat (g)	Cal. from Fat	Sat. Fat (g)	Trans Fat (g)	Chol. (mg)	Sod. (mg)	Carb. (g)	Sugar (g)	Fiber (g)	Prot. (g)	Servings/Exchanges
Dressing, Oil & Vinegar	2 Tbsp	144	16	145	3	0	0	0	<1	<1	0	0	3 fat
Mayonnaise	1 tsp	33	4	35	<1	0	2	26	0	0	0	0	1 fat
Mayonnaise, Light/ Reduced-Fat	1 Tbsp	45	5	45	<1	0	4	120	1	<1	0	0	1 fat
Salad Dressing, Fat-Free	1 Tbsp	21	0	0	0	0	0	136	5	3	0	0	free
Salad Dressing, Reduced-Fat, Cream Based	2 Tbsp	70	4	35	<1	0	0	241	9	5	0	0	1/2 carb, 1 fat
Salad Dressing, Regular	1 Tbsp	69	7	65	<1	0	0	125	2	2	0	0	1 fat
Bernstein's													
Balsamic Italian	2 Tbsp	110	11	100	0.5	0	0	270	2	1	0	0	2 fat
Cheese Fantastico	2 Tbsp	100	10	90	1	0	5	400	2	0	0	1	2 fat
Cheese & Garlic Italian	2 Tbsp	110	11	100	1	0	0	340	2	1	0	1	2 fat
Creamy Caesar	2 Tbsp	120	13	115	1	0	15	200	1	0	0	0	3 fat
Fat Free Cheese & Garlic Italian	2 Tbsp	10	0	0	0	0	0	380	2	1	0	0	free

Herb Garden French	2 Tbsp	130	12	110	1	0	0	260	6	3	0	0	1/2 carb, 2 fat
Light Fantastic Cheese Fantastico	2 Tbsp	25	1.5	15	0.5	0	5	370	3	1	0	1	free
Light Fantastic Parmesan Garlic Ranch	2 Tbsp	50	2.5	25	0.5	0	5	330	6	2	0	1	1/2 carb, 1 fat
Restaurant Recipe Italian	2 Tbsp	120	12	110	1	0	5	360	1	0	0	1	2 fat
Best Foods													
Canola Cholesterol-Free Mayonnaise	1 Tbsp	40	4	40	0	0	0	115	<1	0	0	0	1 fat
Light Mayonnaise	1 Tbsp	35	3.5	30	0	0	<5	135	1	0	0	0	1 fat
Low Fat Mayonnaise Dressing	1 Tbsp	15	1	10	0	0	0	130	2	<1	0	0	free
Mayonnaise Dressing with Olive Oil	1 Tbsp	60	6	50	1	0	5	125	<1	0	0	0	1 fat
Organic Spicy Chipotle Mayonnaise	1 Tbsp	100	11	100	1.5	0	5	90	0	0	0	0	2 fat
Real Mayonnaise	1 Tbsp	100	11	100	1.5	0	5	100	0	0	0	0	2 fat

SALAD DRESSING

	Serving	Calories	Fat (g)	Cal. from Fat	Sat. Fat (g)	Trans Fat (g)	Chol. (mg)	Sod. (mg)	Carb. (g)	Sugar (g)	Fiber (g)	Prot. (g)	Servings/Exchanges
Cardini's													
Balsamic Vinaigrette	2 Tbsp	100	8	80	2	0	0	250	5	4	0	0	2 fat
Caesar Light	2 Tbsp	80	7	60	1	0	30	250	5	1	0	1	1 fat
Fat Free Caesar	2 Tbsp	40	0	0	0	0	0	500	9	3	0	0	1/2 carb
Honey Mustard	2 Tbsp	120	11	100	1.5	0	10	180	6	5	0	0	2 fat
Light Greek Vinaigrette	2 Tbsp	50	4.5	40	1	0	0	280	2	2	0	0	1 fat
Original Caesar	2 Tbsp	160	17	150	3	0	30	240	1	0	0	1	3 fat
Roasted Asian Sesame	2 Tbsp	120	10	90	1.5	0	12	370	6	6	0	0	1/2 carb, 2 fat
Dorothy Lynch													
Fat Free Home Style Dressing	2 Tbsp	55	0	0	0	0	0	180	12	10	2	0	1 carb
Home Style Dressing	2 Tbsp	100	7	60	1	0	0	160	11	8	1	0	1 carb, 1 fat
Girard's													
Caesar	2 Tbsp	120	13	110	2	0	10	320	1	0	0	1	3 fat
Chinese Chicken Salad	2 Tbsp	120	10	90	2	0	0	320	6	6	0	0	1/2 carb, 2 fat

	Amount	Cal.	Fat (g)	Cal. Fat	Sat. Fat (g)	Trans Fat (g)	Chol. (mg)	Sod. (mg)	Carb. (g)	Sugar (g)	Fiber (g)	Prot. (g)	Choices/Exchanges
Greek Feta Vinaigrette	2 Tbsp	100	11	100	2	0	0	260	1	1	0	0	2 fat
Light Caesar	2 Tbsp	80	7	70	0	0	10	370	2	2	0	1	1 fat
Light Champagne	2 Tbsp	60	5	45	5	0	0	470	2	1	0	0	1 fat
Light Creamy Balsamic Vinaigrette	2 Tbsp	45	3	30	0	0	0	230	4	3	0	0	1 fat
Original French	2 Tbsp	120	12	120	2	0	0	410	0	0	0	0	2 fat
Raspberry	2 Tbsp	70	4.5	40	1	0	0	330	7	6	0	0	1/2 carb, 1 fat
Spinach Salad	2 Tbsp	60	1.5	15	0	0	0	250	11	10	0	0	1 carb
Hidden Valley													
Avocado Ranch	2 Tbsp	90	9	80	1.5	0	15	240	2	1	0	0	2 fat
Buttermilk Ranch Light	2 Tbsp	70	5	45	1	0	5	310	3	2	0	1	1 fat
Coleslaw	2 Tbsp	150	15	140	2.5	0	10	170	5	4	0	0	3 fat
Fiesta Salsa Ranch Light	2 Tbsp	60	5	50	1	0	0	240	3	1	0	0	1 fat
Greek Yogurt Cucumber Dill	2 Tbsp	60	5	45	1	0	0	240	3	2	0	1	1 fat
Original Homestyle	2 Tbsp	140	14	120	2.5	0	10	260	2	1	0	0	3 fat
Original Ranch	2 Tbsp	140	14	130	2.5	0	10	260	2	1	0	1	3 fat

SALAD DRESSING

	Serving	Calories	Fat (g)	Cal. from Fat	Sat. Fat (g)	Trans Fat (g)	Chol. (mg)	Sod. (mg)	Carb. (g)	Sugar (g)	Fiber (g)	Prot. (g)	Servings/Exchanges
Pomegranate Vinaigrette	2 Tbsp	60	6	50	0	0	0	100	3	2	0	0	1 fat
Ken's Steak House													
Buttermilk Ranch	2 Tbsp	180	20	180	3	0	5	260	1	1	0	0	4 fat
Country French	2 Tbsp	150	12	100	1.5	0	0	220	10	9	0	0	1/2 carb, 2 fat
Greek with Imported Olive Oil	2 Tbsp	100	11	90	1.5	0	0	270	1	1	0	0	2 fat
Light Caesar	2 Tbsp	80	7	60	1.5	0	10	320	2	1	<1	1	1 fat
Light Olive Oil & Vinegar	2 Tbsp	50	4	35	0.5	0	0	240	3	3	0	0	1 fat
Ranch	2 Tbsp	80	7	70	1	0	5	310	3	2	0	0	1 fat
Kraft													
Buttermilk Ranch	2 Tbsp	120	12	110	2	0	10	290	2	1	0	0	2 fat
Catalina	2 Tbsp	90	6	50	1	0	0	340	9	8	0	0	1/2 carb, 1 fat
Classic Caesar	2 Tbsp	110	12	100	2	0	10	320	2	1	0	0	2 fat
Classic Ranch	2 Tbsp	110	11	100	1.5	0	10	260	2	1	0	0	2 fat

	Serving	Cal.	Fat (g)	Sat. Fat (g)	Chol. (mg)	Sod. (mg)	Carb. (g)	Sugar (g)	Fiber (g)	Prot. (g)	Exchanges
Fat Free Catalina	2 Tbsp	50	0	0	0	350	11	7	0	0	1 carb
Greek Vinaigrette	2 Tbsp	50	7	0.5	0	370	2	<1	0	<1	1 fat
Lite Asian Toasted Sesame	2 Tbsp	45	1.5	0	0	260	7	6	0	<1	1/2 carb
Lite Balsamic Vinaigrette	2 Tbsp	25	1	0	0	210	4	4	0	0	free
Lite Ranch	2 Tbsp	70	4.5	0.5	10	350	7	1	0	0	1/2 carb, 1 fat
Lite Raspberry Vinaigrette	2 Tbsp	30	1	0	0	240	5	5	0	0	1/2 carb
Roka Blue Cheese	2 Tbsp	120	12	2	0	250	1	<1	0	0	2 fat
Thousand Island with Bacon	2 Tbsp	100	8	1	0	190	6	6	0	0	2 fat
Zesty Italian	2 Tbsp	60	4.5	0.5	0	300	3	2	0	0	1 fat
Kraft Miracle Whip/Mayonnaise											
Light Mayonnaise	1 Tbsp	35	3	0	0	95	2	<1	0	0	1 fat
Light Miracle Whip	1 Tbsp	20	1.5	0	5	125	2	<1	0	0	free
Light Olive Oil Mayonnaise	1 Tbsp	50	5	0.5	5	105	1	0	0	0	1 fat
Mayonnaise	1 Tbsp	90	10	1.5	<5	70	0	0	0	0	2 fat

SALAD DRESSING

	Serving	Calories	Fat (g)	Cal. from Fat	Sat. Fat (g)	Trans Fat (g)	Chol. (mg)	Sod. (mg)	Carb. (g)	Sugar (g)	Fiber (g)	Prot. (g)	Servings/Exchanges
Miracle Whip	1 Tbsp	40	3.5	30	0.5	0	<5	100	2	1	0	0	1 fat
Litehouse													
Balsamic Vinaigrette	2 Tbsp	100	10	80	0	0	0	160	4	3	0	0	2 fat
Chunky Bleu Cheese	2 Tbsp	150	16	140	1.5	0	15	220	1	1	0	1	3 fat
Coleslaw	2 Tbsp	110	9	80	0.5	0	5	130	9	8	0	0	1/2 carb, 2 fat
Honey Mustard	2 Tbsp	130	12	110	1	0	10	140	4	4	0	0	2 fat
Lite Ranch	2 Tbsp	60	5	50	0	0	10	210	3	2	0	1	1 fat
Mango Habanero	2 Tbsp	25	0	0	0	0	0	170	6	5	0	0	1/2 carb
Original Bleu Cheese	2 Tbsp	150	16	140	1.5	0	15	230	1	1	0	1	3 fat
Parmesan Caesar	2 Tbsp	100	10	90	1	0	5	220	3	1	0	1	2 fat
Pear Gorgonzola Vinaigrette	2 Tbsp	50	2.5	25	0	0	0	240	7	6	0	0	1 fat
Poppyseed	2 Tbsp	60	4	35	0	0	10	220	6	6	0	0	1/2 carb, 1 fat
Ranch	2 Tbsp	120	12	110	1	0	10	200	2	2	0	0	2 fat

Sesame Ginger	2 Tbsp	40	0	0	5	0	0	270	9	8	0	0	1/2 carb
Sriracha Lime	2 Tbsp	20	0	0	0	0	0	200	5	5	0	0	free

Maple Grove Farms of Vermont

Asiago & Garlic	2 Tbsp	40	3.5	30	0	0	0	260	2	1	0	0	1 fat
Fat Free Balsamic Vinaigrette	2 Tbsp	15	0	0	0	0	0	120	3	2	0	0	free
Fat Free Cranberry Balsamic Vinaigrette	2 Tbsp	35	0	0	0	0	0	220	8	7	0	0	1/2 carb
Fat Free Honey Dijon	2 Tbsp	40	0	0	0	0	0	210	10	9	1	0	1/2 carb
Honey Mustard	2 Tbsp	100	8	70	0.5	0	0	260	8	7	0	<1	1/2 carb, 2 fat
Lite Caesar	2 Tbsp	50	4.5	40	0	0	0	260	4	3	0	0	1 fat
Lite Honey Mustard	2 Tbsp	70	4	35	0	0	0	260	8	7	0	0	1 fat

Marie's

Balsamic Vinaigrette	2 Tbsp	45	4.5	40	0.5	0	0	220	2	2	0	0	1 fat
Basil Pesto Vinaigrette	2 Tbsp	110	11	100	2	0	0	190	2	1	0	1	2 fat
Blue Cheese Vinaigrette	2 Tbsp	120	11	100	2.5	0	5	190	4	4	0	1	2 fat
Caesar	2 Tbsp	170	19	170	3.5	0	15	160	1	1	0	1	4 fat

SALAD DRESSING

	Serving	Calories	Fat (g)	Cal. from Fat	Sat. Fat (g)	Trans Fat (g)	Chol. (mg)	Sod. (mg)	Carb. (g)	Sugar (g)	Fiber (g)	Prot. (g)	Servings/Exchanges
Chunky Blue Cheese	2 Tbsp	160	17	150	3.5	0	15	170	1	0	0	1	3 fat
Creamy Ranch	2 Tbsp	180	19	170	3	0	15	170	1	1	0	0	4 fat
Italian Vinaigrette	2 Tbsp	70	8	70	1.5	0	0	240	3	2	0	0	2 fat
Lite Chunky Blue Cheese	2 Tbsp	60	7	60	1.5	0	5	290	1	1	0	1	1 fat
Lite Creamy Ranch	2 Tbsp	70	6	60	1	0	5	220	6	2	0	1	1/2 carb, 1 fat
Original Coleslaw	2 Tbsp	140	13	110	2	0	10	170	7	7	0	0	1/2 carb, 3 fat
Raspberry Vinaigrette	2 Tbsp	50	3	30	0	0	0	100	7	6	0	0	1/2 carb, 1 fat
Red Wine Vinaigrette	2 Tbsp	60	4.5	40	0.5	0	0	200	6	5	0	0	1/2 carb, 1 fat
Thousand Island	2 Tbsp	150	15	140	2.5	0	10	200	3	3	0	0	3 fat
Yogurt Parmesan Caesar	2 Tbsp	60	5	45	0	0	10	200	2	1	0	1	1 fat
Newman's Own													
Balsamic Vinaigrette	2 Tbsp	90	9	80	1	0	0	280	3	1	0	0	2 fat
Caesar	2 Tbsp	150	16	140	2.5	0	5	340	1	1	0	1	3 fat
Cranberry Walnut	2 Tbsp	70	4.5	40	0.5	0	0	230	9	8	0	0	1/2 carb, 1 fat

Family Recipe Italian	2 Tbsp	130	13	120	2	0	0	320	1	0	0	1	3 fat
Honey Dijon Mustard	2 Tbsp	140	13	120	2	0	0	160	6	6	0	0	3 fat
Light Balsamic Vinaigrette	2 Tbsp	45	4	35	0.5	0	0	310	2	2	0	0	1 fat
Light Caesar	2 Tbsp	70	6	50	1	0	5	380	3	2	0	1	1 fat
Light Sun Dried Tomato Vinaigrette	2 Tbsp	60	4	40	0.5	0	0	380	5	3	0	0	1 fat
Olive Oil & Vinegar	2 Tbsp	150	16	150	2.5	0	0	150	1	1	0	0	3 fat
Ranch	2 Tbsp	150	16	140	2.5	0	10	290	2	1	0	0	3 fat
Rao's Specialty Foods													
8 Star Balsamic Vinaigrette	2 Tbsp	100	10	90	1	0	0	230	<1	<1	0	0	2 fat
Caesar Salad	2 Tbsp	80	8	80	1.5	0	0	310	2	<1	0	2	2 fat
Italian Herb	2 Tbsp	90	9	80	1.5	0	0	370	2	1	0	0	2 fat
Roasted Garlic	2 Tbsp	90	10	90	1	0	5	230	<1	0	0	0	2 fat
Trader Joe's													
Balsamic Vinaigrette	2 Tbsp	80	6	60	0	0	0	60	5	5	0	0	1 fat

SALAD DRESSING

	Serving	Calories	Fat (g)	Cal. from Fat	Sat. Fat (g)	Trans Fat (g)	Chol. (mg)	Sod. (mg)	Carb. (g)	Sugar (g)	Fiber (g)	Prot. (g)	Servings/Exchanges
Fat Free Balsamic Vinaigrette	2 Tbsp	25	0	0	0	0	0	170	6	5	0	0	1/2 carb
Goddess	2 Tbsp	120	12	110	1	0	0	350	2	0	0	1	2 fat
Organic Red Wine & Olive Oil Vinaigrette	2 Tbsp	130	15	130	2	0	0	190	0	0	0	0	3 fat
Organic Sriracha Ranch	2 Tbsp	80	8	70	1	0	5	270	3	2	0	0	2 fat
Raspberry Vinaigrette	2 Tbsp	40	3	25	0	0	0	60	4	4	0	0	1 fat
Romano Caesar	2 Tbsp	180	20	180	1.5	0	1	150	<1	0	0	<1	4 fat
Sesame Soy Ginger Vinaigrette	2 Tbsp	35	0	0	0	0	0	230	9	8	0	0	1/2 carb
Tuscan Italian	2 Tbsp	100	10	90	0.5	0	0	240	3	2	0	0	2 fat
Wish–Bone													
Chunky Blue Cheese	2 Tbsp	150	14	140	2.5	0	5	240	1	<1	0	0	3 fat
Creamy Caesar	2 Tbsp	180	18	160	3	0	10	290	1	<1	0	<1	4 fat
Creamy Italian	2 Tbsp	110	10	90	1.5	0	0	240	4	2	0	<1	2 fat

Deluxe French	2 Tbsp	120	11	100	1.5	0	0	170	5	4	0	0	2 fat
House Italian	2 Tbsp	110	10	90	1.5	0	5	260	3	2	0	0	2 fat
Italian	2 Tbsp	80	7	60	1	0	0	340	4	4	0	0	1 fat
Olive Oil Vinaigrette	2 Tbsp	60	5	45	0.5	0	0	250	4	3	0	0	1 fat
Ranch	2 Tbsp	130	13	120	2	0	0	230	2	1	0	0	3 fat
Raspberry Hazelnut Vinaigrette	2 Tbsp	80	5	45	1	0	0	260	8	5	0	0	1/2 carb, 1 fat
Red Wine Vinaigrette	2 Tbsp	70	5	45	0.5	0	0	230	6	4	0	0	1/2 carb, 1 fat
Russian	2 Tbsp	110	6	50	1	0	0	340	14	6	0	0	1 carb, 1 fat
Sweet & Spicy French	2 Tbsp	140	12	110	2	0	0	330	7	7	0	0	1/2 carb, 2 fat
Thousand Island	2 Tbsp	130	12	110	2	0	10	290	5	4	0	<1	2 fat
Wish-Bone Fat Free													
Chunky Blue Cheese	2 Tbsp	30	0	0	0	0	0	280	7	2	<1	<1	1/2 carb
Italian	2 Tbsp	15	0	0	0	0	0	340	3	2	0	0	free
Ranch	2 Tbsp	30	0	0	0	0	0	270	6	2	0	0	1/2 carb
Western	2 Tbsp	50	0	0	0	0	0	280	12	11	0	0	1 carb

SAUCES, GRAVIES, CONDIMENTS, RELISHES

	Serving	Calories	Fat (g)	Cal. from Fat	Sat. Fat (g)	Trans Fat (g)	Chol. (mg)	Sod. (mg)	Carb. (g)	Sugar (g)	Fiber (g)	Prot. (g)	Servings/Exchanges
Apple Butter	1 Tbsp	29	0	0	0	0	0	3	7	6	<1	0	1/2 carb
Catsup/Ketchup	1 Tbsp	17	0	0	0	0	0	154	5	4	0	0	free
Catsup/Ketchup, Low-Sodium	1 Tbsp	17	0	0	0	0	0	3	5	4	0	0	free
Chutney	1 Tbsp	26	<1	0	<1	0	0	38	7	NA	<1	<1	1/2 carb
Gravy, Au Jus, Canned	1/4 cup	9	<1	0	<1	NA	0	282	2	NA	0	<1	free
Gravy, Beef, Canned	1/4 cup	31	1	10	<1	NA	2	326	3	0	0	2	free
Gravy, Chicken, Canned	1/4 cup	27	2	18	<1	NA	3	222	3	0	0	<1	free
Gravy, Mushroom, Canned	1/4 cup	30	2	18	<1	NA	0	339	3	0	<1	<1	free
Gravy, Turkey, Canned	1/4 cup	30	1	9	<1	NA	1	343	3	0	0	2	free
Guacamole with Tomatoes	1 Tbsp	17	2	17	<1	0	0	27	1	NA	<1	<1	free
Honey	1 Tbsp	64	0	0	0	0	0	<1	17	17	<1	<1	1 carb
Horseradish, Prepared	1 Tbsp	7	<1	0	<1	0	0	47	2	1	<1	<1	free

Food	Serving												
Jam, Cherry/Strawberry	1 Tbsp	56	0	0	0	0	0	6	14	10	<1	0	1 carb
Jam/Marmalade/Preserves, Reduced-Sugar	1 Tbsp	36	<1	<1	0	0	0	5	9	NA	<1	<1	1/2 carb, 2 fat
Jam/Preserves, Artifically Sweetened	1 Tbsp	18	0	0	0	0	0	0	8	5	<1	0	free
Jelly	1 Tbsp	56	0	0	0	0	0	6	15	11	<1	0	1 carb
Jelly, No Sugar	1 Tbsp	23	0	0	0	0	0	1	6	<1	<1	<1	free
Jelly, Reduced-Sugar	1 Tbsp	34	<1	<1	0	0	0	<1	9	9	<1	<1	1/2 carb
Marmalade, Orange	1 Tbsp	49	0	0	0	0	0	11	13	12	<1	<1	1 carb
Mustard, Dijon	1 Tbsp	19	1	<1	9	0	0	379	2	0	<1	<1	free
Mustard, Honey	1 Tbsp	50	3	<1	27	0	0	91	7	NA	<1	<1	1/2 carb
Mustard, Prepared	1 Tbsp	12	<1	<1	0	0	0	196	1	0	<1	<1	free
Olives, Green, Pitted	10	45	5	<1	45	0	0	936	<1	NA	<1	<1	1 fat
Olives, Small Ripe, Canned	10	37	3	<1	27	0	0	279	2	NA	1	<1	1 fat
Olives, Stuffed Green	10	41	5	<1	41	0	0	827	<1	NA	<1	<1	1 fat
Peppers, Pickled Hot Jalapeño	2	8	<1	<1	0	0	0	121	2	NA	<1	<1	free

SAUCES, GRAVIES, CONDIMENTS, RELISHES

	Serving	Calories	Fat (g)	Cal. from Fat	Sat. Fat (g)	Trans Fat (g)	Chol. (mg)	Sod. (mg)	Carb. (g)	Sugar (g)	Fiber (g)	Prot. (g)	Servings/Exchanges
Pickle, Dill	1	12	<1	0	<1	0	0	833	3	NA	<1	<1	free
Pickle, Dill, Low-Sodium	1	12	<1	0	<1	0	0	12	3	NA	<1	<1	free
Pickle Slices, Dill	10	11	<1	0	<1	0	0	769	3	NA	<1	<1	free
Pickle Slices, Dill, Low-Sodium	10	11	<1	0	<1	0	0	11	3	NA	<1	<1	free
Pickle Slices, Fresh Pack	4	22	<1	0	0	0	0	202	5	NA	<1	<1	free
Pickle Slices, Sour	10	8	<1	0	<1	0	0	846	2	NA	<1	<1	free
Pickle, Sour	1	4	<1	0	<1	0	0	423	<1	NA	<1	<1	free
Pickle, Sweet	1 medium	41	<1	0	<1	0	0	329	11	NA	<1	<1	1/2 carb
Relish, Hot Dog	1 Tbsp	14	<1	0	<1	0	0	167	4	NA	<1	<1	free
Relish, Sweet Pickle	1 Tbsp	20	<1	0	<1	0	0	124	5	4	<1	<1	free
Sauce, Bearnaise, Homemade	1/4 cup	161	17	153	10	0	119	222	<1	NA	<1	1	3 fat
Sauce, Black Bean	1/2 cup	129	6	54	1	0	0	1322	14	NA	2	3	1 carb, 1 fat

Sauce, Cheese	1/4 cup	110	8	70	4	0	18	522	4	<1	<1	4	1 med-fat protein, 1 fat
Sauce, Curry	1/2 cup	74	6	54	1	0	0	392	3	NA	<1	3	1 fat
Sauce, Hollandaise, Dry Mix & Water	1/2 cup	119	10	90	6	0	26	783	7	NA	<1	2	1/2 carb, 2 fat
Sauce, Hot Chili/Red Pepper	2 Tbsp	7	<1	0	<1	0	0	8	1	NA	<1	<1	free
Sauce, Hot Green Chili	1 Tbsp	6	<1	0	0	0	0	4	2	NA	<1	<1	free
Sauce, Salsa/Mexican, Homemade	1/2 cup	23	<1	0	<1	0	0	468	5	NA	1	<1	1 vegetable
Sauce, Soy	1 Tbsp	10	<1	0	<1	0	0	1028	2	NA	0	<1	free
Sauce, Spanish-Style Tomato	1/2 cup	40	<1	0	<1	0	0	576	9	NA	2	2	1/2 carb
Sauce, Tartar	1 Tbsp	32	3	27	<1	0	1	100	2	<1	<1	<1	1 fat
Sauce, Teriyaki	1 Tbsp	16	0	0	0	0	0	690	3	3	<1	1	free
Sauce, White, Homemade	1/4 cup	92	7	65	2	0	4	221	6	3	<1	2	1/2 carb, 1 fat
Sauce, Worcestershire	1 Tbsp	13	0	0	0	0	0	167	3	2	0	0	free
Syrup, Maple	1 Tbsp	52	<1	0	0	0	0	2	13	12	0	0	1 carb

SAUCES, GRAVIES, CONDIMENTS, RELISHES

	Serving	Calories	Fat (g)	Cal. from Fat	Sat. Fat (g)	Trans Fat (g)	Chol. (mg)	Sod. (mg)	Carb. (g)	Sugar (g)	Fiber (g)	Prot. (g)	Servings/Exchanges
Syrup, Pancake	1 Tbsp	47	0	0	0	0	0	16	12	4	0	0	1 carb
A.1. Sauce													
Bold & Spicy	1 Tbsp	20	0	0	0	0	0	260	1	3	0	0	free
Marinade, NY Steakhouse	1 Tbsp	20	1	10	0	0	0	230	5	4	0	0	free
Original	1 Tbsp	15	0	0	0	0	0	280	3	2	0	0	free
Thick & Hearty	1 Tbsp	25	0	0	0	0	0	290	2	5	0	0	free
Aunt Jemima													
Butter Lite Syrup	1/4 cup	100	0	0	0	0	0	210	26	25	1	0	2 carb
Butter Rich Syrup	1/4 cup	210	0	0	0	0	0	210	53	29	0	0	3 1/2 carb
Country Rich Lite Syrup	1/4 cup	100	0	0	0	0	0	180	26	25	1	0	2 carb
Country Rich Syrup	1/4 cup	210	0	0	0	0	0	120	53	30	0	0	3 1/2 carb
Lite Syrup	1/4 cup	100	0	0	0	0	0	190	26	25	0	0	2 carb
Original Syrup	1/4 cup	210	0	0	0	0	0	120	52	32	0	0	3 1/2 carb

Betty Crocker

	Serving												
Bac-Os, Salad Topping Bits or Chips	1 1/2 Tbsp	30	1	10	0	0	0	115	2	1	1	3	free

Braswell's

	Serving												
Red Pepper Jelly	1 Tbsp	35	0	0	0	0	0	0	9	0	0	0	1/2 carb

Campbell's

	Serving												
Gravy, Beef	1/4 cup	25	1	10	0.5	0	<5	270	3	<1	0	1	free
Gravy, Chicken	1/4 cup	25	1	10	0.5	0	0	270	3	1	0	1	free
Gravy, Country Style Sausage Gravy	1/4 cup	60	5	45	2	0	5	270	3	0	0	1	1 fat
Gravy, Turkey	1/4 cup	25	1	10	0.5	0	0	270	3	0	0	1	free

Cary's

	Serving												
Syrup, Maple	1/4 cup	210	0	0	0	0	0	5	53	NA	0	0	3 1/2 carb
Syrup, Sugar-Free	1/4 cup	30	0	0	0	0	0	70	11	0	1	0	1 carb

Emeril's

	Serving												
Dijon Mustard	1 tsp	5	0	0	0	0	0	135	0	0	0	0	free

SAUCES, GRAVIES, CONDIMENTS, RELISHES

	Serving	Calories	Fat (g)	Cal. from Fat	Sat. Fat (g)	Trans Fat (g)	Chol. (mg)	Sod. (mg)	Carb. (g)	Sugar (g)	Fiber (g)	Prot. (g)	Servings/Exchanges
Famous Dave's													
BBQ Sauce, Devil's Spit	2 Tbsp	50	0	0	0	0	0	360	12	10	1	1	1 carb
BBQ Sauce, Rich & Sassy	2 Tbsp	60	0	5	0	0	0	360	14	12	0	0	1 carb
BBQ Sauce, Sweet & Zesty	2 Tbsp	70	0	0	0	0	0	320	17	15	0	0	1 carb
Fifty50													
Reduced Calorie Maple Syrup	1/4 cup	70	0	0	0	0	0	80	18	17	0	0	1 carb
Grey Poupon													
Country Dijon Mustard	1 tsp	5	0	0	0	0	0	120	0	0	0	0	free
Hormel													
Real Bacon Bits	1 Tbsp	25	1.5	15	1	0	10	210	0	0	0	3	1 fat
Real Bacon Pieces	1 Tbsp	25	1.5	15	1	0	10	210	0	0	0	3	1 fat

Heinz

Food	Serving	Cal.	Fat (g)	Sat. Fat (g)	Chol. (mg)	Sod. (mg)	Carb. (g)	Sugars (g)	Fiber (g)	Prot. (g)	Exchanges
57 Sauce	1 Tbsp	20	0	0	0	160	4	3	0	0	free
Chili Sauce	1 Tbsp	20	0	0	0	230	5	3	0	0	free
Cocktail Sauce	1/4 cup	70	0	0	0	590	18	12	1	1	1 carb
Gravy, Classic Chicken	1/4 cup	30	2	0.5	20	<5	250	3	0	0	1 fat
Gravy, Fat Free Roasted Turkey	1/4 cup	20	0	0	0	290	4	0	0	1	free
Gravy, Homestyle Savory Beef	1/4 cup	30	1	0.5	<5	390	4	0	0	1	1 fat
Gravy, Rich Mushroom Gravy	1/4 cup	20	0.5	0	0	320	3	0	0	<1	free
Worcestershire Sauce	1 tsp	0	0	0	0	60	0	0	0	0	free

Jack Daniel's

Food	Serving	Cal.	Fat (g)	Sat. Fat (g)	Chol. (mg)	Sod. (mg)	Carb. (g)	Sugars (g)	Fiber (g)	Prot. (g)	Exchanges
BBQ Sauce, Hickory Brown Sugar	2 Tbsp	50	0	0	0	280	12	10	0	0	1 carb
BBQ Sauce, Honey Smokehouse	2 Tbsp	45	0	0	0	280	11	10	0	0	1 carb
Steak Sauce, Original	1 Tbsp	45	0	0	0	300	11	9	0	0	1 carb

SAUCES, GRAVIES, CONDIMENTS, RELISHES

	Serving	Calories	Fat (g)	Cal. from Fat	Sat. Fat (g)	Trans Fat (g)	Chol. (mg)	Sod. (mg)	Carb. (g)	Sugar (g)	Fiber (g)	Prot. (g)	Servings/Exchanges
Karo													
Dark Corn Syrup	2 Tbsp	120	0	0	0	0	0	45	31	11	0	0	2 carb
Karo Lite	2 Tbsp	80	0	0	0	0	0	80	20	7	0	0	1 carb
Light Corn Syrup	2 Tbsp	120	0	0	0	0	0	30	30	10	0	0	2 carb
Pancake Syrup	4 Tbsp	240	0	0	0	0	0	85	63	25	0	0	4 carb
KC Masterpiece													
BBQ Sauce, Original	2 Tbsp	60	0	0	0	0	0	240	15	12	0	0	1 carb
BBQ Sauce, Sweet Roasted Chipotle	2 Tbsp	50	0	0	0	0	0	270	11	9	0	0	1 carb
Kitchen Bouquet													
Browning & Seasoning Sauce	1 tsp	15	0	0	0	0	0	10	3	0	0	0	free
Knott's Berry Farm													
Apricot Preserves	1 Tbsp	50	0	0	0	0	0	0	13	12	0	0	1 carb
Blackberry Preserves	1 Tbsp	50	0	0	0	0	0	0	13	12	0	0	1 carb

Food	Serving												Exchanges
Boysenberry Preserves	1 Tbsp	50	0	0	0	0	0	0	13	12	0	0	1 carb
Orange Marmalade	1 Tbsp	50	0	0	0	0	0	0	13	12	0	0	1 carb
Seedless Red Raspberry Jam	1 Tbsp	50	0	0	0	0	0	0	13	12	0	0	1 carb
Seedless Strawberry Jam	1 Tbsp	50	0	0	0	0	0	0	13	12	0	0	1 carb
Strawberry Preserves	1 Tbsp	50	0	0	0	0	0	0	13	12	0	0	1 carb
Kraft													
BBQ Sauce, Hickory Smoke	2 Tbsp	60	0	0	0	0	0	310	13	11	0	0	1 carb
BBQ Sauce, Honey Hickory Smoke	2 Tbsp	60	0	0	0	0	0	310	13	11	0	0	1 carb
BBQ Sauce, Honey Sweet	2 Tbsp	60	0	0	0	0	0	340	15	13	0	0	1 carb
BBQ Sauce, Original	2 Tbsp	60	0	0	0	0	0	350	15	13	0	0	1 carb
Sauce, Horseradish	2 Tbsp	100	9	80	0	0	0	230	4	3	0	0	2 fat
Sauce, Lemon Herb Tartar	2 Tbsp	60	5	45	0.5	0	<5	200	4	3	0	0	1 fat
Sauce, Tartar	2 Tbsp	60	5	45	0.5	0	<5	200	4	3	0	0	1 fat

SAUCES, GRAVIES, CONDIMENTS, RELISHES

	Serving	Calories	Fat (g)	Cal. from Fat	Sat. Fat (g)	Trans Fat (g)	Chol. (mg)	Sod. (mg)	Carb. (g)	Sugar (g)	Fiber (g)	Prot. (g)	Servings/Exchanges
La Choy													
Sauce, Soy	1 Tbsp	10	0	0	0	0	0	920	<1	<1	0	1	free
Sauce, Soy, Lite	1 Tbsp	15	0	0	0	0	0	550	2	2	0	1	free
Sauce, Sweet & Sour	1 Tbsp	60	0	0	0	0	0	110	14	11	0	0	1 carb
La Victoria													
Enchilada Sauce, Green Chili	1/4 cup	15	0	0	0	0	0	380	3	0	0	0	free
Enchilada Sauce, Red Chili	1/4 cup	15	0	0	0	0	0	430	3	0	0	0	free
Green Taco Sauce	1 Tbsp	5	0	0	0	0	0	95	1	0	0	0	free
Red Taco Sauce	1 Tbsp	5	0	0	0	0	0	90	1	1	0	0	free
Lawry's													
Marinade, Baja Chipotle	1 Tbsp	15	0	0	0	0	0	440	2	1	0	0	free
Marinade, Caribbean Jerk	1 Tbsp	30	0	0	0	0	0	480	7	6	0	0	free
Marinade, Herb & Garlic	1 Tbsp	10	0	0	0	0	0	420	2	1	0	0	free

Marinade, Lemon Pepper	1 Tbsp	10	0	0	0	0	390	2	1	0	0	free
Marinade, Mesquite	1 Tbsp	10	0	0	0	0	340	2	1	0	0	free
Marinade, Sesame Ginger	1 Tbsp	30	0	0	0	0	600	7	6	0	0	1/2 carb
Marinade, Steak & Chop	1 Tbsp	5	0	0	0	0	390	<1	0	0	0	free
Marinade, Teriyaki	1 Tbsp	35	0	0	0	0	460	8	7	0	0	free
Las Palmas												
Enchilada Sauce, Original Style	1/4 cup	15	0.5	5	0	0	0	370	3	2	1	free
Green Chili Enchilada Sauce	1/4 cup	25	1.5	10	0	0	0	350	3	1	0	free
Red Chili Sauce	1/4 cup	15	0.5	5	0	0	0	370	3	2	1	free
Log Cabin												
Lite Syrup	1/4 cup	100	0	0	0	0	0	180	25	22	<1	1 1/2 carb
Original Syrup	1/4 cup	200	0	0	0	0	0	140	53	26	0	3 1/2 carb
Maple Grove Farms Cozy Cottage												
Maple Syrup, Sugar Free	1/4 cup	30	0	0	0	0	0	105	10	0	0	1/2 carb

SAUCES, GRAVIES, CONDIMENTS, RELISHES

	Serving	Calories	Fat (g)	Cal. from Fat	Sat. Fat (g)	Trans Fat (g)	Chol. (mg)	Sod. (mg)	Carb. (g)	Sugar (g)	Fiber (g)	Prot. (g)	Servings/Exchanges
McCormick													
Bac'n Pieces, Bits	1 Tbsp	30	1	10	0	0	0	180	2	NA	0	3	1 fat
Salad Toppins	1 1/3 Tbsp	35	1.5	15	0	0	0	70	3	NA	0	2	1 fat
Mezzetta													
Cocktail Onions	8 pieces	5	0	0	0	0	0	300	1	1	0	0	free
Hot Pepper Rings	1/4 cup	10	0	0	0	0	0	310	2	0	0	0	free
Jalapeño Stuffed Olives	1	10	1	10	0	0	0	140	1	0	0	0	free
Sliced Jalapeño Peppers	1/4 cup	5	0	0	0	0	0	380	1	0	0	0	free
Sweet Bell Pepper Relish	3 pieces	15	0	5	0	0	0	340	2	1	1	1	free
Mrs. Butterworth's													
Lite Syrup	1/4 cup	90	0	0	0	0	0	190	25	9	0	0	1 1/2 carb
Original Syrup	1/4 cup	210	0	0	0	0	0	160	52	47	0	0	3 1/2 carb
Sugar Free Syrup	1/4 cup	20	0	0	0	0	0	160	8	0	0	0	1/2 carb

Mrs. Dash

Garlic Herb Marinade	1 Tbsp	25	0	0	0	0	0	0	3	0	0	free
Lemon Pepper Marinade	1 Tbsp	10	0	0	0	0	0	0	2	1	0	free
Lime Garlic Marinade	1 Tbsp	15	0	0	0	0	0	0	3	1	0	free
Sweet Teriyaki Marinade	1 Tbsp	35	0	0	0	0	0	0	9	8	0	free

Musselman's

Apple Butter	1 Tbsp	30	0	0	0	0	0	0	8	6	0	1/2 carb

Old El Paso

Enchilada Sauce, Green Chili	1/4 cup	25	1.5	10	0	0	0	280	4	1	0	free
Enchilada Sauce, Red Mild	1/4 cup	20	0	0	0	0	0	330	4	1	0	free
Taco Sauce, Medium	1 Tbsp	5	0	0	0	0	0	60	1	0	0	free
Taco Sauce, Mild	1 Tbsp	5	0	0	0	0	0	60	1	1	0	free

Ortega

Salsa, Thick & Chunky Mild	2 Tbsp	10	0	0	0	0	0	170	2	<1	0	free

SAUCES, GRAVIES, CONDIMENTS, RELISHES

	Serving	Calories	Fat (g)	Cal. from Fat	Sat. Fat (g)	Trans Fat (g)	Chol. (mg)	Sod. (mg)	Carb. (g)	Sugar (g)	Fiber (g)	Prot. (g)	Servings/Exchanges
Taco Sauce, Original	1 Tbsp	10	0	0	0	0	0	120	2	<1	0	0	free
Taco Sauce, Sriracha	1 Tbsp	10	0	0	0	0	0	105	2	1	0	0	free
Oscar Mayer													
Bacon Bits	1 Tbsp	25	1.5	15	0.5	0	2	170	0	0	0	2	free
Turkey Bacon Bits	1 Tbsp	20	1.5	15	0	0	0	95	0	0	0	0	free
Polaner													
All Fruit Strawberry Spread	1 Tbsp	35	0	0	0	0	0	0	9	7	0	0	1/2 carb
Strawberry Preserves	1 Tbsp	50	0	0	0	0	0	0	13	8	0	0	1 carb
Sugar Free with Fiber Strawberry Preserves	1 Tbsp	10	0	0	0	0	0	0	5	0	3	0	free
Progresso													
Artichoke Hearts with Liquid	3 pieces	30	0	0	0	0	0	550	5	1	2	1	free

Food	Serving	Cal	Fat (g)	Fat Cal	Sat Fat (g)	Trans Fat (g)	Chol (mg)	Sod (mg)	Carb (g)	Sugar (g)	Fiber (g)	Pro (g)	Exch
Regina													
Red Cooking Wine	1 oz	25	0	0	0	0	0	190	3	1	0	0	free
Red Wine Vinegar	1 Tbsp	0	0	0	0	0	0	0	<1	0	0	0	free
White Cooking Wine	1 oz	20	1	9	0	0	0	190	3	0	0	0	free
White Wine Vinegar	1 Tbsp	0	0	0	0	0	0	0	<1	0	0	0	free
Smucker's													
Apple Jelly	1 Tbsp	50	0	0	0	0	0	0	13	12	0	0	1 carb
Apricot Preserves	1 Tbsp	50	0	0	0	0	0	0	13	12	0	0	1 carb
Apricot-Pineapple Preserves	1 Tbsp	50	0	0	0	0	0	0	13	12	0	0	1 carb
Blueberry Preserves	1 Tbsp	50	0	0	0	0	0	0	13	12	0	0	1 carb
Blueberry Syrup	1/4 cup	200	0	0	0	0	0	0	51	44	0	0	3 1/2 carb
Boysenberry Syrup	1/4 cup	200	0	0	0	0	0	0	51	44	0	0	3 1/2 carb
Cider Apple Butter	1 Tbsp	45	0	0	0	0	0	10	11	10	0	0	1 carb
Concord Grape Jam	1 Tbsp	50	0	0	0	0	0	0	13	12	0	0	1 carb
Fruit & Honey, Blueberry Lemon	1 Tbsp	35	0	0	0	0	0	0	9	8	0	0	1/2 carb

SAUCES, GRAVIES, CONDIMENTS, RELISHES

	Serving	Calories	Fat (g)	Cal. from Fat	Sat. Fat (g)	Trans Fat (g)	Chol. (mg)	Sod. (mg)	Carb. (g)	Sugar (g)	Fiber (g)	Prot. (g)	Servings/Exchanges
Low Sugar Apricot Preserves	1 Tbsp	10	0	0	0	0	0	0	5	0	2	0	free
Low Sugar Concord Grape Jelly	1 Tbsp	25	0	0	0	0	0	0	6	5	0	0	1/2 carb
Low Sugar Strawberry Preserves	1 Tbsp	25	0	0	0	0	0	0	6	5	0	0	1/2 carb
Low Sugar Sweet Orange Marmalade	1 Tbsp	25	0	0	0	0	0	0	6	5	0	0	1/2 carb
Red Raspberry Preserves	1 Tbsp	50	0	0	0	0	0	0	13	12	0	0	1 carb
Seedless Strawberry Jam	1 Tbsp	50	0	0	0	0	0	0	13	12	0	0	1 carb
Simply Fruit Spreadable Fruit, Strawberry	1 Tbsp	40	0	0	0	0	0	0	10	8	0	0	1/2 carb
Squeeze Grape Jelly	1 Tbsp	50	0	0	0	0	0	5	13	12	0	0	1 carb
Squeeze Strawberry Fruit Spread	1 Tbsp	50	0	0	0	0	0	0	13	12	0	0	1 carb

Food	Serving	Cal.	Fat Cal.	Total Fat	Sat. Fat	Trans Fat	Chol.	Sodium	Carb.	Sugars	Fiber	Protein	Carb Choices
Strawberry Preserves	1 Tbsp	50	0	0	0	0	0	0	13	12	0	0	1 carb
Sugar Free Blackberry with Splenda	1 Tbsp	10	0	0	0	0	0	0	5	2	0	0	free
Sugar Free Blueberry Fruit Syrup	1/4 cup	25	0	0	0	0	0	0	8	0	1	0	1/2 carb
Sugar Free Strawberry with Truvia Sweetener	1 Tbsp	15	0	0	0	0	0	0	5	0	0	0	free
Sweet Orange Marmalade Preserves	1 Tbsp	50	0	0	0	0	0	0	13	12	0	0	1 carb
Sweet Baby Ray's													
BBQ Sauce	2 Tbsp	70	0	0	0	0	0	290	18	16	0	0	1 carb
Honey BBQ Sauce	2 Tbsp	70	0	0	0	0	0	300	17	15	0	0	1 carb
Tabasco													
Sauce, Green Pepper	1 tsp	0	0	0	0	0	0	150	0	0	0	0	free
Sauce, Pepper	1 tsp	0	0	0	0	0	0	35	0	0	0	0	free
Trappy's Red Devil													
Cayenne Pepper Sauce	1 tsp	0	0	0	0	0	0	150	0	0	0	0	free

SAUCES, GRAVIES, CONDIMENTS, RELISHES

	Serving	Calories	Fat (g)	Cal. from Fat	Sat. Fat (g)	Trans Fat (g)	Chol. (mg)	Sod. (mg)	Carb. (g)	Sugar (g)	Fiber (g)	Prot. (g)	Servings/Exchanges
Soy Vay, Veri Veri Teriyaki													
Low Sodium Marinade & Sauce	1 Tbsp	50	1.5	10	0	0	0	440	9	7	0	1	1/2 carb
Marinade & Sauce	1 Tbsp	45	1	10	0	0	0	590	8	7	0	1	1/2 carb
Vlasic													
Dill Relish	1 Tbsp	0	0	0	0	0	0	240	<1	0	0	0	free
Sweet Gherkins	1 oz	30	0	0	0	0	0	170	7	7	0	0	1/2 carb
Sweet Relish	1 Tbsp	15	0	0	0	0	0	140	3	3	0	0	free
Welch's													
Chia Concord Grape Spread	1 Tbsp	50	0	0	0	0	0	10	11	10	0	0	1 carb
Concord Grape Jam	1 Tbsp	50	0	0	0	0	0	10	13	13	0	0	1 carb
Concord Grape Jelly	1 Tbsp	50	0	0	0	0	0	15	13	13	0	0	1 carb
Natural Spread Concord Grape	1 Tbsp	30	0	0	0	0	0	15	8	8	0	0	1/2 carb

Reduced Sugar Concord Grape Jelly	1 Tbsp	20	0	0	0	15	5	5	0	0	free
Reduced Sugar Strawberry Spread	1 Tbsp	20	0	0	0	15	5	5	0	0	free
Squeezable Concord Grape Jelly	1 Tbsp	50	0	0	0	10	13	13	0	0	1 carb
Squeezable Strawberry Spread	1 Tbsp	50	0	0	0	10	13	13	0	0	1 carb

SNACKS, CRACKERS, CHIPS, POPCORN, SNACK BARS

	Serving	Calories	Fat (g)	Cal. from Fat	Sat. Fat (g)	Trans Fat (g)	Chol. (mg)	Sod. (mg)	Carb. (g)	Sugar (g)	Fiber (g)	Prot. (g)	Servings/Exchanges
Chips, Bagel	1 oz	128	4	35	2	0	0	66	19	2	1	5	1 carb, 1 fat
Chips, Potato	3/4 oz	114	7	65	2	0	0	171	11	<1	<1	2	1 carb, 1 fat
Chips, Potato, Baked	3/4 oz	82	1	10	0	0	0	112	17	2	1.5	2	1 carb
Crackers, Animal	8	89	3	25	0.5	0	0	79	15	5	0	1	1 carb
Crackers, Graham	3 squares	99	2	20	<1	0	0	142	18	7	<1	2	1 carb
Crackers, Matzoh, Plain	3/4 oz	83	<1	0	<1	0	0	0	18	0	<1	2	1 carb
Crackers, Oysters	20	86	2	20	<1	0	0	214	14	0	<1	2	1 carb
Crackers, Round Butter Type	6	90	5	45	0.5	0	0	152	11	<1	<1	1	1 carb, 1 fat
Crackers, Saltines	6	77	2	20	<1	0	0	193	13	0	0.5	2	1 carb
Crackers, Whole Wheat, Baked	5	89	3.5	30	<1	0	0	132	14	0	2	2	1 carb, 1 fat
Crackers, Whole Wheat, Reduced-Fat	5	80	2	20	<1	0	0	110	15	0	2.5	2	1 carb
Crispbread	2 slices	73	<1	0	0	0	0	53	16	<1	3	2	1 carb

Granola Bar	1 oz	134	6	55	1	0	0	83	18	7	1.5	3	1 carb, 1 fat
Granola Bar, Chewy, Low-Fat	1 oz	109	2	20	0.5	0	0	70	22	10	1	1	1 1/2 carb
Meal Replacement Bar, Medium	2-oz bar	202	5	45	3	0	2	130	27	0	2	12	2 carb, 1 med-fat protein
Melba Toast	4 pieces	78	<1	0	0	0	0	166	15	<1	1	2	1 carb
Oriental Snack Mix	1 oz	143	7	65	1	0	0	117	15	<1	4	5	1 carb, 1 fat
Pita Chips	3/4 oz	86	3	25	1	0	0	246	12	<1	<1	2	1 carb, 1 fat
Popcorn, Microwave, 94% Fat-Free	3 cups	65	1	10	<1	0	0	155	14	0	2.5	2	1 carb
Popcorn, Microwave Butter	3 cups	96	6	55	3	0	0	216	11	0	2	2	1 carb, 1 fat
Popcorn, No Salt or Fat Added	3 cups	93	1	10	0	0	0	2	19	<1	3.5	3	1 carb
Pretzel, Sticks or Rings	3/4 oz	80	<1	0	0	0	0	360	17	<1	<1	2	1 carb
Rice Cakes	2	70	<1	0	0	0	0	59	15	1	<1	2	1 carb
Sandwich Crackers, Cheese Filled	3	100	4	35	1	0	0	294	13	<1	<1	2	1 carb, 1 fat

SNACKS, CRACKERS, CHIPS, POPCORN, SNACK BARS

	Serving	Calories	Fat (g)	Cal. from Fat	Sat. Fat (g)	Trans Fat (g)	Chol. (mg)	Sod. (mg)	Carb. (g)	Sugar (g)	Fiber (g)	Prot. (g)	Servings/Exchanges
Sandwich Crackers, Peanut Butter	3	102	5	45	1	0	0	198	12	1	<1	2	1 carb, 1 fat
Tortilla Chips	3/4 oz	106	6	55	1	0	0	131	13	<1	<1	2	1 carb, 1 fat
Tortilla Chips, Fat-Free	3/4 oz	82	<1	0	0	0	0	111	18	0	3	2	1 carb
Trail Mix	1 oz	131	8	70	1.5	0	0	65	13	NA	NA	4	1 carb, 1 fat
Act II Microwave Popcorn													
94% Fat Free Butter	6 1/2 cups	130	2	20	0.5	0	0	190	27	NA	4	4	2 carb
100 Calorie Butter	5 1/2 cups	100	2.5	25	1	0	0	310	21	NA	4	3	1 1/2 carb, 1 fat
Butter	4 1/2 cups	120	5	45	2	0	0	180	19	NA	3	3	1 carb, 1 fat
Butter Lovers	4 1/2 cups	120	4	40	2	0	0	250	19	NA	2	3	1 carb, 1 fat
Kettle Corn	4 1/2 cups	150	9	80	4	0	0	170	19	NA	3	2	1 carb, 2 fat

Light Butter	6 1/2 cups	130	2.5	20	1	0	0	300	27	NA	3	4	2 carb, 1 fat
Movie Theatre Butter	4 1/2 cups	150	8	70	4	0	0	370	19	NA	3	2	1 carb, 2 fat
Xtreme Butter	4 1/2 cups	120	4	35	2	0	0	170	19	NA	2	3	1 carb, 1 fat
Austin													
Cracker Sandwiches, Cheese Crackers with Cheddar Cheese	1 pkg	190	10	90	2.5	0	0	350	23	5	<1	3	1 1/2 carb, 2 fat
Cracker Sandwiches, Cheese & Peanut Butter	1 pkg	190	10	90	1.5	0	0	330	23	3	1	4	1 1/2 carb, 2 fat
Cracker Sandwiches, Toast Crackers & Peanut Butter	1 pkg	190	9	80	1.5	0	0	300	23	5	1	4	1 1/2 carb, 2 fat
Betty Crocker													
Fruit By The Foot	1 roll	80	1	10	0.5	0	0	50	17	10	0	0	1 carb
Fruit Flavored Shapes	1 pouch	80	0	0	0	0	0	25	19	10	0	0	1 1/2 carb

SNACKS, CRACKERS, CHIPS, POPCORN, SNACK BARS

	Serving	Calories	Fat (g)	Cal. from Fat	Sat. Fat (g)	Trans Fat (g)	Chol. (mg)	Sod. (mg)	Carb. (g)	Sugar (g)	Fiber (g)	Prot. (g)	Servings/Exchanges
Fruit Gushers	1 pouch	90	1	10	0.5	0	0	45	20	10	0	0	1 carb
Fruit Roll-Ups	1	50	1	5	0.5	0	0	50	11	7	0	0	1 carb
Cracker Jack													
Chocolate Caramel	1/2 cup	110	0.5	5	0	0	0	190	25	15	<1	<1	1 1/2 carb
Chocolate Peanut Butter	1/2 cup	100	0.5	5	0	0	0	160	24	17	<1	<1	1 1/2 carb
Original	1/2 cup	120	2	15	0	0	0	70	23	15	1	2	1 1/2 carb
Entenmann's													
Chewy Chocolate Chip Cereal Bar	1 bar	150	6	50	2.5	0	5	110	25	12	2	2	1 1/2 carb, 1 fat
Extend Bar													
Chocolate & Caramel Anytime Bar	1 bar	130	3	30	1	0	0	180	22	0	5	10	1 1/2 carb, 1 lean protein
Franklin													
Crunch 'N Munch, Buttery Toffee	2/3 cup	140	4	35	1	0	<5	160	24	11	<1	2	1 1/2 carb, 1 fat

Frito-Lay

Baken-ets Fried Pork Rind, Traditional	9 pieces	80	5	45	2.5	0	20	300	0	0	0	7	1 med-fat protein
Cheetos, Crunchy	1 oz	160	10	90	1.5	0	0	250	13	1	<1	2	1 carb, 2 fat
Cheetos, Fantastic Flamin' Hot	1 oz	130	5	45	1	0	0	200	20	<1	2	2	1 carb, 1 fat
Cheetos, Flamin' Hot	1 oz	160	11	100	1.5	0	0	250	13	0	<1	1	1 carb, 2 fat
Cheetos, Mix-Ups	1 oz	150	10	90	1.5	0	0	250	13	<1	<1	2	1 carb, 2 fat
Cheetos, Oven Baked	1 oz	130	5	45	1	0	0	230	20	<1	<1	2	1 carb, 1 fat
Cheetos, Puffs	1 oz	150	10	90	1.5	0	0	300	13	1	<1	2	1 carb, 2 fat
Cheetos, Simply White Cheddar Cheese Puffs	1 oz	150	9	80	1.5	0	0	290	16	1	<1	2	1 carb, 2 fat
Chester's Bacon Cheddar Fries	1 oz	150	8	70	1	0	0	210	17	0	<1	2	1 carb, 2 fat
Chester's Cheddar Popcorn	3 cups	150	9	90	1.5	0	0	240	14	1	3	3	1 carb, 2 fat
Doritos, Cool Ranch	1 oz	150	8	70	1	0	0	180	18	<1	2	2	1 carb, 2 fat

SNACKS, CRACKERS, CHIPS, POPCORN, SNACK BARS

	Serving	Calories	Fat (g)	Cal. from Fat	Sat. Fat (g)	Trans Fat (g)	Chol. (mg)	Sod. (mg)	Carb. (g)	Sugar (g)	Fiber (g)	Prot. (g)	Servings/Exchanges
Doritos, Nacho Cheese	1 oz	140	8	70	1	0	0	210	16	0	1	2	1 carb, 2 fat
Doritos, Salsa Verde	1 oz	140	7	70	1	0	0	210	19	1	1	2	1 carb, 1 fat
Doritos, Spicy Nacho	1 oz	140	8	70	1	0	0	190	16	0	1	2	1 carb, 2 fat
Doritos, Toasted Corn	1 oz	140	7	60	1	0	0	120	18	0	1	2	1 carb, 1 fat
Fritos, BBQ	1 oz	150	10	90	1.5	0	0	290	16	<1	1	2	1 carb, 2 fat
Fritos, Chili Cheese	1 oz	160	10	90	1.5	0	0	270	15	1	1	2	1 carb, 2 fat
Fritos, Flamin' Hot	1 oz	160	10	90	1.5	0	0	160	15	<1	1	2	1 carb, 2 fat
Fritos, Flavor Twists, Honey BBQ	1 oz	150	9	80	1.5	0	0	180	16	1	1	2	1 carb, 2 fat
Fritos, Lightly Salted	1 oz	160	10	90	1.5	0	0	80	16	0	1	2	1 carb, 2 fat
Fritos, Original	1 oz	160	10	90	1.5	0	0	170	15	<1	1	2	1 carb, 2 fat
Fritos, Scoops	1 oz	160	10	90	1.5	0	0	110	16	0	1	2	1 carb, 2 fat
Funyuns	1 oz	130	6	60	1	0	0	280	16	<1	<1	2	1 carb, 1 fat
Lay's, BBQ Potato Chips	1 oz	150	9	80	1.5	0	0	150	16	2	2	2	1 carb, 2 fat

Lay's, Classic Potato Chips	1 oz	160	10	90	1.5	0	0	170	15	<1	1	2	1 carb, 2 fat
Lay's, Kettle Cooked, 40% Less Fat	1 oz	130	6	50	1	0	0	140	19	1	2	2	1 carb, 1 fat
Lay's, Kettle Cooked, Original	1 oz	160	9	80	1.5	0	0	90	16	<1	1	2	1 carb, 2 fat
Lay's, Lightly Salted	1 oz	160	10	90	1.5	0	0	85	16	<1	1	2	1 carb, 2 fat
Lay's, Oven Baked Original Potato Chips	1 oz	120	2	20	0	0	0	135	23	2	2	2	1 1/2 carb
Lay's, Oven Baked Sour Cream & Onion Potato Chips	1 oz	120	3	25	0.5	0	0	170	21	3	1	2	1 1/2 carb, 1 fat
Lay's, Salt & Vinegar Potato Chips	1 oz	160	10	90	1.5	0	0	220	15	<1	1	2	1 carb, 2 fat
Lay's, Simply Sea Salted Thick Cut Potato Chips	1 oz	150	10	90	1	0	0	150	15	0	1	2	1 carb, 2 fat
Lay's, Stax, Original	1 oz	150	8	70	2.5	0	0	140	17	<1	1	2	1 carb, 2 fat
Lay's, Wavy Original Potato Chips	1 oz	160	10	90	1.5	0	0	140	15	<1	1	2	1 carb, 2 fat

SNACKS, CRACKERS, CHIPS, POPCORN, SNACK BARS

	Serving	Calories	Fat (g)	Cal. from Fat	Sat. Fat (g)	Trans Fat (g)	Chol. (mg)	Sod. (mg)	Carb. (g)	Sugar (g)	Fiber (g)	Prot. (g)	Servings/Exchanges
Lay's, Wavy Ranch Potato Chips	1 oz	160	10	90	1.5	0	0	330	15	1	1	2	1 carb, 2 fat
Miss Vickie's, Original Sea Salt Kettle Cooked Potato Chips	1 oz	160	9	80	1.5	0	0	90	16	<1	1	2	1 carb, 2 fat
Miss Vickie's, Smokehouse BBQ Kettle Cooked Potato Chips	1 oz	150	8	80	1.5	0	0	140	17	2	1	2	1 carb, 2 fat
Munchies, Flamin' Hot	1 oz	140	7	60	1	0	0	180	18	<1	2	2	1 carb, 1 fat
Munchos	1 oz	160	10	90	1.5	0	0	230	16	0	1	1	1 carb, 2 fat
Rold Gold, Cheddar Tiny Twists Pretzels	1 oz	110	1.5	10	0	0	0	480	22	1	<1	2	1 1/2 carb
Rold Gold, Honey Mustard Tiny Twists Pretzels	1 oz	110	1	10	0	0	0	370	23	2	<1	2	1 1/2 carb
Rold Gold, Pretzel Cracker Sandwiches	1 pkg	100	4	35	1	0	0	150	14	5	<1	1	1 carb, 1 fat

Product	Serving	Cal	Fat (g)		Sat Fat			Sod	Carb				Exchanges/Choices
Rold Gold, Pretzel Thins, Original	1 oz	120	2	20	0	0	0	470	22	0	1	2	1 1/2 carb
Rold Gold, Salted Caramel Glazed Pretzel Bites	1 oz	130	4.5	40	1.5	0	5	340	20	8	1	2	1 carb, 1 fat
Rold Gold, Stick Pretzels	1 oz	100	0	0	0	0	0	490	23	1	1	2	1 1/2 carb
Rold Gold, Tiny Twists Pretzels	1 oz	110	1	10	0	0	0	450	23	<1	1	2	1 1/2 carb
Ruffles, All Dressed Potato Chips	1 oz	150	9	80	1.5	0	0	170	16	1	1	2	1 carb, 2 fat
Ruffles, Cheddar & Sour Cream Potato Chips	1 oz	160	11	90	1.5	0	0	180	15	1	1	2	1 carb, 2 fat
Ruffles, Original Potato Chips	1 oz	160	10	90	1.5	0	0	160	15	<1	1	2	1 carb, 2 fat
Ruffles, Oven Baked, Original	1 oz	120	3	30	0	0	0	135	22	1	2	2	1 1/2 carb, 1 fat
Ruffles, Reduced Fat Potato Chips	1 oz	140	7	60	1	0	0	180	18	0	1	2	1 carb, 1 fat
Ruffles, Simply Sea Salt Reduced Fat	1 oz	140	7	60	0.5	0	0	160	17	0	1	2	1 carb, 1 fat

SNACKS, CRACKERS, CHIPS, POPCORN, SNACK BARS

	Serving	Calories	Fat (g)	Cal. from Fat	Sat. Fat (g)	Trans Fat (g)	Chol. (mg)	Sod. (mg)	Carb. (g)	Sugar (g)	Fiber (g)	Prot. (g)	Servings/Exchanges
Ruffles, Sour Cream & Onion Potato Chips	1 oz	160	11	90	1.5	0	0	140	15	2	1	2	1 carb, 2 fat
Santitas White Corn Tortilla Chips	1 oz	140	6	50	1	0	0	115	19	0	2	2	1 carb, 1 fat
Santitas Yellow Corn Tortilla Chips	1 oz	140	6	50	1	0	0	110	19	0	2	2	1 carb, 1 fat
Smartfood, Delight White Cheddar	1 oz (3 1/2 cups)	130	5	45	1	0	0	200	18	1	3	3	1 carb, 1 fat
Smartfood, Sweet & Salty Kettle Corn	1 oz (1 1/4 cups)	140	6	50	0.5	0	<5	110	20	11	2	<1	1 carb, 1 fat
Smartfood, White Cheddar Cheese Popcorn	1 oz (1 3/4 cups)	160	10	90	2	0	<5	290	14	2	2	3	1 carb, 2 fat
Stacy's, Everything Bagel Chips	1 oz	130	4	35	0.5	0	0	320	19	1	1	4	1 carb, 1 fat

Stacy's, Multigrain Pita Chips	1 oz	140	5	50	0.5	0	270	19	<1	2	3	1 carb, 1 fat
Stacy's, Simply Naked Pita Chips	1 oz	130	5	45	0.5	0	270	19	<1	1	3	1 carb, 1 fat
Sunchips, French Onion	1 oz	140	6	60	1	0	160	18	2	2	2	1 carb, 1 fat
Sunchips, Original	1 oz	140	6	60	1	0	120	18	2	3	2	1 carb, 1 fat
Sunchips, Veggie Harvest	1 oz	140	6	50	0.5	0	120	18	2	2	3	1 carb, 1 fat
Tostitos, Artisan Roasted Garlic & Black Bean	1 oz	140	7	60	1	0	90	18	0	2	2	1 carb, 1 fat
Tostitos, Bite Size	1 oz	140	7	70	1	0	110	18	0	1	2	1 carb, 1 fat
Tostitos, Cantina Thin & Crispy	1 oz	150	8	70	1	0	110	18	0	2	2	1 carb, 2 fat
Tostitos, Crispy Rounds	1 oz	140	7	70	1	0	120	18	0	1	2	1 carb, 1 fat
Tostitos, Multigrain	1 oz	150	7	70	1	0	110	19	<1	2	2	1 carb, 1 fat
Tostitos, Oven Baked Scoops	1 oz	120	3	25	0.5	0	140	22	0	1	1	1 1/2 carb, 1 fat
Tostitos, Restaurant Style	1 oz	140	7	60	1	0	115	19	0	1	2	1 carb, 1 fat
Tostitos, Rolls	1 oz	150	8	70	1	0	115	18	0	1	2	1 carb, 2 fat

SNACKS, CRACKERS, CHIPS, POPCORN, SNACK BARS

	Serving	Calories	Fat (g)	Cal. from Fat	Sat. Fat (g)	Trans Fat (g)	Chol. (mg)	Sod. (mg)	Carb. (g)	Sugar (g)	Fiber (g)	Prot. (g)	Servings/Exchanges
Tostitos, Simply Black Bean	1 oz	140	7	60	1	0	0	115	17	0	5	4	1 carb, 1 fat
Gardetto's													
Snack Mix, Deli-Style Mustard	1/2 cup	130	2.5	25	0	0	0	240	23	<1	<1	3	1 1/2 carb, 1 fat
Snack Mix, Original	1/2 cup	150	6	60	1	0	0	310	21	<1	1	3	1 1/2 carb, 1 fat
Snack Mix, Reduced Fat Original	1/2 cup	130	4	35	0.5	0	0	330	21	<1	1	3	1 1/2 carb, 1 fat
General Mills													
Bugles, Original	1 1/3 cups	160	9	80	8	0	0	310	18	1	<1	1	1 carb, 2 fat
Bugles, Sweet & Salty Caramel	2/3 cup	160	9	80	5	0	0	190	19	10	0	<1	1 carb, 2 fat
Chex Mix, Bold Party Blend	1/2 cup	120	3.5	30	0.5	0	0	210	21	2	1	0	1 1/2 carb, 1 fat

Food	Serving												
Chex Mix, Caramel Crunch	1/2 cup	120	3.5	30	0.5	0	0	125	21	4	1	2	1 1/2 carb, 1 fat
Chex Mix, Cheddar	1/2 cup	120	3.5	35	0.5	0	0	240	22	3	1	2	1 1/2 carb, 1 fat
Chex Mix, Chocolate Peanut Butter	1/2 cup	140	5	45	1.5	0	0	90	22	6	<1	3	1 1/2 carb, 1 fat
Chex Mix, Chocolate Turtle	1/2 cup	130	5	45	2	0	0	105	20	8	<1	2	1 carb, 1 fat
Chex Mix, Hot & Spicy	1/2 cup	120	3.5	30	0.5	0	0	170	21	2	1	2	1 1/2 carb, 1 fat
Chex Mix, Peanut Lovers	1/2 cup	150	6	50	1	0	0	200	21	2	1	4	1 1/2 carb, 1 fat
Chex Mix, Simply Cheddar 70% Less Fat	1/2 cup	120	3	25	0.5	0	0	160	23	4	2	2	1 1/2 carb, 1 fat
Chex Mix, Traditional	1/2 cup	120	3.5	30	0.5	0	0	230	22	2	1	2	1 1/2 carb, 1 fat
Fiber One, 90 Calorie Chocolate Peanut Butter Bar	1 bar	90	2.5	20	1	0	0	80	17	3	5	1	1 carb, 1 fat
Fiber One, Chewy Bars Oats & Caramel	1 bar	140	3.5	30	1.5	0	0	105	30	9	9	2	2 carb, 1 fat

SNACKS, CRACKERS, CHIPS, POPCORN, SNACK BARS

	Serving	Calories	Fat (g)	Cal. from Fat	Sat. Fat (g)	Trans Fat (g)	Chol. (mg)	Sod. (mg)	Carb. (g)	Sugar (g)	Fiber (g)	Prot. (g)	Servings/Exchanges
Health Valley Organic													
Cereal Bars, Strawberry Cobbler	1 bar	130	2.5	20	0	0	0	85	27	16	3	2	2 carb, 1 fat
GG Bran Crispbread Crackers	2 crackers	50	1	10	0	0	0	80	15	0	8	3	1 carb
Jolly Time													
100 Calorie Healthy Pop Butter	5 cups	110	2	20	0.5	0	0	250	25	0	5	3	1 1/2 carb
Blast O Butter	3 1/2 cups	160	12	110	3	4	0	330	14	<1	3	2	1 carb, 2 fat
Healthy Pop Butter	5 cups	110	2	20	0.5	0	0	250	25	0	5	3	1 1/2 carb
Low Sodium 100 Calorie Healthy Pop Butter	5 cups	110	2	20	0.5	0	0	95	23	0	5	4	1 1/2 carb
Mallow Magic	2 1/2 cups	170	12	110	2	3	0	170	16	5	3	1	1 carb, 2 fat

The Big Cheez	3 1/2 cups	160	11	100	2.5	4	0	340	17	<1	6	2	1 carb, 2 fat
Xtra Butter	4 cups	160	11	100	4	0	0	300	16	<1	3	3	1 carb, 2 fat
Kashi													
Blackberry Graham Cereal Bars	1 bar	120	3	30	0	0	0	120	23	10	3	2	1 1/2 carb, 1 fat
Chewy Granola Trail Mix Bars	1 bar	140	5	45	0	0	0	55	21	7	3	5	1 1/2 carb, 1 fat
Chocolate Chip Chia Crunchy Granola & Seed Bars	2 bars	180	7	65	1.5	0	0	100	28	9	3	3	2 carb, 1 fat
Fire Roasted Veggie Crackers	15 crackers	120	3.5	35	0	0	0	200	20	2	3	4	1 carb, 1 fat
GoLean Plant-Powered Peanut Hemp Crunch Bars	1 bar	200	11	100	1.5	0	0	115	20	8	4	8	1 carb, 2 fat
Original 7 Grain Crackers	15 crackers	120	3.5	30	0	0	0	150	20	4	3	4	1 carb, 1 fat
Pita Crisps, Garlic Pesto	11 crisps	120	3	25	0	0	0	180	23	5	2	3	1 1/2 carb, 1 fat

SNACKS, CRACKERS, CHIPS, POPCORN, SNACK BARS

	Serving	Calories	Fat (g)	Cal. from Fat	Sat. Fat (g)	Trans Fat (g)	Chol. (mg)	Sod. (mg)	Carb. (g)	Sugar (g)	Fiber (g)	Prot. (g)	Servings/Exchanges
Kay's Naturals													
Protein Chips, Chili Nacho Cheese	1.2 oz	120	2.5	30	1	0	0	240	15	1	4	12	1 carb, 1 lean protein
Protein Pretzel Sticks, Cinnamon	1.2 oz	120	3.5	30	1.5	0	0	160	15	3	4	12	1 carb, 1 lean protein
Protein Puffs, Veggie Pizza	1.2 oz	110	2.5	23	0.5	0	0	230	16	3	4	12	1 carb, 1 lean protein
Keebler													
Club Crackers, Multi-Grain	4	60	2.5	25	0	0	0	130	10	2	0	1	1/2 carb, 1 fat
Club Crackers, Original	4	70	3	25	0.5	0	0	125	9	1	<1	<1	1/2 carb, 1 fat
Club Crackers, Reduced-Fat	5	70	2	20	0	0	0	150	12	2	<1	1	1 carb
Toasteds, Savory Onion	5	80	3.5	30	0.5	0	0	160	11	2	<1	1	1 carb, 1 fat
Toasteds, Sesame	5	80	4	35	0.5	0	0	140	10	<1	<1	1	1/2 carb, 1 fat

Food													
Town House, Focaccia Rosemary & Olive Oil Crackers	3	70	3.5	30	1	0	0	95	9	0	0	1	1/2 carb, 1 fat
Town House, Original Crackers	5	90	5	45	1	0	0	130	9	1	0	<1	1/2 carb, 1 fat
Town House, Pita Sea Salt Crackers	6	70	2.5	20	0	0	0	140	11	<1	<1	1	1 carb, 1 fat
Town House, Pretzel Thins Oven Baked Parmesan Herb	6	70	3.5	30	0.5	0	0	180	10	1	0	1	1/2 carb, 1 fat
Town House, Reduced Fat Crackers	6	60	1.5	15	0	0	0	130	12	1	<1	1	1 carb
Wheatables, Original Wheat	17	140	6	60	1.5	0	0	210	20	4	1	2	1 carb, 1 fat
Zesta Saltines, Original	5	60	1.5	15	0	0	0	150	11	0	<1	1	1 carb
Zesta Saltines, Whole Wheat	5	60	1.5	15	0	0	0	230	11	0	<1	1	1 carb

SNACKS, CRACKERS, CHIPS, POPCORN, SNACK BARS

	Serving	Calories	Fat (g)	Cal. from Fat	Sat. Fat (g)	Trans Fat (g)	Chol. (mg)	Sod. (mg)	Carb. (g)	Sugar (g)	Fiber (g)	Prot. (g)	Servings/Exchanges
Kellogg's													
Nutri-Grain Apple Cinnamon Breakfast Biscuits	1 pouch	180	6	60	0.5	0	0	125	28	8	3	3	2 carb, 1 fat
Nutri-Grain Fruit & Nut Blueberry Almond Bar	1 bar	150	6	60	1.5	0	0	50	20	11	3	4	1 carb, 1 fat
Nutri-Grain Fruit & Oat Harvest Blueberry Bliss Bar	1 bar	180	5	45	2	0	0	140	34	15	5	4	2 carb, 1 fat
Nutri-Grain Soft Baked Cereal Bars (All Varieties)	1 bar	120	3	30	0.5	0	0	125	24	11	3	2	1 1/2 carb, 1 fat
Nutri-Grain Soft Baked Stawberry Greek Yogurt Bar	1 bar	130	3.5	30	1	0	0	115	25	12	3	2	1 1/2 carb, 1 fat
Rice Krispies Treats, Original	1 bar	90	2	20	0.5	0	0	105	17	8	0	<1	1 carb

Special K Berry Medley Snack Bar	1 bar	100	2	15	1	0	0	30	19	7	1	2	1 carb
Special K Chocolate Caramel Protein Meal Bar	1 bar	170	4.5	40	3.5	0	0	180	23	14	5	12	1 1/2 carb, 1 med-fat protein
Special K Dark Chocolate Protein Granola Bars	1 bar	110	3	25	1.5	0	0	85	17	7	4	4	1 carb, 1 fat
Special K Red Berries Cereal Bar	1 bar	90	1.5	15	1	0	0	85	18	8	3	<1	1 carb
Kraft													
Ritz Bits, Cheese	13	160	9	80	3	0	0	160	19	4	0	2	1 carb, 2 fat
Ritz Bits, Peanut Butter	12	150	8	70	2	0	0	135	18	4	<1	3	1 carb, 2 fat
Ritz Crackers, Hint of Salt	5	80	4	35	1	0	0	30	10	1	0	<1	1/2 carb, 1 fat
Ritz Crackers, Original	5	80	4.5	40	1	0	0	105	10	1	0	<1	1/2 carb, 1 fat
Ritz Crackers, Reduced Fat	5	70	2	20	0	0	0	130	11	2	0	1	1 carb
Ritz Crackers, Whole Wheat	5	70	2.5	25	0.5	0	0	120	10	2	<1	1	1/2 carb, 1 fat

SNACKS, CRACKERS, CHIPS, POPCORN, SNACK BARS

	Serving	Calories	Fat (g)	Cal. from Fat	Sat. Fat (g)	Trans Fat (g)	Chol. (mg)	Sod. (mg)	Carb. (g)	Sugar (g)	Fiber (g)	Prot. (g)	Servings/Exchanges
Nabisco													
Barnum's Animal Crackers	14	130	3.5	30	0.5	0	0	85	23	7	<1	2	1 1/2 carb, 1 fat
Better Cheddars	18	150	8	70	1.5	0	<5	250	17	0	<1	3	1 carb, 2 fat
Chicken-In-A-Biskit	12	160	8	80	1.5	0	0	240	19	2	<1	2	1 carb, 2 fat
Good Thins, Chickpea Garlic & Herb	22	140	5	45	1	0	0	200	20	3	1	2	1 carb, 1 fat
Good Thins, Potato Original	24	130	4	35	0.5	0	0	230	22	1	2	2	1 1/2 carb, 1 fat
Good Thins, Rice Simple Salt	18	130	1.5	15	0	0	0	85	26	0	0	0	2 carb
Honey Maid Honey Graham Crackers	8 crackers (2 sheets)	130	3	25	0	0	0	160	24	8	1	2	1 1/2 carb, 1 fat
Honey Maid Low Fat Cinnamon Graham Crackers	8 crackers (2 sheets)	130	2	15	0	0	0	150	25	8	2	2	1 1/2 carb

Food	Serving												Exchanges
Honey Maid Low Fat Graham Crackers	8 crackers (2 sheets)	140	2	20	0	0	0	180	28	8	2	2	2 carb
Premium Saltine Crackers, Hint of Salt	5	70	1.5	15	0	0	0	60	13	0	0	1	1 carb
Premium Saltine Crackers, Original	5	70	1.5	15	0	0	0	135	12	0	0	0	1 carb
Sociables	5	70	3	30	0	0	0	140	9	<1	0	<1	1/2 carb, 1 fat
Triscuits, Original	6	120	3.5	30	0.5	0	0	160	20	0	3	3	1 carb, 1 fat
Triscuits, Reduced Fat	6	110	2.5	20	0	0	0	150	21	0	3	3	1 1/2 carb, 1 fat
Triscuit Thin Crisps, Original	15	130	4.5	40	0.5	0	0	170	21	0	3	3	1 1/2 carb, 1 fat
Wheat Thins, Hint of Salt	16	150	5	45	1	0	0	55	23	4	3	2	1 carb, 1 fat
Wheat Thins, Original	16	140	5	45	1	0	0	230	22	4	3	2	1 1/2 carb, 1 fat
Wheat Thins, Reduced Fat	16	130	3.5	30	0.5	0	0	230	22	4	3	2	1 1/2 carb, 1 fat
Orville Redenbacher's Gourmet Popping Corn													
Butter	4 cups	170	12	110	6	0	0	260	17	NA	3	2	1 carb, 2 fat

SNACKS, CRACKERS, CHIPS, POPCORN, SNACK BARS

	Serving	Calories	Fat (g)	Cal. from Fat	Sat. Fat (g)	Trans Fat (g)	Chol. (mg)	Sod. (mg)	Carb. (g)	Sugar (g)	Fiber (g)	Prot. (g)	Servings/Exchanges
Cheddar Cheese	4 1/2 cups	180	14	120	6	0	0	340	16	NA	3	2	1 carb, 3 fat
Movie Theatre Butter	4 cups	160	9	80	4	0	0	250	19	NA	3	2	1 carb, 2 fat
Naturals Light, Garlic and Sea Salt	4 1/2 cups	130	5	45	2	0	0	290	20	NA	3	3	1 carb, 1 fat
Naturals Simple Salted	4 1/2 cups	170	11	100	5	0	0	400	17	NA	3	2	1 carb, 2 fat
Pour Over Movie Theatre Butter	3 1/2 cups	180	14	120	4.5	0	0	320	14	NA	2	3	1 carb, 3 fat
Salted Caramel	3 cups	170	8	70	2	1.5	0	35	26	12	2	1	2 carb, 2 fat
SmartPop! Butter	6 1/2 cups	120	2	20	0.5	0	0	290	25	NA	4	4	1 1/2 carb
Pepperidge Farm													
Cracker Trio	3 crackers	60	2	20	0	0	0	85	9	1	<1	1	1/2 carb
Golden Butter Crackers	2	35	1	10	0	0	0	50	5	0	0	1	1 carb, 1 fat

Goldfish, Fudge Brownie	35	140	5	45	1.5	0	0	105	22	10	2	2	1 1/2 carb, 1 fat
Goldfish, Original	55	150	6	55	0.5	0	0	230	20	<1	<1	3	1 carb, 1 fat
Goldfish, Parmesan	60	140	5	45	1	0	<5	280	20	0	<1	3	1 carb, 1 fat
Goldfish, Pizza Flavor	55	140	5	45	1	0	0	230	20	<1	<1	3	1 carb, 1 fat
Goldfish, Pretzels	43	130	2.5	20	0.5	0	0	430	24	<1	<1	3	1 1/2 carb, 1 fat
Goldfish, Whole Grain Cinnamon Grahams	41	140	4	35	1	0	0	150	23	8	2	2	1 1/2 carb, 1 fat
Harvest Wheat Crackers	2	50	2	20	0	0	0	85	7	2	<1	1	1/2 carb
Planters												
Big Nut Double Peanut Bars	1 bar	220	13	110	3	0	0	160	22	12	3	7	1 1/2 carb, 3 fat
Fiddle Faddle	2/3 cup	130	2	20	0.5	0	0	210	26	15	1	<1	2 carb
Fiddle Faddle, Fat-Free	1 cup	110	0	0	0	0	0	210	28	NA	0	2	2 carb
Trail Mix, Nuts & Chocolate	1 oz	150	9	90	2	0	0	5	13	11	2	4	1 carb, 2 fat
Poore Brothers												
Chips, Original	1 oz	140	9	80	2.5	0	0	180	15	<1	1	2	1 carb, 2 fat

SNACKS, CRACKERS, CHIPS, POPCORN, SNACK BARS

	Serving	Calories	Fat (g)	Cal. from Fat	Sat. Fat (g)	Trans Fat (g)	Chol. (mg)	Sod. (mg)	Carb. (g)	Sugar (g)	Fiber (g)	Prot. (g)	Servings/Exchanges
Chips, Salt & Pepper	1 oz	140	9	80	2.5	0	0	336	15	<1	1	2	1 carb, 2 fat
Chips, Salt & Vinegar	1 oz	140	9	80	2.5	0	0	300	15	1	1	2	1 carb, 2 fat
PowerBar													
Harvest Oatmeal Raisin Cookie	1	200	8	70	1.5	0	0	115	23	16	2	10	1 1/2 carb, 2 fat
Performance Energy Bar, Chocolate Peanut Butter	1	240	3.5	35	1	0	0	200	44	26	1	9	3 carb, 1 fat
Performance Energy Bar, Vanilla Crisp	1	240	3.5	35	0.5	0	0	200	45	26	1	8	3 carb, 1 fat
Protein Plus, Reduced Sugar Lemon Poppy Seed	1	200	7	60	2.5	0	<5	130	25	3	5	20	1 1/2 carb, 2 lean protein
Pringles													
Baked Stix Cheese	1 pkg	80	3	30	1.5	0	0	150	10	1	0	2	1/2 carb, 1 fat
Lightly Salted	1 oz	150	9	90	2.5	0	0	75	16	0	<1	1	1 carb, 2 fat

Multigrain Original	1 oz	140	7	70	2	0	0	140	18	<1	<1	1	1 carb, 1 fat
Original	1 oz	150	9	90	2.5	0	0	150	15	0	<1	1	1 carb, 2 fat
Original, Reduced Fat	1 oz	140	7	70	2	0	0	135	17	0	1	1	1 carb, 1 fat
Sour Cream & Onion	1 oz	150	9	80	2.5	0	0	180	15	1	1	1	1 carb, 2 fat
Sour Cream & Onion, Reduced Fat	1 oz	140	7	70	2	0	0	170	17	1	1	1	1 carb, 1 fat
Tortillas Nacho Cheese	1 oz	150	8	70	2.5	0	0	240	17	1	<1	2	1 carb, 2 fat
Quaker													
25% Less Sugar Chocolate Chip Chewy Granola Bar	1 bar	100	3.5	30	1	0	0	75	17	5	3	1	1 carb, 1 fat
Big Chewy Chocolate & Salted Caramel Granola Bar	1 bar	170	6	50	3	0	0	115	29	12	3	2	2 carb, 1 fat
Chewy 90 Calorie Oatmeal Raisin Granola Bar	1 bar	90	1.5	15	0	0	0	80	19	7	1	1	1 carb

SNACKS, CRACKERS, CHIPS, POPCORN, SNACK BARS

	Serving	Calories	Fat (g)	Cal. from Fat	Sat. Fat (g)	Trans Fat (g)	Chol. (mg)	Sod. (mg)	Carb. (g)	Sugar (g)	Fiber (g)	Prot. (g)	Servings/Exchanges
Chewy Dipps Caramel Nut Granola Bar	1 bar	140	6	50	3.5	0	0	65	21	13	1	2	1 carb, 1 fat
Chewy Granola Bar Chocolate Chip	1 bar	100	3.5	30	1.5	0	0	70	17	7	1	1	1 carb, 1 fat
Mini Rice Cakes, Apple Cinnamon	1 cake	50	0	0	0	0	0	0	11	3	0	1	1 carb
Popped Caramel Corn Crisps	13 pieces	110	0.5	5	0	0	0	310	26	9	1	1	2 carb
Popped Multigrain Wild Blueberry Fiber Crisps	13 pieces	110	1.5	15	0	0	0	135	23	6	3	2	1 1/2 carb
Popped Tortilla Style Cheesy Nacho Chips	15 chips	130	5	45	0.5	0	0	330	19	1	<1	2	1 carb, 1 fat
Popped White Cheddar & Herb Hummus Chips	16 chips	130	5	45	0.5	0	0	210	19	3	3	4	1 carb, 1 fat
Protein Baked Peanut Butter Chocolate Bar	1 bar	190	7	60	1.5	0	0	180	24	13	2	10	1 1/2 carb, 1 fat

Quinoa Chocolate Nut Medley Granola Bar	1 bar	150	6	50	2	0	0	95	24	9	1	2	1 1/2 carb, 1 fat
Pop-Secret Microwave Popcorn													
94% Fat Free, Butter	4 cups	100	1.5	15	0.5	0	0	270	20	0	2	3	1 carb
Butter	3 1/2 cups	160	10	90	5	0	0	300	16	0	2	2	1 carb, 2 fat
Homestyle	3 1/2 cups	150	9	80	4.5	0	0	340	16	0	2	2	1 carb, 2 fat
Kettlecorn	4 cups	160	11	100	6	0	0	95	13	0	2	2	1 carb, 2 fat
Light Butter	4 cups	120	4.5	40	2	0	0	290	18	0	2	2	1 carb, 1 fat
Movie Theater Butter	4 cups	150	9	80	4.5	0	0	290	16	0	2	2	1 carb, 2 fat
Sweet 'n Crunchy Cinnamon Roll	2 cups	150	10	90	5	0	0	100	17	0	1	1	1 carb, 2 fat
Ry Krisp													
Crackers, Natural	2	50	0	0	0	0	0	60	11	0	3	1	1 carb
Crackers, Sesame Rye	2	50	0	0	0	0	0	90	9	0	3	1	1/2 carb
Snyder's of Hanover													
Buttersnaps	24	120	1	10	0	0	0	290	25	<1	<1	3	1 1/2 carb

SNACKS, CRACKERS, CHIPS, POPCORN, SNACK BARS

	Serving	Calories	Fat (g)	Cal. from Fat	Sat. Fat (g)	Trans Fat (g)	Chol. (mg)	Sod. (mg)	Carb. (g)	Sugar (g)	Fiber (g)	Prot. (g)	Servings/Exchanges
Honey Mustard & Onion Pieces	1 oz	140	7	60	3	0	0	240	19	3	<1	2	1 carb, 1 fat
Hot Buffalo Wing Pieces	1/3 cup	140	7	60	3	0	0	380	17	0	<1	2	1 carb, 1 fat
Milk Chocolate Mini Pretzel Dips	1 oz	140	6	50	3.5	0	<5	100	19	11	<1	2	1 carb, 1 fat
Mini Pretzels	20	110	0	0	0	0	0	250	25	<1	<1	3	1 1/2 carb
Original Pretzel Poppers	21	120	1.5	15	0	0	0	400	23	<1	1	3	1 1/2 carb
Pretzel Rods	3	120	1	10	0	0	0	290	24	<1	1	3	1 1/2 carb
S'mores Sweet & Salty Pieces	1 oz	140	8	70	3.5	0	0	70	16	3	<1	2	1 carb, 2 fat
Unsalted Mini Pretzels	20	110	0	0	0	0	0	75	25	<1	<1	3	1 1/2 carb
Sunshine													
Cheez-It, Extra Toasty Crackers	27	150	8	70	2	0	0	230	17	0	<1	3	1 carb, 2 fat
Cheez-It, Grooves	18	140	6	50	1.5	0	0	260	19	0	<1	3	1 carb, 1 fat

Cheez-It, Original	27	150	8	70	2	0	0	230	17	0	<1	3	1 carb, 2 fat
Cheez-It, Reduced Fat	29	130	4.5	40	0	0	0	250	20	0	<1	4	1 carb, 1 fat
Cheez-It, Snack Mix	1/2 cup	140	4.5	40	1	0	0	260	20	<1	1	3	1 carb, 1 fat
Cheez It, White Cheddar	25	150	8	70	2	0	0	210	19	0	<1	3	1 carb, 2 fat
Krispy Saltine Crackers, Original	5	60	1.5	15	0	0	0	150	11	0	<1	1	1 carb

SOUPS, STEWS, CHILIS

	Serving	Calories	Fat (g)	Cal. from Fat	Sat. Fat (g)	Trans Fat (g)	Chol. (mg)	Sod. (mg)	Carb. (g)	Sugar (g)	Fiber (g)	Prot. (g)	Servings/Exchanges
READY-TO-SERVE CANNED SOUP													
Campbell's Chunky													
Baked Potato with Cheddar & Bacon Bits	1 cup	190	9	80	3	0	10	790	23	3	4	4	1 1/2 carb, 2 fat
Beef & Dumplings with Hearty Vegetable	1 cup	130	2.5	25	1	0	35	790	20	8	3	8	1 carb, 1 lean protein
Beef Burrito	1 cup	170	6	50	3	0	25	790	19	2	2	9	1 carb, 1 med-fat protein
Chicken Broccoli Cheese & Potato	1 cup	190	12	110	2.5	0	20	890	14	1	3	7	1 carb, 1 med-fat protein, 1 fat
Classic Chicken Noodle	1 cup	120	3	30	1	0	30	790	14	2	1	8	1 carb, 1 med-fat protein
Creamy Chicken & Dumplings	1 cup	160	8	70	2	0	30	890	16	3	3	6	1 carb, 1 med-fat protein, 1 fat
Grilled Chicken & Sausage Gumbo	1 cup	150	4	40	1	0	10	850	21	4	2	7	1 1/2 carb, 1 med-fat protein

	Serving											Exchanges
Hearty Bean + Ham	1 cup	170	1.5	15	0.5	0	10	780	30	6	8	8	2 carb, 1 lean protein
Hearty Beef Barley	1 cup	140	1	10	0.5	0	10	790	24	6	4	8	1 1/2 carb, 1 lean protein
Hearty Chicken & Vegetable	1 cup	90	1	10	0.5	0	10	830	15	4	3	6	1 carb, 1 lean protein
Mushroom Swiss Burger	1 cup	160	7	60	2.5	0	20	790	16	2	1	8	1 carb, 1 med-fat protein
New England Clam Chowder	1 cup	180	10	90	2.5	0	5	890	18	1	3	5	1 carb, 2 fat
Roasted Beef Tip with Vegetable	1 cup	110	1	10	0.5	0	15	790	18	4	3	7	1 carb, 1 lean protein
Salisbury Steak Mushrooms & Onions	1 cup	130	3.5	30	1.5	0	15	790	19	7	2	6	1 carb, 1 med-fat protein
Steak & Potato	1 cup	110	2	20	0.5	0	15	890	17	1	2	7	1 carb, 1 lean protein
Campbell's Healthy Request												
Beef with Country Vegetables	1 cup	110	2	20	0.5	0	15	410	17	4	3	6	1 carb, 1 lean protein
Chicken Corn Chowder	1 cup	140	3	30	1	0	10	410	22	5	3	6	1 1/2 carb, 1 med-fat protein

SOUPS, STEWS, CHILIS

	Serving	Calories	Fat (g)	Cal. from Fat	Sat. Fat (g)	Trans Fat (g)	Chol. (mg)	Sod. (mg)	Carb. (g)	Sugar (g)	Fiber (g)	Prot. (g)	Servings/Exchanges
Homestyle Chicken Noodle	1/2 cup	60	2	20	1	0	10	410	8	1	1	3	1/2 carb
New England Clam Chowder	1 cup	130	3	30	1	0	10	410	20	2	2	5	1 carb, 1 fat
Old Fashioned Vegetable Beef	1 cup	130	3	25	1	0	15	410	19	4	3	6	1 carb, 1 med-fat protein
Sirloin Burger with Country Vegetables	1 cup	120	1.5	15	1	0	15	410	20	4	3	7	1 carb, 1 lean protein
Split Pea + Ham	1 cup	160	2.5	25	1	0	10	410	22	4	5	12	1 1/2 carb, 1 lean protein
Vegetable	1 cup	90	1	10	0	0	0	410	19	5	3	2	1 carb
Campbell's Low Sodium													
Chicken Broth	1 can	30	1	10	0.5	0	5	140	1	1	0	3	free
Chicken with Noodle	1 can	160	6	50	2	0	30	120	17	4	5	10	1 carb, 1 med-fat protein
Cream of Mushroom	1 can	160	11	100	2.5	0	15	45	12	4	3	2	1 carb, 2 fat

Campbell's Homestyle

Light Baked Potato with Bacon & Cheddar	1 cup	100	3	25	1.5	10	690	15	1	1	3	1 carb
Light Chicken & Dumpling	1 cup	90	2.5	25	0.5	25	790	12	1	2	6	1 carb, 1 fat
Light Chicken Noodle	1 cup	70	1	10	0	15	790	9	2	1	6	1/2 carb, 1 lean protein
Light Creamy Chicken Alfredo	1 cup	90	2	20	1	15	690	11	1	1	6	1 carb
Health Valley Organic												
Black Bean, No Added Salt	1 cup	140	1.5	15	0	0	30	29	4	6	7	2 carb
Chicken Noodle, 40% Less Sodium	1 cup	80	2.5	25	0	15	480	11	1	3	4	1 carb, 1 fat
Cream of Chicken	1 cup	110	3	25	1	5	480	15	5	3	7	1 carb, 1 med-fat protein
Garden Vegetable, 40% Less Sodium	1 cup	80	0	0	0	0	480	18	6	4	3	1 carb
Lentil, No Added Salt	1 cup	140	1.5	15	0	0	30	27	5	8	9	2 carb

SOUPS, STEWS, CHILIS

	Serving	Calories	Fat (g)	Cal. from Fat	Sat. Fat (g)	Trans Fat (g)	Chol. (mg)	Sod. (mg)	Carb. (g)	Sugar (g)	Fiber (g)	Prot. (g)	Servings/Exchanges
Minestrone, No Added Salt	1 cup	90	2	20	0	0	50	50	16	5	3	4	1 carb
Split Pea, No Added Salt	1 cup	140	2.5	25	1	0	0	85	26	4	8	8	2 carb, 1 fat
Tomato, No Added Salt	1 cup	100	2.5	25	1	0	5	60	19	13	3	1	1 carb, 1 fat
Vegetable, No Added Salt	1 cup	100	2.5	25	0	0	0	50	18	4	4	3	1 carb, 1 fat
Healthy Choice													
Bean & Ham	1 cup	180	2.5	25	1	0	10	480	28	3	6	11	2 carb, 1 lean protein
Chicken & Dumpling	1 cup	150	3	25	1	0	25	480	22	2	3	8	1 1/2 carb, 1 lean protein
Chicken Noodle	1 cup	90	1	10	0	0	15	390	12	2	1	8	1 carb, 1 lean protein
Chicken & Rice	1 cup	110	2	20	1	0	10	390	17	<1	2	6	1 carb, 1 lean protein
Chicken Tortilla	1 cup	140	1.5	15	0	0	15	390	23	3	6	9	1 1/2 carb, 1 lean protein
Country Vegetable	1 cup	100	0	0	0	0	<5	480	19	3	4	4	1 carb
Garden Vegetable	1 cup	130	0.5	5	1	0	<5	450	24	4	4	5	1 1/2 carb
Hearty Chicken	1 cup	130	2	20	0.5	0	15	480	18	2	3	8	1 carb, 1 lean protein

New England Clam Chowder	1 cup	110	1.5	10	1	0	10	480	20	3	3	4	1 carb
Split Pea & Ham	1 cup	160	2.5	25	1	0	10	470	27	3	6	12	2 carb, 1 lean protein
Tomato Basil	1 cup	100	0	0	0	0	0	450	22	10	3	2	1 1/2 carb
Vegetable Beef	1 cup	130	1.5	10	0	0	10	420	21	4	4	9	1 1/2 carb, 1 lean protein
Zesty Gumbo with Chicken & Sausage	1 cup	100	2	20	0.5	0	10	460	15	2	2	5	1 carb
Progresso													
Beef & Vegetable	1 cup	100	2	15	0.5	0	10	690	16	4	1	5	1 carb
Chicken & Wild Rice	1 cup	110	1	10	0	0	10	650	22	2	2	6	1 1/2 carb
Chicken Corn Chowder	1 cup	190	8	70	2	0	10	870	23	5	1	6	1 1/2 carb, 2 fat
Chicken Noodle	1 cup	110	2.5	25	0.5	0	20	690	14	1	1	7	1 carb, 1 lean protein
Creamy Mushroom	1 cup	150	10	90	2.5	0	<5	830	11	2	1	2	1 carb, 2 fat
Hearty Penne	1 cup	70	0	0	0	0	0	670	14	1	1	3	1 carb
Hearty Penne in Chicken Broth	1 cup	70	0	0	0	0	0	670	14	1	1	3	1 carb

SOUPS, STEWS, CHILIS

	Serving	Calories	Fat (g)	Cal. from Fat	Sat. Fat (g)	Trans Fat (g)	Chol. (mg)	Sod. (mg)	Carb. (g)	Sugar (g)	Fiber (g)	Prot. (g)	Servings/Exchanges
High Fiber Chicken Tuscany	1 cup	110	1	10	0	0	10	690	16	1	5	8	1 carb
Italian-Style Wedding	1 cup	120	4	35	1.5	0	10	690	16	2	1	6	1 carb, 1 med-fat protein
Lentil	1 cup	160	2	20	0.5	0	0	810	30	2	5	9	2 carb, 1 lean protein
Lentil, 99% Fat Free	1 cup	100	0.5	5	0	0	0	690	20	1	4	6	1 carb, 1 lean protein
Light Beef Pot Roast	1 cup	80	1.5	10	0	0	5	480	12	3	2	6	1 carb
Light Chicken Noodle	1 cup	70	1	10	0	0	15	690	9	1	1	5	1/2 carb, 1 lean protein
Light New England Clam Chowder	1 cup	100	2.5	20	0.5	0	5	690	15	1	2	3	1 carb, 1 fat
Light Vegetable	1 cup	70	0	0	0	0	0	470	15	4	4	2	1 carb
Macaroni & Bean	1 cup	160	3.5	30	1	0	0	690	25	2	6	8	1 1/2 carb, 1 med-fat protein
Minestrone	1 cup	100	2	15	0.5	0	0	690	20	3	4	4	1 carb
Minestrone, 99% Fat Free	1 cup	100	1	10	0	0	0	600	19	4	5	5	1 carb

New England Clam Chowder	1 cup	180	8	70	2	0	15	890	20	2	1	6	1 1/2 carb, 2 fat
Split Pea	1 cup	130	1	10	0	0	5	690	23	2	4	8	1 1/2 carb, 1 lean protein
Tomato Basil	1 cup	150	3	30	0.5	0	0	690	28	15	2	3	2 carb, 1 fat
Turkey Noodle	1 cup	70	0.5	5	0	0	10	690	11	1	<1	5	1 carb
Vegetable	1 cup	80	0	0	0	0	0	600	16	4	3	3	1 carb
Vegetarian Vegetable with Barley	1 cup	90	0	0	0	0	0	670	19	5	3	3	1 carb

CONDENSED CANNED SOUP

Campbell's Condensed

Bean & Bacon	1/2 cup	160	3	30	1	0	5	870	26	4	8	7	2 carb, 1 fat
Beef Broth	1/2 cup	15	0	0	0	0	0	860	1	1	0	2	free
Beef Consommé	1/2 cup	20	0	0	0	0	0	790	1	1	0	5	free
Beef Noodle	1/2 cup	70	2	20	0.5	0	10	820	8	1	1	4	1/2 carb, 1 lean protein
Beef with Vegetables & Barley	1/2 cup	80	1	10	0.5	0	5	890	15	2	3	3	1 carb

SOUPS, STEWS, CHILIS

	Serving	Calories	Fat (g)	Cal. from Fat	Sat. Fat (g)	Trans Fat (g)	Chol. (mg)	Sod. (mg)	Carb. (g)	Sugar (g)	Fiber (g)	Prot. (g)	Servings/Exchanges
Broccoli Cheese	1/2 cup	100	5	45	1	0	5	870	11	3	1	2	1 carb, 1 fat
Chicken Alphabet	1/2 cup	70	2	20	0.5	0	5	480	12	1	1	2	1 carb
Chicken Broth	1/2 cup	20	2	20	0	0	5	450	1	1	0	0	free
Chicken Gumbo	1/2 cup	70	1.5	15	0.5	0	5	660	12	2	1	2	1 carb
Chicken Noodle	1/2 cup	60	2	20	0.5	0	15	890	8	1	1	3	1/2 carb
Chicken & Stars	1/2 cup	70	2	20	0.5	0	15	790	10	1	1	3	1 carb
Chicken Won Ton	1/2 cup	50	1	10	0.5	0	5	870	8	1	0	3	1/2 carb
Cream of Aspargus	1/2 cup	100	7	60	1.5	0	5	870	8	2	2	1	1/2 carb, 1 fat
Cream of Broccoli	1/2 cup	90	5	50	1	0	5	790	9	3	1	1	1/2 carb, 1 fat
Cream of Celery	1/2 cup	100	7	60	1	0	0	850	8	1	3	1	1/2 carb, 1 fat
Cream of Chicken	1/2 cup	130	9	80	2.5	0	10	870	9	0	2	3	1/2 carb, 2 fat
Cream of Mushroom	1/2 cup	90	6	50	1	0	5	870	8	1	2	1	1/2 carb, 1 fat
Fiesta Nacho Cheese	1/2 cup	120	6	50	2	0	10	870	14	5	1	2	1 carb, 1 fat
French Onion	1/2 cup	70	1.5	15	0.5	0	0	780	13	8	1	2	1 carb

Golden Mushroom	1/2 cup	90	3.5	30	0.5	0	0	750	11	1	1	2	1 carb, 1 fat
Green Pea	1/2 cup	180	3	30	1	0	0	870	28	6	4	9	2 carb, 1 med-fat protein
Manhattan Clam Chowder	1/2 cup	60	0.5	5	0.5	0	0	890	12	2	1	2	1 carb
Mega Noodle	1/2 cup	70	2	20	0.5	0	15	790	11	1	1	3	1 carb
Minestrone	1/2 cup	100	1	10	0.5	0	5	890	18	3	3	4	1 carb
Old Fashioned Tomato Rice	1/2 cup	130	1.5	15	0.5	0	0	770	26	12	1	2	2 carb
Split Pea with Ham & Bacon	1/2 cup	180	2	20	2	0	5	850	29	4	5	11	2 carb, 1 lean protein
Tomato	1/2 cup	90	0	0	0	0	0	480	20	12	1	2	1 carb
Tomato Bisque	1/2 cup	120	2.5	25	1.5	0	10	870	22	16	1	2	1 1/2 carb, 1 fat
Vegetarian Vegetables	1/2 cup	90	0.5	5	0	0	0	650	18	6	3	3	1 carb
Campbell's Healthy Request Condensed												
Chicken Noodle	1/2 cup	60	2	20	0.5	0	10	410	8	1	1	3	1/2 carb
Chicken Rice	1/2 cup	80	2	20	0.5	0	5	410	13	1	1	2	1 carb

SOUPS, STEWS, CHILIS

	Serving	Calories	Fat (g)	Cal. from Fat	Sat. Fat (g)	Trans Fat (g)	Chol. (mg)	Sod. (mg)	Carb. (g)	Sugar (g)	Fiber (g)	Prot. (g)	Servings/Exchanges
Cream of Celery	1/2 cup	60	2	20	0.5	0	5	410	10	2	1	1	1/2 carb
Cream of Chicken	1/2 cup	60	2	20	0.5	0	5	410	9	1	0	2	1/2 carb
Cream of Mushroom	1/2 cup	60	2	20	0.5	0	5	410	10	2	1	1	1/2 carb
Homestyle Chicken Noodle	1/2 cup	60	2	20	1	0	10	410	8	1	1	3	1/2 carb
Minestrone	1/2 cup	90	0.5	5	0	0	0	410	19	5	3	4	1 carb
Tomato	1/2 cup	90	1.5	15	0.5	0	0	410	17	10	1	2	1 carb
Vegetable	1/2 cup	90	1	10	0	0	0	410	19	5	3	2	1 carb
Vegetable Beef	1/2 cup	90	1	10	0.5	0	5	410	15	2	3	4	1 carb
READY-TO-SERVE SINGLE SERVING SOUP													
Campbell's GO Soups													
Creamy Red Pepper with Smoked Gouda	1 cup	210	14	130	9	0.5	50	780	14	9	2	6	1 carb, 3 fat

	Serving	Cal	Fat (g)	Cal from Fat	Sat Fat (g)	Trans Fat (g)	Chol (mg)	Sodium (mg)	Carb (g)	Sugars (g)	Fiber (g)	Protein (g)	Choices/Exchanges
Creamy Thai Style Chicken with Rice	1 cup	240	14	130	6	0	20	770	22	9	2	7	1 1/2 carb, 3 fat
Smoked Ham & Potato with Cheese	1 cup	210	11	100	3	0	20	790	20	4	2	7	1 carb, 1 med-fat protein, 1 fat
Campbell's Microwave Classic Bowls													
Creamy Tomato	1 cup	170	6	50	0	0	5	760	25	16	2	3	1 1/2 carb, 1 fat
Homestyle Chicken Noodle	1 cup	70	2	20	0.5	0	5	890	10	1	1	3	1/2 carb
Vegetable Beef	1 cup	80	0.5	5	0.5	0	5	880	15	2	3	5	1 carb
Healthy Choice Microwaveable Bowls													
Beef Pot Roast	1 cup	110	1.5	10	0	0	10	470	17	2	2	6	1 carb, 1 lean protein
Chicken with Rice	1 cup	90	2	15	0.5	0	10	390	13	<1	1	6	1 carb, 1 lean protein
Country Vegetable	1 cup	100	0	0	0	0	0	480	20	4	4	4	1 1/2 carb
Tomato Basil	1 cup	130	0	0	0	0	0	390	19	11	3	2	1 carb
Trader Joe's													
Butternut Squash	1 cup	90	2	20	0	0	0	550	16	4	3	2	1 carb
Butternut Squash, Low Sodium	1 cup	70	0	0	0	0	0	95	19	7	2	1	1 carb

SOUPS, STEWS, CHILIS

	Serving	Calories	Fat (g)	Cal. from Fat	Sat. Fat (g)	Trans Fat (g)	Chol. (mg)	Sod. (mg)	Carb. (g)	Sugar (g)	Fiber (g)	Prot. (g)	Servings/Exchanges
Carrot Ginger Soup	1 cup	80	1	10	0	0	0	320	17	6	1	1	1 carb
Chicken Noodle Soup, Low Fat	1 cup	90	1	10	0.5	0	20	730	14	1	1	6	1 carb
Chicken Noodle Soup with Veggies	1 cup	100	1	40	0	0	10	600	16	3	1	7	1 carb, 1/2 lean protein
Clam Chowder	1/2 cup	80	2	20	0	0	10	600	11	<1	<1	5	1 carb
Creamy Corn & Roasted Pepper	1 cup	110	2	20	0	0	0	590	23	11	2	3	1 1/2 carb
Latin Style Black Bean	1 cup	70	1	10	0	0	0	520	12	3	4	4	1 carb
Lentil	1 cup	160	1	10	0	0	0	660	29	3	6	9	2 carb
Minestrone	1 cup	120	2.5	20	0.5	0	0	610	19	5	5	5	1 carb, 1 fat
Organic Creamy Tomato	1 cup	100	2	20	1.5	0	10	750	16	10	1	5	1 carb
Organic Creamy Tomato, Low Sodium	1 cup	90	3.5	30	2	0	15	140	15	8	1	2	1 carb, 1 fat

	Serving	Cal	Fat (g)	Fat Cal	Sat Fat (g)	Trans Fat (g)	Chol (mg)	Sodium (mg)	Carb (g)	Fiber (g)	Sugar (g)	Protein (g)	Exchanges
Organic Lentil & Roasted Red Pepper	1 cup	100	2	20	1.5	0	10	750	16	10	1	5	1 carb
Organic Lentil Vegetable	1 cup	100	0	0	0	0	0	680	24	4	8	7	1/2 carb
Organic Split Pea	1 cup	130	0	0	0	0	0	670	24	4	7	9	1 1/2 carb, 1 lean protein
Sweet Potato Bisque	1 cup	130	1	10	0	0	0	410	28	7	1	2	2 carb

SINGLE-SERVING SOUP MIX

Lipton Cup-a-Soup

	Serving	Cal	Fat (g)	Fat Cal	Sat Fat (g)	Trans Fat (g)	Chol (mg)	Sodium (mg)	Carb (g)	Fiber (g)	Sugar (g)	Protein (g)	Exchanges
Chicken Noodle	1 envelope	50	1	10	0	0	10	520	8	0	0	2	1/2 carb

Maruchan Noodle Cups

	Serving	Cal	Fat (g)	Fat Cal	Sat Fat (g)	Trans Fat (g)	Chol (mg)	Sodium (mg)	Carb (g)	Fiber (g)	Sugar (g)	Protein (g)	Exchanges
Chicken	1 container	290	12	110	6	0	0	1190	39	2	2	7	2 1/2 carb, 2 fat

Maruchan Ramen Noodle Soup

	Serving	Cal	Fat (g)	Fat Cal	Sat Fat (g)	Trans Fat (g)	Chol (mg)	Sodium (mg)	Carb (g)	Fiber (g)	Sugar (g)	Protein (g)	Exchanges
Chicken	1/2 block	190	7	70	3.5	0	0	830	26	1	<1	4	2 carb, 1 fat

SOUPS, STEWS, CHILIS

	Serving	Calories	Fat (g)	Cal. from Fat	Sat. Fat (g)	Trans Fat (g)	Chol. (mg)	Sod. (mg)	Carb. (g)	Sugar (g)	Fiber (g)	Prot. (g)	Servings/Exchanges
Nissin Top Ramen Noodle Soup													
Chicken	1/2 block	190	7	60	3.5	0	0	910	26	<1	2	5	2 carb, 1 fat
CHILI & STEW													
Amy's Organic													
Light in Sodium Medium Chili	1 cup	280	9	80	1	0	0	340	35	5	7	16	2 carb, 1 med-fat protein, 1 fat
Low Fat Medium Black Bean Chili	1 cup	200	3	30	0	0	0	680	31	3	13	13	2 carb, 1 lean protein
Medium Chili	1 cup	280	9	80	1	0	0	680	35	5	9	16	2 carb, 2 med-fat protein
Medium Chili with Vegetables	1 cup	200	6	50	0.5	0	0	590	29	6	8	7	2 carb, 1 fat
Spicy Chili	1 cup	280	9	80	1	0	0	680	35	5	7	15	2 carb, 1 med-fat protein, 1 fat

Campbell's

	Serving	Cal											Exchanges/Choices
Beef & Bean Roadhouse Chili	1 cup	240	7	60	3	0	20	870	30	5	7	14	2 carb, 1 med-fat protein
Grilled Steak Chunky Chili with Beans	1 cup	200	3	25	1	0	20	870	27	9	7	16	2 carb, 1 lean protein
Hold the Beans Chili	1 cup	310	20	180	8	0.5	35	770	15	7	4	17	1 carb, 2 med-fat protein, 2 fat
Hot & Spicy Beef & Bean Firehouse Chili	1 cup	240	7	60	3	0	20	870	30	5	7	14	2 carb, 1 med-fat protein

Dennison's

	Serving	Cal											Exchanges/Choices
Chunky Con Carne with Beans	1 cup	320	9	80	3	0	20	1020	40	3	13	19	2 1/2 carb, 2 med-fat protein
Original Chili Con Carne with Beans	1 cup	330	13	120	5	0.5	30	940	35	2	11	20	2 carb, 2 med-fat protein, 1 fat
Turkey Chili with Beans	1 cup	230	4	35	1	0	45	760	32	2	11	16	2 carb, 2 lean protein

Dinty Moore

	Serving	Cal											Exchanges/Choices
Beef Stew	1 cup	200	10	90	4	0	30	990	17	3	1	10	1 carb, 1 med-fat protein, 1 fat

SOUPS, STEWS, CHILIS

	Serving	Calories	Fat (g)	Cal. from Fat	Sat. Fat (g)	Trans Fat (g)	Chol. (mg)	Sod. (mg)	Carb. (g)	Sugar (g)	Fiber (g)	Prot. (g)	Servings/Exchanges
Hormel Chili													
Chili with Beans	1 cup	260	7	60	2.5	0	35	990	29	4	7	19	2 carb, 2 lean protein
Chunky Chili with Beans	1 cup	260	7	60	3	0	30	1080	33	5	7	16	2 carb, 1 med-fat protein
Chunky Chili No Beans	1 cup	210	8	70	3	0	50	1130	19	6	3	16	1 carb, 2 med-fat protein
Hot Chili with Beans	1 cup	260	7	60	3	0	30	1060	33	5	7	16	2 carb, 1 med-fat protein
Hot Chili No Beans	1 cup	220	9	80	4	0	40	970	18	3	3	16	1 carb, 2 med-fat protein
Hot & Spicy Chili with Beans	1 cup	260	7	60	3	0	25	1120	33	5	7	16	2 carb, 1 med-fat protein
Less Sodium Chili with Beans	1 cup	260	7	60	3	0	30	670	33	5	7	16	2 carb, 1 med-fat protein
Turkey Chili No Beans	1 cup	190	3	30	1	0	80	1230	16	4	3	23	1 carb, 3 lean protein

	Serving	Cal	Fat (g)	Fat cal	Sat (g)	Trans (g)	Chol (mg)	Sod (mg)	Carb (g)	Fiber (g)	Sugar (g)	Prot (g)	Exchanges
Vegetarian Chili with Beans	1 cup	190	1	10	0	0	0	780	35	6	10	11	2 carb, 1 lean protein
White Chicken Chili with Beans	1 cup	220	8	70	4	0	50	990	17	5	4	19	1 carb, 2 med-fat protein
Health Valley Organic Chili													
Vegetarian 3 Bean Chipotle Chili	1 cup	200	3	25	0	0	0	470	37	8	8	11	2 1/2 carb, 1 lean protein
Vegetarian No Salt Added Tame Tomato Chili	1 cup	210	2.5	25	0	0	0	70	41	11	8	10	2 1/2 carb, 1 med-fat protein
Vegetarian Spicy Tomato Chili	1 cup	190	3	25	0	0	0	470	36	9	8	10	2 carb, 1 lean protein
Shelton's													
Mild Turkey Chili	1 cup	220	4.5	40	1.5	0	30	950	27	5	7	18	2 carb, 2 lean protein
Spicy Turkey Chili	1 cup	220	4.5	40	1.5	0	30	950	27	5	7	18	2 carb, 2 lean protein
Stagg Chili													
Chili Con Carne No Beans	1 cup	410	30	270	13	1.5	65	1000	18	3	4	17	1 carb, 2 med-fat protein, 4 fat

SOUPS, STEWS, CHILIS

	Serving	Calories	Fat (g)	Cal. from Fat	Sat. Fat (g)	Trans Fat (g)	Chol. (mg)	Sod. (mg)	Carb. (g)	Sugar (g)	Fiber (g)	Prot. (g)	Servings/Exchanges
Classic Chili with Beans	1 cup	290	13	120	5	0	35	810	30	7	6	14	2 carb, 1 med-fat protein, 2 fat
Country Brand Chili with Beans	1 cup	330	17	150	7	1	40	1020	28	5	6	16	2 carb, 1 med-fat protein, 2 fat
Laredo Chili with Beans	1 cup	300	15	140	5	0	30	1100	26	3	7	14	2 carb, 1 med-fat protein, 2 fat
Silverado Beef Chili with Beans	1 cup	250	7	60	3	0	30	860	30	6	6	17	2 carb, 2 lean protein
Trader Joe's													
99% Fat Free Beef Chili with Beans	1 cup	210	3	30	1.5	0	55	880	28	7	6	18	2 carb, 2 lean protein
Chicken Chili with Beans	1 cup	290	9	80	3	0	50	810	32	6	6	19	2 carb, 2 med-fat protein
Organic Vegetarian Chili	1 cup	260	9	80	1	0	0	690	34	4	8	15	2 carb, 1 med-fat protein, 1 fat
Turkey Chili with Beans	1 cup	240	4.5	40	1.5	0	35	800	30	6	7	19	2 carb, 2 lean protein

Wolf Brand

	Serving	Cal											Exchanges
Chili with Beans	1 cup	350	18	160	7	0.5	40	920	28	3	8	17	2 carb, 2 med-fat protein, 2 fat
Chili Hot Dog Sauce	2 Tbsp	30	1	10	0	0	0	170	5	0	1	<1	1/2 carb
Chili No Beans	1 cup	400	29	260	11	1.5	50	990	18	2	6	19	1 carb, 2 med-fat protein, 4 fat
Homestyle with Beans	1 cup	330	17	160	7	0.5	35	880	27	3	8	17	2 carb, 2 med-fat protein, 1 fat
Lean Beef Chili No Beans	1 cup	220	6	60	2.5	0	40	750	17	3	5	23	1 carb, 3 lean protein
Turkey Chili with Beans	1 cup	250	5	50	1.5	0	25	910	33	3	8	17	2 carb, 2 lean protein
Turkey Chili No Beans	1 cup	230	8	80	2	0	45	810	21	3	5	18	1 1/2 carb, 2 med-fat protein

SWEET BREADS, MUFFINS, PASTRIES, DONUTS

	Serving	Calories	Fat (g)	Cal. from Fat	Sat. Fat (g)	Trans Fat (g)	Chol. (mg)	Sod. (mg)	Carb. (g)	Sugar (g)	Fiber (g)	Prot. (g)	Servings/Exchanges
Baklava	2 x 2-inch piece	333	23	207	9	NA	26	291	29	NA	2	5	2 carb, 4 fat
Bread, Banana	1 slice	196	6	54	1	NA	34	181	33	NA	<1	3	2 carb, 1 fat
Bread, Date Nut	1 slice	217	10	90	2	NA	28	140	30	NA	<1	3	2 carb, 2 fat
Bread, Fruit, No Nuts	1 slice	150	6	54	2	NA	22	109	23	NA	<1	2	1 1/2 carb, 1 fat
Cream Puff with Custard Filling	1	335	20	180	5	NA	174	375	30	NA	<1	9	2 carb, 4 fat
Crepe/French Pancake	1	239	13	117	4	NA	163	274	22	NA	<1	9	1 1/2 carb, 3 fat
Croissant, Cheese	1 medium	236	12	108	6	NA	37	316	27	7	2	5	2 carb, 2 fat
Danish Pastry, Cinnamon	1 (4-inch) pastry	262	15	135	4	NA	14	241	29	NA	<1	5	2 carb, 3 fat
Danish Pastry, Fruit-Filled	1	263	13	115	3.5	NA	81	251	34	20	1	4	2 carb, 3 fat
Doughnut, Cake	1	174	10	100	4	NA	4	191	19	7	2	2	1 carb, 2 fat

Doughnut, Cake, with Chocolate Icing	1	194	11	100	6	NA	8	178	22	12	<1	2	1 1/2 carb, 2 fat
Doughnut, Cake, Sugared/Glazed	1	192	10	90	2	NA	14	181	23	NA	<1	2	1 1/2 carb, 2 fat
Doughnut, Custard-Filled with Icing	1	261	13	117	6	NA	21	125	34	NA	1	3	2 carb, 3 fat
Doughnut, Yeast, Creme-Filled	1	307	21	189	6	NA	20	263	26	12	<1	5	2 carb, 4 fat
Doughnut, Yeast, Glazed	1	269	15	135	6	NA	19	202	31	15	1	4	2 carb, 3 fat
Doughnut, Yeast, Jelly-Filled	1	289	16	144	4	NA	22	190	33	18	<1	5	1 1/2 carb, 3 fat
Eclair, Chocolate with Custard Filling	1	377	21	189	8	NA	75	299	42	25	1	5	3 carb, 4 fat
Muffin	1 small	133	5	45	1	NA	18	210	19	NA	1	3	1 carb, 1 fat
Muffin, Cheese	1 small	184	8	72	3	NA	30	274	23	NA	<1	5	1 1/2 carb, 2 fat
Muffin, Chocolate Chip	1 small	190	9	81	3	NA	25	186	27	NA	1	4	2 carb, 2 fat
Muffin, Cranberry Nut	1 small	164	5	45	2	NA	39	326	25	NA	<1	4	1 1/2 carb, 1 fat
Muffin, Oat Bran	1 small	175	8	70	1	NA	0	444	55	NA	5	8	3 1/2 carb, 2 fat

SWEET BREADS, MUFFINS, PASTRIES, DONUTS

	Serving	Calories	Fat (g)	Cal. from Fat	Sat. Fat (g)	Trans Fat (g)	Chol. (mg)	Sod. (mg)	Carb. (g)	Sugar (g)	Fiber (g)	Prot. (g)	Servings/Exchanges
Muffin, Pumpkin with Raisins & Nuts	1 small	181	4	36	<1	NA	26	154	34	NA	1	3	2 carb, 1 fat
Muffin, Wheat Bran	1 small	161	7	63	2	NA	19	335	24	NA	2	4	1 1/2 carb, 1 fat
Muffin, Whole-Wheat	1 small	142	6	54	2	NA	21	283	20	NA	3	4	1 carb, 1 fat
Muffin, Zucchini with Nuts	1 small	210	11	99	2	NA	37	169	26	NA	<1	3	2 carb, 2 fat
Pannetone or Italian Sweetbread	1 slice	86	2	18	1	NA	19	96	15	NA	<1	2	1 carb
Sweet Roll	1 roll	264	12	110	2	NA	47	272	36	NA	2	4	2 1/2 carb, 2 fat
Sweet Roll, Cheese	1	238	12	108	4	NA	40	236	29	NA	<1	5	2 carb, 2 fat
Sweet Roll, Cinnamon Raisin	1	223	10	90	2	NA	40	230	31	19	1	4	2 carb, 2 fat
Sweet Roll, Cinnamon with Raisins & Nuts, Homemade	1	196	7	63	2	NA	13	185	30	NA	1	4	2 carb, 1 fat

Betty Crocker

Muffin Mix, Banana Nut	1	170	8	72	1.5	0	35	190	22	11	0	1	1 1/2 carb, 2 fat
Muffin Mix, Chocolate Chip	1	190	8	70	2.5	0	35	190	27	16	<1	2	2 carb, 2 fat
Muffin Mix, Cinnamon Streusel	1	190	8	70	2	0	35	200	26	15	0	1	2 carb, 2 fat
Muffin Mix, Wild Blueberry	1	160	7	60	1.5	0	35	190	24	13	<1	2	1 1/2 carb, 1 fat

Duncan Hines Simple Mornings

Muffin Mix, Apple Cinnamon	1/12 mix	220	10	90	2.5	0	35	210	29	13	3	3	2 carb, 2 fat
Muffin Mix, Blueberry Streusel	1/12 mix	200	8	70	1.5	0	35	200	30	15	3	3	2 carb, 2 fat
Muffin Mix, Triple Chocolate Chunk	1/12 mix	240	13	120	4.5	0	35	250	30	17	3	4	2 carb, 3 fat

Entenmann's

Apple Puffs	1	290	14	130	7	0	0	260	39	20	1	3	2 1/2 carb, 3 fat
Cheese Topped Buns	1	320	15	140	6	0	55	320	40	19	1	6	2 1/2 carb, 3 fat

SWEET BREADS, MUFFINS, PASTRIES, DONUTS

	Serving	Calories	Fat (g)	Cal. from Fat	Sat. Fat (g)	Trans Fat (g)	Chol. (mg)	Sod. (mg)	Carb. (g)	Sugar (g)	Fiber (g)	Prot. (g)	Servings/Exchanges
Cherry Cheese Danish	1/8	180	6	50	2.5	0	20	120	28	14	<1	3	2 carb, 1 fat
Cinnamon Swirl Buns	1	320	14	130	5	0	45	280	44	19	2	5	3 carb, 3 fat
Coffee Cake, Crumb	1/10	260	13	120	4	0	15	210	34	13	1	3	2 carb, 3 fat
Danish, Cheese Twist	1/8	230	12	110	5	0	25	210	29	15	<1	3	2 carb, 2 fat
Danish Pastry Twist, Raspberry	1/8	220	11	100	4.5	0	15	170	29	15	<1	3	2 carb, 2 fat
Donuts, Crumb Mini	2	250	14	130	6	0	<5	220	29	12	<1	2	2 carb, 3 fat
Donuts, Frosted Devil Food	1	310	18	160	12	0	10	170	36	24	2	3	2 1/2 carb, 4 fat
Donuts, Frosted Popems	4	320	23	210	14	0	10	180	28	16	1	2	2 carb, 5 fat
Donuts, Glazed Popems	4	230	13	120	6	0	15	160	28	17	0	2	2 carb, 3 fat
Donuts, Rich Frosted	1	300	20	180	13	0	10	190	30	17	1	2	2 carb, 4 fat
Little Bites Banana Chocolate Chip Muffins	1 pkg	180	8	70	1.5	0	25	150	26	17	0	2	2 carb, 2 fat

												Exchanges
Little Bites Blueberry Muffins	1 pkg	180	8	70	1.5	0	25	190	25	14	0	2	1 1/2 carb, 2 fat
Hostess													
Pecan Danish Twist	1/6	260	16	140	5	0	20	190	27	11	2	3	2 carb, 3 fat
Coffee Cake, Cinnamon Streusel	1.5 oz	160	5	45	1.5	0	10	135	26	18	0	1	2 carb, 1 fat
Donettes, Mini Maple Glazed	3	190	8	80	4	0	5	105	27	18	0	1	2 carb, 2 fat
Donettes, Mini Powdered	4	240	12	100	5	0	15	230	31	15	<1	2	2 carb, 2 fat
Muffins, Mini Blueberry	1 pkg	160	6	60	1	0	30	135	24	15	1	2	1 1/2 carb, 1 fat
Muffins, Mini Chocolate Chip	1 pkg	170	8	70	1.5	0	25	115	24	14	1	2	1 1/2 carb, 2 fat
Jiffy													
Muffin Mix, Banana	1/4 cup mix	150	4.5	45	2	0	<5	310	25	10	<1	2	1 1/2 carb, 1 fat
Muffin Mix, Blueberry	1/4 cup mix	170	6	50	2.5	0	<5	350	29	12	0	2	2 carb, 1 fat

SWEET BREADS, MUFFINS, PASTRIES, DONUTS

	Serving	Calories	Fat (g)	Cal. from Fat	Sat. Fat (g)	Trans Fat (g)	Chol. (mg)	Sod. (mg)	Carb. (g)	Sugar (g)	Fiber (g)	Prot. (g)	Servings/Exchanges
Muffin Mix, Chocolate	1/4 cup mix	170	6	50	2.5	0.5	<5	280	27	14	1	2	2 carb, 1 fat
Muffin Mix, Oatmeal	1/4 cup mix	150	4.5	40	2	0	<5	290	25	8	<1	2	1 1/2 carb, 1 fat
Muffin Mix, Raspberry	1/4 cup mix	190	6	60	2.5	0	<5	350	29	12	0	2	2 carb, 1 fat
Kellogg's													
Pop-Tarts Pastry, Blueberry	1	200	5	45	1.5	0	0	170	38	16	<1	2	2 1/2 carb, 1 fat
Pop-Tarts Pastry, Brown Sugar Cinnamon	1	210	7	60	2.5	0	0	170	35	15	<1	2	2 carb, 1 fat
Pop-Tarts Pastry, Cherry, Frosted	1	200	5	45	1.5	0	0	170	38	17	<1	2	2 1/2 carb, 1 fat
Pop-Tarts Pastry, Chocolate Chip Cookie Dough	1	190	5	45	2	0	0	190	35	18	<1	2	2 carb, 1 fat

Pop-Tarts Pastry, Chocolate Fudge, Frosted	1	200	5	45	1.5	0	0	230	37	18	1	3	2 1/2 carb, 1 fat
Pop-Tarts Pastry, Frosted A&W Root Beer	1	200	5	45	1.5	0	0	170	36	15	<1	2	2 1/2 carb, 1 fat
Pop-Tarts Pastry, Gone Nutty Chocolate Peanut Butter	1	200	5	45	2	0	0	240	36	19	<1	2	2 1/2 carb, 1 fat
Pop-Tarts Pastry, Gone Nutty PB&J Strawberry	1	190	4.5	40	2	0	0	220	37	17	<1	2	2 1/2 carb, 1 fat
Pop-Tarts Pastry, Raspberry, Frosted	1	200	5	45	1.5	0	0	160	38	16	<1	2	2 1/2 carb, 1 fat
Pop-Tarts Pastry, S'mores, Frosted	1	200	5	45	1.5	0	0	210	36	19	<1	3	2 1/2 carb, 1 fat
Pop-Tarts Pastry, Strawberry, Frosted	1	200	5	45	1.5	0	0	170	38	16	<1	2	2 1/2 carb, 1 fat
Krusteaz													
Muffin Mix, Banana Nut	1/4 cup	150	5	45	1	0	0	220	25	14	<1	1	1 1/2 carb, 1 fat
Muffin Mix, Cinnamon Swirl	1/4 cup	210	5	45	1.5	1	0	270	39	25	<1	1	2 1/2 carb, 1 fat

SWEET BREADS, MUFFINS, PASTRIES, DONUTS

	Serving	Calories	Fat (g)	Cal. from Fat	Sat. Fat (g)	Trans Fat (g)	Chol. (mg)	Sod. (mg)	Carb. (g)	Sugar (g)	Fiber (g)	Prot. (g)	Servings/Exchanges
Muffin Mix, Wild Blueberry	1/4 cup	150	3.5	30	1	0	0	210	28	15	<1	1	2 carb, 1 fat
Little Debbie													
Donuts, Mini Frosted	4	280	16	140	10	0	15	230	32	18	1	3	2 carb, 3 fat
Donuts, Mini Powdered	4	220	11	100	6	0	15	220	29	15	0	2	2 carb, 2 fat
Honey Buns	1	230	16	120	6	0	<5	150	26	13	<1	2	2 carb, 3 fat
Muffin, Little Bites Blueberry	1 pouch	180	8	70	1.5	0	30	200	27	15	0	2	2 carb, 2 fat
Muffin, Little Bites Chocolate Chip	1 pouch	200	9	80	2.5	0	25	50	29	18	1	2	2 carb, 2 fat
Muffin, Little Bites S'mores	1 pouch	190	8	70	2	0	25	150	28	18	0	2	2 carb, 2 fat
Martha White													
Muffin Mix, Blueberry	1/4 cup mix	150	3.5	30	1.5	0	5	200	31	15	0	2	2 carb, 1 fat

Muffin Mix, Blueberry Whole Grain	1/4 cup mix	160	3.5	35	1.5	0	5	180	30	16	1	2	2 carb, 1 fat
Muffin Mix, Chocolate Chip	1/4 cup mix	170	4.5	40	2	0	5	190	31	16	0	2	2 carb, 1 fat
Muffin Mix, Fat Free Cranberry Orange	1/4 cup mix	140	0	0	0	0	0	290	33	17	2	1	2 carb
Pepperidge Farm Puff Pastry													
Apple Turnover	1	260	13	110	7	0	0	230	31	11	1	4	2 carb, 3 fat
Cherry Turnover	1	260	13	110	7	0	0	230	31	10	1	4	2 carb, 3 fat
Chocolate Turnover	1	350	22	200	9	0	<5	190	35	14	4	5	2 carb, 4 fat
Raspberry Turnover	1	270	13	110	7	0	0	230	34	13	2	4	2 carb, 3 fat
Pillsbury (Refrigerated)													
Apple Toaster Strudel	1	180	7	60	3	0	0	180	26	8	1	2	2 carb, 1 fat
Boston Cream Pie Toaster Strudel	1	180	7	60	3	0	0	180	25	8	1	3	1 1/2 carb, 1 fat
Cinnabon Cinnamon Rolls with Icing	1	140	4.5	40	2.5	0	0	350	23	9	<1	2	1 1/2 carb, 1 fat

SWEET BREADS, MUFFINS, PASTRIES, DONUTS

	Serving	Calories	Fat (g)	Cal. from Fat	Sat. Fat (g)	Trans Fat (g)	Chol. (mg)	Sod. (mg)	Carb. (g)	Sugar (g)	Fiber (g)	Prot. (g)	Servings/Exchanges
Cinnabon Mini Pull-Aparts	1	140	7	60	3	0	0	240	19	10	0	1	1 carb, 1 fat
Cinnamon Roll Toaster Strudel	1	180	7	60	3	0	0	200	27	9	1	2	2 carb, 1 fat
Cinnamon Rolls with Icing, Reduced Fat	1	130	3	30	2	0	0	340	24	9	<1	2	1 1/2 carb, 1 fat
Flaky Cinnamon Rolls with Buttercream Frosting	1	160	7	60	3	0	0	330	23	10	<1	2	1 1/2 carb, 1 fat
Flaky Cinnamon Twists	1	160	7	60	3	0	0	340	23	9	1	2	1 1/2 carb, 1 fat
Grands Caramel Rolls	1	190	8	70	3.5	0	0	520	53	23	1	5	3 1/2 carb, 2 fat
Grands Cinnamon Rolls with Icing	1	360	16	150	7	0	0	530	48	20	1	4	3 carb, 3 fat

VEGETABLES & VEGETABLE JUICES

	Serving	Calories	Fat (g)	Cal. from Fat	Sat. Fat (g)	Trans Fat (g)	Chol. (mg)	Sod. (mg)	Carb. (g)	Sugar (g)	Fiber (g)	Prot. (g)	Servings/Exchanges
Alfalfa Sprouts	1 cup	8	<1	0	0	0	0	2	<1	0	<1	1	free
Artichoke Hearts, Canned, Drained	1/2 cup	30	0	0	0	0	0	240	6	<1	1	2	1 vegetable
Artichokes, Cooked	1/2 artichoke	30	<1	0	0	0	0	57	7	<1	<1	3	1 vegetable
Arugula, Raw	1 cup	5	0	0	0	0	0	6	<1	<1	0	<1	free
Asparagus, Canned, Drained	1/2 cup	23	<1	0	0	0	0	347	3	1	2	3	1 vegetable
Asparagus, Fresh, Cooked	4 spears	13	0	0	0	0	0	8	2.5	<1	1	1	free
Asparagus, Frozen, Cooked	1/2 cup	25	<1	0	0	0	0	4	4	1	1	3	1 vegetable
Baby Corn, Canned	1/2 cup	20	0	0	0	0	0	10	5	3	2	1	1 vegetable
Bamboo Shoots, Canned	1/2 cup	12	0	0	0	0	0	5	2	1	<1	1	free

VEGETABLES & VEGETABLE JUICES

	Serving	Calories	Fat (g)	Cal. from Fat	Sat. Fat (g)	Trans Fat (g)	Chol. (mg)	Sod. (mg)	Carb. (g)	Sugar (g)	Fiber (g)	Prot. (g)	Servings/Exchanges
Bamboo Shoots, Sliced, Raw	1 cup	41	<1	0	<1	0	0	6	8	5	3	4	1 vegetable
Bean Sprouts, Fresh, Cooked	1/2 cup	13	0	0	0	0	0	6	3	2	<1	1	free
Beans, Green or Wax, Canned	1/2 cup	14	0	0	0	0	0	178	3	1	1	<1	1 vegetable
Beans, Green, Fresh, Cooked	1/2 cup	22	0	0	0	0	0	1	5	1	2	1	1 vegetable
Beans, Green, Frozen	1/2 cup	19	0	0	0	0	0	1	4	1	2	<1	1 vegetable
Beets, Canned	1/2 cup	26	0	0	0	0	0	165	6	5	1	<1	1 vegetable
Beets, Harvard, Diced	1/2 cup	90	4	36	0	0	0	200	22	NA	3	1	1 carb, 1 vegetable, 1 fat
Beets, Pickled	1/2 cup	74	<1	0	<1	0	0	301	19	13	1	<1	1 carb, 1 vegetable
Bitter Melon Gourd, Cooked	1/2 cup	12	0	0	0	0	0	4	3	1	1	<1	1 vegetable
Bok Choy	1 cup	9	0	0	0	0	0	46	2	<1	<1	1	free

Food	Serving										
Broccoli, Fresh, Cooked	1/2 cup	22	0	0	0	20	4	1	2	2	1 vegetable
Broccoli, Frozen, Cooked	1/2 cup	26	0	0	0	22	5	1	3	3	1 vegetable
Brussels Sprouts, Frozen, Cooked	1/2 cup	33	0	0	0	18	7	2	3	3	1 vegetable
Cabbage, Fresh, Cooked	1/2 cup	17	0	0	0	6	3	1	2	<1	1 vegetable
Cabbage, Raw, Green	1 cup	18	0	0	0	13	4	2	2	1	1 vegetable
Cabbage, Red, Cooked	1/2 cup	22	0	0	0	21	5	2.5	2	1	1 vegetable
Carrot Juice, Canned	1/2 cup	47	<1	0	<1	34	11	4	<1	1	2 vegetable
Carrots, Canned	1/2 cup	28	0	0	0	295	7	3	2	<1	1 vegetable
Carrots, Fresh, Cooked	1/2 cup	35	0	0	0	51	8	3	3	<1	1 vegetable
Carrots, Raw, Strips or Slices	1 cup	50	0	0	0	84	12	6	4	1	2 vegetable
Cassava, Cooked	1/3 cup	70	0	0	0	7	17	<1	<1	<1	1 carb
Cassava, Raw	1/4 cup	83	0	0	0	7	20	<1	1	1	1 carb
Cauliflower, Fresh, Raw	1 cup	25	0	0	0	30	5	2	3	2	1 vegetable
Cauliflower, Frozen, Cooked	1/2 cup	17	0	0	0	16	3	1	2	1	1 vegetable
Celery, Fresh, Cooked	1/2 cup	14	0	0	0	68	3	2	1	<1	1 vegetable

VEGETABLES & VEGETABLE JUICES

	Serving	Calories	Fat (g)	Cal. from Fat	Sat. Fat (g)	Trans Fat (g)	Chol. (mg)	Sod. (mg)	Carb. (g)	Sugar (g)	Fiber (g)	Prot. (g)	Servings/Exchanges
Celery, Fresh, Raw	1 cup	17	0	0	0	0	0	99	4	2	2	<1	1 vegetable
Chard, Swiss, Fresh, Cooked	1/2 cup	18	0	0	0	0	0	158	4	1	2	2	1 vegetable
Chayote Squash, Cooked	1/2 cup	19	0	0	0	0	0	1	4	1	2	<1	1 vegetable
Coleslaw Mix	1/2 cup	17	0	0	0	0	0	15	3	<1	2	0	1 vegetable
Collard Greens, Fresh, Cooked	1/2 cup	26	0	0	0	0	0	15	6	<1	3	1	1 vegetable
Corn, Canned	1/2 cup	66	<1	0	0	0	0	175	15	2	2	2	1 carb
Corn, Frozen, Cooked	1/2 cup	66	<1	0	0	0	0	4	16	1.5	2	2	1 carb
Corn on the Cob, Cooked	1/2 large ear	66	<1	0	0	0	0	3	16	2	2	2	1 carb
Cucumber, Raw	1 cup	16	0	0	0	0	0	2	4	2	<1	<1	1 vegetable
Eggplant, Fresh, Cooked	1/2 cup	17	0	0	0	0	0	0	4	2	1	<1	1 vegetable
Endive/Escarole, Raw	1 cup	8	0	0	0	0	0	12	2	0	2	<1	1 vegetable

Food	Amount												
French Fries, Frozen, Oven-Heated	10	109	4	36	2	0	0	140	17	NA	2	2	1 carb, 2 fat
Green Onions (Scallions), Raw	1 cup	32	0	0	0	0	0	16	7	2	3	2	1 vegetable
Heart of Palm, Canned	1/2 cup	20	0.5	5	0	0	0	311	3	0	2	2	1 vegetable
Hominy, Yellow, Canned	1/2 cup	90	1	10	0	0	0	157	18	2	3	2	1 carb
Jicama	1/2 cup	30	0	0	0	0	0	3	7	1	3	<1	1 vegetable
Kale, Fresh, Cooked	1/2 cup	18	0	0	0	0	0	15	4	<1	1	1	1 vegetable
Kohlrabi, Cooked	1/2 cup	24	0	0	0	0	0	17	6	4	<1	2	1 vegetable
Leeks, Cooked	1/2 cup	16	0	0	0	0	0	5	4	<1	<1	<1	1 vegetable
Lettuce, Butterhead, Raw	1 cup	7	0	0	0	0	0	3	1	<1	<1	0	1 vegetable
Lettuce, Iceberg, Raw	1 cup	8	0	0	0	0	0	6	1	1	<1	<1	1 vegetable
Lettuce, Romaine, Chopped	1 cup	8	0	0	0	0	0	4	2	<1	1	<1	free
Lima Beans, Frozen, Cooked	1/2 cup	94	0	0	0	0	0	26	18	1	5	6	1 carb
Luffa, Cooked	1/2 cup	20	0	0	0	0	0	12	4	2	2	2	1 vegetable

VEGETABLES & VEGETABLE JUICES

	Serving	Calories	Fat (g)	Cal. from Fat	Sat. Fat (g)	Trans Fat (g)	Chol. (mg)	Sod. (mg)	Carb. (g)	Sugar (g)	Fiber (g)	Prot. (g)	Servings/Exchanges
Mixed Vegetables (No Corn, Peas, or Pasta)	1/2 cup	20	0	0	0	0	0	15	3	1	1	1	1 vegetable
Mixed Vegetables with Corn, Frozen, Cooked	1 cup	80	0	0	0	0	0	80	18	5	4	4	1 carb, 2 fat
Mixed Vegetables with Pasta, Frozen, Cooked	1 cup	80	0	0	0	0	0	39	15	3	5	3	1 carb
Mung Bean Sprouts, Cooked	1/2 cup	13	0	0	0	0	0	6	3	2	<1	1	1 vegetable
Mushrooms, Canned	1/2 cup	20	0	0	0	0	0	332	4	2	2	1	1 vegetable
Mushrooms, Fresh	1 cup	15	0	0	0	0	0	4	2	1	<1	2	free
Mustard Greens, Fresh, Cooked	1/2 cup	10	0	0	0	0	0	11	2	<1	1	2	1 vegetable
Okra, Frozen, Cooked	1/2 cup	34	0	0	0	0	0	3	5	2	3	2	1 vegetable
Onions, Fresh	1 cup	67	0	0	0	0	0	5	16	7	2	2	3 vegetable
Onions, Fresh, Cooked	1/2 cup	46	0	0	0	0	0	3	11	7	2	1	2 vegetable

Food	Serving										
Oriental Radish, Fresh	1 cup	21	0	0	0	24	5	3	2	<1	1 vegetable
Palm Hearts, Cooked	1/2 cup	20	0	0	0	311	3	NA	2	2	1 carb
Parsnips, Fresh, Cooked	1/2 cup	63	0	0	0	8	15	3	3	1	1 carb
Pea Pods, Fresh, Cooked	1/2 cup	34	0	0	0	3	6	3	2	3	1 vegetable
Pea Pods, Raw	1 cup	26	0	0	0	3	5	2.5	2	2	2 vegetable
Peas, Green, Canned	1/2 cup	72	<1	0	0	229	13	4	4	4	1 carb
Peas, Green, Fresh, Cooked	1/2 cup	67	0	0	0	2	13	4	4	4	1 carb
Peas, Green, Frozen, Cooked	1/2 cup	40	<1	0	0	193	7	3.5	2.5	3	1 carb
Peas, Sugar Snap, Frozen, Uncooked	1/2 cup	30	0	0	0	3	5	3	2	2	1 vegetable
Peppers, Green, Fresh	1 cup	18	0	0	0	3	4	2	2	<1	1 vegetable
Peppers, Hot Green Chili, Canned	1/2 cup	25	0	0	0	565	3	0	3	0	1 vegetable
Peppers, Red, Fresh, Cooked	1/2 cup	19	0	0	0	1	5	2	<1	<1	1 vegetable

VEGETABLES & VEGETABLE JUICES

	Serving	Calories	Fat (g)	Cal. from Fat	Sat. Fat (g)	Trans Fat (g)	Chol. (mg)	Sod. (mg)	Carb. (g)	Sugar (g)	Fiber (g)	Prot. (g)	Servings/Exchanges
Plantains, Cooked	1/3 cup	59	0	0	0	0	0	3	16	7	1	<1	1 carb
Potatoes, Baked with Skin	3 oz	79	0	0	0	0	0	9	18	1	2	2	1 carb
Potatoes, French-Fried, Frozen, Baked	1 cup	98	3	25	0.5	0	0	18	16	<1	2	2	1 carb, 1 fat
Potatoes, Fresh, Mashed, Made with Milk	1/2 cup	85	<1	0	0	0	0	250	19	1	2	2	1 carb
Potatoes, White, Cooked, Peeled	3 oz	73	0	0	0	0	0	4	17	1	2	2	1 carb
Pumpkin, Canned	1 cup	83	0	0	0	0	0	12	20	8	7	3	1 carb
Radicchio, Raw	1 cup	9	0	0	0	0	0	9	2	<1	0	0	1 vegetable
Radishes, Raw	1 cup	20	0	0	0	0	0	28	4	3	2	<1	1 vegetable
Rutabagas, Fresh, Cooked	1/2 cup	33	0	0	0	0	0	17	7	5	2	1	1 vegetable
Sauerkraut, Canned	1/2 cup	23	0	0	0	0	0	471	5	2	3	1	1 vegetable

Soybean Sprouts, Cooked	1/2 cup	38	2	20	0	0	5	3	<1	4	1 vegetable
Spinach, Canned	1/2 cup	25	0	0	0	0	29	4	0	3	1 vegetable
Spinach, Frozen, Cooked	1/2 cup	32	<1	0	0	0	92	5	<1	4	1 vegetable
Spinach, Raw	1 cup	7	0	0	0	0	24	1	0	<1	1 vegetable
Squash, Summer, Fresh, Cooked	1/2 cup	18	0	0	0	0	1	4	2	1	1 vegetable
Squash, Summer, Raw	1 cup	18	0	0	0	0	2	4	2.5	3	1 vegetable
Squash, Winter, Cooked	1 cup	39	<1	0	0	0	1	9	3	3	1/2 carb
Succotash, Frozen, Cooked	1/2 cup	79	<1	0	0	0	38	17	2	4	1 carb
Tomato Juice	1/2 cup	21	0	0	0	0	440	5	4	<1	1 vegetable
Tomato Paste, Canned	1/2 cup	110	1	9	<1	0	1034	25	NA	6	5	1 carb, 1 vegetable
Tomato Sauce	1/2 cup	37	0	0	0	0	738	9	6	2	2	1 vegetable
Tomatoes, Canned	1/2 cup	24	0	0	0	0	250	6	4	1	1	1 vegetable
Tomatoes, Raw	1 cup	32	0	0	0	0	9	7	5	2	2	1 vegetable
Tossed Green Salad	3/4 cup	19	0	0	<1	0	11	4	NA	1	<1	1 vegetable
Turnip Greens, Fresh, Cooked	1/2 cup	14	0	0	0	0	21	3	<1	3	1 vegetable

VEGETABLES & VEGETABLE JUICES

	Serving	Calories	Fat (g)	Cal. from Fat	Sat. Fat (g)	Trans Fat (g)	Chol. (mg)	Sod. (mg)	Carb. (g)	Sugar (g)	Fiber (g)	Prot. (g)	Servings/Exchanges
Turnips, Fresh, Cooked	1/2 cup	17	0	0	0	0	0	12	4	2	2	<1	1 vegetable
Vegetable Juice	1/2 cup	25	0	0	0	0	0	310	6	4	<1	<1	1 vegetable
Vegetable Juice Cocktail	1/2 cup	23	0	0	0	0	0	214	5	3.5	<1	1	1 vegetable
Water Chestnuts, Canned	1/2 cup	40	0	0	0	0	0	18	9	2	3	<1	1 vegetable
Watercress, Raw	1 cup	4	0	0	0	0	0	14	<1	<1	<1	<1	1 vegetable
Yams, Cooked	1/2 cup	79	0	0	0	0	0	5	19	<1	3	1	1 carb
Yard-Long Beans, Fresh, Cooked	1/2 cup	24	0	0	0	0	0	2	5	<1	2	1	1 vegetable
Zucchini, Fresh, Cooked	1/2 cup	14	0	0	0	0	0	3	4	1.5	1	<1	1 vegetable
Zucchini, Raw	1 cup	18	0	0	0	0	0	11	4	2	1	1	1 vegetable
Betty Crocker													
Mashed Potatoes, Four Cheese	2/3 cup	150	7	30	4	0	20	45	19	2	1	3	1 carb, 1 fat
Mashed Potatoes, Roasted Garlic	2/3 cup	150	7	30	4	0.5	20	460	19	2	1	3	1 carb, 1 fat

Potatoes, Au Gratin	1/2 cup	150	6	50	3.5	1	15	500	23	2	1	3	1 1/2 carb, 1 fat
Potatoes, Cheesy Scalloped	1/2 cup	140	5	45	3	0	15	480	22	1	1	3	1 1/2 carb, 1 fat
Potatoes, Julienne	2/3 cup	140	5	50	3.5	0	15	510	21	2	1	2	1 1/2 carb, 1 fat
Potatoes, Loaded Au Gratin Casserole	2/3 cup	150	6	50	3.5	0	15	500	23	3	1	3	1 1/2 carb, 1 fat
Potatoes, Three Cheese	2/3 cup	130	3.5	30	2	0	10	480	24	2	1	3	1 1/2 carb, 1 fat

Bird's Eye Sauced & Seasoned

California Blend & Cheddar Cheese Sauce	1/2 cup	70	4	35	2	0	5	345	7	3	1	2	1 vegetable, 1 fat
Peas & Pearl Onions in Lightly Seasoned Sauce	2/3 cup	75	0.5	5	0	0	0	600	14	7	3.5	4	1 carb
Roasted Potatoes & Broccoli	2/3 cup	90	2.5	25	1	0	0	435	14	2	1	2	1 carb, 1 fat
Sweet Corn & Butter Sauce	3/4 cup	112	2	20	0.5	0	0	200	22	6	1	2	1 1/2 carb
Szechuan Vegetables in Sesame Sauce	1 cup	55	1.5	15	0	0	0	420	8	5	1	1	2 vegetable

VEGETABLES & VEGETABLE JUICES

	Serving	Calories	Fat (g)	Cal. from Fat (g)	Sat. Fat (g)	Trans Fat (g)	Chol. (mg)	Sod. (mg)	Carb. (g)	Sugar (g)	Fiber (g)	Prot. (g)	Servings/Exchanges
Tuscan Vegetables in Herb Tomato Sauce	1 cup	45	2	15	0	0	0	165	6	2	2	<1	1 vegetable
Campbell's													
Tomato Juice	8 oz	50	0	0	0	0	0	670	10	6	2	2	2 vegetable
V8 Essential Antioxidants	8 oz	50	0	0	0	0	0	480	10	7	2	2	2 vegetable
V8 High Fiber	8 oz	60	0	0	0	0	0	480	13	7	5	2	1 carb
V8 Low Sodium	8 oz	50	0	0	0	0	0	140	10	7	2	2	2 vegetable
V8 Spicy Hot	8 oz	50	0	0	0	0	0	650	10	7	2	2	2 vegetable
V8 Vegetable Juice	8 oz	50	0	0	0	0	0	640	10	6	2	2	2 vegetable
Contadina													
Tomato Paste	2 Tbsp	30	0	0	0	0	0	20	6	3	1	2	1 vegetable
Tomato Paste, Italian	2 Tbsp	35	0.5	5	0	0	0	290	7	4	1	1	1 vegetable
Tomato Purée	1/4 cup	30	0	0	0	0	0	15	4	1	<1	<1	1 vegetable
Tomato Sauce	1/4 cup	15	0.5	0	0	0	0	280	3	1	<1	<1	1 vegetable

Tomato Sauce, Italian	1/4 cup	15	0	0	0	0	320	4	2	1	<1	1 vegetable
Tomato Sauce, Thick & Zesty	1/4 cup	20	0.5	0	0	0	340	3	2	1	1	1 vegetable
Tomatoes, Crushed	1/4 cup	20	0	0	0	0	150	4	2	1	1	1 vegetable
Tomatoes, Italian Stewed	1/2 cup	35	0	0	0	0	260	8	7	1	1	1 vegetable

Green Giant

Steamers Bagged Vegetables

Baby Brussels Sprouts & Butter Sauce	1 cup	70	2	20	0	5	320	11	3	3	4	2 vegetable
Basil Vegetable Medley	1 1/3 cups	45	0	0	0	0	270	10	5	2	2	2 vegetable
Broccoli, Carrots, Cauliflower & Cheese Sauce	1 cup	50	1	10	0	0	370	8	4	2	2	2 vegetable
Broccoli & Cheese Sauce	1 cup	50	1	10	0	0	420	8	4	2	2	2 vegetable
Corn & Butter Sauce	3/4 cup	100	2	20	0	0	220	18	6	2	3	1 carb
Cut Green Beans	3/4 cup	30	0	0	0	0	0	6	2	2	1	1 vegetable
Market Blend	1 cup	40	1	10	0	0	210	7	3	2	1	1 vegetable

VEGETABLES & VEGETABLE JUICES

	Serving	Calories	Fat (g)	Cal. from Fat	Sat. Fat (g)	Trans Fat (g)	Chol. (mg)	Sod. (mg)	Carb. (g)	Sugar (g)	Fiber (g)	Prot. (g)	Servings/Exchanges
Mixed Vegetables	2/3 cup	50	0	0	0	0	0	35	12	4	2	2	2 vegetable
Niblets Corn	2/3 cup	90	1	10	0	0	0	35	19	4	2	2	1 carb
Sugar Snap Peas	3/4 cup	35	0	0	0	0	0	0	8	3	1	2	1 vegetable
Valley Blend	1 1/4 cups	40	1	10	0	0	0	270	7	3	2	2	2 vegetable
Steamers Boxed Vegetables													
Baby Brussels Sprouts & Butter Sauce	1/2 cup	60	1	10	0	0	5	340	9	3	3	3	2 vegetable
Broccoli, Cauliflower, Carrots & Cheese Sauce	2/3 cup	60	2	20	1	0	5	430	8	3	2	2	2 vegetable
Broccoli Spears & Butter Sauce	4 oz	40	1	10	1	0	5	360	6	3	2	2	1 vegetable
Cream Style Corn	1/2 cup	80	1	10	0	0	0	340	17	9	2	2	1 carb
Teriyaki Vegetables	1 1/4 cups	40	0	0	0	0	0	400	8	5	2	2	2 vegetable

Sautés

Food	Serving											Exchanges
Brussels Sprouts with Bacon	1 1/3 cups	130	3.5	30	1	0	5	440	18	5	6	9	1 carb, 1 fat
Herb Butternut Squash Medley	3/4 cup	35	1	10	0	0	0	280	7	3	2	1	1 vegetable
Parmesan Garden Medley	2/3 cup	70	1	10	0	0	0	60	6	3	2	2	1 vegetable

Idahoan

Food	Serving											Exchanges
Mashed Potatoes, Applewood Smoked Bacon	1/2 cup	100	2	15	1	0	0	540	20	2	1	2	1 carb
Mashed Potatoes, Baby Red Flavored	1/2 cup	110	2.5	25	2	0	0	390	21	2	1	2	1 1/2 carb, 1 fat
Mashed Potatoes, Butter & Herb Flavored	1/2 cup	110	3	25	1	0	0	520	20	2	1	2	1 carb, 1 fat
Mashed Potatoes, Four Cheese	1/2 cup	110	2.5	25	1	0	0	590	20	2	1	2	1 carb, 1 fat
Mashed Potatoes, Fully Loaded Nacho Cheese	1/2 cup	100	2	20	1	0	0	780	20	2	1	2	1 carb

VEGETABLES & VEGETABLE JUICES

	Serving	Calories	Fat (g)	Cal. from Fat	Sat. Fat (g)	Trans Fat (g)	Chol. (mg)	Sod. (mg)	Carb. (g)	Sugar (g)	Fiber (g)	Prot. (g)	Servings/Exchanges
Libby's													
Bavarian Style Sauerkraut	2 Tbsp	10	0	0	0	0	0	200	3	2	<1	0	free
Pumpkin, Solid Pack, Canned	1/2 cup	40	0.5	5	0	0	0	5	9	4	5	2	2 vegetable
Ore-Ida													
Crispy Crowns	11 pieces	170	10	90	2	0	0	480	19	<1	2	2	1 1/2 carb, 2 fat
Extra Crispy Easy Fries	4.75 oz	120	8	70	1.5	0	0	430	12	1	2	2	1 carb, 2 fat
Extra Crispy Fast Food Fries	3 oz	150	6	50	1	0	0	440	24	<1	2	2	1 1/2 carb, 1 fat
Extra Crispy Golden Crinkles	3 oz	160	7	60	1.5	0	0	410	22	<1	2	2	1 1/2 carb, 1 fat
Extra Crispy Seasoned Crinkles	3 oz	150	6	60	1	0	0	450	22	<1	2	2	1 1/2 carb, 1 fat
Golden Fries	3 oz	130	3.5	30	1	0	0	290	21	<1	2	2	1 1/2 carb, 1 fat

Mashed Potato Bites	2.5 oz	200	13	120	6	0	30	340	20	3	2	3	1 carb, 3 fat
Potatoes O'Brien	3/4 cup	60	0	0	0	0	0	30	13	<1	2	2	1 carb, 2 fat
Shoestrings	3 oz	140	5	45	1	0	0	290	22	<1	2	2	1 1/2 carb, 1 fat
Steak Fries	3 oz	110	3	25	0.5	0	0	290	19	<1	2	2	1 carb, 1 fat
Steam n' Mash Russet Potatoes	3/4 cup	70	0	0	0	0	0	260	16	0	2	2	1 carb
Sweet Potato Straight Fries	3 oz	160	8	60	1.5	0	0	160	21	6	2	1	1 carb, 2 fat
Tater Tots	3 oz	160	8	70	1.5	0	0	440	20	<1	2	2	1 carb, 2 fat
Waffle Fries	3 oz	150	6	60	1	0	0	360	11	<1	2	2	1 carb, 1 fat

VEGETARIAN FOODS

	Serving	Calories	Fat (g)	Cal. from Fat	Sat. Fat (g)	Trans Fat (g)	Chol. (mg)	Sod. (mg)	Carb. (g)	Sugar (g)	Fiber (g)	Prot. (g)	Servings/Exchanges
Edamame, Frozen, Unprepared	1/2 cup	64	3	27	0	0	0	4	5	2	3	7	1 med-fat protein
Falafel, Home Prepared	1 patty	57	3	27	0.51	0	0	50	5	0	0	2	1 fat
Miso	1/2 cup	272	8	72	1.5	0	0	5126	35	9	7	16	2 1/2 carb, 1 med-fat protein, 1 fat
Tempeh (Bean Cake)	1/4 cup	80	5	45	1	0	0	4	3	0	0	8	1 med-fat protein
Tofu, Firm, Raw	1/2 cup	181	11	99	1.5	0	0	11	2	0	2	14	2 med-fat protein
Tofu, Regular, Raw	1/2 cup	94	6	54	1	0	0	9	2	<1	<1	10	1 med-fat protein
Tofu Yogurt	1 cup	246	5	45	<1	0	0	92	42	3	<1	9	3 carb, 1 fat
Amy's													
Bowls & Pot Pies													
Baked Ziti Bowl	9.5 oz	390	12	110	2	0	0	590	62	8	6	9	4 carb, 2 fat
Brown Rice, Black-Eyed Peas & Veggies Bowl	9 oz	290	11	100	1.5	0	0	580	38	5	8	11	2 1/2 carb, 1 med-fat protein, 1 fat
Brown Rice & Vegetable Bowl	10 oz	260	9	80	1	0	0	550	36	7	5	9	2 1/2 carb, 2 fat

Dairy Free Vegetable Pot Pie	7.5 oz	390	14	120	1.5	0	0	680	56	3	6	12	3 1/2 carb, 3 fat
Gluten Free Vegetable Pot Pie	7.6 oz	490	24	220	10	0	0	580	60	3	5	8	4 carb, 5 fat
Light & Lean Quinoa & Black Beans with Butternut Squash & Chard	8 oz	240	5	45	0.5	0	0	440	38	6	11	10	2 1/2 carb, 1 med-fat protein
Light in Sodium Brown Rice & Veggies Bowl	10 oz	260	9	80	1	0	0	270	36	7	5	9	2 1/2 carb, 2 fat
Light in Sodium Mexican Casserole Bowl	9.5 oz	370	16	140	0.5	0	0	390	48	4	7	12	3 carb, 1 med-fat protein, 1 fat
Mexican Tamale Pie	8.1 oz	170	4.5	40	0	0	0	590	27	2	4	5	2 carb, 1 fat
Shepherd's Pie	8 oz	160	4	35	0	0	0	590	27	5	5	5	2 carb, 1 fat
Teriyaki Bowl	9.5 oz	290	4.5	40	0.5	0	0	780	52	15	6	12	3 1/2 carb, 1 fat

Entrées & Meals

Asian Noodles Stir Fry	10 oz	300	7	60	1	0	0	630	50	16	5	9	3 carb, 1 fat
Black Bean Tamale Verde	10.3 oz	340	10	90	1	0	0	780	55	6	12	7	3 1/2 carb, 2 fat
Black Bean Vegetable Enchilada Meal	4.75 oz	160	6	50	0.5	0	0	390	22	2	4	5	1 1/2 carb, 1 fat

VEGETARIAN FOODS

	Serving	Calories	Fat (g)	Cal. from Fat	Sat. Fat (g)	Trans Fat (g)	Chol. (mg)	Sod. (mg)	Carb. (g)	Sugar (g)	Fiber (g)	Prot. (g)	Servings/Exchanges
Breakfast Scramble	8.4 oz	360	20	180	2.5	0	0	780	27	8	5	18	2 carb, 2 med-fat protein, 2 fat
Gluten Free Dairy Free Vegetable Lasagna	7.6 oz	300	14	120	3	0	0	680	39	7	4	9	2 1/2 carb, 3 fat
Gluten Free Rice Mac & Cheese	9 oz	400	16	140	10	0	50	640	47	6	1	16	3 carb, 1 med-fat protein, 2 fat
Indian Mattar Tofu	9.5 oz	280	8	70	1	0	0	680	40	5	5	12	2 1/2 carb, 1 med-fat protein, 1 fat
Indian Vegetable Korma	9.5 oz	310	12	110	3.5	0	0	680	41	7	7	9	2 1/2 carb, 2 fat
Light in Sodium Vegetable Black Bean Enchilada	4.8 oz	160	6	50	0.5	0	0	190	22	2	4	5	1 1/2 carb, 1 fat
Roasted Vegetable Tamale	9.8 oz	350	11	100	3.5	0	15	680	47	9	4	16	3 carb, 1 med-fat protein, 1 fat
Thai Stir-Fry	9.5 oz	310	11	100	7	0	0	420	45	2	5	8	3 carb, 2 fat

Burritos & Wraps

Bean & Rice Burrito, No Dairy	6.1 oz	320	8	70	1	0	0	580	52	2	8	10	3 1/2 carb, 2 fat
Black Bean Vegetable Burrito	6.1 oz	290	8	80	0.5	0	0	680	45	3	6	8	3 carb, 2 fat
Breakfast Burrito	6 oz	270	8	70	1	0	0	540	38	3	6	12	2 1/2 carb, 1 med-fat protein, 1 fat
Gluten Free Non Dairy Burrito	5.6 oz	240	6	60	0.5	0	0	430	38	3	5	7	2 1/2 carb, 1 fat
Gluten Free Teriyaki Wrap	5.5 oz	250	6	50	0.5	0	0	540	38	7	3	9	2 1/2 carb, 1 fat
Gluten Free Tofu Scramble in a Pocket Sandwich	5.6 oz	300	13	120	1.5	0	0	460	35	4	3	11	2 carb, 1 med-fat protein, 2 fat
Indian Samosa Wrap	5 oz	250	9	80	1	0	0	680	35	2	4	8	2 carb, 2 fat
Light in Sodium Bean & Rice Burrito, Dairy Free	6.1 oz	320	8	70	1	0	0	290	52	2	8	10	3 1/2 carb, 2 fat

VEGETARIAN FOODS

	Serving	Calories	Fat (g)	Cal. from Fat	Sat. Fat (g)	Trans Fat (g)	Chol. (mg)	Sod. (mg)	Carb. (g)	Sugar (g)	Fiber (g)	Prot. (g)	Servings/Exchanges
Veggie Burgers, Sausages													
All American Veggie Burger	2.5 oz	140	3.5	30	0	0	0	390	14	2	4	13	1 carb, 1 med-fat protein
Bistro Burger	2.5 oz	110	3	30	0	0	0	330	15	1	2	5	1 carb, 1 fat
California Veggie Burger	2.5 oz	150	5	45	0.5	0	0	500	21	2	4	6	1 1/2 carb, 1 fat
Light in Sodium California Veggie Burger	2.5 oz	110	4	35	0	0	0	250	16	1	3	5	1 carb, 1 fat
Quarter Pound Veggie Burger	4 oz	210	3.5	30	0.5	0	0	600	24	6	6	20	1 1/2 carb, 2 lean protein
Veggie Sausages	4 links	110	3	27	0	0	0	320	13	1	2	7	1 carb, 1 med-fat protein
Beyond Meat													
Beast Burger	1 patty (4 oz)	260	16	140	2	0	0	480	7	0	4	23	1/2 carb, 3 med-fat protein
Beefy Crumble	1/2 cup (2 oz)	100	5	40	0	0	0	340	3	1	2	13	2 lean protein

Feisty Buffalo Poppers	6 poppers (3 oz)	210	10	90	1	0	0	480	16	0	2	13	1 carb, 1 med-fat protein, 1 fat
Grilled Strips	6 strips (3 oz)	120	5	30	0	0	0	340	3	1	1	20	3 lean protein
Homestyle Tenders	3 tenders (3 oz)	220	11	100	1	0	0	450	15	0	2	13	1 carb, 2 med-fat protein
Italian Meatballs	4 balls (3 oz)	200	12	110	2	0	0	350	6	0	3	18	1/2 carb, 3 lean protein
Swedish Meatballs	4 balls (3 oz)	200	12	110	2	0	0	350	6	0	3	18	1/2 carb, 3 lean protein
Boca													
All American Classic	2.5 oz	90	2	20	0.5	0	<5	350	6	0	6	15	1/2 carb, 2 lean protein
Spicy Chik'n Veggie Pattie	2.5 oz	150	6	50	0.5	0	0	430	12	<1	3	12	1 carb, 1 med-fat protein
Caroline's													
Chik'n Chunks	1.5 oz drained	45	0	0	0	0	0	210	5	1	0	6	1 lean protein

VEGETARIAN FOODS

	Serving	Calories	Fat (g)	Cal. from Fat	Sat. Fat (g)	Trans Fat (g)	Chol. (mg)	Sod. (mg)	Carb. (g)	Sugar (g)	Fiber (g)	Prot. (g)	Servings/Exchanges
Chik'n Patty	1 (2.3-oz) patty	60	1.5	15	0	0	0	270	3	<1	2	10	1 lean protein
Fishless Tuna	1.5 oz drained	60	1	10	0	0	0	140	5	<1	0	7	1 lean protein
Taco Filling	1/4 cup (2 oz)	80	3.5	30	0.5	0	0	200	6	1	2	7	1/2 carb, 1 high-fat protein
Cedarlane													
Baked Stacked Eggplant	9.5 oz	230	10	90	4.5	0	30	540	21	9	5	14	1 1/2 carb, 1 med-fat protein, 1 fat
Burrito Grande with Salsa Roja	5.1 oz	240	9	80	4.5	0	20	540	31	2	3	10	2 carb, 1 med-fat protein, 1 fat
Chili & Cheese Tamales	5.1 oz	270	14	120	7	0	30	420	31	6	7	9	2 carb, 3 fat
Eggplant Parmesan	10 oz	280	13	120	5	0	25	590	26	13	5	13	2 carb, 1 med-fat protein, 2 fat
Low Fat Beans, Rice & Cheese Style Burrito	1	260	1	10	0	0	0	490	48	2	7	13	3 carb, 1 lean protein

Food	Serving	Cal											Exchanges
Low Fat Garden Vegetable Enchilada	4.5 oz	140	3	25	1.5	0	10	350	19	3	2	9	1 carb, 1 med-fat protein
Low Fat Garden Vegetable Lasagna	5 oz	140	3	25	1.5	0	10	400	21	4	4	8	1 1/2 carb, 1 med-fat protein
Quinoa & Vegetable Enchiladas	9 oz	340	15	130	6	0	30	800	44	5	7	12	3 carb, 3 fat
Roasted Chili Relleno	10 oz	380	20	170	10	0	50	660	34	6	11	23	2 carb, 2 med-fat protein, 2 fat
Spinach & Mushroom Egg White Omelette	1	270	12	110	6	0	30	670	18	5	2	23	1 carb, 3 lean protein
Three Layer Enchilada Pie	11 oz	380	14	130	7	0	35	850	45	7	9	20	3 carb, 2 med-fat protein, 1 fat
Uncured Turkey Bacon Egg White Omelette	1	300	13	120	7	0	45	640	21	3	1	24	1 1/2 carb, 3 med-fat protein
Field Roast Grain Meat Company													
Celebration Roast	4 oz	280	10	90	0.5	0	0	710	16	5	6	31	1 carb, 4 lean protein
Classic Meatloaf	4 oz	340	21	190	7	0	0	420	9	0	5	30	1/2 carb, 4 med-fat protein

VEGETARIAN FOODS

	Serving	Calories	Fat (g)	Cal. from Fat	Sat. Fat (g)	Trans Fat (g)	Chol. (mg)	Sod. (mg)	Carb. (g)	Sugar (g)	Fiber (g)	Prot. (g)	Servings/Exchanges
FieldBurger	3.25 oz	340	24	220	8	0	0	510	9	<1	2	22	1/2 carb, 3 med-fat protein, 2 fat
Frankfurters	1	180	8	70	2	0	0	690	6	2	4	21	1/2 carb, 3 lean protein
Smoked Apple Sage Sausage	2	100	3.5	35	0	0	0	320	7	3	2	10	1/2 carb, 1 med-fat protein
Smoked Tomato Loaf	2 oz	90	1.5	10	0	0	0	290	7	2	3	14	1/2 carb, 2 lean protein
Wild Mushroom Loaf	2 oz	110	1.5	10	0	0	0	300	9	2	2	15	1/2 carb, 2 lean protein
Gardein													
Barbecue Chick'n Wings	4 wings (2.6 oz)	110	5	45	0	0	0	300	4	0	2	14	2 lean protein
Beefless Ground	3/4 cup (3.1 oz)	120	2	15	0	0	0	350	8	2	4	18	1/2 carb, 2 lean protein
Chick'n Sliders with Bun	1 (2.9-oz) slider	180	5	45	0.5	0	0	270	25	4	1	10	1 1/2 carb, 1 med-fat protein
Chipotle Black Bean Burger	1 (3-oz) burger	150	7	60	0	0	0	390	20	3	6	6	1 carb, 1 med-fat protein

Food	Serving												Exchanges
Garden Veggie Burger	1 (3-oz) burger	140	4.5	40	0		0	310	19	1	3	5	1 carb, 1 med-fat protein
Golden Fishless Filet	2 pieces (3.4 oz)	180	10	90	0.5		0	340	14	0	3	9	1 carb, 1 med-fat protein, 1 fat
Meatless Meatballs	3 meatballs (3.2 oz)	150	7	60	0.5		0	340	9	1	4	15	1/2 carb, 2 lean protein
Meatless Meatloaf	2 pieces (5 oz)	220	8	70	0.5		0	620	18	2	5	19	1 carb, 2 med-fat protein
Mini Crabless Cakes	1 cake (2.7 oz)	130	6	50	0		0	300	11	1	1	9	1 carb, 1 med-fat protein
Seven Grain Crispy Tenders	2 pieces (1.8 oz)	100	4.5	40	0		0	230	8	0	1	8	1/2 carb, 1 med-fat protein
Ultimate Beefless Burger	1 burger (3 oz)	140	5	45	0		0	330	8	1	3	15	1/2 carb, 2 lean protein
Gardenburger													
Black Bean Chipotle Veggie Burger	2.5 oz	90	3	25	0		0	390	16	3	4	5	1 carb, 1 fat
Portabella Burger	2.5 oz	100	2.5	20	1	0	<5	450	16	<1	5	4	1 carb, 1 fat

VEGETARIAN FOODS

	Serving	Calories	Fat (g)	Cal. from Fat	Sat. Fat (g)	Trans Fat (g)	Chol. (mg)	Sod. (mg)	Carb. (g)	Sugar (g)	Fiber (g)	Prot. (g)	Servings/Exchanges
The Original Veggie Burger	2.5 oz	110	3	30	1.5	0	5	490	16	0	4	5	1 carb, 1 fat
Healthy Choice Vegetarian Entrées													
Asian Potstickers	10 oz	330	3.5	45	1	0	<5	560	67	18	5	7	4 1/2 carb, 1 fat
Portabella Spinach Parmesan	9.9 oz	230	5	45	1	0	<5	570	38	3	5	8	2 1/2 carb, 1 fat
Pumpkin Squash Ravioli	9.6 oz	260	6	50	2	0	<5	520	44	9	6	8	3 carb, 1 fat
Tortellini Primavera Parmesan	9.6 oz	250	4.5	40	2.5	0	10	460	42	10	8	11	3 carb, 1 fat
Kashi Frozen Entrées													
Amaranth Polenta Plantain Bowl	10.1 oz	340	9	80	1	0	0	390	59	19	7	9	4 carb, 2 fat
Black Bean Mango Bowl	10.1 oz	330	9	80	1	0	0	270	56	12	11	10	3 1/2 carb, 2 fat
Chimichurri Quinoa Bowl	9.1 oz	260	8	70	1.5	0	0	350	42	5	10	10	3 carb, 2 fat
Sweet Potato Quinoa Bowl	9.1 oz	300	8	80	1.5	0	0	440	50	9	7	9	3 carb, 2 fat

Lightlife

Garden Veggie Tempeh Burger	1	100	3	25	0	0	490	10	2	3	9	1/2 carb, 1 lean protein
Gimme Lean Beef	2 oz	60	0	0	0	0	330	7	<1	3	8	1/2 carb, 1 lean protein
Gimme Lean Breakfast Patties	1 patty (1.5 oz)	40	0	0	0	0	270	5	0	2	6	1 lean protein
Gimme Lean Sausage	2 oz	60	0	0	0	0	310	7	<1	3	7	1/2 carb, 1 lean protein
Smart Bacon	1 slice (0.4 oz)	20	1	10	0	0	150	<1	0	0	2	free
Smart Cutlets, Original	1 cutlet (3 oz)	110	1	10	0	0	360	7	<1	3	17	1/2 carb, 2 lean protein
Smart Dogs	1 (1.5-oz) link	50	2	20	0	0	330	2	0	1	7	1 lean protein
Smart Ground Mexican	1/3 cup (2 oz)	60	0	0	0	0	230	6	<1	3	10	1/2 carb, 1 lean protein
Smart Ground Original	1/3 cup (2 oz)	70	0	0	0	0	320	6	<1	3	11	1/2 carb, 1 lean protein

VEGETARIAN FOODS

	Serving	Calories	Fat (g)	Cal. from Fat	Sat. Fat (g)	Trans Fat (g)	Chol. (mg)	Sod. (mg)	Carb. (g)	Sugar (g)	Fiber (g)	Prot. (g)	Servings/Exchanges
Smart Menu Veggie Meatballs	3 meatballs (2.7 oz)	100	1.5	10	0	0	0	370	9	1	4	13	1/2 carb, 2 lean protein
Smart Patties Black Bean Burger	2.5 oz	100	2.5	20	0	0	0	330	11	2	4	10	1 carb, 1 lean protein
Smart Patties Original Burger with Quinoa	2.5 oz	100	2.5	20	0	0	0	300	10	2	3	10	1/2 carb, 1 lean protein
Smart Sausage, Chorizo	1 (3-oz) link	150	9	80	1.5	0	0	500	4	0	2	14	2 med-fat protein
Smart Sausage, Harvest Apple	1 (3-oz) link	170	9	80	1.5	0	0	880	13	4	1	16	1 carb, 2 med-fat protein
Smart Sausage, Italian	1 (3-oz) link	140	7	60	1	0	0	560	7	<1	1	13	1/2 carb, 2 lean protein
Smart Strips, Chick'n	3 oz	80	0	0	0	0	0	350	5	0	4	14	2 lean protein
Smart Tenders, Savory Chick'n	3 tenders (3 oz)	110	0	0	0	0	0	370	7	0	5	18	1/2 carb, 2 lean protein

Smart Wings, Buffalo	4 wings (3 oz)	110	2.5	20	0	0	580	6	<1	4	13	1/2 carb, 2 lean protein
Tofu Pups	1 (1.5-oz) link	50	2.5	25	0	0	300	0	0	<1	7	1 lean protein
Loma Linda											
Big Franks	1 (1.8-oz) link	110	6	60	1	0	220	3	0	2	11	2 lean protein
Chik'n Chunks	1.5 oz drained	45	0	0	0	0	210	5	1	0	6	1 lean protein
Chorizo	2 oz	90	4	35	0.5	0	130	6	1	<1	7	1/2 carb, 1 med-fat protein
Fishless Tuna	1.5 oz drained	60	1	10	0	0	140	5	<1	0	7	1 lean protein
Little Links	2 (1.6-oz) links	90	5	45	0.5	0	250	3	0	2	8	1 med-fat protein
Low Fat Big Franks	1 (1.8-oz) link	80	2.5	20	0.5	0	240	3	0	2	12	2 lean protein
Redi-Burger	3 oz	120	2.5	25	0	0	450	7	1	4	18	1/2 carb, 2 lean protein
Sloppy Joe	2 oz	60	0.5	10	0	0	170	8	4	<1	5	1/2 carb, 1 lean protein

VEGETARIAN FOODS

	Serving	Calories	Fat (g)	Cal. from Fat	Sat. Fat (g)	Trans Fat (g)	Chol. (mg)	Sod. (mg)	Carb. (g)	Sugar (g)	Fiber (g)	Prot. (g)	Servings/Exchanges
Super Links	1 (1.7-oz) link	110	8	70	1	0	0	350	2	0	1	7	1 med-fat protein, 1 fat
Taco Filling	1/4 cup (2 oz)	80	3.5	30	0.5	0	0	220	6	1	2	7	1/2 carb, 1 med-fat protein
Tender Bites	3 oz	120	4	35	0.5	0	0	440	7	0	3	13	1/2 carb, 2 lean protein
Vege Burger	1/4 cup (2 oz)	60	0.5	5	0	0	0	130	2	0	2	12	2 lean protein
Vegetable Skallops	1/2 cup (3 oz)	90	1	10	0	0	0	390	4	0	3	17	2 lean protein
Morningstar Farms													
Burgers													
Garden Veggie Patties	1 (2.4-oz) pattie	110	3.5	30	0.5	0	0	350	9	1	3	10	1/2 carb, 1 lean protein
Grillers California Turk'y Burger	1 (2.3-oz) pattie	100	5	45	0.5	0	0	440	8	1	5	10	1/2 carb, 1 med-fat protein

	Serving Size												
Grillers Original	1 (2.3-oz) pattie	130	6	50	1	0	0	260	5	<1	2	15	2 lean protein
Grillers Prime Burger	1 (2.5-oz) pattie	170	9	80	1	0	0	360	4	0	2	17	2 med-fat protein
Spicy Black Bean Burger	1 (2.4-oz) burger	110	4	35	0.5	0	0	330	13	1	4	10	1 carb, 1 med-fat protein
Tomato & Basil Pizza Burger	1 (2.4-oz) pattie	110	6	50	1.5	0	10	280	9	2	6	10	1/2 carb, 1 med-fat protein
White Bean Chili Burger	1 (2.4-oz) burger	150	9	80	1	0	0	400	14	1	6	8	1 carb, 1 med-fat protein, 1 fat
Veggie Classics & Patties													
Buffalo Chik Patties	1 (2.5-oz) patty	180	9	80	1.5	0	0	540	18	2	4	9	1 carb, 1 med-fat protein, 1 fat
Buffalo Wings Veggie Wings	5 wings (3 oz)	200	9	80	1.5	0	0	550	19	2	4	12	1 carb, 1 med-fat protein, 1 fat
Chik'n Nuggets	4 nuggets (3 oz)	180	8	70	1	0	0	350	18	2	4	12	1 carb, 1 med-fat protein, 1 fat

VEGETARIAN FOODS

	Serving	Calories	Fat (g)	Cal. from Fat	Sat. Fat (g)	Trans Fat (g)	Chol. (mg)	Sod. (mg)	Carb. (g)	Sugar (g)	Fiber (g)	Prot. (g)	Servings/Exchanges
Corn Dog	1 (2.5-oz) dog	150	2.5	25	0.5	0	0	470	26	8	3	8	2 carb, 1 fat
Garden Veggie Nuggets	5 nuggets (2.9 oz)	160	10	90	1	0	0	340	14	3	6	8	1 carb, 1 med-fat protein, 1 fat
Original Chik Patties	1 (2.5-oz) patty	160	6	60	1	0	0	320	19	2	3	9	1 carb, 1 med-fat protein
Veggie Dogs	1 (1.4-oz) link	50	0.5	0	0	0	0	430	4	2	<1	7	1 lean protein
Veggie Bowls													
Mushroom & Asparagus Orzo Bowl	9.1 oz	250	9	80	5	0	0	610	38	2	10	14	2 1/2 carb, 1 med-fat protein, 1 fat
Spicy Black Bean Enchilada Bowl	9.1 oz	310	13	120	4	0	15	430	40	5	7	15	2 1/2 carb, 1 med-fat protein, 2 fat
Thai Yellow Curry Bowl	9.3 oz	230	8	70	5	0	0	530	35	8	7	9	2 carb, 1 med-fat protein, 1 fat

Food	Serving	Cal.	Fat (g)	Cal. from Fat	Sat. Fat (g)	Trans Fat (g)	Chol. (mg)	Sod. (mg)	Carb. (g)	Fiber (g)	Sugar (g)	Prot. (g)	Exchanges/Choices
Tuscan Greens and Beans	8.6 oz	270	15	140	7	0	30	390	28	6	9	14	2 carb, 1 med-fat protein, 2 fat
Meal Starters													
Chik'n Strips	12 (3 oz)	150	4.5	40	0.5	0	0	460	4	0	2	23	3 lean protein
Chipotle Black Bean Crumbles	1/2 cup (2 oz)	70	2.5	20	0	0	0	280	6	<1	2	8	1/2 carb, 1 lean protein
Grillers Recipe Crumbles	1/2 cup (1.8 oz)	70	2	20	0	0	0	220	4	<1	3	9	1 lean protein
Hickory BBQ Riblets with Sauce	1 (5-oz) riblet	210	3.5	30	0	0	0	620	35	24	6	16	1 1/2 carb, 2 lean protein
Original Sausage Patties	1 (1.4-oz) patty	70	3	25	0	0	0	260	3	0	1	9	1 lean protein
Steak Strips	12 (3 oz)	150	4.5	40	0.5	0	0	430	6	0	2	23	1/2 carb, 3 lean protein
Trader Joe's													
Beef-less Ground Beef	1/3 cup (2 oz)	60	1	10	0	0	0	270	4	<1	3	9	1 lean protein
Chicken-less Crispy Tenders	3 tenders (2.8 oz)	150	7	60	0.5	0	0	360	12	2	2	12	1 carb, 1 med-fat protein

VEGETARIAN FOODS

	Serving	Calories	Fat (g)	Cal. from Fat	Sat. Fat (g)	Trans Fat (g)	Chol. (mg)	Sod. (mg)	Carb. (g)	Sugar (g)	Fiber (g)	Prot. (g)	Servings/Exchanges
Chicken-less Mandarin Orange Morsels	1/2 bag with sauce	320	11	100	1	0	0	570	39	17	2	16	2 1/2 carb, 1 med-fat protein, 1 fat
Chicken-less Strips	9 strips (2.7 oz)	110	1.5	15	0	0	0	330	3	1	1	20	2 lean protein
Dr. Praeger's California Veggie Burger	2.5 oz	120	5	45	0.5	0	0	240	14	1	4	5	1 carb, 1 fat
Italian Sausage-less Sausage	1 (3-oz) link	140	7	60	1	0	0	560	7	<1	1	13	1/2 carb, 2 lean protein
Meatless Corn Dogs	2.5 oz	160	3.5	35	0.5	0	0	510	23	6	2	9	1 1/2 carb, 1 med-fat protein
Pizza Veggie Burger	2.4 oz	130	7	60	1	0	5	360	7	2	4	9	1/2 carb, 1 med-fat protein
Quinoa Cowboy Veggie Burger	3.3 oz	180	8	70	1	0	0	280	22	2	6	5	1 1/2 carb, 2 fat
Soy Chorizo	2.5 oz	160	10	90	2	0	0	730	9	1	2	11	1/2 carb, 1 med-fat protein, 1 fat

Thai Sweet Chili Veggie Burger	2.5 oz	150	6	50	0	0	0	270	17	5	3	8	1 carb, 1 med-fat protein
Tofurky Original Italian Sausage	3.5 oz	280	14	130	1.5	0	0	620	8	3	1	30	1/2 carb, 4 med-fat protein
Vegetable Masala Burger	2.5 oz	140	8	70	0.5	0	0	390	17	1	3	2	1 carb, 2 fat

Yves Veggie Cuisine

Good Dog	2 oz	70	3.5	30	0	0	0	430	1	<1	0	8	1 med-fat protein
Hot Dog	1.6 oz	50	0.5	5	0	0	0	400	2	<1	0	10	1 lean protein
Meatless Beef Burger	2.7 oz	110	4	35	0	0	0	440	8	<1	2	14	1/2 carb, 2 lean protein
Meatless Beef Strips	3 oz	120	1	10	0	0	0	870	4	<1	1	23	3 lean protein
Meatless Breakfast Pattie	2 patties (2 oz)	80	2	15	0	0	0	350	4	1	2	11	2 lean protein
Meatless Canadian Bacon	3 slices (2 oz)	80	0.5	5	0	0	0	400	2	<1	0	17	2 lean protein
Meatless Chicken Burger	2.7 oz	100	3	25	0	0	0	420	5	<1	2	15	2 lean protein
Meatless Chicken Strips	3 oz	110	1	10	0	0	0	440	8	1	<1	22	1/2 carb, 3 lean protein
Meatless Ground Round	1/3 cup (2 oz)	60	0.5	5	0	0	0	270	5	1	2	10	1 lean protein

VEGETARIAN FOODS

	Serving	Calories	Fat (g)	Cal. from Fat	Sat. Fat (g)	Trans Fat (g)	Chol. (mg)	Sod. (mg)	Carb. (g)	Sugar (g)	Fiber (g)	Prot. (g)	Servings/Exchanges
Meatless Ground Taco Stuffers	1/3 cup (2 oz)	90	2.5	20	0	0	0	300	5	1	2	11	2 lean protein
Meatless Ground Turkey	1/3 cup (2 oz)	60	1	10	0	0	0	330	4	0	2	14	2 lean protein
Meatless Lemon Herb Chicken Skewers	1 (2.9-oz) skewer	100	1	10	0	0	0	450	7	2	4	15	1/2 carb, 2 lean protein
Tofu Dogs	1.4 oz	45	1	5	0	0	0	300	2	0	0	8	1 lean protein
Veggie Brat Classic	3.4 oz	160	5	50	0	0	0	840	9	2	1	19	1/2 carb, 3 lean protein
Veggie Shrimp	3 oz	50	1.5	15	1	0	0	240	8	<1	5	2	1/2 carb
Veggie Tuna Steak	3.5 oz	250	20	180	2	0	0	510	8	3	4	8	1/2 carb, 1 med-fat protein, 3 fat

Index

Note: Page numbers in **bold** refer to tables.